# OSTEOPATHY FOR THE OVER 50s

# OSTEOPATHY FOR THE OVER 50s
## The maintenance of function and the treatment of dysfunction

## Nicette Sergueef

DO, France, Associate Professor, Department of Osteopathic Manipulative Medicine, Chicago College of Osteopathic Medicine, Midwestern University, USA

## Kenneth Nelson

DO, Professor, Department of Osteopathic Manipulative Medicine, Family Medicine and Biochemistry, Chicago College of Osteopathic Medicine, Midwestern University, USA

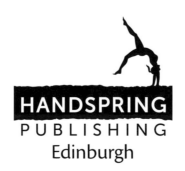

**HANDSPRING**
PUBLISHING
Edinburgh

HANDSPRING PUBLISHING LIMITED
The Old Manse, Fountainhall,
Pencaitland, East Lothian
EH34 5EY, United Kingdom
Tel: +44 1875 341 859
Website: www.handspringpublishing.com

First published 2014 in the United Kingdom by Handspring Publishing

ISBN 978-1-909141-09-4

**British Library Cataloguing in Publication Data**
A catalogue record for this book is available from the British Library

**Important notice**

It is the responsibility of the clinician/practitioner, employing a range of sources of information, their personal experience, and their understanding of the particular needs of the patient/client, to determine the best approach to treatment.

Neither the publishers nor the authors will be liable for any loss or damage of any nature occasioned to or suffered by any person or property in regard to product liability, negligence or otherwise, or through acting or refraining from acting as a result of adherence to the material contained in this book.

**Commissioning Editor** Sarena Wolfaard
**Design** by Designers Collective
**Artwork** by Designers Collective
**Cover** design by Bruce Hogarth, kinesis-creative.com
**Typeset** by DiTech Process Solutions
**Printed** in the Czech Republic by Finidr Ltd

The
Publisher's
policy is to use
paper manufactured
from sustainable forests

# CONTENTS

This text is written with the express intent of describing the application of osteopathic principles to the healthcare of aging patients, as delineated by Andrew Taylor Still and those who followed him including: John Martin Littlejohn, William Garner Sutherland, Harrison H. Fryette, Rollin E. Becker, Walford A. Schwab, and Norman J. Larson.

It lists a broad spectrum of clinical conditions that untowardly impact older patients. It explains the rationale for the care of these patients in the context of thoroughly researched and referenced functional anatomy and physiology and goes on to describe how dysfunction can be responsible for, or contributory to, diseases of the elderly.

Although we employ a systems based approach here, we have attempted to provide the reader with diagnostic and therapeutic methods that synthesize patient care into a holistic approach directed at the individual patient. We discuss the entire spectrum of osteopathic manipulative treatment (OMT) procedures available, and consider them in the context of a dosage continuum.

It is, however, precisely because of the potential fragility of elder patients that we have intentionally elected to choose indirect OMT procedures as the predominant type of treatment considered here. Osteopathic manipulative treatment dosage is extremely important and whereas one can always progressively increase the dosage of OMT once the level of patient tolerance has been exceeded, nothing can be done to undo an overdose except wait for the patient to recuperate, and then to start over. Wherever possible we provide instructions for patient participation that empower the patient and integrate them into the healthcare team to participate in the self healing process that is fundamental to osteopathic medicine.

Over the past 140 years osteopathic principles and practice have served as a foundation for medical reformation. Where 50 years ago osteopathy was viewed as a cult of medical eccentrics, osteopathic medicine now occupies a prominent position in the mainstream of medical science. Osteopathy—the distinctive foundation of osteopathic medicine—has from its inception selectively considered the different aspects of medical practice, choosing methods that are effective and rejecting harmful practices, as exemplified by most of the pharmacopeia of the nineteenth century. As such, osteopathic medicine represents, possibly, the first organized form of integrative medical practice.

As originally conceived, osteopathy was intended to replace the practice of medicine. However, since that time, tremendous strides have been made in medical science, and it is questionable that if what is known today in the treatment of infectious diseases had been known in 1864, when Still's children succumbed to spinal meningitis, he may not have considered becoming a medical reformer.

Further, osteopathy with its origins in the heartland of the nineteenth-century United States has grown to become a global phenomenon, and as such is practiced by a very diverse community of healthcare providers. Traditionally, medical practitioners have been trained to identify pathology and not as much to recognize dysfunction. Practitioners of osteopathic medicine look at the relationship between structure and function and for the impact of dysfunction resulting from structural imbalance. It is now, in the twenty-first century, that we must look at how osteopathic principles, as applied by the many different types of practitioners throughout the world, are integrated into medical practice and may be employed to benefit all of our patients. It is imperative to unite the two, either as the practice of osteopathic medicine, or through the integration of osteopaths into the community of contemporary healthcare providers.

The contents of this text are intended to provide insight into the appropriate care of aging individuals, specifically in the context of the application of osteopathic principles. This text is not intended to provide training in the psychomotor skill of OMT. Individuals who use the information contained here within should be trained, qualified healthcare providers and must recognize that OMT is used specifically only in the treatment of somatic dysfunction. Osteopathic manipulative treatment is not specific treatment for organic pathology. It may, however, be integratively employed as a complementary therapy in the presence of organic pathology. The elimination or reduction of the influence of somatic dysfunction, from a mechanical, neurophysiological, and circulatory perspective, facilitates the body's inherent capacity for self-healing. Osteopathic manipulative treatment, therefore, may be used integratively for its complementary contribution in the treatment of essentially all clinical conditions. Osteopathic manipulative treatment should, however, never be employed without a complete medical diagnosis or exclusively as an alternative to accepted standards of medical practice.

The use of OMT is specifically determined by the precise diagnosis of the somatic dysfunction to be treated in the context of the patient's overall health status. In most instances, OMT is employed to alleviate the motion restriction that is found in association with somatic dysfunction. It is, therefore, inappropriate to manipulate structurally unstable areas of the body. Individuals who employ the information in this text must recognize that when any intervention is applied to another human being, it inevitably carries with it inherent risk. Therefore, to the fullest extent of the law, the authors assume no liability for injury or damage to persons stemming from, or related to, the use of the material presented within this text. It is the full responsibility of the treating practitioner, based upon their independent expertise and knowledge of the patient, to determine in each instance the most appropriate treatment and its proper method of application.

As time passes, other changes have occurred as well. The vocabulary of anatomy continues to evolve, and in some instances the vocabulary of osteopathy has not kept pace. Although the new anatomic nomenclature refers to the spheno-occipital, instead of sphenobasilar, synchondrosis we have elected to keep the old nomenclature which is so familiar to most osteopathic practitioners. In the same manner, we have kept the terms external and internal rotation for motion descriptions of the craniosacral mechanism, although for other motions we use the new nomenclature which is lateral rotation or medial rotation, while external rotation or internal rotation is kept to describe motions occurring inside a cavity (e.g., internal rotation of the fetus inside the uterine cavity).

We would like to acknowledge and thank our perennial associate, Tom Glonek, PhD, for his consultations during the production of this text. We hope it will contribute to the understanding and intelligent use of osteopathic principles in the provision of healthcare by you, our colleagues throughout the world.

Nicette Sergueef, DO (France)
Kenneth E. Nelson, DO, FAAO, FACOFP(Dist)
Lyon, France and Chicago, Illinois, USA
May 12, 2013

# Abbreviations

AASM - American Academy of Sleep Medicine
ACh - acetylcholine
ACR - American College of Rheumatology
ACTH - adrenocorticotropin hormone
AHI - apnea-hypopnea index
ANS - autonomic nervous system
AP - anteroposterior
ASIS - anterior superior iliac spine
ATP - adenosine 5´-triphosphate
AVP - arginine vasopressin
BLT - balanced ligamentous tension
BP - blood pressure
BPH - benign prostatic hyperplasia
BPPV - benign paroxysmal positional vertigo
CAL - coracoacromial ligament
CAP - community-acquired pneumonia
CC - chief complaint
CDC - Centers for Disease Control and Prevention
CFS - chronic fatigue syndrome
CHF - congestive heart failure
CN - cranial nerve
CNS - central nervous system
COPD - chronic obstructive pulmonary disease
CR - cranial treatment
CRH - corticotropin-releasing hormone
CRI - cranial rhythmic impulse
CRPS1 - complex regional pain syndrome 1
CS - counterstrain
CSF - cerebrospinal fluid
CSK - cytoskeleton
CT - connective tissue
CTS - carpal tunnel syndrome
CVD - cardiovascular disease
CVLM - caudal ventrolateral medulla
CV4 - compression of the fourth ventricle
DMNV - dorsal motor nucleus of the vagus
ECM - extracellular matrix
ENS - enteric nervous system
EOM - extraocular muscles
FM - fibromyalgia
FOR - facilitated oscillatory release technique
FPR - facilitated positional release
GAG - glycosaminoglycan
GEJ - gastroesophageal junction

GER - gastroesophageal reflux
GI - gastrointestinal
GVA - general visceral afferent
HEENT - head, eyes, ears, nose, & throat
HF - heart failure
HPA - hypothalamic-pituitary-adrenal (axis)
HPI - history of present illness
HR - heart rate
HRV - heart rate variability
HTN - hypertension
HVLA - high velocity, low amplitude
IBS - irritable bowel syndrome
ICC - interstitial cells of Cajal
ILA - inferolateral angle
IL-6 - interleukin 6
IL-1 β - interleukin-1 beta
INR - integrated neuromusculoskeletal release
IOP - intraocular pressure
LAS - ligamentous articular strain technique
LD - light-dark
LDL - low-density lipoprotein
LES - lower esophageal sphincter
LLI - leg length inequality
LUTD - lower urinary-tract dysfunctions
LV - left ventricular
LVP - levator veli palatini
ME - muscle energy
MFR - myofascial release
MSC - mesenchymal stem cells
MUI - mixed urinary incontinence
NO - nitric oxide
NREM - non-rapid eye-movement
NSAIDs - non-steroidal anti inflammatory drugs
NTS - nucleus tractus solitarius
OA - osteoarthritis
OCF - osteopathy in the cranial field
OM - occipitomastoid
OMT - osteopathic manipulative treatment
OSA - obstructive sleep apnea
PFH - past family history
PG - proteoglycans
PINS - progressive inhibition of neuromuscular structures
PMH - past medical history

PNS - parasympathetic nervous system
PRM - primary respiratory mechanism
PSIS - posterior superior iliac spine
RD - retinal detachment
RHT - retinohypothalamic tract
ROM - range of motion
ROS - review of systems
RTM - reciprocal tension membrane
RVLM - rostral ventrolateral medulla
SBS - sphenobasilar synchondrosis
SCN - suprachiasmatic nucleus
SH - social history
SI - sacroiliac (joint)
SNS - sympathetic nervous system
SS - stomatognathic system
SS - symptom severity

ST - soft tissue
SUI - stress urinary incontinence
SVA - special visceral afferent
SWS - slow-wave sleep
TLESR - transient lower esophageal sphincter relaxation
TMJ - temporomandibular joint
TNF - tumor necrosis factor
TVP - tensor veli palatini
UES - upper esophageal sphincter
UUI - urge urinary incontinence
VIS - visceral manipulation
VNC - vestibular nuclear complex
VOR - vestibulo-ocular reflex
WPI - widespread pain index

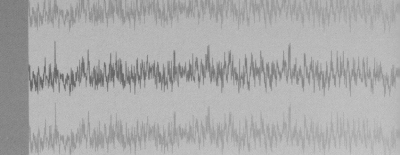

# SECTION 1

# Osteopathy, fascia, fluid, and the primary respiratory mechanism

*The more I study Osteopathy, the more it seems to boil down to a Highly Intelligent fluid surrounded and held in shape by fascial membranes.*

*Allow the fascial strains to correct what might be present, allow the fluid to resume its normal TIDAL mechanism, and all associated pathologies in the muscle, skin, blood vessels, or nerves will correct themselves. 'Bend to the oar' through the fascia, and 'ride the TIDE to the shore' by way of the fluid.*

—R. E. Becker[1]

*Tensegrity refers to a system that stabilizes itself mechanically because of the way in which tensional and compressive forces are distributed and balanced within the structure.*

—D. E. Ingber[2]

## Fascia

The importance of the fascia in the maintenance of the body's structural integrity and consequently upon structure, function, and dysfunction on both mechanical and fluid levels has been recognized as fundamental to osteopathic practice since its inception. The tensile and elastic properties of the body's fascial superstructure modulate the fluid sol-gel nature of the interstitium contributing greatly to the dynamic status of the primary respiratory mechanism (PRM). This is a prime example of anatomic tensegrity.

Aging, the normal process of growing old, is associated with a decline in cell, tissue, and organ system function. Impairments of the musculoskeletal system are among the most prevalent and symptomatic chronic complaints of middle and old age.[3] Osteopathic practitioners provide distinctive care, particularly in the treatment of musculoskeletal dysfunction, and through their interventions can reduce restriction of motion and

pain, and consequently help to prevent decrease in strength and disability. Also, because age-related deterioration of musculoskeletal tissues and function do not progress inevitably, appropriate osteopathic treatment can restore and maintain optimal musculoskeletal function.

Among the different tissues that form the musculoskeletal system, the fascia holds a significant place. As Andrew Taylor Still stated: "Thus a knowledge of the universal extent of the fascia is almost imperative, and is one of the greatest aids to the person who seeks cause of disease."[4] Fascia is considered to be a connective tissue (CT), but some controversy exists regarding which CT structures should be considered to be 'fascia,' and how fascia should be classified. The text that follows will provide a definition of fascia, with the different structures considered as fascia; then, histological components of fascia, terminologies of fascia, the role of fascia, and its evolution through aging, dysfunction, or both will be discussed.

## Definition

Fascia, or fasciola, in Roman antiquity was a fillet, or band of cloth, worn around the head as a diadem (an indication of royalty), over the breast by women (fascia pectoralis) or around the legs and feet.[5] From this origin the term fascia was applied to anatomical structures to designate the CT surrounding more specialized structures such as the muscles, blood vessels, and nerves, binding these structures together or establishing a packing material between them. These anatomical terms were in Latin, however, and when translated into other languages, they took different meanings.

As an illustration, 'Tela subcutanea' was translated into 'superficial fascia' in English speaking countries, whereas in French, it was 'tissu sous-cutané' (subcutaneous tissue).[6] Per se, the 'superficial fascia' described in English is not considered as a fascia in French speaking countries, where 'fascia' begins at the level of the fascia superficialis, a membranous layer located underneath the subcutaneous tissue and associated fatty layer.

Recently, the term fascia has been defined as "masses of connective tissue large enough to be visible to the unaided eye. Its structure is highly variable but, in general, collagen fibers in fascia tend to be interwoven and seldom show the compact, parallel orientation seen in tendons and aponeuroses."[7] De facto, tendons and aponeuroses are consequently not considered as fascia in this definition. For many practitioners of manual therapies, such as acupuncture, massage, chiropractic, and osteopathy, however, the term fascia "extends to all fibrous connective tissues, including aponeuroses, ligaments, tendons, retinacula, joint capsules, organ and vessel tunics, the epineuria, the meninges, the periosteum, and all the endomysial and intermuscular fibers of the myofasciae."[8] From these two definitions, it appears that although fascia is considered as a CT by the majority, all CTs are not always regarded as fascia.

From an anatomical point of view, since the collagen fibers in fascia tend to be interwoven without any specific design, precise descriptions of fascial structures are scarce. Descriptions tend to represent portions of fascia for particular areas in the human body, such as the 'thoracolumbar fascia,' or they tend to define anatomic entities, for example the intermuscular septa, interosseal membrane, periosteum, neurovascular tract, epimysium, intra- and extramuscular aponeurosis, perimysium, or endomysium.[9] Some authors suggest that the term 'fascia' in itself is incomplete. They propose to define fascia from the arrangement of its histological components, for instance 'dense CT' or 'non-dense (areolar) CT,' or to consider the topographic relationships of the fascia with respect to the skin, such as with the 'superficial' or 'deep' fasciae.

In order to better understand these differences, we will review the histological components of fascia. Next, we will consider the description of fascia based upon its components, and then, the description of fascia based upon its topography i.e., superficial fascia and deep fascia, which are the two main layers typically described.

## Histological components of fascia in the context of connective tissue

Classically, four types of tissues are described in the adult: epithelial, muscular, nervous, and connective. CT is the tissue that establishes a structural framework of the body. It supports, permeates, and binds together all other types of tissue into functioning groups of cells such as organs or muscles. Fascia is usually considered as a CT.[10]

CT is derived from the mesenchyme arising from the embryonic mesoderm with a large contribution from neural crest mesenchyme in the cephalic region. Mesenchyme consists of fusiform or stellate cells enclosed in a jelly-like matrix from where all the CTs arise.

Classification of CT is influenced by its composition. Sometimes loosely organized and highly cellular, it may be extremely fibrous or it may present with a predominance of ground substance. Several varieties of CT are described: areolar or loose, adipose, dense, regular or irregular, white fibrous, elastic, or mucous. Cartilage and bone are considered as special skeletal types of CT.

The peripheral blood cells, lymphoid tissues, and their precursors are also regarded as CTs because of their similar mesenchymal origins. Additionally, numerous defensive cells of the blood are part of the migrating cells found in CT.

According to local needs, the proportions of CT components differ in the various parts of the body. However, it always consists of an amorphous ground substance called the extracellular matrix (ECM), in which numerous cells and resident or migrating and extracellular fibers are found.

### Extracellular matrix

ECM is the main constituent of CT and consists of all the extracellular components of CTs. It provides the foundation for the different cells present in the ECM, and dissipates mechanical stresses placed upon tissues.

ECM consists of a transparent and amorphous ground substance, with the consistency of a semi-fluid gel containing adhesive glycoproteins. These glycoproteins regulate interactions between cells and other components of the ECM, in particular cell-matrix adhesion and matrix-cell signaling. Among them, proteoglycans (PG) are some of the major components of the ECM; they include hyaluronan (hyaluronic acid), chondroitin sulfate, dermatan sulfate, keratan sulfate, and heparin sul-

fate. PG may undergo extensive post-translational modifications that include the addition of glycosaminoglycan (GAG or mucopolysaccharide) chains. Because they are highly hydrated, PG and GAG may constitute a firm gel that tolerates compressive forces, for example, those occurring in cartilage.

### Connective tissue cells

Cells of CT are embedded in the ECM and can be either resident cells such as the fibroblasts, myofibroblasts, adipocytes, and mesenchymal stem cells, or migrant cells, with various defensive functions, such as the macrophages, lymphocytes, neutrophils, eosinophils, and mast cells.

#### Fibroblasts

Fibroblasts are usually the main components of CT cells. At the end of their existence, somewhat inactive fibroblasts are referred to as fibrocytes. Fusiform or spindle-shaped, the fibroblast cells display one large nucleus, several nucleoli, and multiple extended processes that communicate with the processes of other fibroblasts.

Fibroblasts are very resilient and active. They contribute to the secretion of proteins and synthesize most of the elements that constitute the ECM: collagen, elastin, and enzymes responsible for the

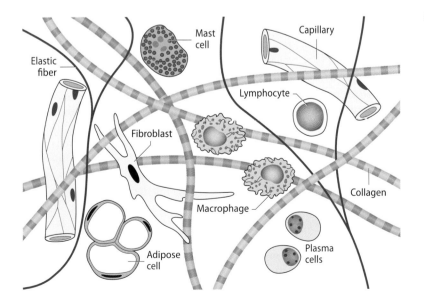

Figure 1.1: Connective tissue cells

degradation of ECM cells. Under the influence of cytokines, they can be differentiated into osteoblasts or chondroblasts. Multiple factors affect fibroblastic activity, in particular mechanical stresses, dietary habits, or hormonal concentrations.

Fibroblasts respond to tensions in the CT by changing shape, from a spindle shape as seen in the inactive state, to a more round or stellate form when submitted to mechanical stress. Mechanical stretching of fibroblasts increases their proliferation and biochemically adjusts their environment by influencing their synthesis of ECM proteins. In fact, in vitro, fibroblasts react within minutes to stretch, pressure, traction, or shear forces with cellular responses such as modifications in intracellular calcium and ATP release, or signaling pathway activation, actin polymerization, and gene expression.[11]

### Myofibroblasts

Myofibroblasts resemble fibroblasts, but they also contain actin-myosin complex, giving them several characteristics of smooth muscle with contractile properties that can produce long lasting isometric contractions. Most myofibroblasts arise from regular fibroblasts modified under the influence of mechanical tension and particular cytokines. They can also be derived from epithelial cells, endothelial cells, smooth muscle cells, pericytes, hepatic perisinusoidal cells, mesenchymal stem cells, and bone marrow-derived cells.[12] Once developed, myofibroblasts' contractile apparatus forms a mechanotransduction system distributing the force produced by its stress fibers to the surrounding ECM and thereby resulting in a local contraction of the matrix. Following this the deposition of ECM, especially collagen, stabilizes the contraction that may become permanent.[13]

During wound repair, myofibroblasts are believed to be responsible for contracture of the edges of the wounds and synthesis of new ECM.[14] [15] In the presence of excessive scar formation and chronic fascial contractures, as seen in frozen shoulder or Dupuytren's disease, an increased presence of myofibroblasts has been shown to be a contributing factor.[16] [17]

Of interest, as it relates to the concept of the PRM, it has been demonstrated that myofibroblasts exhibit periodic oscillations periods of approximately 100 seconds.[18] This is a frequency essentially identical to the six cycles in ten minutes attributed to the slow tide by Rollin E. Becker.[19]

### Adipocytes

Adipocytes, or fat cells, are found in many CTs, alone or organized into groups. They form the adipose tissue, and although spread throughout the body, this tissue constitutes one of the body's biggest organs. With some variations, in males, adipocytes constitute 15 to 20% of total body weight and in females, 20 to 25%. Adipose tissue is one of the greatest reservoirs of energy and also contributes to thermal insulation. It is continuously being modified under the influence of nervous or hormonal control. Normally, the mobilization of fat is induced by noradrenaline released at sympathetic nerve endings.

While adipose tissue is normally white or slightly yellow, another form of adipose tissue, the brown fat, is found in embryos and neonates. In neonates it is mainly found in the neck and interscapular region, where it contributes to the regulation of body temperature. Its distribution is quite limited in adults, with a small amount found around the adrenal glands.

### Mesenchymal stem cells

"Mesenchymal stem cells (MSC) are a heterogeneous population of stem/progenitor cells with pluripotent capacity to differentiate into mesodermal and non-mesodermal cell lineages, including osteocytes, adipocytes, chondrocytes, myocytes, cardiomyocytes, fibroblasts, myofibroblasts, epithelial cells, and neurons."[20]

MSC maintain a continuous renewal and repair of tissues, contributing to tissue regeneration and homeostasis. Quantity and quality of stem cells are of paramount important. They are influenced by the cellular environment and aging when MSC demonstrate a weakening in differentiation potential and proliferation rate. This may reflect the erosion of telomeres, the distal end of chromosome arms.[21] Because of their specific properties, MSC along with bone marrow stem cells are interesting targets for potential therapeutic use in regenerative medicine and tissue engineering.[22]

## Macrophages

Macrophages and neutrophils are the first line of defense against infections. They attack and destroy invading bacteria, viruses, and other damaging agents. Macrophages begin their life as blood monocytes, which are immature cells with modest capacity to fight infectious agents. After they enter the tissues they are referred to as macrophages. Thus, their role is to initiate the immune response with an inflammatory reaction, to phagocytize and kill pathogens, and to recruit natural killer cells.

Aging has an extreme influence on the phenotype and functions of these cells. Modification of the expression, function, or both, of innate immunity receptors and signal transduction decreases their activation with a decline in chemotaxis, phagocytosis, and intracellular killing of pathogens.[23]

## Lymphocytes, neutrophils, and eosinophils

Normally, there are six types of leukocytes (white blood cells) in the blood. They are the polymorphonuclear neutrophils, polymorphonuclear eosinophils, polymorphonuclear basophils, monocytes, lymphocytes, and, occasionally, plasma cells. Because of the granular appearance of their cytoplasm, the polymorphonuclear cells are also called granulocytes. In association with the monocytes they play a significant role, predominantly by phagocytosis, in the defense against invading agents. The lymphocytes and plasma cells contribute to the function of the immune system.

Granulocytes, monocytes, and some lymphocytes are produced in the bone marrow whereas remaining lymphocytes and plasma cells are produced in the lymphoid tissue. From their respective sites of origin they travel in the blood to areas of infection and inflammation.

Most of the lymphocytes are found in the lymph nodes, others are located in lymphoid tissues such as the spleen, submucosal areas of the gastrointestinal tract, thymus, and bone marrow. They are classified into two groups: T lymphocytes and B lymphocytes. Both develop from pluripotent hematopoietic stem cells in the embryo. One group travels to the thymus gland to form activated T lymphocytes in charge of cell-mediated immunity.

The B lymphocytes travel to the liver during mid-fetal life, and to the bone marrow thereafter, to form antibodies. Because they were first identified in the bursa of Fabricius, a site of hematopoiesis in birds, they are named B lymphocytes, after bursa.[24]

Over the extent of the individual's life, the thymus evolves. Located in the superior mediastinum and lower part of the neck, it achieves its maximum relative weight soon after birth and its maximum absolute weight at puberty. After that, it involutes and much of the lymphoid tissue turns into fat. As a consequence its output of T lymphocytes decreases. This, combined with the decline of hematopoietic stem cells' ability to replicate, could have a significant effect on the immune system of the aging individual.[25]

## Mast cells

Mast cells are part of the group of CT traveling cells. They develop from multi-potential hematopoietic precursor cells that travel from the bone marrow to diverse tissues where they differentiate. Mast cells are predominantly found immediately under the skin and within lymph nodes, near blood vessels and nerves.

Often compared to sentinels, mast cells respond to invaders with the release of histamine, leukotrienes (fatty signaling molecules), prostaglandins, proteases, and cytokines, which then have a rapid and remarkable immunomodulatory effect upon T cells, dendritic cells, and B cells.[26] In fact, mast cells can increase or block out inflammation and immune responses according to conditions and surroundings.

For a long time, mast cells were thought to be essentially related to allergy and the pathologic response to antigens. Current evidence, however, suggests that mast cells exert a multitude of functions during inflammation and cellular proliferation, and may be implicated in the pathogenesis of rheumatoid arthritis, scleroderma, and multiple sclerosis.[27]

## *Connective tissue extracellular fibers*

Extracellular fibers are mainly produced by the fibroblasts through the generation of proteins consisting of long peptide chains. The number of different extracellular fibers varies according to CT structural requirements. Different varieties exist, including collagen fibers, elastic fibers, and reticular fibers.

### Collagen fibers

Collagen is the most abundant protein in the human body and the most abundant protein in the animal kingdom. As such, collagen fibers are the most common and the strongest extracellular fiber of the ECM and CT, providing structural support.

Tropocollagen molecules, the precursors of collagen, consist of three polypeptide chains helically arranged around each other. They aggregate and cross-link to form collagen fibrils, which in turn assemble to produce mature collagen fibers.

To date, 28 distinct types of collagen are recognized, each serving a specific function. Collagen types I, II, and III are the most frequently encountered. Type I is found in the dermis, fascia, bones, tendons, ligaments, blood vessels, and sclera of the eyeball. Type II is present in cartilage and the vitreous body of the eye, and type III is found in multiple tissues. With age the amount of type I collagen usually increases, while type III decreases.[28]

Each layer of fascia displays a different spatial orientation of collagen fibers. Because of anisotropy, the property of being directionally dependent, fascia may be considered a composite material. This property reinforces the strength of the CT.

Because collagens serve to help tissues withstand stretching, collagen fibers are found in various proportions, according to the density of the tissue. As such, they are abundant in dense CT, whereas they are sparse in loose CT. Furthermore, collagen fibers are arranged in accordance with local structural needs. For instance, in tendons and ligaments the fibers are organized in parallel collection for tensile strength, whereas around blood vessels or the intestines they surround the long axes of these tubular structures.

### Elastic fibers

Elastic fibers, also named yellow fibers because of their color, consist of elastin proteins. They are produced by fibroblasts and smooth muscle cells. Less often encountered than collagen and frequently

thinner, elastic fibers are, however, found in some thick structures, like the ligamenta flava and ligamentum nuchae.

While collagen fibers resist tension, elastic fibers, with the capacity to recoil after being stretched, provide some resilience to deformation. They are found, as such, in tissues like the mesenteries that must adjust to changes in shape and volume of the gut or the aorta that must adapt to hydrostatic forces with every beat of the heart.

### Reticular fibers

Before the use of electron microscopy, a group of particular CT fibers were described as the reticular fibers because of their frequent arrangement in a spider web manner. They are now recognized, indeed, as being collagen fibrils, principally type III collagen. Reticular fibers form the supporting mesh framework of the cellular components of glands such as the liver, the kidney, and lymphoreticular tissues including the lymph nodes and spleen.

## Description of fascia based upon its histological components

Histological components present in the CTs lead to a description based upon their distribution. This terminology is suggested to facilitate communication.

### Dense connective tissue

Dense CT is characterized by a great number of closely packed fibers interspersed with a relatively small proportion of cells, predominantly fibroblasts, and vasculature. Its function is predominantly mechanical, and the orientation of its fibers corresponds to the direction of load applied to the tissue. As such, when stretch is applied in many directions, the fibers form a web, and the CT is referred to as *dense irregular*. When the tensile loading is mainly in one or a few directions, fiber orientation follows the direction of the load put upon the tissue, and the CT is referred to as *dense regular*.

Dense irregular CT is found for instance in the dermis and meninges, where multidirectional orientation of the fibers offers a significant resistance in all directions, therefore protecting the structures surrounded. Dense regular CT forms most tendons, ligaments and aponeuroses, providing a resistance to the load accommodated by such structures.

Collagen fibers are thick and the most abundant in dense CT where they provide high tensile strength. Elastic fibers may, however, also be present, and when profuse the CT is referred to as elastic CT.

### Non-dense connective tissue

Non-dense CT consists of areolar, adipose, and reticular tissues. Areolar tissue, also named 'loose CT,' is the most common. It contains sparse, irregularly arranged collagen fibers with a profusion of ground substance. Neurovascular bundles and small branches of sensory nerves traverse this tissue. In fact, peripheral nerves and blood and lymph vessels are surrounded by the loose packing of areolar tissue as they pass between other structures. Areolar tissue fills the spaces between organs as well, where it provides flexibility and permits some amount of shear deformation between adjacent dense CT layers. As an example, under normal conditions, the areolar tissue located between the thoracolumbar fascial layers of dense CT lets these dense layers glide past one another during motion of the trunk.[29]

Adipose tissue consists mostly of adipocytes and due to the presence of these fat vacuoles, seems 'empty.' Adipose tissue is found throughout the body where it forms protective cushions and plays a major role in the storage of energy.

In reticular tissue the collagenous fibers create a stable network. Thus it provides support and stability to underlying tissue or to organs, forming their stroma.

## Description of fascia based upon its topography

### Superficial fascia

The superficial fascia that completely covers the body is a fine, three-dimensional meshwork containing loose areolar CT and fat.[30] It combines with the deep aspect of the dermis superficially and extends underneath to the deep muscle fascia. Sometimes, when fibrous bands bind the skin to the deep fascia, sheets of dense CT may be present in the superficial fascia.[31] The thickness of the superficial fascia depends upon its adipose content, the panniculus adiposus. This adipose content varies among individuals and contributes to mobility of skin, storage of energy and thermal insulation. Appearance of the superficial fascia differs depending on the anatomic region. In the limbs and the perineum, it is clearly distinct. It is very thin over the dorsal aspects of the hands and feet,[32] while in the scalp, palms, and soles, the superficial fascia is especially dense and connected to underlying structures.

In the head and neck, several striated muscles, including the platysma or the occipitofrontalis, are embedded in the superficial fascia. They are a vestige of musculature, the panniculus carnosus, present in other mammals and participate in facial expression in humans. Other muscles found in the superficial fascia include the palmaris brevis and the smooth muscles that constitute the subareolar muscle of the nipple, the dartos sheet of the scrotum, and the corrugator cutis ani. One of the characteristics of all of these muscles is that one end is fixed to the skin while the other attaches to the deep fascia or bone.

In many regions of the body, the inner portion of the superficial fascia consists of from one to several thin, horizontal membranous layers. These fascial layers are usually thicker on the posterior aspects of the body than they are anteriorly.[33] Subcutaneous nerves, blood vessels, and lymphatic vasculature pass through the superficial fascia to and from the skin. The relationship between these structures and the membranous layers of the superficial fascia is of interest in clinical practice. For instance, the major subcutaneous veins of the upper and lower extremities are encased in special compartments between the membranous layers of the superficial fascia and the deep muscular fascia underneath. On each side of these veins, the two fascial layers fuse. A fibrous lamina, compared to a 'ligament' fastens the vessel to the compartment wall.[34] In pathologic conditions, venous muscular pumping may be modified by alteration of the wall of the main venous compartment. Varicosities may result from a lack of constraint upon the vein in its interfascial course. This takes place most frequently in the superficial tributary veins where fascial sheathing is less developed.[35]

The fibrous bands located in the superficial fascia fix the skin to the deep fascia. Thus, the superficial fascia constitutes an interconnecting system holding the skin onto the underlying tissues. With aging, the skin and underlying layers of superficial fascia stretch. The superficial fascial system is compromised and tends to cause ptotic soft tissues, pseudo-fat deposit deformity, and cellulite.[36]

### Deep fascia

The deep fascia, also referred to as the investing fascia, is located under the superficial fascia. It is a layer of variable thickness where collagenous fibers are organized in a dense layout, quite often in an ordered arrangement close to aponeuroses. Externally, it is blended with the superficial fascia. Internally, it surrounds the skeletal muscles forming their endo- and epimysia.

The deep fascia also contributes to the constitution of the peritendinous portion of tendons, and to the periosteum of bone, to which it is always strongly attached. Particularly well developed in limbs, where collagen fibers are organized in a longitudinal or transverse pattern, it creates their intermuscular septa and forms inelastic sheaths around the musculature. In addition to the investing layer of deep fascia on the surface of the body, there are several additional fascial layers in deeper parts, of widely differing dispositions.

The thickness of the deep fascia varies, however, among the different parts of the body. Particularly well developed in the iliotibial tract, deep fascia is scarce in the face. Moreover, differences exist in the fasciae surrounding different muscles. Over non-expansile muscles such as those found in the prevertebral musculature, the surrounding fascia is strongly developed, whereas over expansile muscles such as the musculature of the cheek, it consists of thin loose areolar tissue. In some places, several fascial layers exist in the deep fascia surrounding the muscles, consisting of a number of layers of dense CT and areolar CT with adipose content.

Because deep fascia forms thin sheets of tissue between adjacent muscles, it plays an important role in movement, permitting individual fibers, or entire muscles, to move separately. When they lengthen and shorten, muscles can slide along underneath deep fascia, apart from some areas where they are fixed to the deep fascia.

## Innervation of fascia

"No doubt nerves exist in the fascia that change the fluid to gas, and force it through the spongy and porous system as a delivery by the vital chain of wonders, that go on all the time to keep nerves wholly pure."[37]

Different studies describe free nerve endings and encapsulated mechanoreceptors, including Ruffini and Pacinian corpuscles, in fascia such as the thoracolumbar fascia,[38] and the antebrachial and brachial fasciae.[39] Such findings suggest a role in nociception and a proprioceptive capacity of the deep fascia, so that fascia may be considered as a sensory organ.[40 41] Debate exists, however, as to whether deep fascia is itself innervated or the nerve fibers supply associated areolar or adipose tissues.[42]

Autonomic nervous fibers have also been described within fascia.[43] Because they are often found in association with blood vessels, it is assumed that these nerves have a strong vasomotor component. However, these unmyelinated autonomic fibers may have motor functions affecting myofibroblasts as well as other autonomic nervous system functions. As such, the stimulation of intrafascial sympathetic afferent neurons, as produced through manual therapy, may cause adjustments in global tone of the autonomic nervous system.[44] "Any intervention on fascia is also an intervention on the autonomics."[45]

## Functions of fascia

Fascial functions and dysfunctions occupy a large space in the legacy of Still. As stated:

> The fascia gives one of, if not the greatest problems to solve as to the part it takes in life and death. It belts each muscle, vein, nerve, and

all organs of the body. It is almost a network of nerves, cells, and tubes, running to and from it; it is crossed and filled with, no doubt, millions of nerve centers and fibers to carry on the work of secreting and excreting fluid vital and destructive. By its action we live, and by its failure we shrink, or swell, and die.[46]

Since Still's time, the functions of fascia have been emphasized by multiple osteopaths. Among them, William Garner Sutherland, Harold Ives Magoun Sr, Angus G. Cathie, Rollin E. Becker, and Alan R. Becker are the most well-known. They all insist upon the role of fascia in health and disease. Changes take place within the fascia as functional pathologies before the recognition of a more serious disorder and trained practitioners must be able to recognize and address these changes as soon as possible. Knowledge of fascial functions allows one to recognize fascial dysfunctions that may then be addressed, thereby avoiding potentially catastrophic outcomes or, if pathologic changes have already occurred, augmenting the body's self healing capacity.

## Physical properties

In healthy individuals, the mechanical properties of fascia reflect the abundance of its different components. In tissues rich in collagen fibers, fascia may resist tension, whereas the presence of elastin provides resilience to deformation by stretching. In areas that must absorb compressive forces such as cartilages, the proteoglycans and glycosaminoglycans of the ECM produce a stiff gel to tolerate these forces.

### Creep, relaxation, hysteresis, and viscoelasticity

Globally, fasciae demonstrate several mechanical properties that allow one to adapt to the environment. These properties include creep, relaxation, hysteresis, and viscoelasticity and are defined as follows:

- Creep is a time-dependent strain that occurs in response to the application of a force or stress. It results from long-term exposure to high levels of stress that are below the yield strength of the material.
- Relaxation is the release of tension and return to equilibrium.
- Hysteresis is the dependence on both existing and past environment.
- Viscoelasticity is the ability to exhibit both viscous and elastic properties when undergoing deformation. Viscoelastic tissues possess time dependent or rate sensitive stress-strain relations.

Environmental variation in factors, such as temperature, pH, and ionic content, influences fascial viscosity.[47] The state of hydration has been shown to affect creep in ligaments, with decreased hydration decreasing creep and increased hydration increasing creep.[48]

### Elasticity

Elasticity is a quality that protects a structure from physical disruption when it is stretched. Elasticity also allows the stretched structure to act as a capacitor, absorbing the energy from the stretching forces to later release that energy as recoil. This is an important quality for tissues to possess in their contribution to the PRM. Tissue capacitance is also significant in the context of direct manipulative procedures.

When elastic fibers predominate, fascia demonstrates elasticity. The walls of the arteries and of the bronchial tree demonstrate this property. As life progresses, fascial elasticity decreases and potentially contributes to disorders related to aging. For instance, increased arterial stiffness is associated with the development of cardiovascular disease.

### Contractility

The capacity of the fascia to manifest inherent contractility is of extreme significance to the dynamic model of osteopathic function and dysfunction. In 1946, Thomas L. Northup stated: "that possibly the connective tissues of the body were capable of contraction and relaxation and that these functions were under the control of the autonomic nervous system."[49] Furthermore in 1974, Cathie declared: "Its (fascia) outstanding properties are contractility and elasticity." He went on to say that: "The contractile phase persists throughout life but the elasticity decreases with age. The contractile phase not only persists but supersedes all other qualities of fascia."[50]

Since then, spontaneous contraction of CT has been observed.[51] Cells with smooth muscle characteristics and contractile properties have been described in the crural fascia, suggesting a role of pre-stress in the collagen scaffold, the 'ectoskeleton', described further below.[52] (See below: 'Mechanotransduction,' p. 12.)

Myofibroblasts are the contractile, smooth muscle-like cells within the fascia. They develop their extremely contractile cytoskeletal apparatus only above a certain ECM stiffness limit.[53] In this process, chemical factors, such as cytokines, are also involved in the regulation of the myofibroblasts.

Thus, when fascia is being subjected to mechanical force, myofibroblasts contract to provide resistance. It has been suggested "that intramuscular connective tissues, particularly the perimysium and especially in tonic muscles, may be able to actively contract and thereby adapt muscle stiffness to altered tensional demands."[54]

Fascial contractility may also be influenced by the vascular and autonomic nervous systems, as implied by the great number of autonomic nerves and rich intrafascial supply of capillaries.[55] Conversely, dysfunction in the apparatus involved in fascial contractility leads to increased passive muscle stiffness and fibroses. (See below: 'Connective tissues and aging,' p. 14.)

## Protection

Fascia supports, binds, and packs together the other tissues and organs of the body. Each structure of the body is surrounded with some fascial envelope, and all the different envelopes are wrapped together in one bigger envelope that is the superficial fascia.

As such, muscles are enveloped with fascia that assists their function, exerting tension and pressure upon their surfaces to prevent them from tearing and forming hernias during muscular contraction. When fascia surrounds groups of muscles, it coordinates their function. As an example, the deeper lamina of the posterior layer of thoracolumbar fascia surrounds the paraspinal muscles that all together stabilize the spine when upright. Actually, thoracolumbar fascial constraint of radial expansion of the erector spinae muscles augments their power by up to 30%.[56]

Viscera, as well, are enclosed in fascia that suspends the organs within their cavities. Fascia protects every organ and for some of them provides sufficient elasticity to allow changes in shape and motility.

Fascia is referred to as our 'organ of form.'[57] Hypothetically, if we were to remove all of our organs, muscles, and bones from our body, we would still be able to conserve the shape of the body through the fascial three-dimensional complex.[58]

## Continuity

In the establishment of a holistic model of healthcare the presence of structural continuity is fundamental. Fascia is ubiquitous. Fascia permeates the human body and establishes a structural and functional continuity between the different regions and tissues of the body. Fascia is a tensegral structure (see below: 'Tensegrity,' p. 13) from the histologic level to the whole-body gross anatomic level. Thus the body is a holistic structure in which every part is united with every other part through this network of tissue. Fascia surrounds every structure. Forces exerted by anatomic structures, whose shape is defined by their respective fascial envelopes, load their surrounding fascia. These forces are in turn transmitted to adjacent and distant fascia determining the alignment of component collagen and elastic fibers.

With its multiple connections, the thoracolumbar fascia is a good example of functional fascial continuity. Attached to the spinous processes of the lumbar and sacral vertebrae, the transverse processes of the lumbar vertebrae, the iliac crest, the 12th rib, the supraspinous, intertransverse, lumbocostal, and iliolumbar ligaments, the thoracolumbar fascia forms the lateral arcuate ligament of the diaphragm and the aponeurotic origin of the transversus abdominis. Therefore, each time muscles such as the latissimus dorsi, gluteus maximus, and erector spinae contract, the superficial lamina of the posterior layer of the thoracolumbar fascia is tensed, while contraction of the biceps femoris tense the deep lamina.[59] The thoracolumbar fascia integrates the activity and promotes continuity in load transfer to different regions, in this case, the lower limb, upper limb, spine, and pelvis.

Continuity between muscles fibers and fascia is frequent. In the foot, a study showed that only eight of the 69 interossei muscles studied demonstrated attachments that were limited to bone. Most of the time, the muscles had widespread attachments to ligaments and fascia.[60]

Quite often muscles originate from the deep surface of fascia and are invested by fascia. For instance, the gluteus maximus arises from the ilium, sacrum, and coccyx, but also from the aponeurosis of erector spinae, the sacrotuberous ligament, and the gluteal fascia, the fascia that covers the gluteus medius. Then, the fibers descend laterally, with the upper part and superficial portion of the lower part attaching to the iliotibial tract of the fascia lata. Only the deeper portion of the lower part of the muscle attaches to the gluteal tuberosity. This explains why patients with ilium dysfunction may complain of pain in their knee. Imbalance among structures at a particular site is transmitted through fascial continuity to a distant site, where it contributes to produce a secondary dysfunction.

Because muscles attach to fascia as well as to bone, there is a whole-body connection between the bones, muscles, and fascia. To capture this concept, Frederic Wood Jones coined the term 'ectoskeleton' or 'soft tissue skeleton,' thus describing the role of fascia as a significant site of muscle attachment.[61]

Fascia forms a three-dimensional pattern of structural support taking part in the transmission of forces between adjacent and distant parts of the body. Nevertheless, there are more than just mechanical fascial relations between muscles, bones, ligaments, and other body parts. Fascia establishes cellular connections as well that may represent a body-wide signaling network.[62] (See below: 'Mechanotransduction,' p. 12 and 'Tensegrity,' p. 13.)

## Postural implications

An immediate indication of somatic function status is the overall quality of an individual's posture. Thus an understanding of fascial anatomy, physiology, and its contribution to the dynamics of human posture is of diagnostic importance.

Several studies report the presence of nerve fibers within fascia.[63 64 65 66 67] Free nerve endings and encapsulated receptors, in particular, Ruffini and Pacinian corpuscles have been found. Regional differences are present probably reflecting variations in functional significance. The fact that nerves are observable, however, does not attest that these nerves innervate the fascia. They may just be in transit on their way to the muscle, or skin, or they may simply be lying upon the fascia.[68]

Nevertheless, fascia is considered to be involved in proprioception.[69] In particular, myelinated nerve endings found in fascia are suggestive of a proprioceptive function.[70] As well, Pacinian corpuscles located near the superficial fascia may contribute to exteroceptive sensations when deep pressure is applied to the body. This in turn may affect posture.

Definite stress bands can be observed within fasciae, emphasizing their role in postural control.[71] In fact, some of the fasciae are described as 'postural fascia': the thoracolumbar fascia, the iliotibial band of the fascia lata, the gluteal fascia, and the cervical fascia.[72] They contribute to postural stabilization and, simultaneously, permit motion initiated by muscular activity. They are among the first to demonstrate alterations in the presence of postural defects. In such circumstances, fascia may play a role in nociception. A study suggests that the nociceptive input from the thoracolumbar fascia contributes to the pain in low back pain patients.[73]

Trauma or cumulative microtrauma affects fascia and can lead to postural defects. Damage to spinal ligaments and mechanoreceptors embedded in these ligaments and fascia is described as a source of muscle control dysfunction. As a result, corrupted mechanoreceptor signals are hypothesized to produce higher stress, muscle fatigue, neural and connective tissue inflammation, and over time, chronic back pain.[74]

## Circulatory support

"It (connective tissue) is an integral portion of every body structure and serves as the pathway through which all nourishment and nerve supply reach the specialized cells and through which all cellular lymphatic drainage occurs."[75]

In the context of a system that synchronizes cellular respiration on a total-body level, the

PRM, the role of the circulatory system is fundamental. Fascia helps to adjust circulation; it affects in particular the function of the venous and lymphatic systems. The deep fascia that surrounds muscles is tough, thick, and resistant. During muscular contraction, the fine-walled veins and lymphatics inside the muscles are compressed and as a result, blood and lymph are directed toward the heart. Muscles and fascia, particularly in the lower extremities, act as a pump moving venous blood and lymph against the force of gravity.

### Homeostasis

Physiological homeostasis is the ultimate outcome of a perfectly functioning holistic anatomy. CTs create a total-body network that envelops and permeates every muscle, organ, and tissue. Among ECM cells, the fibroblasts are interconnected collectively via their cytoplasmic processes to form a reticular arrangement encompassing the entire body.[76] Under specific circumstances fibroblasts form gap junctions at points of contact between cells that allow responses to stressors such as mechanical load.[77] This cellular network within the CT establishes a direct communication throughout the body, as well as potentially an indirect communication via the nervous system.[78] This is, in turn, likely to influence other physiological systems contributing to homeostasis.

In particular, CTs demonstrate defensive roles wherein their cellular components play a central part. ECM and its numerous cells are constantly interacting in order to regulate their metabolism, proliferation and motility. According to Cathie: "Fascia (connective tissue) is the arena for inflammation," and "infections and fluid often track along fascial planes."[79] When inflammation occurs, part of the inflammatory response is a buildup of the CT migrant inflammatory cells in tissues. They produce lymphokines, such as the interleukins, and other factors, to attract other migrant CT immune cells such as macrophages and other lymphocytes in order to produce an immune response that ultimately launches an adaptive response of the whole organism.

### Mechanotransduction

Mechanotransduction is the capacity of the cell to sense, process, and respond to mechanical stimuli. Thus, mechanical stresses placed upon the cell are transduced into chemical information that influences cellular physiology. Cells possess a cytoskeleton (CSK), a cellular 'skeleton,' within their cytoplasm. It consists of various proteins that form an intricate network. The CSK acts as a support to stiffen cells, making it possible for the cells to assume irregular shapes. It supplies support for projections from the cell surface (microvilli and cilia) and fixes them into the cytoplasm. It also plays important roles in intracellular transport and cellular division.[80]

Cells are intricately connected to the external environment through their CSK. Connection could be direct with contiguous cells or indirect through the dense meshwork of the ECM.[81] In particular, fibroblasts connect with one another through their elongated processes, developing a three-dimensional network within CT.

The cells and the ECM are interdependent, and the mechanical properties of the ECM affect cytoskeletal organization and cell behavior while cells synthesize, secrete, modify, and degrade ECM constituents.[82] As such, fibroblasts sense any modification in physical conditions of the ECM, such as when a tissue is stretched or compressed. Signals from the ECM are perceived through special receptors located on the cell membrane surfaces known as integrins. Such transmembrane mechanoreceptors that form a bridge between the ECM and the cells' CSK are gathered in complexes referred to as 'focal adhesions.'[83] When signals are perceived by the integrins, they are directed to the cell nuclei of the fibroblasts.[84] They are then transduced into chemical information, indications that are integrated with growth factor derived stimuli to complete specific changes in gene expression.[85] This process defines mechanotransduction that is the conversion of a physical signal into a biological or chemical response.[86] Mechanotransduction signaling has a significant function in the protection of many mechanically stressed tissues such as muscle, bone, cartilage, and blood vessels and is inseparably related to the concept of biological tensegrity.

## Tensegrity

The structural basis of cellular mechanotransduction is derived from the architectural concept of tensegrity.[87] Richard Buckminster Fuller ('Bucky'), an American architect, and design genius, coined the term combining the words 'tension' and 'integrity'.[88] "Tensegrity refers to a system that stabilizes itself mechanically because of the way in which tensional and compressive forces are distributed and balanced within the structure."[89]

A wide variety of structural systems from the molecular, (see Buckyballs, the geodesic arrangement of carbon atoms) to the organization of the cellular CSK and interfibroblastic relationships, on through to gross anatomic interrelationships, demonstrate the architectural principles of tensegrity. That is, structural integrity is dynamically maintained by the interrelationship between compression-bearing rigid 'girders' that stretch flexible, tension-bearing 'cables,' while simultaneously the tension-bearing 'cables' compress the rigid 'girders.'

On the microscopic level, the structure demonstrated by most cells is established by a tensegrital state of balance. This occurs not only from within the cell as the result of the CSK, but also from without through the influence of the ECM.

The CSK, the infrastructure of the cell, consists of a complex mesh of contractile microfilaments that extend throughout the cell's interior. These microfilaments act like cables to exert tension that pull the cell wall and everything within the cell, toward the cell's nucleus. In opposition to this centripetal force there are, within the cell, microtubules and cytoskeletal cross-linked bundles of microfilaments that behave like girders to resist the compressive tensions exerted by the microfilaments.

A third component of the tensegral structure of the CSK consists of intermediate filaments that integrate the resistance to compression exerted by the microtubules and the centripetal forces of the contractile microfilaments. These intermediate filaments also unite the cell's nucleus with the cell wall. As such, they function as guy wires to maintain the central position of the nucleus. While the CSK is covered by an exterior cellular membrane and filled with cytoplasm, the cell's shape is ultimately determined by this architectural linkage between intracellular 'girders' and 'cables.'

The component from outside the cell is the result of compressive forces exerted upon the cell wall by the ECM. This aspect, the result of pressures within the extracellular compartment, is produced by the macro tensegral influence of gross anatomy (discussed below) further modulated by the osmotic influence upon the interstitium of arterial supply, venous and lymphatic drainage, and biochemical variations in the molecular content of the ECM. Pathologic states like diabetes mellitus and renal failure have been demonstrated to exert a palpable change upon interstitial fluid content.[90] [91]

On the gross anatomic level, the constituent bones of the human skeleton are vertically stabilized and supported against gravity as the result of tensions exerted by muscles and tendons, ligaments and the total-body fascial envelope. The bones constitute the compression 'girders,' and muscles, tendons, ligaments, and fascia are the tension-bearing 'cables.' Ultimately the human body stabilizes critical articulations through the imposition of internal tension, composed of opposing tension and compressive elements, to reduce any tendency for instability. The force of gravity additionally influences this tensegral relationship by increasing the internal tension exerted upon skeletal 'girders' from the musculotendinous, ligamentous, and fascial 'cables.'

Therefore, because of the principles of tensegrity, the application of mechanical forces through procedures like osteopathic manipulative treatment (OMT), applied on a gross anatomic level, is directed through the load-bearing qualities of the ECM of the body to cellular adhesion sites that physically couple the CSK to the ECM.[92]

The integrins act as mechanoreceptors and are among the first molecular structures on the cell surface to sense a mechanical signal. They, then, transmit the information across the cell membrane where it induces alterations in cellular biochemistry and genetic expression.[93]

Thus a tension-dependent architectural system, through mechanical forces applied at the gross anatomic level, alters cellular level biochemistry and genetic expression. As such, this provides a plausible explanation as to how the application of OMT may influence cellular activities, including cellular physiology, and conceivably even cellular immune responses critical to the maintenance of health.[94]

## Connective tissues and aging

The normal process of growing old, which can only be arrested by early death, brings on inevitable physical alterations. The structure and properties of CTs change. Normally, a constant interaction exists between the CT cells and the ECM. The cells synthesize, secrete, modify, and degrade ECM constituents and the ECM adjusts cell metabolism, proliferation, and motility. As the individual gets older, adjustments occur that may contribute to the decline in cell function and mechanical properties, such as modification of cell metabolism, changes in the responsiveness of cells to hormones and growth factors, reduction of proliferative capacity, and variation in ECM composition and organization. Additionally, diminished vascular perfusion decreases nutritional supply to CT and a lifetime of ultraviolet light exposure, mechanical wear and tear, and inflammation contribute to the aging process of the CT.

Under normal physiological conditions, a balance exists at the cellular level between the internal forces exerted by the CSK and the external forces exerted by osmotic pressures and the physical adhesions of the cell to the ECM and other cells. Tissue homeostasis depends upon this dynamic state of balance. Cell growth, differentiation, polarity, motility, contractility, and apoptosis are under the influence of cellular deformation through the influence of the cellular ECM adhesions.[95] As such, tissue reactions to abnormal mechanical stress and atypical cells may well play a role in the clinical presentation of lower back pain, and in the etiology of multiple significant diseases, including: atherosclerosis, cancer progression, cardiomyopathies, diabetes, and osteoporosis.[96][97]

Mechanotransduction seems to change with age.[98] Concomitantly, changes in mechanotransduction may promote aging.[99] Mechanotransduction may be altered through changes in cell mechanics, ECM structure, or by deregulation of the molecular mechanisms by which the cells sense mechanical signals or convert them into chemical responses.[100] Normally, even in the absence of external loading, the ECM is under tension that stimulates mechanochemical transduction. With age, changes occur in this state of tension, the degree of stiffness of human fibroblasts decreases, and that may, in turn, influence the cells' responses to mechanical stimulations.[101]

In biology, from bacteria to mammals, physical force is a primary regulator of life's form and function, and mechanical stress can modify physiological processes at the molecular, cellular, and systemic level. Mechanical stress may result from gravity or physical movement. Mechanical loading is transmitted at a tissue level to each cell through cellular adhesions to the ECM, or by the opening of ion channels in the cell membrane in response to applied forces. Mechanical loading may also result as a consequence of pressure, as with blood pressure, or from shear forces, as with blood flow over vascular endothelial cells. Interestingly, reduction of mechanical loading is one of the factors that can trigger apoptosis.[102]

When CT length is modified, an immediate reorganization of the fibroblasts' CSK occurs. This has been shown to transform the stiffness and viscosity of areolar CT.[103] In fact, cellular realignment depends upon the conditions of applied strain, i.e., static or cyclic, and upon strain magnitude, frequency, and duration.[104] Strain direction also contributes to fibroblastic responses.[105] Changes in CT tensions modulate the growth, ion conductance, and gene expression of fibroblasts. It also affects organ-specific cell populations present within the CT complex, such as the vascular, nervous, and immune cells.[106] Somatic dysfunction and associated postural disorders are quite common in older individuals. Such dysfunction modifies the transmission of forces through tissues, contributing to unbalanced tissue tensions that can, in turn, affect mechanotransduction and predispose to multiple pathological conditions.[107]

There are strong indications that as part of the aging process pro-inflammatory physiology is underlying the development of age-related diseases.[108]

Thus, inflammation can also promote pathologic tissue damage and activation of fibroblasts. Indeed, besides their role in contributing to the ECM, when inflammation is present fibroblasts respond in a highly complex fashion, releasing cytokines and conditioning the cellular environment. Inflammation can, at least momentarily, modify the gene expression profiles of the fibroblasts.[109] In fact, as immunoregulatory cells, fibroblasts are described as resident sentinel cells.[110] Fibroblasts are also considered to play an active role in the persistence of chronic inflammatory reactions.[111]

Dysfunction of fibroblasts leads to the dysregulation of their anabolic and catabolic processes, disruption of the control of biosynthesis, and degradation of CT components. As a consequence, ECM deposition and inappropriate tissue contraction result in fibrosis. When stimulated by the influence of mechanical tension and specific cytokines, fibroblasts can differentiate into myofibroblasts. Normally, the regulated temporary activation of myofibroblasts contributes to tissue repair, as exemplified by cutaneous scar formation or the healing of a ruptured tendon. Typically, as the healing process is completed, the number of myofibroblasts is reduced by apoptosis. Under extreme and prolonged myofibroblastic activity, however, the normal constructive function becomes damaging, with resultant fibrosis formation.[112 113] Chronic fascial contractures as seen in Morbus Dupuytren, plantar fibromatosis, or frozen shoulder, for instance, seem to be associated with the occurrence of an increased number of myofibroblasts.[114]

When CT becomes dysfunctional, because of mechanical stresses or inflammation, myofascial relationships, muscle balance, and proprioception are altered. Sliding of the muscles as they lengthen and shorten beneath the deep fascia can be affected, as can be seen in the thoracolumbar fascia in patient suffering of low back pain.[115] Adhesions in scars of CTs are described as a source of dysfunction either locally, or at a distance from the scar.[116] As such, abdominal scars may be associated with low back pain that can be reduced with treatment of the scar.[117]

Dysfunctional CT affects vascular and lymphatic drainage as well, causing passive interstitial congestion and cellulite. Congestion, in turn, affects the vasa nervorum and vasa vasorum, further compromising efficient tissue perfusion.

## Clinical applications

"When you deal with the fascia, you deal and do business with the branch offices of the brain, and under the general corporation law, the same as the brain itself, and why not treat it with the same degree of respect?"[118]

Multiple mechanoreceptors have been identified within fascia. These include free nerve endings and encapsulated mechanoreceptors, including Pacinian and Ruffini corpuscles. Pacinian corpuscles, located beneath the skin and in the depths of fascial tissues, respond in a few hundredths of a second to rapid local compression, repetitive stimuli, and vibrations of the tissues. Thus, they may be implicated in high-velocity manipulation or vibratory techniques.[119] On the other hand, Ruffini's endings are located in joint capsules and in the CT. They register mechanical change within joints and respond very slowly to sustained, deep pressure, and in particular slow, lateral stretches upon tissues.[120] Additionally, stimulation of pressure receptors causes an increase in vagal efferent activity, possibly through the activation of vagal afferent fibers.[121] Studies show that moderate pressure massage compared to light pressure massage increases the high frequency component of heart rate variability implying increased vagal efferent activity.[122] By experience the application of slow deep tissue procedures, indeed, tends to foster patient relaxation.

Application of manual techniques on fascia have been shown to demonstrate improvement of different clinical conditions, including fibromyalgia,[123 124] rheumatoid arthritis,[125] Raynaud's phenomenon,[126] venous insufficiency,[127] neck and low back pain,[128] and lateral epicondylitis.[129] It should be noted, that although reduction of pain and improvement of quality of life in patients with these conditions seem to follow treatments, improvements do not last. The beneficial effects, do however, return with repeated manipulative treatment sessions.[130]

Favorable patient response substantiates osteopathic principles. Treatment of somatic dysfunction is intended to improve neuroendocrine and autonomic functions, fluidic flow through the tissues, cellular metabolism, and reduce pain. The following illustrates these conclusions.

Fibroblasts play a significant part in the maintenance and repair of CT, and modification of the mechanical environment in which the fibroblasts reside is of great influence on cell signaling, gene expression, and matrix adhesion, all of which may contribute to the results of manual therapies. Mechanical load upon fibroblasts can change cellular morphology in an expected fashion and biochemically modify their environment.[131]

Studies show that cultured human fibroblasts adapt distinctively to mechanical loading in fashions dependent upon strain magnitude, duration, and frequency of the application of load. This affects myoblast differentiation, suggesting that when myofascial release is applied to a fibroblast-rich tissue after an injury, it may assist muscle repair.[132] The resulting better muscular and fascial function enhances venous and lymphatic flow through the tissue that in turn restores normal oxygenation, nutrient transport to the cells, and eliminates toxins and inflammatory products. Increased interstitial fluid flow also increases collagen production and alignment, and fibroblast proliferation.[133]

In vitro, when human fibroblasts are experimentally strained unequally along two axes, secretion of proinflammatory interleukin 6 (IL-6) and nitric oxide is increased, with distinct modifications in cellular structure and intracellular actin activity.[134] Equal biaxial strain direction when compared to unequal biaxial strain direction, however, produced a significant decrease in proliferation, inflammatory IL-6 secretion, and macrophage-derived chemoattractant/chemokine secretion.[135] When OMT (experimentally modeled counterstrain and myofascial release) was applied upon strained human fibroblasts, reversal of the strain effects is observed, suggesting that proliferation of fibroblasts and expression and secretion of anti-inflammatory interleukins may contribute to the efficacy of OMT.[136][137][138] Strain direction, frequency,

and duration are important factors affecting fibroblastic functions such as mediation of pain, decrease of edema, and inflammation. The recognition that fibroblast strain direction (unequal biaxial versus equal biaxial) has a distinct influence upon differentiating cellular cytokine secretion and proliferative responses to OMT, suggests the existence of optimal therapeutic strain application patterns for the treatment of somatic dysfunctions. Thus the effective treatment of somatic dysfunction is predicated upon correct diagnosis of dysfunctional patterns.[139]

Experiments done either ex vivo or in vivo, where areolar tissue is stretched, demonstrate that fibroblasts change in shape and remodeling of their CSK occurs.[140] Cytoskeletal remodeling is associated with important changes in cellular and tissue biochemistry such as signal transduction, gene expression, and matrix adhesion. As a result, depending on the length of the tissue, connective tissue may become more or less loose. Change in fibroblast nuclear shape has been demonstrated when mouse subcutaneous tissue is stretched.[141] In spite of this, in dense connective tissue and stiff cross-linked gel, tissue stretch does not demonstrate cytoskeletal remodeling.[142] This suggests that although fibroblastic nuclear shape may be affected by exogenous forces, the extent of this influence is determined by the histological environment of the cells.

The presence of myofibroblasts in fascia is well documented.[143][144] They adapt to change in tension with contraction, and through mechanotransduction transmit the stress forces to the surrounding ECM. As a result, ECM tonicity is increased with deposition of collagen that stabilizes the contraction that, under pathologic conditions, may become permanent.[145] Evaluation of fascial tone is part of an osteopathic assessment. In order to avoid an increase of fascial tonicity, indirect procedures, with constant listening to the tissue, are recommended. (See 'Section 2: Osteopathic assessment,' p. 37.)

Viscosity of the ECM may change with the application of fascial techniques. In the 1930s Ida Rolf developed a treatment system known as 'Rolfing.' This approach applied the gel-to-sol concept described in physics to fascia. The application of energy, such as heat or mechanical pressure, can change ground substance from a more dense colloidal gel into sol i.e., a more fluid state.[146] Indeed, interstitial mechanoreceptors within the fascia involved in efferent control of the vasodilatation and plasma extravasation,[147] may, when stimulated, initiate ECM viscosity change.[148] OMT is thought to contribute to the restoration of the acidic, gel-like character of CT resulting in a healthy, fluid quality that allows optimal nervous function, blood flow, and lymphatic drainage.[149]

OMT applied to vascular and nervous tissue increased nitric oxide (NO) concentration on a cellular level within the blood.[150] NO is an important signaling molecule that, when expressed by nerves, conveys information from one nerve to another.[151] This finding may, in part, explain the therapeutic effects of OMT. As stated by Still: "all diseases are mere effects, the cause being a partial or complete failure of the nerves to properly conduct the fluids of life."[152]

Other signaling molecules are also found within the blood, particularly the endocannabinoids (eCB). The eCB system takes part in fascial reorganization by remodeling fibroblasts. Endocannabinoids also diminish nociception and reduce inflammation in myofascial tissues. Studies have demonstrated a strong possibility that the physiological effects of OMT may be in part the result of stimulation of the cannabinoid receptors.[153] [154]

After OMT, consisting of articulatory treatment system, muscle energy, soft tissue, and strain-counterstrain techniques directed to specific sites of somatic dysfunction, the concentration of several circulatory nociceptive biomarkers has been shown to decrease with statistical significance in patients with chronic low back pain.[155]

Many different types of OMT have been described for the treatment of somatic dysfunction. (See 'Section 3: Treatment of the patient,' p. 79.) Osteopathic manipulative treatment, however, can be simply classified into two fundamental groups of treatment procedures: direct and indirect techniques. Most of the time, somatic dysfunction involves fluidic, cellular, neural, fascial, ligamentous, muscular, osseous, and visceral structures more or less simultaneously. As the objective of the practitioner is to treat somatic dysfunction and to 'find health,' treatment must intervene upon any of these structures, or any combination of them as necessary, even if fascia is the focus of this chapter.

When treating fascia with direct procedures, the treatment can be done by applying low load along the lines of maximal fascial restriction. The pressure is sustained over the skin, without allowing the hands to slide for a minimum of 90–120 seconds. Stretches must be long duration stretches in the direction of restriction, until the barrier is felt and tissue release occurs. Then, pressure is maintained while the practitioner's hands follow the direction of the fascial release.[156]

With indirect procedures, the dysfunctional body part is moved away from the restrictive barrier. This unloads the tissue and decreases neural activity, possibly resetting sensory input to the facilitated spinal cord area. Subsequent adjustments may occur, including changes in the tonus of associated striated muscle, local vasodilatation with change in local fluid dynamics, modification of the viscoelastic properties of CTs, and lowered tonus of intrafascial smooth muscle cells.

In the case of fascial dysfunctions that are quite established, a 'pumping' procedure may be applied. As with direct procedures, low load is applied, with long duration stretches in the direction of restriction, without engaging the dysfunctional barrier. The practitioner then lets the tissue return to a position of ease, and slowly repeats the 'pumping' process. Each stretch must be done 'listening' to the tissue, i.e., without engaging a barrier. For best results, the rhythm of the 'pumping' can follow the inner rhythms of the patient, such as the PRM.

Another approach to reset fascial tone would be to instruct the patient to actively, but very gently, move the body area to be treated in the direction of the restriction, while the practitioner opposes, using a very minimal resistance. The movement and forces applied should be as small as possible. During the relaxation phase, it is appropriate to wait for a few (3–5) seconds during which time the practitioner should evaluate the quality of the return to the initial position. This procedure is repeated several times until the practitioner feels a return of good quality and relaxation in the fascial tone.

The PRM, among various internal rhythms, may also be employed whenever possible to treat CT. Whatever the procedures, we suggest that CT be treated with great respect, considering its potential effect on the neuroendocrine and autonomic systems, and cellular metabolism. Treatment must be designed according to the specificity of every patient, as stated by Still, "To find health," because "Anyone can find disease."[157]

# The primary respiratory mechanism

A mechanism is defined as the fundamental processes involved in, or responsible for, an action, reaction, or natural phenomenon.[158] In 1939, Sutherland first proposed his concept of a primary respiratory mechanism (PRM).[159] This hypothesis was further delineated to consist of five components including:[160]

1. The inherent motility of the central nervous system (CNS) with its resultant effect upon the four remaining components:
2. Fluctuation of the cerebrospinal fluid;
3. Articular mobility of the cranial bones;
4. Mobility of the intracranial and intraspinal membranes;
5. Involuntary mobility of the sacrum between the ilia.

The first component may reasonably be considered as the energy source driving components two through five. Following in the footsteps of Still, and consistent with the works of the eighteenth-century neuroanatomist and theologian Emanuel Swedenborg,[161] [162] Sutherland proposed a system for the PRM that is anatomically focused. The PRM, he stated, is tidal in nature; a biphasic phenomenon consisting of inspiration and expiration.[163] The inspiratory phase of primary respiration manifests flexion of midline structures with coupled external rotation of bilaterally paired structures. While the expiratory phase respectively manifests extension and internal rotation.

The palpable motion of the cranial bones under the influence of the PRM was later referred to as the cranial rhythmic impulse (CRI) by Woods and Woods.[164] Becker went on to identify various frequencies of activity within the PRM. He identified what he referred to as a 'fast tide' with a frequency of 8–12 cpm (0.13–0.20 Hz) and a 'slow tide' of approximately six cycles in ten minutes (0.01 Hz).[165]

It must be recognized that this approach describes the mechanism. It fails, however, to provide a physiological origin for the motility, beyond referring to the inherent motility of the CNS, and ascribing it to Spirit.

In 1902 John Martin Littlejohn, an ardent osteopathic physiologist, addressed the issue of CNS motion.[166] He states that:

In "...the therapeutic plane we are dealing with the nexus of spirit and body, and, therefore, with those vibrations or fluxions that lie at the foundation of the force called vital."

In "...the brain...we find certain rhythmical movements... corresponding, (1) with systole and diastole of the heart, (2) with inspiratory and expiratory changes, and (3) with vascular variations of vasomotion."

The 'vascular variations of vasomotion' that Littlejohn refers to were originally described by Ludwig Traube[167] in the mid-nineteenth century, later to be corroborated by Ewald Hering[168] and further delineated by Siegmund Mayer.[169] They are found in the 0.5–12 cpm (0.009–0.20 Hz) frequency range. In human cardiovascular physiology the frequency range between 0.5 and 120 cpm (0.009–2.0 Hz) shows consistent areas of activity at:[170]

60–120 cpm (1.0–2.0 Hz) associated with heart rate.*

15–25 cpm (0.25–0.42 Hz) associated with pulmonary respiration.

6–12 cpm (0.10–0.20 Hz) associated with baroreflex and vagal activity.

0.5–1.2 cpm (0.009–0.02 Hz) associated with thermal regulation and endothelially-mediated vasomotion.

*It should be noted that although heart rate normally occurs within the 1.0–2.0 Hz range, it also demonstrates frequency modulations at each of the lower listed frequencies.

The frequencies reported throughout the text that follows may vary slightly from the above ranges. This is because of differences in sensitivity of measurement methods employed by different researchers.

These physiological oscillations, specifically at the 6–12 cpm (0.10–0.20 Hz) and 0.5–1.2 cpm (0.009–0.02 Hz) frequencies, have been clearly linked to cranial osteopathy.[171 172 173 174] It is of interest to note that oscillatory phenomena of microvascular origin occupying the same frequency ranges as Becker's slow and fast tides have been identified. The wave frequency interval of 0.009–0.02 Hz, occupying the same frequency band as the slow tide is attributed to vascular endothelial activity, mediated by nitric oxide (NO) and the wave frequency interval of 0.06–0.20 Hz, fast tide frequency, is related to the myogenic activity of the baroreflex upon the microvessel wall.[175] Activity in these same frequency bands is also demonstrable in blood pressure[176] and heart rate variability.[177]

A complex interrelationship of tonic activities, reflecting phasic input from the brainstem and the humoral effect of renin-angiotensin, gives rise to these systemic cardiovascular oscillations.[178] The neural activity is generated in the nucleus of the tractus solitarius (NTS) located in the floor of the fourth ventricle. Within the NTS, there are lateral vasoconstriction and medial vasodilatation areas that exhibit inherent automaticity.[179 180] The vagus nerve (CN X) located within the medulla immediately adjacent to the NTS, contributes to the cardiovascular oscillations through its cardio-inhibitory efferent fibers.

## Homeostasis and the primary respiratory mechanism

Magoun, in his description of Sutherland's PRM, stated that it was a means whereby "...every cell in the body receives not only the inspired oxygen but also the nutrition, the enzymes, the hormones and whatever else contributes to high level wellness.

Included in this internal respiration is the elimination of waste metabolites through the proper emunctories."[181]

There is a range that physiological parameters must, necessarily, be within for bodily equilibrium, the continuation of life, and the maintenance of health. The earliest unicellular organisms interacted directly with the external environment, and early in the evolutionary process, developed mobility as a method of adjusting to change within their environment. As multicellular organisms evolved, and became more and more complex, the individual cells became sequestered within the organism, isolated from the external environment. As such, it became necessary for the organism to regulate its internal environment. This regulation resulted from the need to maintain cellular homeostasis, the product of multiple processes through which bodily equilibrium is maintained.[182] The low frequency oscillations, discussed above, are recognized for their contribution to the maintenance of homeostasis.[183]

Physiology is continually modulating the internal environment, to maintain the organism within the necessary range of viability. In the process of maintaining the state of balance between opposing pressures, over time, dynamic systems will tend to drift. In order to maintain stability they must, therefore, continuously be reset. The resultant correction of drift causes the system to, in turn, drift in the direction of the correction. Thus the repeated correction of drift causes the system to oscillate within the vitally acceptable range set by homeostatic parameters.

## Inherent physiological rhythms, capacitance, frequency modulation, and the primary respiratory mechanism

Oscillating physiological systems may maintain themselves through capacitance. Energy is stored in the physiological equivalent of a capacitor and released intermittently thereby maintaining the oscillation. Signal variation with time is indicative of frequency modulation among interacting signals[184] and implies the presence of a capacitor in the responsible physiological mechanism. [185] [186] [187] This occurs among the cardiovascular frequencies with the heart rate and the baroreflex demonstrating frequency modulations at the lower frequencies. Similarly, the oscillating PRM, as manifest by the CRI, exhibits a 20% frequency modulation.[188] [189] There must, therefore, be physiological capacitors within the PRM.

## Fluctuation of the cerebrospinal fluid and motion of the central nervous system

Sutherland stated that:

> "According to my present hypothesis...the brain involuntarily and rhythmically moves within the skull. This involuntary rhythmical movement involves dilation and contraction of the ventricles, during respiratory periods. The ventricle dilation and contraction in turn effects (sic) cerebrospinal fluid circulatory activity; and the circulatory activity effects movement of the arachnoid and dural membranes; and through the special reciprocal tension membrane...effects mobility of the basilar articulations.... The hypothesis does not include dilation nor (sic) contraction of the spinal canal. The spinal canal merely moves upward and downward.... The cerebrospinal fluid throughout the vertebral column fluctuates by way of the arachnoid membrane; the membrane being hung from above, with only one attachment, and that at the sacrum."[190]

The first four components of the PRM: the inherent motility of the CNS, the fluctuation of the cerebrospinal fluid (CSF), and the mobility of the cranial bones and the intracranial and intraspinal membranes are readily explained in the context of the low frequency cardiovascular oscillations.

Motion of the cranium, in compensation for fluid volume changes within the cranial cavity, has been demonstrated using X-ray and NMR tomography. Periodic movement with a frequency of 6–14 cpm (0.10–0.23 Hz) was observed and changes in frontal and sagittal dimensions with mean amplitude of $0.38 \pm 0.21$ mm, and maximum deviation of up to 1 mm, were recorded.[191]

Complex motions of the brain[192] and CSF, [193] [194] in the same frequency range as the cardiovascular oscillations and bony motion described above, have been confirmed by magnetic resonance velocity imaging. The images demonstrate that, during cardiac systole, there is inflow of blood into the cranial cavity, causing the brain to expand in volume, moving complexly. The volume change within the cranial cavity displaces the central portion of the brain in a caudal direction. The CSF within the lateral ventricles of the cerebral cortex is displaced medially into the third ventricle, and from there, caudally into the fourth ventricle. Ultimately, an amount of CSF equaling the brain volume change moves in a caudal direction from the cranial cavity into the spinal canal. This increases the pressure in the dural sac surrounding the spinal cord. During diastole, with lower intracranial pressure, the caudal displacement of the brain recoils, and the motion direction of the CSF reverses.

As blood flow velocity and blood pressure fluctuations have been demonstrated at the low frequency cardiovascular oscillations, so too, low frequency volume oscillations in the brains of conscious healthy human subjects have been measured using ultrasound[195] and bioimpedance.[196] The 0.10–0.20 Hz CSF oscillation, C waves, demonstrates amplitude from barely discernible to 20 mm Hg. The lower frequency B waves, at 0.009–0.02 Hz, have amplitude as great as 50 mm Hg.[197]

Using exposure times that were too slow to assess cardiac and baroreflex synchronous motions (<0.1 Hz), computerized tomography has been employed to observe movement of the lateral and third ventricles in the normal brain. It was shown that the brain, rostral to the foramen of Monro, demonstrates a complex rolling peristaltic motion with a rate (26 second to several minutes in duration) in the range of the B waves, or that of the slow tide.[198]

Thus, the motion of the cranium, brain, and CSF, synchronous with the cardiac cycle, continues at the rate of the low frequency cardiovascular oscillations. These pulsatile motions can, therefore, be considered to act as a pump energized, at least in part, by the volumetric fluctuations of circulating blood and CSF. As the intracranial blood volume increases, the cranium changes shape compliantly, and CSF moves through the ventricular system, and is displaced into the extracranial subarachnoid space thereby increasing the amount of CSF in the spinal dural sac. As intracranial blood volume decreases, the tension of the distended spinal dural sac facilitates the return of CSF back into the skull. Thus, synchronous with, and, at least partially because of the low frequency cardiovascular oscillations, the CSF is 'ebbing and flowing.'

For this to occur effectively, tension placed upon the spinal dural sac during periods of increased intracranial pressure, provides the required capacitance to return the CSF back into the cranium as intracranial pressure drops. This explains the PRM in the context of a craniosacral mechanism. It does not, however, satisfactorily provide insight into a whole-body PRM.

## The whole-body primary respiratory mechanism

At the outset of this discussion it is important that the reader understands the physical process of entrainment between oscillating systems. Entrainment occurs when two systems are oscillating at close frequency, one to the other. The dominant frequency will force the second oscillation to assume, in synchrony, the same frequency as the dominant input.[199] [200] [201] [202] [203] This is how diverse systems within human physiology are proposed to come together in a holistic manner.

Heart rate, blood pressure, and blood flow velocity demonstrate low frequency oscillations within the 0.009 to 0.20 Hz range. The peripheral vascular system, and consequently tissue perfusion, is therefore entirely under the influence of these oscillations.[204] [205] [206] [207] [208] [209] [210] [211] [212] [213] [214] [215] [216] [217] [218] [219] [220] [221] Circulatory and body core temperature homeostasis is maintained by the low frequency oscillations.[222] [223] [224] [225] Efficient cellular respiration, the purpose of the PRM, is dependent upon effective tissue perfusion.

### Cellular respiration

Occurring through a series of intracellular metabolic pathways, cellular respiration results in the conversion of nutrient derived biochemical energy into adenosine triphosphate (ATP), and the release of cellular waste products into the interstitium. Cytochrome oxidase, within the mitochondria, is the terminal enzyme in the respiratory electron transport chain. The electron transport chain produces a transmembrane electrochemical potential that is used by ATP synthase to produce ATP. The ensuing stored energy may then be employed for processes including biosynthesis, motility, and molecular transport across the cell membrane. This process is possibly the best physical representation of what Becker referred to as the "Breath of Life"[226] and what Magoun attributed to the actions of the PRM.[227]

Consistent in frequency with the PRM, 'oxygen availability waves' within the CNS have been recognized for years.[228] [229] [230] [231] [232] [233] [234] [235] It has been demonstrated, using reflectance spectrophotometry of the cortical cytochrome oxidase redox state, that cortical metabolism oscillates in the same frequency range as the baroreflex. Cyclic increases in cortical oxidative metabolism within the range of 7–10 cpm (0.11–0.17 Hz) represent the source of the local vascular oscillations, thereby effecting tissue perfusion.[236] [237] [238]

The redox state of cytochrome oxidase is linked with endothelial vasomotion induced by NO that is generated, among other sites, in arteriolar walls by endothelial nitric oxide synthase. The generation and release of NO occurs as the result of shear forces exerted by the flow of the blood against the vessel wall. Vasoconstriction increases shear forces, releasing NO, causing vasodilatation. Thus generated, NO is also released into the interstitium where it enters the cell, binds to, and reversibly inhibits, mitochondrial cytochrome oxidase, with resultant reduction of cellular oxygen consumption. The NO-mediated inhibition of cellular oxygen consumption may be modulated in part by the redox state of cytochrome oxidase in the mitochondria.[239] It is also of interest to note that NO has been demonstrated to act as a mediator of the baroreflex in the NTS.[240]

Interhemispheric synchrony of the slow oscillations of cortical blood volume and cytochrome oxidase redox state has been demonstrated.[241] [242] Although this process is independent of baroreflex physiology, it is not unreasonable to conclude that the overlapping frequencies of the cytochrome oxidase redox and baroreflex oscillations allow these two vasoactive processes to become entrained, thus linking local tissue perfusion with central vasomotor control.[243] [244] [245] [246] It is further reasonable to hypothesize that, because mitochondrial activity is primordial, similar cellular physiology occurs throughout the body.

For cellular respiration to occur in a coordinated fashion on the level of complexity of a multicellular organism, an equally complex circulatory apparatus has to be functioning. Consequently a whole-body PRM model may be proposed in the context of the physiology of peripheral circulation. It is therefore appropriate to consider cellular respiration in the context of each component of peripheral circulatory anatomy: the arterial resistance vessels, the capillary bed and its interface with the interstitium, the extravascular compartment as defined by fascia, the lymphatic and venous return, and how this all comes together, in association with pulmonary respiration and renal physiology, to function as the PRM.

### The arterial resistance vessels

The arterial system is the active location of blood pressure and flow velocity modulation. This occurs, to a great extent, through baroreflex control of arterial vasomotor tone. [247] [248] [249] [250] Stretch receptors, located in the aortic arch, brachiocephalic artery bifurcation, common carotid arteries, and carotid sinuses, continuously monitor systemic arterial pressure. Afferent neurons transmit information regarding the status of the blood pressure (increasing or decreasing) to the NTS where neural activity producing the baroreflex oscillation originates. Within the NTS pressor and depressor areas exhibit inherent automaticity.[251] [252] Efferent myelinated vasoconstrictor fibers under the control of the NTS descend within the spinal cord to the thoracolumbar sympathetic ganglia to synapse with unmyelinated post-ganglionic fibers

that carry vasoconstrictor activity to the periphery. Even though, in humans, oscillating sympathetic activity demonstrates frequency content from as low as 0.5 cpm (0.009 Hz) to heart rate, 60–120 cpm (1.0–2.0 Hz), the arterial vasculature, acting as low-pass filters, responds with significant gain only to modulation of sympathetic stimuli in the 6–12 cpm (0.10–0.20 Hz) frequency range or lower.[253] This response of rhythmic tonic activity, reflecting the phasic input from the NTS, results in the baroreflex oscillation of blood pressure and flow velocity.[254]

Arteriolar motion physically drives fluid into the interstitium. Oscillating changes in arteriolar diameter, the result of local influences and central vasomotor activity, in combination with the length of the active vessels, causes an equivalent displacement of the tissue mass and interstitial fluid.[255] [256]

### The capillary bed and its interface with the interstitium

The blood flow and pressure oscillations, demonstrable in the thicker walled arterial system, become less constrained as the blood passes into the thinner walled capillaries and venous system. The capacitance of these thinner walled vessels allows for greater volume fluctuation with proportionate displacement of the adjacent interstitium. In some tissues the capillary beds demonstrate local contractility in response to distension.[257] It has been suggested that the low frequency blood flow and pressure oscillations, the result of associated arteriolar and venular vasomotion, aid in the distribution and mixing of extravascular fluids and mechanically augment the passage of fluid through the capillary and lymphatic walls. [258]

Capillary, and as a result cellular, perfusion is determined by the interplay between central regulation and local requirements. Blood flow through the peripheral tissues demonstrates periods of underperfusion alternating with increased perfusion. This allows for blood flow through individual capillaries that satisfies local metabolic tissue demands. Such variation in tissue perfusion has been demonstrated to occur in discrete groups of from 10–15 capillaries. Consistent with the relationship between the interaction of mitochondrial cytochrome oxidase, NO, and vasomotion (7–10 cpm or 0.11–0.17 Hz)[259] [260] [261], the control of this local fluctuation in blood flow velocity is presumed to be at the level of the supply arterioles.[262]

With the low pass suppression of pressure oscillations above the pulmonary respiratory frequency (0.25–0.42 Hz), independently occurring local blood flow oscillations, at 7–10 cpm (0.11–0.17 Hz), are thought to be coordinated by the central baroreflex oscillation through entrainment of frequency.[263] [264] [265] [266] [267] Thus, although regulated by local tissue requirements, the oscillating arteriolar vasomotion is synchronized by the NTS.

This oscillation also has significant effects upon Starling's equilibrium (Table 1.1: Starling's equilibrium). Arteriolar vasomotion causes capillary hematocrit changes in such a way that during periods of vasodilatation, with increased blood flow velocity, there is increased local hematocrit and, therefore, increased transcapillary pressure gradients. During the alternate vasoconstrictive phase, the hematocrit decreases, and intracapillary pressure drops to the level of adjacent venules facilitating reabsorption from the interstitium.[268]

## Fascia and the interstitium

The fascia surrounds and supports all other tissues and organs of the body. Every structure within the body, from the histologic level to the gross anatomic level, is surrounded by envelopes of fascia, and all of these envelopes are held together by the superficial fascia, acting as one big envelope. Thus fascia divides the body into compartments within compartments within compartments, delineating all structures and spaces, including the interstitium. This structural arrangement protects, while providing sufficient elasticity to accommodate for changes in shape and motility.

This compartmentalization of areas within the body would initially appear to physically isolate those areas. In fact the compartmental contents can become swollen from a myriad of causes with potentially life threatening results.[269] This having been recognized, the anatomy of the fascia plays a vital role in the hypothetical model for the PRM.

As fascia permeates the body it establishes a structural and functional continuity that links the smallest components with the anatomic and functional whole. In part, because of this, the body functions as a holistic structure in which every part is united with every other part through the network of fascia. Forces exerted by anatomic structures, whose shape is defined by their respective fascial envelopes, load their surrounding fascia. These forces are in turn transmitted to adjacent and distant fascia determining the alignment of component collagen and elastic fibers and the gross structure of the body.

The fascial envelopes are in a tensegrital relationship with their contents. The human body is approximately 60% water.[270] As such, water constitutes the single largest component within the fascial envelopes. As fluid moves from the intravascular space into the interstitium, under the influence of the low frequency oscillations of vasomotion, blood flow, and blood pressure, interstitial pressure increases. This presumably occurs, at least in part, because of the physical restraint of fascial compartmentalization.

The capacity of the fascia to manifest inherent contractility[271] is of extreme significance in this model. Myofibroblasts, smooth muscle-like cells within the fascia, exhibit periodic oscillations periods of approximately 100 seconds.[272] This is a frequency of 0.01 Hz and is located at the low end of the 0.009–0.02 Hz frequency band of the slow tide oscillation. Spontaneous contractions in some areas of fascia, suggest a role of pre-stress in the collagen scaffold.[273] Thus, when fascia is distended, the myofibroblasts contract to provide resistance. This is known to occur in the fascial perimysium.[274]

Table 1.1: Starling's equilibrium

| Forces moving fluid out of the vascular compartment | |
| --- | --- |
| Mean capillary pressure: | 17.0 mm Hg |
| Mean negative interstitial pressure: | 7.0 mm Hg |
| Interstitial fluid colloid osmotic pressure: | 4.5 mm Hg |
| **Total outward pressure:** | **28.5 mm Hg** |
| **Forces drawing fluid into the vascular compartment** | |
| **Total colloid osmotic pressure:** | **28.0 mm Hg** |
| **The summation of these forces results in a net outward force of:** | **0.5 mm Hg** |

Fascial contractility may also be influenced by the vascular and autonomic nervous systems, as implied by the great number of autonomic nerves and the rich intrafascial supply of capillaries.[275]

So, as interstitial fluid volume increases, the investing fascia is distended and, in a manner similar to that of the spinal dura described above, can behave as a capacitor. The fascia then contracts, in synchrony with the low frequency pressure oscillations, facilitating the return of fluid into the intravascular space, and compressing the terminal lymphatic sacs (see below).

Fascia further mechanically contributes to venous and lymphatic central return. The deep fascia that surrounds muscles is tough, thick, and resistant. During muscular contraction, the fine-walled veins and lymphatic vessels inside the muscles are compressed and as a result, blood and lymph is propelled in the direction of the heart. Muscles and fascia, particularly in the lower extremities, act as a pump moving venous blood and lymph against the force of gravity. It is of interest to note here that sympathetic tone to the muscles also oscillates in the low (0.009 to 0.42 Hz) frequency range.[276]

### Lymphatic return

Sutherland suggested an association between the PRM and lymphatic circulation. "Compression was applied around the head with the intent to limit all basilar activity. The experiment resulted in an immediate change of the movement of the diaphragmatic respiratory mechanism, as well as an indication of a change throughout the systemic lymph channels; the indication in the lymph activity being greater in its manifestation than the author has thus been able to secure through the application of the lymphatic pump method."[277]

As blood flows through the capillaries, fluid filters out into the interstitium. In a resting adult, approximately 15 ml/min leaves the vascular space and 12 to 13.5 ml/min (or 80–90%) returns. This results in 1.5 to 3 ml/min, or 2 to 4 L/24 hr, carrying 80–200 gm of protein that remains in the interstitium and, therefore, must be removed by the lymphatic system each day.[278]

Effective lymphatic drainage requires that fluid moves efficiently through the interstitium.

Essentially all of the fluid within the interstitium is in a gel-like state. Proteoglycan filaments form weak cross-links with each other, with collagen fibers, and with protein molecules to give the interstitial content its gel-like consistency. Consequently, fluid does not flow freely through the interstitium.[279] The interstitial gel, however, demonstrates tensegral elasticity. [280] An oscillation of this gel matrix with a more fluid sol state in synchrony with the PRM has been proposed.[281] Tissue fluid pressure is a determinant of fluid transfer between the blood and the tissue spaces, and between the tissue spaces and the terminal lymphatic sacs.[282] It is probable that the 6–12 cpm (0.10–0.20 Hz) baroreflex-mediated pressure changes induce this fluid movement through the interstitial matrix.

The primary force driving lymphatic filling is volume change within the terminal lymphatic sacs. The cells of the terminal lymphatic sacs are arranged in an overlapping shingle fashion, thus allowing interstitial fluid to enter the vessel. Due to one-way valves in the proximal lymph vessels that prevent retrograde flow, volume increases in the terminal lymphatic sacs can occur only when fluid traverses the interstitium and crosses the lymphatic endothelium.

Hydrostatic pressure within the terminal lymphatic sacs is presumed to be similar to that of the interstitial fluid, with transient differences between the two compartments being quickly equilibrated.[283] The negative interstitial pressure (-7 mm Hg) of Starling's equilibrium (Table 1.1: Starling's equilibrium, p. 23.) results in interstitial fluid being drawn into the terminal lymphatic sacs. This negative interstitial pressure is maintained by the removal of protein from the interstitium by the lymphatic flow.[284] Additionally intermittent motion in the tissues associated with the baroreflex-mediated arteriolar vasomotion causes pulses of fluid to move into the terminal lymphatic sacs.[285] The baroreflex-driven fluctuating intracapillary pressure and hematocrit further adds to this mechanism.

When the terminal lymphatic sacs have become filled to capacity, augmented by the drop in interstitial pressure from arteriolar vasomotion and fluctuating intracapillary pressure and hematocrit, the overlapping cells approximate one another. This causes the terminal lymphatic vessel to become distended and prevents fluid return back into the interstitium.

Lymph is then propelled centrally by movement of the surrounding tissues and by contraction of the lymphatic endothelial cells induced by the low frequency oscillations in interstitial pressure and the recoil of the fascial capacitor. Vascular distension may be the stimulus for the release of prostaglandin H2 and thromboxane, both mediators of lymphatic vasomotion.[286] [287] Lymph endothelial cells contain actin or actomyosin filaments that, when stretched, are capable of causing the cells to contract.[288] Lymph vessels demonstrate spontaneous contractions, varying in frequency from 1 to 30 cpm (0.017–0.50 Hz).[289] [290] [291] [292] [293] [294] [295] [296] [297] Spontaneous lymphatic vascular contractility, independent of arterial pulse rate, respiration, and body movement, has also been recorded at 1 to 9 (average 4) cpm (0.017–0.15 Hz).[298] This spontaneous contractility is potentially subject to entrainment with the low frequency arteriolar, capillary, and interstitial pressure oscillations.

Lymphatic vessels proximal to the terminal lymphatic sacs and lymphatic capillaries consist of a series of individual units: lymphangia. A lymphangion is that portion of a lymphatic vessel delineated by two adjacent one-way valves. The presence of the valves in the lymphatic vessels, and low resistance along the vascular walls, ensures that any volume decrease of the terminal lymphatic vasculature must occur because of the displacement of fluid centrally.[299] Similar to the terminal lymphatic sacs, and lymphatic capillaries, each lymphangion is also capable of spontaneous independent contractility. The pacemaker for these contractions appears to be located in the lymphangion wall just proximal to the distal valve.[300] Although lymphangia may contract randomly, they function more efficiently when contracting synchronously. Lymphatic vessels tend to develop synchronous activity easily.[301] Again entrainment, mediated by the low frequency pressure oscillations, probably ensures optimal efficiency of this aspect of the mechanism.

## Venous return

Of the fluid from the capillary bed that enters the interstitium, 10–20% returns to the general circulation via the lymphatic system. The majority, 80–90% however, re-enters the capillary bed, exiting through the venous system.

In comparison to the arterioles, the venules, of relatively greater diameter with thinner muscular walls, are also innervated by the sympathetic nervous system. Their walls contract and relax, contributing greatly to vascular capacitance and regulation of tissue perfusion,[302] [303] and to the observed frequency modulation of the low frequency waveforms.[304] [305] As post-capillary resistance vessels, the venules help to regulate capillary hydrostatic pressure and contribute to fluid exchange in the capillaries.[306] As pre-capillary arterioles constrict, there is a resultant intracapillary hematocrit decrease and a drop in intracapillary pressure to the level of adjacent venules, facilitating reabsorption from the interstitium.[307] It is probable that post-capillary resistance control lies in the larger venules up to 300 micrometers in diameter.[308]

The thin walled veins in their role as a capacitance system hold up to 80% of systemic blood.[309] Reflex changes in sympathetic tone affect the diameter of the veins and the compliance of their walls, as such adjusting the size of the venous capacitor.[310] The resultant changes in venous capacitance impact both the nature (selection of coupled frequencies) and degree (magnitude of the coupling) to which frequency modulation contributes to changing the blood flow and pressure waveform, and its impact upon any associated systems.

The venous capacitor, in concert with arterial resistance, contracts slowly and regularly, fluctuating at the low frequencies.[311] [312] [313] This fluctuation facilitates the return of venous blood to the heart, while it augments fluid movement through the interstitium and lymphatic circulation. Vasomotion at the low frequencies accounts for the negative interstitial pressure of Starling's equilibrium (Table 1.1: Starling's equilibrium, p. 23.). General anesthesia and certain drugs (calcium channel blockers) disrupt these oscillations, resulting in peripheral edema.[314]

The venous system is also involved in thermal regulation, by the controlled shifting of blood between the compliant splanchnic veins, typically containing up to 30% of blood volume, and the cutaneous veins.[315] Thermal regulation is under the control of the sympathetic and parasympathetic components of the autonomic nervous system in concert with renin-angiotensin.[316 317 318 319] It manifests in the 0.5–2.0 cpm (0.009–0.02 Hz) frequency range,[320 321 322 323 324 325] the same frequency range as Becker's 'slow tide.'[326]

## Pulmonary respiration and renal physiology

The final obligation of the PRM, as stated by Magoun, is "the elimination of waste metabolites through the proper emunctories."[327] The waste products of aerobic (water and $CO_2$) and anaerobic (nitrite, succinate, sulfide, methane, and acetate) cellular respiration are predominantly disposed of through the lungs and kidneys. Pulmonary respiration and renal physiology are consequently of importance in the context of the PRM.

The mechanics of pulmonary respiration physically provide the final step in the return of venous blood and lymph to the chest where the lungs act to expel waste products and oxygenate the blood. The thoracic cage, thoracoabdominal diaphragm, and abdominal cavity in concert form a two-chambered pump that actively pull blood and lymph back into the chest.

During pulmonary inspiration, as the thoracoabdominal diaphragm descends, intrathoracic pressure drops and intra-abdominal increases, pulling venous blood and lymph into the chest from the abdomen, pelvis, upper extremities, and head and neck. The liver and spleen, two organs of significant circulatory sequestration and immune function, are compressed by the combination of thoracoabdominal diaphragm descent and intra-abdominal pressure increase. Conversely during pulmonary expiration, as the thoracoabdominal diaphragm ascends, intrathoracic pressure increases and intra-abdominal pressure drops, pulling venous blood and lymph into the abdomen from the lower extremities.

Pulmonary respiration is recognized as closely associated with, yet independent of, the PRM.[328]

[329 330 331] Patient respiratory cooperation is often employed in association with cranial treatment.[332] [333 334 335 336] Cranial manipulation is said to affect pulmonary respiration.[337 338] Spontaneous deep sighing respiration is reported to be coincidental with the therapeutic end point of cranial manipulation.[339] Fourier analysis of blood pressure and blood flow velocity shows that the low frequency oscillations, the 0.5–1.2 cpm (0.009–0.02 Hz) thermal and endothelial vasomotion frequency, the 6–12 cpm (0.10–0.20 Hz) baroreflex and vagal frequency, and the 15–25 cpm (0.25–0.42 Hz) pulmonary frequency are each distinct frequency bands. [340 341 342] The thermal and endothelial vasomotion frequency and baroreflex and vagal frequency components are, however, closely linked to, and potentially modulated by, pulmonary respiration through frequency entrainment.[343 344]

Although pulmonary respiration typically occurs at the 15–25 cpm (0.25–0.42 Hz) frequency, respiration may be voluntarily slowed. When individuals breathe at 5 to 7 breaths per minute (0.08–0.12 Hz) the 0.1 Hz baroreflex component entrains with respiration with a proportionate increase in the power of the resultant oscillation and an effect upon cardiovascular physiology at that frequency.[345 346 347] Examples of such entrainment include chanting and singing. [348 349] Thus through entrainment of frequencies, controlled pulmonary respiration increases the power of the cardiovascular oscillations.

The kidneys also act to clear the blood of the waste products of cellular respiration. The pressure of the arterial blood perfusing the kidneys is oscillating complexly within the 0.5 and 120 cpm (0.009–2.0 Hz) frequency range. As blood pressure drops the juxtaglomerular cells within the kidneys secrete renin into the circulation where it hydrolyzes hepatic angiotensinogen to form angiotensin I. In the lungs, angiotensin converting enzyme catalyses the conversion of angiotensin I to form the potent vasoconstrictor angiotensin II. The 0.5–2.0 cpm (0.009–0.02 Hz) frequency oscillation, at the same frequency as Becker's 'slow tide'[350] is regulated by the sympathetic and parasympathetic nervous systems in concert with the renin-angiotensin system.[351 352]

## Conclusion

The comparison of descriptions of the PRM from the osteopathic literature along with current information about low frequency physiological oscillations within the 0.009 to 0.20 Hz range demonstrates much more than coincidental similarity. It is proposed here that there is sufficient evidence to conclude that the 6–12 cpm (0.10–0.20 Hz) oscillation, associated with baroreflex and vagal physiology, is the Sutherland wave, or Becker's 'fast tide', and that the 0.5–1.2 cpm (0.009–0.02 Hz) oscillation, associated with thermal regulation and endothelially-mediated vasomotion, is Becker's 'slow tide'. It follows therefore, that a hypothetical description of the PRM can be logically provided in the context of oscillations within the 0.5–12 cpm (0.009–0.20 Hz) range, and their associated physiology and biochemistry. Using these oscillations to study and understand the PRM provides a holistic model that unites the CNS with every cell in the body through the sympathetic and parasympathetic branches of the autonomic nervous system, the cardiovascular system, the fascia, and the physiology of cellular respiration.

The NTS, and possibly the vagal nuclei, in the floor of the fourth ventricle provides the zeitgeber for the 6–12 cpm (0.10–0.20 Hz) fast tide and the 0.5–1.2 cpm (0.009–0.02 Hz) slow tide frequencies. These oscillations in cardiovascular physiology, synchronized with the metabolic requirements of individual brain cells provide, at least in part, for the motion of the CNS that, in turn, drives the circulation of the CSF. The oscillation of intracranial pressure at these frequencies displaces CSF into the spinal dural sac that, demonstrating capacitance, returns the displaced CSF back into the skull as intracranial pressure decreases. This oscillation demonstrable as motion of the brain and fluctuation of the CSF is occurring at the rates attributed to the fast and slow tides of the PRM. The PRM, as a total-body phenomenon however, must include more than just an oscillation of the CNS. It is, therefore, proposed to occur as follows:

- The heart, under the central influence of the brainstem, beats with a rhythm, the frequency of which fluctuates at the 6–12 cpm (0.10–0.20 Hz) fast tide, and 0.5–1.2 cpm (0.009–0.02 Hz) slow tide frequencies. It pumps blood that arrives in *all* of the capillary beds in the body via arteries and arterioles whose walls are contracting at those same frequencies. Blood pressure, capillary blood flow rate, capillary hematocrit, and venous capacitance are all oscillating at these frequencies.

- The 6–12 cpm (0.10–0.20 Hz) fast and 0.5–1.2 cpm (0.009–0.02 Hz) slow tide oscillations are less constrained, as the blood traverses the low pass filter capillaries and enters the venous system, than they are in the thicker walled arterial system. The capacitance of these thin walled veins allows for significantly greater volume fluctuation with proportionate displacement of adjacent structures. The arteriolar and venular vasomotion and blood pressure and hematocrit fluctuation that result from the 6–12 cpm (0.10–0.20 Hz) fast and 0.5–1.2 cpm (0.009–0.02 Hz) slow tide oscillations, are augmented by fascial capacitance, aiding in the distribution and mixing of extravascular fluids and mechanically facilitating the passage of fluid through capillary and lymphatic walls.

- Locally, the metabolism of the individual cell, regulated by the respiratory activity of its mitochondria, is oscillating independently, with essentially the same frequency as the 6–12 cpm (0.10–0.20 Hz) fast tide component of the PRM. Cellular respiration regulates local arteriolar tone. Oscillating hematocrit and blood flow velocity, in turn, results in oscillating shear forces affecting the vascular epithelium with resultant modulation of NO synthesis. Increasing NO liberation results in local vasodilatation and the inhibition of mitochondrial activity.

- Capillary hematocrit, and consequently Starling's equilibrium (Table 1.1: Starling's equilibrium, p. 23.), fluctuates under this influence. Cellular metabolic exchange occurs within the interstitial gel medium. Fluid, that will not move as freely through this gel as it can in a purely liquid medium, is pumped in and out of the intravascular compartment and through the interstitium by the oscillating pressures. The central PRM blood flow and pressure oscillations act to entrain the local metabolically-induced oscillations.

- Fluid, proteins, and particulate matter, not returned to the arteriovenous system are removed from the interstitium via the lymphatic circulation. End lymphatic filling and fluid transport through subsequent lymphangia is subject to spontaneous vascular contractility. Again, efficiency of the system is enhanced through entrainment by the central brainstem zeitgeber at the frequencies of the 6–12 cpm (0.10–0.20 Hz) fast and 0.5–1.2 cpm (0.009–0.02 Hz) slow tides.

- Fluid returned to the capillaries is transported back to the heart through the thin walled veins. The capacitance of the veins permits variable sequestration of blood in the periphery and facilitates thermal regulation. Oscillation of the venous system at the rate of the 6–12 cpm (0.10–0.20 Hz) fast and 0.5–1.2 cpm (0.009–0.02 Hz) slow tide frequencies facilitates the efficient return of blood to the heart. Oscillation at the 0.5–1.2 cpm (0.009–0.02 Hz) slow tide frequency maintains body core temperature by shifting blood back and forth between the splanchnic and cutaneous veins.

- The coordinating effect upon the lymphatic and venous systems of the 6–12 cpm (0.10–0.20 Hz) fast and 0.5–1.2 cpm (0.009–0.02 Hz) slow tide oscillations may be thought of as a 'peripheral heart' functioning to efficiently return lymph and blood centrally.

- Thus, local and central control mechanisms act synergistically to satisfy the metabolic demands of the peripheral tissues and to remove waste products to be disposed of by the lungs and kidneys. Locally, the activity of the musculature of the vascular bed is modified and integrated by changes in the composition of the extracellular fluid. Neural control is exercised via specialized sensory endings of peripheral afferent neurons within the integrative centers of the CNS. Response occurs to varying levels of oxygen, carbon dioxide, and hydrogen ion concentration and temperature of the blood and extracellular fluid. Or as Magoun proposed of the PRM, the low frequency physiological oscillations within the 0.009 to 0.20 Hz range facilitate "dynamic metabolic interchange in every cell, with each phase of action."

# References

1. Becker RE. The stillness of life. Brooks RE, editor. Portland, OR: Stillness Press; 2000:178.
2. Ingber DE. The architecture of life. Sci Am. 1998 Jan;278(1):48-57.
3. Jette AM, Branch LG, Berlin J. Musculoskeletal impairments and physical disablement among the aged. J Gerontol. 1990 Nov;45(6):M203-8.
4. Still AT. Philosophy of Osteopathy. Kirksville, MO: A.T. Still; 1899. Reprinted, Indianapolis, IN: American Academy of Osteopathy; 1971:167.
5. Dictionary of Greek and Roman antiquities. Smith W, ed. New York, NY: Harpers & Brothers; 1843:431.
6. Wendell-Smith CP. Fascia: an illustrative problem in international terminology. Surg Radiol Anat. 1997;19(5):273-7.
7. Standring S, ed. Gray's Anatomy The anatomical basis of clinical practice. 39th ed. Edinburgh: Churchill Livingstone; 2004.
8. Lloyd TN. A Massage Therapist's Perspective on the Fascia Research Congresses. Int J Ther Massage Bodywork. 2011;4(4):48-9.
9. Langevin HM, Huijing PA. Communicating about fascia: history, pitfalls, and recommendations. Int J Ther Massage Bodywork. 2009 Dec 7;2(4):3-8.
10. Merriam-Webster on-line dictionary .Available at http://www.merriam-webster.com/medical/fascia. Accessed May 17, 2012.
11. Stoltz JF, Dumas D, Wang X, Payan E, Mainard D, Paulus F, Maurice G, Netter P, Muller S. Influence of mechanical forces on cells and tissues. Biorheology. 2000;37(1-2):3-14.
12. Hinz B, Gabbiani G. Fibrosis: recent advances in myofibroblast biology and new therapeutic perspectives. F1000 Biol Rep. 2010 Nov;2:78.
13. Gabbiani G. The myofibroblast in wound healing and fibrocontractive diseases. J Pathol. 2003 Jul;200(4):500-3.
14. Tomasek JJ, Gabbiani G, Hinz B, Chaponnier C, Brown RA. Myofibroblasts and mechano-regulation of connective tissue remodelling. Nat Rev Mol Cell Biol. 2002 May;3(5):349-63.
15. Mayrand D, Laforce-Lavoie A, Larochelle S, Langlois A, Genest H, Roy M, Moulin VJ. Angiogenic properties of myofibroblasts isolated from normal human skin wounds. Angiogenesis. 2012 Jun;15(2):199-212.
16. Schleip R, Naylor IL, Ursu D, Melzer W, Zorn A, Wilke HJ, Lehmann-Horn F, Klingler W. Med Hypotheses. 2006;66(1):66-71.
17. Findley TW. Second international fascia research congress. Int J Ther Massage Bodywork. 2009 Jun 29;2(2):1-6.
18. Castella LF, Buscemi L, Godbout C, Meister JJ, Hinz B. A new lock-step mechanism of matrix remodelling based on subcellular contractile events. J Cell Sci. 2010 May 15;123(Pt 10):1751-60.
19. Becker RE. Life in Motion. Brooks RE, editor. Portland, OR: Rudra Press; 1997.
20. Liu ZJ, Zhuge Y, Velazquez OC. Trafficking and differentiation of mesenchymal stem cells. J Cell Biochem. 2009 Apr 15;106(6):984-91.
21. Fehrer C, Lepperdinger G. Mesenchymal stem cell aging. Exp Gerontol. 2005 Dec;40(12):926-30.
22. Reiser J, Zhang XY, Hemenway CS, Mondal D, Pradhan L, La Russa VF. Potential of mesenchymal stem cells in gene therapy approaches

for inherited and acquired diseases. Expert Opin Biol Ther. 2005 Dec;5(12):1571-84.

23. Solana R, Tarazona R, Gayoso I, Lesur O, Dupuis G, Fulop T. Innate immunosenescence: Effect of aging on cells and receptors of the innate immune system in humans. Semin Immunol. 2012 Oct;24(5):331-41.

24. Ribatti D, Crivellato E, Vacca A. The contribution of Bruce Glick to the definition of the role played by the bursa of Fabricius in the development of the B cell lineage.Clin Exp Immunol. 2006 Jul;145(1):1-4.

25. Linton PJ, Dorshkind K.Age-related changes in lymphocyte development and function. Nat Immunol. 2004 Feb;5(2):133-9.

26. Sigal LH. Basic science for the clinician 53: mast cells. J Clin Rheumatol. 2011 Oct;17(7):395-400.

27. Sigal LH. Basic science for the clinician 53: mast cells. J Clin Rheumatol. 2011 Oct;17(7):395-400.

28. Mays PK, Bishop JE, Laurent GJ. Age-related changes in the proportion of types I and III collagen. Mech Ageing Dev. 1988 Nov 30;45(3):203-12.

29. Langevin HM, Fox JR, Koptiuch C, Badger GJ, Greenan-Naumann AC, Bouffard NA, Konofagou EE, Lee WN, Triano JJ, Henry SM. Reduced thoracolumbar fascia shear strain in human chronic low back pain. BMC Musculoskelet Disord. 2011 Sep 19;12:203.

30. Langevin HM, Stevens-Tuttle D, Fox JR, Badger GJ, Bouffard NA, Krag MH, Wu J, Henry SM. Ultrasound evidence of altered lumbar connective tissue structure in human subjects with chronic low back pain. BMC Musculoskelet Disord. 2009 Dec 3;10:151.

31. McMinn R.M.H. Last's anatomy: regional and applied. 9th ed. Edinburgh: Churchill Livingstone; 1994.

32. Standring S, ed. Gray's Anatomy: The anatomical basis of clinical practice. 39th ed. Edinburgh : Churchill Livingstone; 2004.

33. Abu-Hijleh MF, Roshier AL, Al-Shboul Q, Dharap AS, Harris PF. The membranous layer of superficial fascia: evidence for its widespread distribution in the body. Surg Radiol Anat. 2006 Dec;28(6):606-19.

34. Caggiati A.Fascial relationships of the short saphenous vein. J Vasc Surg. 2001 Aug;34(2):241-6.

35. Abu-Hijleh MF, Roshier AL, Al-Shboul Q, Dharap AS, Harris PF. The membranous layer of superficial fascia: evidence for its widespread distribution in the body. Surg Radiol Anat. 2006 Dec;28(6):606-19.

36. Lockwood TE. Superficial fascial system (SFS) of the trunk and extremities: a new concept. Plast Reconstr Surg. 1991 Jun;87(6):1009-18.

37. Still AT. Philosophy of Osteopathy. Kirskville, MO: A.T. Still; 1899. Reprinted, Indianapolis, IN: American Academy of Osteopathy; 1971:23.

38. Yahia L, Rhalmi S, Newman N, Isler M. Sensory innervation of human thoracolumbar fascia. An immunohistochemical study. Acta Orthop Scand. 1992 Apr;63(2):195-7.

39. Stecco C, Porzionato A, Macchi V, Tiengo C, Parenti A, Aldegheri R, Delmas V, De Caro R. Histological characteristics of the deep fascia of the upper limb. Ital J Anat Embryol. 2006 Apr-Jun;111(2):105-10.

40. Stecco C, Gagey O, Belloni A, Pozzuoli A, Porzionato A, Macchi V, Aldegheri R, De Caro R, Delmas V. Anatomy of the deep fascia of the upper limb. Second part: study of innervation. Morphologie. 2007 Mar;91(292):38-43.

41. Tesarz J, Hoheisel U, Wiedenhöfer B, Mense S. Sensory innervation of the thoracolumbar fascia in rats and humans. Neuroscience. 2011 Oct 27;194:302-8.

42. Benjamin M. The fascia of the limbs and back--a review. J Anat. 2009 Jan;214(1):1-18.

43. Staubesand J, Baumbach KU, Li Y. La structure fine de l'aponévrose jambière. Phlébologie. 1997;50(1):105-13.

44. Schleip R. Fascial plasticity – a new neurobiological explanation. Part 1. J Bodyw Mov Ther. 2003;7(1):11-9.

45. An Interview with Prof. Dr. med. J. Staubesand. Available at http:www.somatics.de/somatics-06. Accessed August 23, 2012.

46. Still AT. Philosophy of Osteopathy. Kirskville, MO: A.T. Still; 1899. Reprinted, Indianapolis, IN: American Academy of Osteopathy; 1971:164.

47. Yahia LH, Pigeon P, DesRosiers EA. Viscoelastic properties of the human lumbodorsal fascia. J Biomed Eng. 1993 Sep;15(5):425-9.

48. Thornton GM, Shrive NG, Frank CB. Altering ligament water content affects ligament prestress and creep behaviour. J Orthop Res. 2001 Sep;19(5):845-51.

49. Northup TL. Osteopathic cranial technic and its influence on hypertension. Year Book of the Academy of Applied Osteopathy. American Academy of Osteopathy. Indianapolis, IN. 1948:70-7.

50. Cathie AG. The fascia of the body in relation to function and manipulative therapy. Year Book of the American Academy of Osteopathy. Indianapolis, IN. 1974:81-4.

51. Yahia LH, Pigeon P, DesRosiers EA. Viscoelastic properties of the human lumbodorsal fascia. J Biomed Eng. 1993 Sep;15(5):425-9.

52. Staubesand J, Baumbach KU, Li Y. La structure fine de l'aponévrose jambière. Phlébologie. 1997;50(1):105–13.

53. Hinz B, Phan SH, Thannickal VJ, Prunotto M, Desmoulière A, Varga J, De Wever O, Mareel M, Gabbiani G. Recent developments in myofibroblast biology: paradigms for connective tissue remodeling. Am J Pathol. 2012 Apr;180(4):1340-55.

54. Schleip R, Naylor IL, Ursu D, Melzer W, Zorn A, Wilke HJ, Lehmann-Horn F, Klingler W. Passive muscle stiffness may be influenced by active contractility of intramuscular connective tissue. Med Hypotheses. 2006;66(1):66-71.

55. Staubesand J, Baumbach KU, Li Y. La structure fine de l'aponévrose jambière. Phlébologie. 1997;50(1):105–13.

56. Hukins DW, Aspden RM, Hickey DS. Thoracolumbar fascia can increase the efficiency of the erector spinae muscles. Clin. Biomech. 1990;5:30-34.

57. Varela FJ, Frenk S. The organ of form: towards a theory of biological shape. J Soc Biol Struct. 1987;10(1): 73–83.

58. Snyder GE. Fasciae - Applied Anatomy and Physiology. Year Book of the Academy of Applied Osteopathy. American Academy of Osteopathy. Indianapolis, IN. 1956:65-75.

59. Vleeming A, Pool-Goudzwaard AL, Stoeckart R, van Wingerden JP, Snijders CJ. The posterior layer of the thoracolumbar fascia. Its function in load transfer from spine to legs. Spine (Phila Pa 1976). 1995 Apr 1;20(7):753-8.

60. Kalin PJ, Hirsch BE. The origins and function of the interosseous muscles of the foot. J Anat. 1987 Jun;152:83-91.

61. Wood Jones F. Structure and function as seen in the foot. London: Baillière, Tindall and Cox; 1944.

62. Langevin HM. Connective tissue: a body-wide signaling network? Med Hypotheses. 2006;66(6):1074-7.

63. Yahia L, Rhalmi S, Newman N, Isler M. Sensory innervation of human thoracolumbar fascia. An immunohistochemical study. Acta Orthop Scand. 1992 Apr;63(2):195-7.

64. Staubesand J, Baumbach KU, Li Y. La structure fine de l'aponévrose jambière. Phlébologie. 1997;50(1):105-13.

65. Stecco C, Gagey O, Belloni A, Pozzuoli A, Porzionato A, Macchi V, Aldegheri R, De Caro R, Delmas V. Anatomy of the deep fascia of the upper limb. Second part: study of innervation. Morphologie. 2007 Mar;91(292):38-43.

66. Benjamin M. The fascia of the limbs and back--a review. J Anat. 2009 Jan;214(1):1-18.

67. Tesarz J, Hoheisel U, Wiedenhöfer B, Mense S. Sensory innervation of the thoracolumbar fascia in rats and humans. Neuroscience. 2011 Oct 27;194:302-8.

68. Benjamin M. The fascia of the limbs and back--a review. J Anat. 2009 Jan;214(1):1-18.

69. Stecco C, Gagey O, Belloni A, Pozzuoli A, Porzionato A, Macchi V, Aldegheri R, De Caro R, Delmas V. Anatomy of the deep fascia of the upper limb. Second part: study of innervation. Morphologie. 2007 Mar;91(292):38-43.

70. Schleip R, Zorn A, Klingler W. Biomechanical Properties of Fascial Tissues and Their Role as Pain Generators. J Musculoskelet Pain. 2010;18(4):393-5.

71. Stecco C, Gagey O, Belloni A, Pozzuoli A, Porzionato A, Macchi V, Aldegheri R, De Caro R, Delmas V. Anatomy of the deep fascia of the upper limb. Second part: study of innervation. Morphologie. 2007 Mar;91(292):38-43.

72. Cathie AG. The fascia of the body in relation to function and manipulative therapy. Year Book of the American Academy of Osteopathy. Indianapolis, IN. 1974:81-4.

73. Hoheisel U, Taguchi T, Treede RD, Mense S. Nociceptive input from the rat thoracolumbar fascia to lumbar dorsal horn neurones. Eur J Pain. 2011 Sep;15(8):810-5.

74. Panjabi MM. A hypothesis of chronic back pain: ligament subfailure injuries lead to muscle control dysfunction. Eur Spine J. 2006 May;15(5):668-76.

75. Becker AR. Connective tissue and osteopathy. Resume of Lectures Given by Charles H. Kauffman, D.O. MSC at Denver Polyclinic and Postgraduate Course August 1944. Year Book of the Academy of Applied Osteopathy. American Academy of Osteopathy. Indianapolis, IN. 1945:57-62.

76. Langevin HM, Cornbrooks CJ, Taatjes DJ. Fibroblasts form a body-wide cellular network. Histochem Cell Biol. 2004 Jul;122(1):7-15.

77. Ko K, Arora P, Lee W, McCulloch C. Bio-chemical and functional characterization of intercellular adhesion and gap junctions in fibroblasts. Am J Physiol Cell Physiol. 2000 Jul;279(1):C147-57.

78. Langevin HM. Connective tissue: a body-wide signaling network? Med Hypotheses. 2006;66(6):1074-7.

79. Cathie AG. The fascia of the body in relation to function and manipulative therapy. Year Book of the American Academy of Osteopathy. Indianapolis, IN. 1974:81-4.

80. Standring S, ed. Gray's Anatomy: The anatomical basis of clinical practice. 40th ed. Edinburgh: Churchill Livingstone; 2008.

81. Fletcher DA, Mullins RD. Cell mechanics and the cytoskeleton. Nature. 2010 Jan 28;463(7280):485-92.

82. Discher DE, Janmey P, Wang YL. Tissue cells feel and respond to the stiffness of their substrate. Science. 2005 Nov 18;310(5751):1139-43.

83. Ingber DE. Mechanobiology and diseas-es of mechanotransduction. Ann Med. 2003;35(8):564-77.

84. Kragstrup TW, Kjaer M, Mackey AL. Struc-tural, biochemical, cellular, and functional changes in skeletal muscle extracellular matrix with aging. Scand J Med Sci Sports. 2011 Dec;21(6):749-57.

85. Chiquet M, Gelman L, Lutz R, Maier S.From mechanotransduction to extracellular matrix gene expression in fibroblasts. Biochim Biophys Acta. 2009 May;1793(5):911-20.

86. Ingber DE. Tensegrity: the architectural basis of cellular mechanotransduction. Annu Rev Physiol. 1997;59:575-99.

87. Ingber DE. Tensegrity: the architectural basis of cellular mechanotransduction. Annu Rev Physiol. 1997;59:575-99.

88. Fuller B. Tensegrity. Portfolio & ARTnews annual. 1961;4:112-27.

89. Ingber DE. The architecture of life. Sci Am. 1998 Jan;278(1):48-57.

90. Tarr R, Nelson K, Vatt R, Richardson D. Palpa-tory findings associated with the diabetic state. J Am Osteopath Assoc. 1985;85(9):604-5.

91. Nelson K, Mnabhi A, Glonek T. The Accuracy of Diagnostic Palpation: The Comparison of Soft Tissue Findings with Random Blood Sugar in Diabetic Patients. Osteopathic Family Physician Nov-Dec 2010 2(6):165-9.

92. Ingber DE. Tensegrity and mechanotransduc-tion. J Bodyw Mov Ther. 2008 Jul;12(3):198-200.

93. Ingber DE. Tensegrity and mechanotransduc-tion. J Bodyw Mov Ther. 2008 Jul;12(3):198-200.

94. Ingber DE. Tensegrity and mechanotransduc-tion. J Bodyw Mov Ther. 2008 Jul;12(3):198-200.

95. Ingber DE. Mechanobiology and diseas-es of mechanotransduction. Ann Med. 2003;35(8):564-77.

96. Ingber DE. Mechanobiology and diseas-es of mechanotransduction. Ann Med. 2003;35(8):564-77.

97. Jaalouk DE, Lammerding J.Mechanotransduc-tion gone awry. Nat Rev Mol Cell Biol. 2009 Jan;10(1):63-73.

98. Wu M, Fannin J, Rice KM, Wang B, Blough ER.Effect of aging on cellular mechanotrans-duction. Ageing Res Rev. 2011 Jan;10(1):1-15.

99. Silver FH, DeVore D, Siperko LM. Invited Review: Role of mechanophysiology in aging of ECM: effects of changes in mechano-chemical transduction. J Appl Physiol. 2003 Nov;95(5):2134-41.

100.Ingber DE. Mechanobiology and diseas-es of mechanotransduction. Ann Med. 2003;35(8):564-77.

101.Zahn JT, Louban I, Jungbauer S, Bissinger M, Kaufmann D, Kemkemer R, Spatz JP. Age-de-pendent changes in microscale stiffness and mechanoresponses of cells. Small. 2011 May 23;7(10):1480-7.

102.Grinnell F, Zhu M, Carlson MA, Abrams JM. Release of mechanical tension triggers apoptosis of human fibroblasts in a model of regressing granulation tissue. Exp Cell Res. 1999 May 1;248(2):608-19.

103.Langevin HM, Bouffard NA, Badger GJ, Iatridis JC, Howe AK. Dynamic fibroblast cytoskeletal response to subcutaneous tissue stretch ex vivo and in vivo. Am J Physiol Cell Physiol. 2005 Mar;288(3):C747-56.

104.Faust U, Hampe N, Rubner W, Kirchgessner N, Safran S, Hoffmann B, Merkel R. Cyclic stress at mHz frequencies aligns fibroblasts in direction of zero strain. PLoS One. 2011;6(12):e28963.

105.Wang JH, Yang G, Li Z, Shen W. Fibroblast responses to cyclic mechanical stretching depend on cell orientation to the stretching direction. J Biomech. 2004 Apr;37(4):573-6.

106.Langevin HM, Bouffard NA, Fox JR, Palmer BM, Wu J, Iatridis JC, Barnes WD, Badger GJ, Howe AK. Fibroblast cytoskeletal remodeling contributes to connective tissue tension. J Cell Physiol. 2011 May;226(5):1166-75.

107.Kolahi KS, Mofrad MR.Mechanotransduction: a major regulator of homeostasis and devel-opment. Wiley Interdiscip Rev Syst Biol Med. 2010 Nov-Dec;2(6):625-39.

108.Chung HY, Lee EK, Choi YJ, Kim JM, Kim DH, Zou Y, Kim CH, Lee J, Kim HS, Kim ND, Jung JH, Yu BP. Molecular inflammation as an underlying mechanism of the aging process and age-related diseases. J Dent Res. 2011 Jul;90(7):830-40.

109.McAnulty RJ. Fibroblasts and myofi-broblasts: their source, function and role in disease. Int J Biochem Cell Biol. 2007;39(4):666-71.

110.Smith RS, Smith TJ, Blieden TM, Phipps RP. Fibroblasts as sentinel cells. Synthesis of chemokines and regulation of inflammation. Am J Pathol. 1997 Aug;151(2):317-22.

111.Parsonage G, Falciani F, Burman A, Filer A, Ross E, Bofill M, Martin S, Salmon M, Buckley CD. Global gene expression profiles in fibroblasts from synovial, skin and lymphoid tissue reveals distinct cytokine and chemokine expression patterns. Thromb Haemost. 2003 Oct;90(4):688-97.

112.Gabbiani G. The myofibroblast in wound healing and fibrocontractive diseases. J Pathol. 2003 Jul;200(4):500-3.

113.Hinz B, Phan SH, Thannickal VJ, Prunotto M, Desmoulière A, Varga J, De Wever O, Mareel M, Gabbiani G. Recent developments in

myofibroblast biology: paradigms for con-nective tissue remodeling. Am J Pathol. 2012 Apr;180(4):1340-55.

114.Findley TW. Int J Ther Massage Bodywork. 2009 Jun 29;2(2):1-6.

115.Langevin HM, Fox JR, Koptiuch C, Badger GJ, Greenan-Naumann AC, Bouffard NA, Konofagou EE, Lee WN, Triano JJ, Henry SM. Reduced thoracolumbar fascia shear strain in human chronic low back pain. BMC Mus-culoskelet Disord. 2011 Sep 19;12:203.

116.Lewit K, Olsanska S. Clinical importance of active scars: abnormal scars as a cause of myofascial pain. J Manipulative Physiol Ther. 2004 Jul-Aug;27(6):399-402.

117.Kobesova A, Morris CE, Lewit K, Safarova M. Twenty-year-old pathogenic "active" postsurgical scar: a case study of a patient with persistent right lower quadrant pain. J Manipulative Physiol Ther. 2007 Mar-Apr;30(3):234-8.

118.Still AT. Philosophy of Osteopathy. Kirksville, MO: A.T. Still; 1899. Reprinted, Indianapolis, IN: American Academy of Osteopathy; 1971:167.

119.Schleip R. Fascial plasticity – a new neurobio-logical explanation. Part 2. J Bodyw Mov Ther. 2003;7(2):104-16.

120.Kruger L. Cutaneous sensory system. In: Adelman G, ed. Encyclopedia of Neuroscience. Vol 1. Boston, MA: Birkhäuser; 1987:293-4.

121.Diego MA, Field T. Moderate pressure mas-sage elicits a parasympathetic nervous system response. Int J Neurosci. 2009;119(5):630-8.

122.Diego MA, Field T. Moderate pressure mas-sage elicits a parasympathetic nervous system response. Int J Neurosci. 2009;119(5):630-8.

123.Castro-Sánchez AM, Matarán-Peñarrocha GA, Arroyo-Morales M, Saavedra-Hernán-dez M, Fernández-Sola C, Moreno-Lorenzo C. Effects of myofascial release techniques on pain, physical function, and postural stability in patients with fibromyalgia: a randomized controlled trial. Clin Rehabil. 2011 Sep;25(9):800-13.

124.Castro-Sánchez AM, Matarán-Peñarrocha GA, Granero-Molina J, Aguilera-Manrique G, Quesada-Rubio JM, Moreno-Lorenzo C. Bene-fits of massage-myofascial release therapy on pain, anxiety, quality of sleep, depression, and quality of life in patients with fibromyalgia. Evid Based Complement Alternat Med. 2011;2011:561753.

125.Cubick EE, Quezada VY, Schumer AD, Davis CM. Sustained release myofascial release as treatment for a patient with complications of rheumatoid arthritis and collagenous colitis: a case report. Int J Ther Massage Bodywork. 2011;4(3):1-9.

126.Walton A. Efficacy of myofascial release techniques in the treatment of primary Raynaud's phenomenon. J Bodyw Mov Ther. 2008 Jul;12(3):274-80.

127.Ramos-González E, Moreno-Lorenzo C, Matarán-Peñarrocha GA, Guisado-Barrilao R, Aguilar-Ferrándiz ME, Castro-Sánchez AM. Comparative study on the effectiveness of myofascial release manual therapy and physical therapy for venous insufficiency in postmenopausal women. Complement Ther Med. 2012 Oct;20(5):291-8.

128. Tozzi P, Bongiorno D, Vitturini C. Fascial release effects on patients with non-specific cervical or lumbar pain. J Bodyw Mov Ther. 2011 Oct;15(4):405-16.

129. Ajimsha MS, Chithra S, Thulasyammal RP. Effectiveness of myofascial release in the management of lateral epicondylitis in computer professionals. Arch Phys Med Rehabil. 2012 Apr;93(4):604-9.

130. Cubick EE, Quezada VY, Schumer AD, Davis CM. Sustained release myofascial release as treatment for a patient with complications of rheumatoid arthritis and collagenous colitis: a case report. Int J Ther Massage Bodywork. 2011;4(3):1-9.

131. Eastwood M, McGrouther DA, Brown RA. Fibroblast responses to mechanical forces. Proc Inst Mech Eng H. 1998;212(2):85-92.

132. Hicks MR, Cao TV, Campbell DH, Standley PR. Mechanical strain applied to human fibroblasts differentially regulates skeletal myoblast differentiation. J Appl Physiol. 2012 Aug;113(3):465-72.

133. Willard FH. The Fascial System of the Body. Chapt 7. In: Chila AG. ed. Foundations of Osteopathic Medicine. 3rd ed. Philadelphia: Wolters Kluwer/Lippincott Williams and Wilkins. 2011:85.

134. Dodd JG, Good MM, Nguyen TL, Grigg AI, Batia LM, Standley PR. In vitro biophysical strain model for understanding mechanisms of osteopathic manipulative treatment. J Am Osteopath Assoc. 2006 Mar;106(3):157-66.

135. Eagan TS, Meltzer KR, Standley PR. Importance of strain direction in regulating human fibroblast proliferation and cytokine secretion: a useful in vitro model for soft tissue injury and manual medicine treatments. J Manipulative Physiol Ther. 2007 Oct;30(8):584-92.

136. Dodd JG, Good MM, Nguyen TL, Grigg AI, Batia LM, Standley PR. In vitro biophysical strain model for understanding mechanisms of osteopathic manipulative treatment. J Am Osteopath Assoc. 2006 Mar;106(3):157-66.

137. Meltzer KR, Standley PR. Modeled repetitive motion strain and indirect osteopathic manipulative techniques in regulation of human fibroblast proliferation and interleukin secretion. J Am Osteopath Assoc. 2007 Dec;107(12):527-36.

138. Standley PR, Meltzer K. In vitro modeling of repetitive motion strain and manual medicine treatments: potential roles for pro- and anti-inflammatory cytokines. J Bodyw Mov Ther. 2008 Jul;12(3):201-3.

139. Standley PR, Meltzer K. In vitro modeling of repetitive motion strain and manual medicine treatments: potential roles for pro- and anti-inflammatory cytokines. J Bodyw Mov Ther. 2008 Jul;12(3):201-3.

140. Langevin HM, Bouffard NA, Badger GJ, Iatridis JC, Howe AK. Dynamic fibroblast cytoskeletal response to subcutaneous tissue stretch ex vivo and in vivo. Am J Physiol Cell Physiol. 2005 Mar;288(3):C747-56.

141. Langevin HM, Storch KN, Snapp RR, Bouffard NA, Badger GJ, Howe AK, Taatjes DJ. Tissue stretch induces nuclear remodeling in connective tissue fibroblasts. Histochem Cell Biol. 2010 Apr;133(4):405-15.

142. Abbott RD, Koptiuch C, Iatridis JC, Howe AK, Badger GJ, Langevin HM. Cytoskeletal remodeling of connective tissue fibroblasts in response to static stretch is dependent on matrix material properties. J Cell Physiol. 'Accepted Article,' doi:10.1002/jcp.24102.

143. Gabbiani G. The myofibroblast in wound healing and fibrocontractive diseases. J Pathol. 2003 Jul;200(4):500-3.

144. Hinz B, Gabbiani G. Fibrosis: recent advances in myofibroblast biology and new therapeutic perspectives. F1000 Biol Rep. 2010 Nov 11;2:78.

145. Gabbiani G. The myofibroblast in wound healing and fibrocontractive diseases. J Pathol. 2003 Jul;200(4):500-3.

146. Rolf IP. Rolfing: The Integration of Human Structures. Santa Monica, CA: Dennis-Landman; 1977:42.

147. Kruger L. Cutaneous sensory system. In: Adelman G, ed. Encyclopedia of Neuroscience. Vol 1. Boston, MA: Birkhäuser; 1987:293-4.

148. Schleip R. Fascial plasticity a new neurobiological explanation. Part 2. J. Bodyw Mov Ther. 2003; 7 (2), 104-16.

149. Lee RP. Still's concept of connective tissue: lost in "translation"? J Am Osteopath Assoc. 2006 Apr;106(4):176-7.

150. Salamon E, Zhu W, Stefano GB. Nitric oxide as a possible mechanism for understanding the therapeutic effects of osteopathic manipulative medicine. Int J Mol Med. 2004 Sep;14(3):443-9.

151. Garthwaite J. Concepts of neural nitric oxide-mediated transmission. Eur J Neurosci. 2008 Jun;27(11):2783-802.

152. Still AT. Autobiography of Andrew T, Still. Kirskville, MO: A.T. Still; 1908. Reprinted, Colorado Springs, CO: American Academy of Osteopathy; 1981:94.

153. McPartland JM, Giuffrida A, King J, Skinner E, Scotter J, Musty RE. Cannabimimetic effects of osteopathic manipulative treatment. J Am Osteopath Assoc. 2005 Jun;105(6):283-91.

154. McPartland JM. Expression of the endocannabinoid system in fibroblasts and myofascial tissues. J Bodyw Mov Ther. 2008 Apr;12(2):169-82.

155. Degenhardt BF, Darmani NA, Johnson JC, Towns LC, Rhodes DC, Trinh C, McClanahan B, DiMarzo V. Role of osteopathic manipulative treatment in altering pain biomarkers: a pilot study. J Am Osteopath Assoc. 2007 Sep;107(9):387-400.

156. Barnes JF, Marzano A. Myofascial Release: The Search for Excellence. Paoli, PA: Rehabilitation Services Inc.; 1990.

157. Still AT. Philosophy of Osteopathy. Kirskville, MO: A.T. Still; 1899. Reprinted, Indianapolis, IN: American Academy of Osteopathy; 1971:28.

158. Merriam-Webster on-line dictionary. Available at http://www.merriam-webster.com/dictionary. Accessed March 30, 2013.

159. Sutherland WG. The cranial bowl. Mankato, MN: Free Press Company; 1939. Reprinted: Indianapolis, IN: American Academy of Osteopathy; 1986.

160. Magoun HI. Osteopathy in the cranial field. Kirskville, MO: The Journal Printing Company; 1951.

161. Swedenborg E. The Brain. Edited, translated and annotated by Tafel R.L. James Spiers London; 1882.

162. Fuller D. Osteopathy and Swedenborg. Swedenborg Scientific Assn Press, Bryn Athyn PA. 2012.

163. Sutherland WG. The cranial bowl. Mankato, MN: Free Press Company; 1939. Reprinted: Indianapolis, IN: American Academy of Osteopathy; 1986.

164. Woods JM, Woods RH. A physical finding related to psychiatric disorders. J Am Osteopath Assoc. 1961 Aug;60:988-93.

165. Becker RE. Life in Motion. Brooks RE, editor. Portland, OR: Rudra Press; 1997.

166. Littlejohn JM. The physiological basis of the therapeutic law. J Am Osteopath Assoc, 1902; 2:42-60.

167. Traube L. Über periodische Tätigkeitsänderungen des Vasomotorischen und Hemmungs-Nervenzentrums. Cbl Med Wiss 1865;56:881-5.

168. Hering E. Über Athembewegungen des Gefässsystems. Sitzungs d k Akad d W math naturw 1869;60:829-56-Table III.

169. Mayer S. Über spontane Blutdruckschwankungen. Sitzungb d k Akad d W math naturw 1876;67:281-305.

170. Stefanovska, A., Bracic, M., Kvernmo, K., Wavelet analysis of oscillations in the peripheral blood circulation measured by laser Doppler technique. IEEE Trans. Biomed. Eng. 1999. 46:1230–9.

171. Nelson KE, Sergueef N, Lipinski CM, Chapman AR, Glonck T. Cranial rhythmic impulse related to the Traube-Hering-Mayer oscillation: comparing laser-Doppler flowmetry and palpation. J Am Osteopath Assoc. 2001 Mar;101(3):163-73.

172. Sergueef N, Nelson KE, Glonek T. The effect of cranial manipulation on the Traube-Hering-Mayer oscillation as measured by laser-Doppler flowmetry. Altern Ther Health Med. 2002 Nov-Dec;8(6):74-6.

173. Nelson KE, Sergueef N, Glonek T. Cranial Manipulation Induces Sequential Changes in Blood Flow Velocity on Demand. AAO Journal. September 2004:14(3):15-17.

174. Nelson KE, Sergueef N, Glonek T. The effect of an alternative medical procedure upon low-frequency oscillations in cutaneous blood flow velocity. J Manipulative Physiol Ther. 2006 Oct;29(8):626-36.

175. Stefanovska, A., Bracic, M., Kvernmo, K., Wavelet analysis of oscillations in the peripheral blood circulation measured by laser Doppler technique. IEEE Trans. Biomed. Eng. 1999. 46:1230-9.

176. Akselrod S, Gordon D, Madwed JB, Snidman NC, Shannon DC, Cohen RJ. Hemodynamic regulation: investigation by spectral analysis. Am J Physiol. 1985 Oct;249(4 Pt 2):H867-75.

177. Akselrod S, Gordon D, Ubel FA, Shannon DC, Berger AC, Cohen RJ. Power spectrum analysis of heart rate fluctuation: a quantitative probe of beat-to-beat cardiovascular control. Science. 1981 Jul 10;213(4504):220-2.

178. Akselrod S, Gordon D, Ubel FA, Shannon DC, Berger AC, Cohen RJ. Power spectrum analysis of heart rate fluctuation: a quantitative probe

of beat-to-beat cardiovascular control. Science. 1981 Jul 10;213(4504):220-2.

179. Kitney RI. An analysis of the nonlinear behavior of the human thermal vasomotor control system. J Theor Biol 1975;52:231-48.

180. Barron DH. Chapt. 31, Vasomotor Regulation. In: Ruch TC, Fulton JF, editors. Medical Physiology and Biophysics, 18th ed. Philadelphia: W.B. Saunders Co, 1960:691-707.

181. Magoun HI. Osteopathy in the cranial field. 2nd ed. Kirksville, MO: The Journal Printing Company; 1966:34.

182. Stedman's Medical Dictionary, 28th Ed. Baltimore, MD: Wolters Kluwer/Lippincott Williams & Wilkins, 2005.

183. Hyndman BW. The role of rhythms in homeostasis. Kybernetik 1974;15:227-36.

184. Hyndman BW, Kitney RI, Sayers BMcA. Spontaneous rhythms in physiological control systems. Nature 1971;233:339-41.

185. Kitney RI. An analysis of the nonlinear behavior of the human thermal vasomotor control system. J Theor Biol 1975;52:231-48.

186. Hyndman BW. The role of rhythms in homeostasis. Kybernetik 1974;15:227-36.

187. Infeld E. An exact theory of direct capacitance frequency modulation. J. Phys. D: Appl. Phys. 1977 10(11):1405-12.

188. Nelson KE, Sergueef N, Lipinski CM, Chapman AR, Glonek T. Cranial rhythmic impulse related to the Traube-Hering-Mayer oscillation: comparing laser-Doppler flowmetry and palpation. J Am Osteopath Assoc. 2001 Mar;101(3):163-73.

189. Lockwood MD, Degenhardt BF. Cycle-to-cycle variability attributed to the primary respiratory mechanism. J Am Osteopath Assoc. 1998 Jan;98(1):35-6, 41-3.

190. Sutherland WG. The cranial bowl. Mankato, MN: Free Press Company; 1939. Reprinted: Indianapolis, IN: American Academy of Osteopathy; 1986:51-3.

191. Moskalenko YE, Kravchenko TI, Gaidar BV, Weinstein GB, et. al. Periodic mobility of cranial bones in humans. Human Physiology. 1999 25(1):51-58.

192. Enzmann DR, Pelc NJ. Normal flow patterns of intracranial and spinal cerebrospinal fluid defined with phase-contrast cine MR imaging. Radiology. 1991 Feb;178(2):467-74.

193. Enzmann DR, Pelc NJ. Normal flow patterns of intracranial and spinal cerebrospinal fluid defined with phase-contrast cine MR imaging. Radiology. 1991 Feb;178(2):467-74.

194. Feinberg DA, Mark AS. Human brain motion and cerebrospinal fluid circulation demonstrated with MR velocity imaging. Radiology. 1987 Jun;163(3):793-9.

195. Jenkins CO, Campbell JK, White DN. Modulation resembling Traube-Hering waves recorded in the human brain. Euro Neurol 1971;5:1-6.

196. Moskalenko YE, Kravchenko TI, Vainshtein GB, Halvorson P, Feilding A, Mandara A, et al. Slow-wave oscillations in the craniosacral space: a hemoliquorodynamic concept of origination. Neurosci Behav Physiol. 2009 May;39(4):377-81.

197. Hara K, Nakatani S, Ozaki K, Ikeda T, Mogami H. Detection of the B waves in the oscillation of intracranial pressure by fast Fourier

transform. Med Inform (Lond). 1990 Apr-Jun;15(2):125-31.

198. Podlas H, Allen KL, Bunt EA. Computed tomography studies of human brain movements. S Afr J Surg. 1984 Feb-Mar;22(1):57-63.

199. Kitney RI. An analysis of the nonlinear behavior of the human thermal vasomotor control system. J Theor Biol 1975;52:231-48.

200. Hyndman BW. The role of rhythms in homeostasis. Kybernetik 1974;15:227-36.

201. Bachoo M, Polosa C. Properties of the inspiration-related activity of sympathetic preganglionic neurones of the cervical trunk in the cat. J Physiol. 1987 Apr;385:545-64.

202. Mearns AJ, Harness JB, Stockman AG, Zarneh A. Forcing frequency testing, a new approach to physiologic measurement. In: Orlebeke JF, Mulder G, Van Doorman LJP, eds. Psychophysiology of cardiovascular control models, methods, and data. New York: Plenum Press, 1985:425-36.

203. Nasimi SG, Harness JB, Marjanović DZ, Knight T, Mearns AJ. Periodic posture stimulation of the baroreceptors and the local vasomotor reflexes. J Biomed Eng. 1992 Jul;14(4):307-12.

204. Traube L. Über periodische Tätigkeitsänderungen des Vasomotorischen und Hemmungs-Nervenzentrums. Cbl Med Wiss 1865;56:881-5.

205. Hering E. Über Athembewegungen des Gefässsystems. Sitzungb d k Akad d W math naturw 1869;60:829-56-Table III.

206. Mayer S. Über spontane Blutdruckschwankungen. Sitzungb d k Akad d W math naturw 1876;67:281-305.

207. Akselrod S, Gordon D, Madwed JB, Snidman NC, Shannon DC, Cohen RJ, Hemodynamic regulation: Investigation by spectral analysis. Amer J Physiol 1985;249:H867-H875.

208. Akselrod S, Gordon D, Ubel FA, Shannon DC, Barger AC, Cohen RJ. Power spectrum analysis of heart rate fluctuation: A quantitative probe of beat-to-beat cardiovascular control. Science 1981;213:220-1.

209. Barron DH. Chapt. 31, Vasomotor Regulation. In: Ruch TC, Fulton JF, editors. Medical Physiology and Biophysics, 18th ed. Philadelphia: W.B. Saunders Co, 1960:691-707.

210. Hyndman BW. The role of rhythms in homeostasis. Kybernetik 1974;15:227-36.

211. Hara K, Nakatani S, Ozaki K, Ikeda T, Mogami H. Detection of the B waves in the oscillation of intracranial pressure by fast Fourier transform. Med Inform (Lond). 1990 Apr-Jun;15(2):125-31.

212. Peñáz J. Mayer Waves: History and methodology. Automedica 1978;2:135-41.

213. Fuller BF. The effects of stress-anxiety and coping styles on heart rate variability. Int J Psychophysiol. 1992 Jan;12(1):81-6.

214. Negoescu R, Filcescu V, Boantă F, Dincă-Panaitescu S, Popovici C. Hypobaric hypoxia: dual sympathetic control in the light of RR and QT spectra. Rom J Physiol. 1994 Jan-Dec;31(1-4):47-53.

215. Szidon JP, Cherniack NS, Fishman AP. Traube-Hering waves in the pulmonary circulation of the dog. Science 1969 Apr 4;164(3875):75-6.

216. White DN. The early development of neurosonology: III. Pulsatile echoencephalography

and Doppler techniques. Ultrasound Med Biol. 1992;18(4):323-76.

217. Clarke MJ, Lin JC. Microwave sensing of increased intracranial water content. Invest Radiol. 1983 May-Jun;18(3):245-8.

218. Chess GF, Tam RM, Calaresu FR. Influence of cardiac neural inputs on rhythmic variations of heart period in the cat. Am J Physiol. 1975 Mar;228(3):775-80.

219. Burch GE, Cohn AE, Neumann C. A study by quantitative methods of the spontaneous variations in volume of the finger tip, toe tip, and posterior-superior portion of the pinna of resting normal white adults. Amer J Physiol 1942;136:433-47.

220. Burton AC, Taylor RM. A study of the adjustment of peripheral vascular tone to the requirements of the regulation of body temperature. Amer J Physiol 1940;129:565-77.

221. Bornmyr S, Svensson H, Lilja B, Sundkvist G. Skin temperature changes and changes in skin blood flow monitored with laser Doppler flowmetry and imaging: a methodological study in normal humans. Clin Physiol. 1997 Jan;17(1):71-81.

222. Akselrod S, Gordon D, Madwed JB, Snidman NC, Shannon DC, Cohen RJ. Hemodynamic regulation: investigation by spectral analysis. Am J Physiol. 1985 Oct;249(4 Pt 2):H867-75.

223. Kitney RI. An analysis of the nonlinear behavior of the human thermal vasomotor control system. J Theor Biol 1975;52:231-48.

224. Hyndman BW. The role of rhythms in homeostasis. Kybernetik 1974;15:227-36.

225. Peñáz J. Mayer Waves: History and methodology. Automedica 1978;2:135-41.

226. Becker RE. Life in Motion. Brooks RE, editor. Portland, OR: Rudra Press; 1997.

227. Magoun HI. Osteopathy in the cranial field. 2nd ed. Kirksville, MO: The Journal Printing Company; 1966:34.

228. Davies PW, Bronk DW, Oxygen tension in mammalian brain. Fed Proc. 1957 Sep;16(3):689-92.

229. Clark LC Jr, Misrahy G, Fox RP, Chronically implanted polarographic electrodes. J Appl Physiol. 1958 Jul;13(1):85-91.

230. Marczynski TJ. Badania nad wahsniami zawartosci tlenu w niekotorych osrodkach mozgu krolika. Acta Physiol Pol 1960;11:819.

231. Moskalenko YY. Regional cerebral blood flow and its control at rest and during increased functional activity. In: Ingvar DH, Lassen NA, eds. Brain Work. Copenhagen, Munksgaard; 1975:343-51.

232. Gretchin VB. Some data on oxygen dynamics in subcortical structures of the human brain. Electroencephalogr Clin Neurophysiol. 1969 May;26(5):546-7.

233. Seylaz J, Mamo H, Caron JP, Hondart R. Pathophysiological behavior of cortical blood flow as measured in man by a semiquantitative, continuous and circumscribed method. In: Taveras JM, Fishgold H, Dilenge D, eds. Recent Advances in the Study of Cerebral Circulation. Springfield, IL. Charles C Thomas; 1970:70-82.

234. Cooper R, Crow HJ. Changes of cerebral oxygenation during motor and mental tasks. In: Ingvar DH, Lassen NA, eds. Brain Work. Copenhagen, Munksgaard; 1975:189-392.

235. Dymond AM, Crandall PH. Oxygen availability and blood flow in the temporal lobes during

spontaneous epileptic seizures in man. Brain Res. 1976 Jan 30;102(1):191-6.

236. Vern BA, Schuette WH, Leheta B, Juel VC, Radulovacki M. Low-frequency oscillations of cortical oxidative metabolism in waking and sleep. J Cereb Blood Flow Metab. 1988 Apr;8(2):215-26.

237. Vern BA, Leheta BJ, Juel VC, LaGuardia J, Graupe P, Schuette WH. Interhemispheric synchrony of slow oscillations of cortical blood volume and cytochrome aa3 redox state in unanesthetized rabbits. Brain Res. 1997 Nov 14;775(1-2):233-9.

238. Vern BA, Leheta BJ, Juel VC, LaGuardia J, Graupe P, Schuette WH. Slow oscillations of cytochrome oxidase redox state and blood volume in unanesthetized cat and rabbit cortex. Interhemispheric synchrony. Adv Exp Med Biol. 1998;454:561-70.

239. Forfia PR, Hintze TH, Wolin MS, Kaley G. Role of nitric oxide in the control of mitochondrial function. Adv Exp Med Biol. 1999;471:381-8.

240. Umans JG, Levi R. Nitric oxide in the regulation of blood flow and arterial pressure. Annu Rev Physiol. 1995;57:771-90.

241. Vern BA, Leheta BJ, Juel VC, LaGuardia J, Graupe P, Schuette WH. Interhemispheric synchrony of slow oscillations of cortical blood volume and cytochrome aa3 redox state in unanesthetized rabbits. Brain Res. 1997 Nov 14;775(1-2):233-9.

242. Vern BA, Leheta BJ, Juel VC, LaGuardia J, Graupe P, Schuette WH. Slow oscillations of cytochrome oxidase redox state and blood volume in unanesthetized cat and rabbit cortex. Interhemispheric synchrony. Adv Exp Med Biol. 1998;454:561-70.

243. Kitney RI. An analysis of the nonlinear behavior of the human thermal vasomotor control system. J Theor Biol 1975;52:231-48.

244. Hyndman BW. The role of rhythms in homeostasis. Kybernetik 1974;15:227-36.

245. Bachoo M, Polosa C. Properties of the inspiration-related activity of sympathetic preganglionic neurones of the cervical trunk in the cat. J Physiol. 1987 Apr;385:545-64.

246. Mearns AJ, Harness JB, Stockman AG, Zarneh A. Forcing frequency testing, a new approach to physiologic measurement. In: Orlebeke JF, Mulder G, Van Doorman LJP, eds. Psychophysiology of cardiovascular control models, methods, and data. New York: Plenum Press, 1985:425-36.

247. Akselrod S, Gordon D, Madwed JB, Snidman NC, Shannon DC, Cohen RJ. Hemodynamic regulation: investigation by spectral analysis. Am J Physiol. 1985 Oct;249(4 Pt 2):H867-75.

248. Hyndman BW, Kitney RI, Sayers BMcA. Spontaneous rhythms in physiological control systems. Nature 1971;233:339-41.

249. Peñáz J. Mayer Waves: History and methodology. Automedica 1978;2:135-41.

250. Sayers BM. Analysis of heart rate variability. Ergonomics. 1973 Jan;16(1):17-32.

251. Kitney RI. An analysis of the nonlinear behavior of the human thermal vasomotor control system. J Theor Biol 1975;52:231-48.

252. Barron DH. Chapt. 31, Vasomotor Regulation. In: Ruch TC, Fulton JF, editors. Medical Phys-iology and Biophysics, 18th ed. Philadelphia: W.B. Saunders Co, 1960:691-707.

253. Saul JP, Rea RF, Eckberg DL, Berger RD, Cohen RJ. Heart rate and muscle sympathetic nerve variability during reflex changes of autonomic activity. Am J Physiol. 1990 Mar;258(3 Pt 2):H713-21.

254. Best and Taylor. West JB, ed. Physiologic Basis of Medical Practice, 12th ed. Baltimore: Williams &Wilkins, 1990:127.

255. Intaglietta M, Gross JF. Vasomotion, tissue fluid flow and the formation of lymph. Int J Microcirc Clin Exp. 1982;1(1):55-65.

256. Parsons RJ, McMaster PD. The effect of the pulse upon the formation and flow of lymph. J Exp Med. 1938 Aug 31;68(3):353-76.

257. Best and Taylor. West JB, ed. Physiologic Basis of Medical Practice, 12th ed. Baltimore: Williams &Wilkins, 1990:127.

258. Parsons RJ, McMaster PD. The effect of the pulse upon the formation and flow of lymph. J Exp Med. 1938 Aug 31;68(3):353-76.

259. Vern BA, Schuette WH, Leheta B, Juel VC, Radulovacki M. Low-frequency oscillations of cortical oxidative metabolism in waking and sleep. J Cereb Blood Flow Metab. 1988 Apr;8(2):215-26.

260. Vern BA, Leheta BJ, Juel VC, LaGuardia J, Graupe P, Schuette WH. Interhemispheric synchrony of slow oscillations of cortical blood volume and cytochrome aa3 redox state in unanesthetized rabbits. Brain Res. 1997 Nov 14;775(1-2):233-9.

261. Vern BA, Leheta BJ, Juel VC, LaGuardia J, Graupe P, Schuette WH. Interhemispheric synchrony of slow oscillations of cortical blood volume and cytochrome aa3 redox state in unanesthetized rabbits. Brain Res. 1997 Nov 14;775(1-2):233-9.

262. Intaglietta M. Arteriolar vasomotion: Normal physiologic activity of defense mechanism? Diabetes and Metabolism 1988; 14(4bis):489-94.

263. Kitney RI. An analysis of the nonlinear behavior of the human thermal vasomotor control system. J Theor Biol 1975;52:231-48.

264. Hyndman BW. The role of rhythms in homeostasis. Kybernetik 1974;15:227-36.

265. Bachoo M, Polosa C. Properties of the inspiration-related activity of sympathetic preganglionic neurones of the cervical trunk in the cat. J Physiol. 1987 Apr;385:545-64.

266. Mearns AJ, Harness JB, Stockman AG, Zarneh A. Forcing frequency testing, a new approach to physiologic measurement. In: Orlebeke JF, Mulder G, Van Doorman LJP, eds. Psychophysiology of cardiovascular control models, methods, and data. New York: Plenum Press, 1985:425-36.

267. Nasimi SG, Harness JB, Marjanović DZ, Knight T, Mearns AJ. Periodic posture stimulation of the baroreceptors and the local vasomotor reflexes. J Biomed Eng. 1992 Jul;14(4):307-12.

268. Intaglietta M. Arteriolar vasomotion: Normal physiologic activity of defense mechanism? Diabetes and Metabolism 1988; 14(4bis):489-94.

269. American College of Surgeons. Injuries to the Extremities: Compartment Syndrome and Fasciotomy. Available at http:// www.operationgivingback.facs.org/stuff/contentmgr/files. Accessed March 17, 2013.

270. EFSA Panel on Dietetic Products, Nutrition, and Allergies (NDA); Scientific Opinion on Dietary reference values for water. EFSA Journal 2010; 8(3):1459. Available at http://www.efsa. europa.eu/en/scdocs/doc/1459.pdf Accessed March 17, 2013.

271. Yahia LH, Pigeon P, DesRosiers EA. Viscoelastic properties of the human lumbodorsal fascia. J Biomed Eng. 1993 Sep;15(5):425-9.

272. Castella LF, Buscemi L, Godbout C, Meister JJ, Hinz B. A new lock-step mechanism of matrix remodelling based on subcellular contractile events. J Cell Sci. 2010 May 15;123(Pt 10):1751-60.

273. Staubesand J, Baumbach KU, Li Y. La structure fine de l'aponévrose jambière. Phlébologie. 1997;50(1):105-13.

274. Schleip R, Naylor IL, Ursu D, Melzer W, Zorn A, Wilke HJ, Lehmann-Horn F, Klingler W. Passive muscle stiffness may be influenced by active contractility of intramuscular connective tissue. Med Hypotheses. 2006;66(1):66-71.

275. Staubesand J, Baumbach KU, Li Y. La structure fine de l'aponévrose jambière. Phlébologie. 1997;50(1):105–13.

276. Eckberg DL, Nerhed C, Wallin BG. Respiratory modulation of muscle sympathetic and vagal cardiac outflow in man. J Physiol. 1985 Aug;365:181-96.

277. Sutherland WG. The cranial bowl. Mankato, MN: Free Press Company; 1939. Reprinted: Indianapolis, IN: American Academy of Osteopathy; 1986:55.

278. Johnston MG, editor. Experimental Biology of the Lymphatic Circulation. Amsterdam: Elsevier, 1985:5.

279. Johnston MG, editor. Experimental Biology of the Lymphatic Circulation. Amsterdam: Elsevier, 1985:6.

280. Johnston MG, editor. Experimental Biology of the Lymphatic Circulation. Amsterdam: Elsevier, 1985:15.

281. Lee RP. The primary respiratory mechanism beyond the craniospinal axis. AAO Journal 2001;11(1):24-34.

282. Johnston MG, editor. Experimental Biology of the Lymphatic Circulation. Amsterdam: Elsevier, 1985:16.

283. Johnston MG, editor. Experimental Biology of the Lymphatic Circulation. Amsterdam: Elsevier, 1985:62.

284. Johnston MG, editor. Experimental Biology of the Lymphatic Circulation. Amsterdam: Elsevier, 1985:19.

285. Johnston MG, editor. Experimental Biology of the Lymphatic Circulation. Amsterdam: Elsevier, 1985:7.

286. Johnston MG, Kanalec A, Gordon JL. Effects of arachidonic acid and its cyclo-oxygenase and lipoxygenase products on lymphatic vessel contractility in vitro. Prostaglandins. 1983 Jan;25(1):85-98.

287. Johnston MG, Gordon JL. Regulation of lymphatic contractility by arachidonate metabolites. Nature. 1981 Sep 24;293(5830):294-7.

288. Johnston MG, editor. Experimental Biology of the Lymphatic Circulation. Amsterdam: Elsevier, 1985:25.

289. Johnston MG, editor. Experimental Biology of the Lymphatic Circulation. Amsterdam: Elsevier, 1985.

290. McHale NG, Roddie IC. The effect of transmural pressure on pumping activity in isolated bovine lymphatic vessels. J Physiol. 1976 Oct;261(2):255-69.

291. Olszewski WL, Engeset A. Lymphatic contractions. N Engl J Med. 1979 Feb 8;300(6):316.

292. Ohhashi T, Azuma T, Sakaguchi M. Active and passive mechanical characteristics of bovine mesenteric lymphatics. Am J Physiol. 1980 Jul;239(1):H88-95.

293. Olszewski WL, Engeset A. Intrinsic contractility of prenodal lymph vessels and lymph flow in human leg. Am J Physiol. 1980 Dec;239(6):H775-83.

294. Mislin H. Chapt. 3, The lymphangion. In: Földi M, Casley-Smith JR, ed. Lymphangiology. Stutgart, New York: F. K. Schatauer-Verlag, 1983:165-75.

295. Reddy NP, Staub NC. Intrinsic propulsive activity of thoracic duct perfused in anesthetized dogs. Microvasc Res. 1981 Mar;21(2):183-92.

296. Armenio S, Cetta F, Tanzini G, Guercia C. Spontaneous contractility in the human lymph vessels. Lymphology. 1981 Dec;14(4):173-8.

297. Hogan RD. Chapt 16, The initial lymphatics and interstitial pressure. In: Hargens AR, ed. Tissue Fluid Pressure and Composition. Baltimore: Williams and Wilkins, 1981:155-63.

298. Olszewski WL, Engeset A. Lymphatic contractions. N Engl J Med. 1979 Feb 8;300(6):316.

299. Johnston MG, editor. Experimental Biology of the Lymphatic Circulation. Amsterdam: Elsevier, 1985:58.

300. Ohhashi T, Azuma T, Sakaguchi M. Active and passive mechanical characteristics of bovine mesenteric lymphatics. Am J Physiol. 1980 Jul;239(1):H88-95.

301. Ohhashi T, Azuma T, Sakaguchi M. Active and passive mechanical characteristics of bovine mesenteric lymphatics. Am J Physiol. 1980 Jul;239(1):H88-95.

302. Best and Taylor. West JB, ed. Physiologic Basis of Medical Practice, 12th ed. Baltimore: Williams &Wilkins, 1990:111.

303. Gretchin VB. Some data on oxygen dynamics in subcortical structures of the human brain. Electroencephalogr Clin Neurophysiol. 1969 May;26(5):546-7.

304. Nelson KE, Sergueef N, Lipinski CM, Chapman AR, Glonek T. Cranial rhythmic impulse related to the Traube-Hering-Mayer oscillation: comparing laser-Doppler flowmetry and palpation. J Am Osteopath Assoc. 2001 Mar;101(3):163-73.

305. Kobayashi M, Musha T. 1/f fluctuation of heartbeat period. IEEE Trans Biomed Eng. 1982 Jun;29(6):456-7.

306. Best and Taylor. West JB, ed. Physiologic Basis of Medical Practice, 12th ed. Baltimore: Williams &Wilkins, 1990:118.

307. Intaglietta M. Arteriolar vasomotion: Normal physiologic activity of defense mechanism? Diabetes and Metabolism 1988; 14(4bis):489-94.

308. Best and Taylor. West JB, ed. Physiologic Basis of Medical Practice, 12th ed. Baltimore: Williams &Wilkins, 1990:127.

309. Best and Taylor. West JB, ed. Physiologic Basis of Medical Practice, 12th ed. Baltimore: Williams &Wilkins, 1990:150.

310. Best and Taylor. West JB, ed. Physiologic Basis of Medical Practice, 12th ed. Baltimore: Williams &Wilkins, 1990:124.

311. Akselrod S, Gordon D, Madwed JB, Snidman NC, Shannon DC, Cohen RJ. Hemodynamic regulation: investigation by spectral analysis. Am J Physiol. 1985 Oct;249(4 Pt 2):H867-75.

312. Peñáz J. Mayer Waves: History and methodology. Automedica 1978;2:135-41.

313. Shoukas AA, Sagawa K. Control of total systemic vascular capacity by the carotid sinus baroreceptor reflex. Circ Res. 1973 Jul;33(1):22-33.

314. Intaglietta M. Arteriolar vasomotion: Normal physiologic activity of defense mechanism? Diabetes and Metabolism 1988; 14(4bis):489-94.

315. Rowell LB, Johnson JM. Role of splanchnic circulation in reflex control of the cardiovascular system. In: Physiology of intestinal circulation. Shepherd AP, Granger DN, eds. Raven Press 1984:153-63.

316. Kitney RI. An analysis of the nonlinear behavior of the human thermal vasomotor control system. J Theor Biol 1975;52:231-48.

317. Hyndman BW. The role of rhythms in homeostasis. Kybernetik 1974;15:227-36.

318. Burton AC, Taylor RM. A study of the adjustment of peripheral vascular tone to the requirements of the regulation of body temperature. Amer J Physiol 1940;129:565-77.

319. Bornmyr S, Svensson H, Lilja B, Sundkvist G. Skin temperature changes and changes in skin blood flow monitored with laser Doppler flowmetry and imaging: a methodological study in normal humans. Clin Physiol. 1997 Jan;17(1):71-81.

320. Akselrod S, Gordon D, Madwed JB, Snidman NC, Shannon DC, Cohen RJ. Hemodynamic regulation: investigation by spectral analysis. Am J Physiol. 1985 Oct;249(4 Pt 2):H867-75.

321. Akselrod S, Gordon D, Ubel FA, Shannon DC, Berger AC, Cohen RJ. Power spectrum analysis of heart rate fluctuation: a quantitative probe of beat-to-beat cardiovascular control. Science. 1981 Jul 10;213(4504):220-2.

322. Kitney RI. An analysis of the nonlinear behavior of the human thermal vasomotor control system. J Theor Biol 1975;52:231-48.

323. Barron DH. Chapt. 31, Vasomotor Regulation. In: Ruch TC, Fulton JF, editors. Medical Physiology and Biophysics, 18th ed. Philadelphia: W.B. Saunders Co, 1960:691-707.

324. Hyndman BW. The role of rhythms in homeostasis. Kybernetik 1974;15:227-36.

325. Chess GF, Tam RM, Calaresu FR. Influence of cardiac neural inputs on rhythmic variations of heart period in the cat. Am J Physiol. 1975 Mar;228(3):775-80.

326. Becker RE. Life in Motion. Brooks RE, editor. Portland, OR: Rudra Press; 1997.

327. Magoun HI. Osteopathy in the cranial field. 2nd ed. Kirksville, MO: The Journal Printing Company; 1966:35.

328. Sutherland WG. The cranial bowl. Mankato, MN: Free Press Company; 1939. Reprinted:

Indianapolis, IN: American Academy of Osteopathy; 1986.

329. Magoun HI. Osteopathy in the cranial field. 2nd ed. Kirksville, MO: The Journal Printing Company; 1966.

330. Frymann VM. A study of the rhythmic motions of the living cranium. J Am Osteopath Assoc. 1971 May;70(9):928-45

331. Sergueef N. Le B.A.BA du crânien. Paris: SPEK, 1986.

332. Sutherland WG. The cranial bowl. Mankato, MN: Free Press Company; 1939. Reprinted: Indianapolis, IN: American Academy of Osteopathy; 1986.

333. Magoun HI. Osteopathy in the cranial field. 2nd ed. Kirksville, MO: The Journal Printing Company; 1966.

334. Wales AL. Osteopathic dynamics. Yearbook of the Academy of Applied Osteopathy. American Academy of Osteopathy. Indianapolis, IN. 1946:38-42.

335. Lippincott HA. Respiratory technique. Yearbook of the Academy of Applied Osteopathy. American Academy of Osteopathy. Indianapolis, IN. 1948:31-33.

336. Kimberly PE. The application of the respiratory principle to osteopathic manipulative procedures. J Am Osteopath Assoc. 1949;48(7):331-4.

337. Lee RP. Primary and secondary respiration, Part II. AAO Journal 1993;3(1):17-19,27.

338. Younozai R, Frymann VM, Nardell BE, Pryor MJ, Senicki M. Effects of temporal manipulation on respiration. J Amer Osteopath Assoc 1981;80:751-EOA.

339. Sergueef N. Le B.A.BA du crânien. Paris: SPEK, 1986.

340. Akselrod S, Gordon D, Madwed JB, Snidman NC, Shannon DC, Cohen RJ. Hemodynamic regulation: investigation by spectral analysis. Am J Physiol. 1985 Oct;249(4 Pt 2):H867-75.

341. Akselrod S, Gordon D, Ubel FA, Shannon DC, Berger AC, Cohen RJ. Power spectrum analysis of heart rate fluctuation: a quantitative probe of beat-to-beat cardiovascular control. Science. 1981 Jul 10;213(4504):220-2.

342. Peñáz J. Mayer Waves: History and methodology. Automedica 1978;2:135-41.

343. Barman SM, Gebber GL. Basis for synchronization of sympathetic and phrenic nerve discharges. Am J Physiol. 1976 Nov;231(5 Pt. 1):1601-7.

344. Ahmed AK, Harness JB, Mearns AJ. Respiratory control of heart rate. Euro J Appl Physiol Occupation Physiol 1982(50):95-104.

345. Bachoo M, Polosa C. Properties of the inspiration-related activity of sympathetic preganglionic neurones of the cervical trunk in the cat. J Physiol. 1987 Apr;385:545-64.

346. Ahmed AK, Harness JB, Mearns AJ. Respiratory control of heart rate. Euro J Appl Physiol Occupation Physiol 1982(50):95-104.

347. Tharion E, Samuel P, Rajalakshmi R, Gnanasenthil G, Subramanian RK. Influence of deep breathing exercise on spontaneous respiratory rate and heart rate variability: a randomised controlled trial in healthy subjects. Indian J Physiol Pharmacol. 2012 Jan-Mar;56(1):80-7.

348. Bernardi L, Sleight P, Bandinelli G, Cencetti S, Fattorini L, Wdowczyc-Szulc J, Lagi A. Effect of rosary prayer and yoga mantras on autonomic cardiovascular rhythms: comparative study. BMJ. 2001 Dec 22-29;323(7327):1446-9.

349. Niu NN, Perez MT, Katz JN. Singing intervention for preoperative hypertension prior to total joint replacement: a case report. Arthritis Care Res (Hoboken). 2011 Apr;63(4):630-2. doi: 10.1002/acr.20406.

350. Becker RE. Life in Motion. Brooks RE, editor. Portland, OR: Rudra Press; 1997.

351. Akselrod S, Gordon D, Madwed JB, Snidman NC, Shannon DC, Cohen RJ. Hemodynamic regulation: investigation by spectral analysis. Am J Physiol. 1985 Oct;249(4 Pt 2):H867-75.

352. Akselrod S, Gordon D, Ubel FA, Shannon DC, Berger AC, Cohen RJ. Power spectrum analysis of heart rate fluctuation: a quantitative probe of beat-to-beat cardiovascular control. Science. 1981 Jul 10;213(4504):220-2.

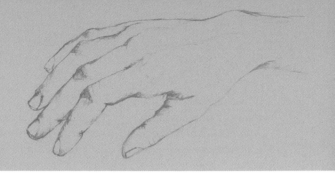

# SECTION 2
# Osteopathic assessment

*Our art has always been ahead of our science. It will always be. But the nearer we can bring them together, the most effectively we can practice osteopathy.*

—A. Willard[1]

The description of the process necessary for a complete history and physical examination of the aging patient exceeds the scope of this text. What follows in this chapter is a description of what is distinctive in the osteopathic approach to the diagnosis and treatment of somatic dysfunction in the aging patient. This assessment is a valuable addition to the complete history and physical, and not intended to replace it.

Assessment consists of the gathering of information for the purpose of evaluating an individual's health status and needs. It is typically focused by a chief complaint; the expressed reason for the patient to seek healthcare. The chief complaint directs the questions that follow to obtain a focused understanding of the complaint. This is often followed by a generalized history of the patient's health status. Following the acquisition of historical information, the physical examination is performed. Evaluation of the information obtained from the history and physical examination is used to identify a diagnosis and formulate a treatment intervention.

Allopathic medical practice focuses predominantly upon the identification of pathology. Osteopathy seeks not only the diagnosis of such pathology, but also stresses the interrelationship between structure and function, and the impact of somatic dysfunction, associated with structural imbalances independently or as a contributing factor to the patient's ability to respond to, or compensate for any organic pathology.

## Somatic dysfunction

Somatic dysfunction is defined as "impaired or altered function of related components of the somatic (body framework) system: skeletal, arthrodial, and myofascial structures and their related vascular, lymphatic, and neural elements."[2] It is the recognition of the contribution of somatic dysfunction to the overall status of the individual and its specific treatment with osteopathic manipulation that makes osteopathy distinctive.

The classification of somatic dysfunction may be further subdivided by considering the dysfunctional anatomic structures that are predominantly involved. As such, somatic dysfunction may be primarily osseous (intraosseous), articular (interosseous), ligamentous, membranous, fascial, muscular, or any combination of these structures. Additionally somatic dysfunction can affect, either mechanically or neuro-reflexly, visceral, neural, lymphatic, and vascular structures.

Intraosseous dysfunctions can occur because infants' and children's bones consist of multiple growth centers united by flexible cartilaginous or membranous tissue. Until complete ossification occurs, this relationship is subject to the impact of exogenous forces upon the bone, with the resultant development of intraosseous dysfunction. These dysfunctions are often not found until later in life when they result in symptomatic compensations. As such intraosseous dysfunction is best treated earlier in life because the longer it persists, the more recalcitrant it becomes. While intraosseous dysfunction occurs within the structure of a single bone, interosseous dysfunction occurs between adjacent bones and involves the articular relationship between the bones and any associated soft tissues.

Somatic dysfunction may also be classified etiologically as: physiologic dysfunction within the normal range of motion of the involved structures; non-physiologic dysfunction—the effect of exogenous forces upon the involved structures; and reflex dysfunction that is a neurologically-mediated response to conditions elsewhere in the body.

Any of the above subdivisions of somatic dysfunction may be described in terms of the motion pattern demonstrated by the dysfunctional structure. These motions include flexion, extension, rotation, sidebending, anteroposterior (AP) translation, lateral translation, compression, distraction, lateral (external) rotation, medial (internal) rotation, torsion, and primary and pulmonary respiration.

All components of the body must move freely, each in its individually complex spatial pattern. Understanding dysfunction in this context may be simplified by defining it in terms of four dimensions, the three cardinal axes and planes, and time. During the physical examination, palpation is employed to assess the movement of a structure around the three cardinal axes, in the three cardinal planes, and in the context of its relationship in time as exemplified by the biphasic primary respiratory mechanism (PRM).

Anatomic structures typically demonstrate complex motion patterns. Somatic dysfunction as described in the context of the three cardinal axes and planes will often exhibit motion in one plane at greater amplitude to that in the other planes. This is referred to as the major motion of the structure, and the two other components of variable amplitude in the two remaining planes are the minor motions. It is important to recognize that, although the terms major and minor are being applied to the description of the dysfunction, this description refers to the amplitude of the motion, and not necessarily its significance in the context of the dysfunction and its treatment. When diagnosing somatic dysfunction, all of the aspects of motion must be taken equally into consideration. Frequently, however, the solution to effective treatment lies in the recognition of the contribution of a minor movement.

In this text, somatic dysfunction, as a diagnosis, is named for the direction of the freest motion. Thus, if a rib moves freely into exhalation and is restricted in inhalation, it will be described as an exhaled rib.

Somatic dysfunction may further be classified as primary or secondary, depending upon whether it exists independently or is mechanically or reflexly compensatory for adjacent or distant dysfunction(s). Additionally, it may be classified according to duration as: acute, less than 30 days since the cause of the dysfunction; sub acute, present from one to six months; or chronic, present for longer than six months.

Frequently somatic dysfunction is associated with physical discomfort. This discomfort is neurologically most often a manifestation of nociception. Nociceptive activity from the area of dysfunction affects the central nervous system (CNS). This results in a state of irritability, referred to as facilitation, at the anatomic level of the CNS supplied by the stimulated nociceptive neurons. This irritability is the source of the neurological, viscerosomatic, somatovisceral, somatosomatic, and viscerovisceral reflex manifestations of somatic dysfunction and through the ascending spinal pathway, the spinal segmental facilitation of somatic dysfunction can manifest somatoemotionally.

As the individual experiences the physiological changes of aging with the resultant loss of flexibility and narrowing of their homeostatic base, and more and more conditions, including somatic dysfunction, become chronic, they become vulnerable. The state of facilitation is also chronically present, thus, lowering the individual threshold for discomfort from additional stimuli. As such, diagnostic palpation and manipulative treatment must be employed with the greatest gentility in order to avoid physical distress and potential increase in inflammatory response.

Somatic dysfunction should be considered in the context of its untoward effect upon body mechanics. It must also be considered from the perspective of its impact upon body energy. It requires the expenditure of energy for any area of the body to move. The presence of somatic dysfunction necessitates that the individual works harder and, consequently, expends greater energy to achieve the same level of function as could be present in the absence of somatic dysfunction. Consequently assessment for somatic dysfunction must be defined both mechanically and energetically.

# Diagnosis of somatic dysfunction

The diagnosis of somatic dysfunction, as with any other clinical diagnosis, is based upon the acquisition of a complete history and physical examination. The physical examination may be further subdivided to include the evaluation of all relevant body systems for organic pathology and the assessment of the functional status of the body. A thorough functional assessment may be performed by first observing for static position, then for active motion, and lastly by palpation for structural anomalies and subtle functional restrictions. Somatic dysfunction is ultimately defined by the precise palpatory identification of functional restriction. When one palpates simply for structure, one gets information only about structural size, shape, and asymmetry and not necessarily the result of reversible somatic dysfunction.

It should be recognized that observation and palpation for structure may reveal asymmetries that are the result of intraosseous dysfunction. Such a dysfunction typically is established, between different parts of a bone before its ossification, early in life. For instance, in the first years of life, the sacrum consists of five vertebral segments that are not fused. If a two year old child falls forcefully on the side of their bottom, a dysfunctional intraosseous torsion between the upper and the lower parts of the sacrum may result. As a consequence of this, later in life, the individual may develop a compensatory somatic dysfunction between L5 and S1. This secondary dysfunction can be alleviated with osteopathic manipulative treatment. It will, however, tend to reoccur because of the underlying intraosseous sacral dysfunction. In the aged patient, although intraosseous dysfunction may be addressed, the potential for resolution is greatly reduced by complete ossification. As such, compensatory therapeutic interventions like orthotics and exercise may be added to the treatment protocol to provide the desired therapeutic outcomes.

## General principles
### Observation

"The basis of science is observation."[3]

Observation, or visual assessment, can be employed to define structure (static) and function (dynamic). To effectively observe structure requires a detailed understanding of anatomy. This knowledge allows the practitioner to identify landmarks and consequently variations from structurally normal configuration and position. At this time, it is also appropriate to observe for other physical signs including respiration and cutaneous features such as pallor, hyperemia, lesions, scars, and hair distribution. These changes may be the result of altered neurophysiology found in association with somatic dysfunction. As such they can direct the observant practitioner to identify underlying somatic dysfunction.

Dynamic observation, the study of the quality and quantity of gross and minor movements, requires knowledge of the motion available in the area examined. It can be of value here to observe the patient as they undress for the physical examination to follow. Is the patient capable of symmetrically executed activities, with full amplitude of normally available motion, or does their performance demonstrate asymmetry, stiffness or discoordination?

With experience, combined static and dynamic observations allow one to identify the area of dysfunction. As when you observe a tree, you can see how that tree is being, or has been, blown by the wind. Your observation provides information as to the strength and direction of the wind. Such information about external forces is contained within any structure, including the patient, and is available by observing their structure and how they move.

## Palpation for structure

Palpation for structure necessitates respect for the patient's willingness to be touched and the need for warm, clean hands. Begin by palpating the skin. Is it soft and smooth or rough, oily, moist, or dry? Note the skin's temperature. Somatic dysfunction can result in areas of autonomic dysfunction acting upon vasomotor tone, causing altered skin temperature.

Employing the lightest touch, next, palpate through the skin for the feel of the subcutaneous tissues. As the individual ages, the quality of tissue feel loses it flexibility and softness. Depending on the individual, fascia is more or less dense. To identify somatic dysfunction through palpation, the practitioner must recognize discrete areas where the tissues demonstrate diminished flexibility.

It is also important to note here that generalized changes in tissue flexibility are recognized in the presence of systemic illness. Hypothyroidism if insufficiently addressed results in palpable subcutaneous fullness: myxedema. Diabetes mellitus has been shown to demonstrate subcutaneous edema that is proportionate to hyperglycemia.[4] Renal failure produces subcutaneous tissue texture changes that are distinctively similar to that of diabetes.[5] It is probable that the majority if not all systemic illnesses create discernible generalized tissue texture changes that may be identified by skilled palpation.

Now, in order to palpate muscle, palpate deeper for texture, tone, volume, and shape, looking for areas of tissue inconsistency that might be indicative of somatic dysfunction. Applying increased pressure through the layers of tissue will focus your attention to bone and articular relationships.

The application of graduated pressure allows one to palpate the differentiation between skin, connective tissue, muscles, bones, and joints. With discerning palpation it is possible to identify shape, size, and position in space of structures within the area under consideration. It is further possible to compare the feel of that area with normal palpatory findings for the same area and age group of the individual patient. Paired structures may be compared with the same structure on the other side.

Somatic dysfunction demonstrates alteration of shape, position, and tissue texture. The palpatory assessment of these qualities allows for the differentiation between normal and abnormal, and provides the practitioner with an appreciation of the level of the patient's health.

## Palpation for function

Diagnostic impressions drawn from observation and palpation for structure should be confirmed by palpating for function. Somatic dysfunction results in the functional compromise of normal physiology and anatomic mobility and consequently acts as a drain upon body energy. Osteopathic manipulation may be employed to enhance body energy, but it also specifically treats somatic dysfunction by re-establishing normal motion. In order to most effectively accomplish both of these issues, motion restrictions must be precisely diagnosed. This is the role of palpation for function.

The appreciation of the amount, pattern, and amplitude of available motion covers a continuum from the potency of the subtlest inherent motility present in all living tissue to the grossest movement of large areas of the body. Consequently, diagnostic palpation for function must employ a similar continuum from the subtlest test of listening to range of motion testing. While the test of listening passively monitors the potency and pattern of motion, range of motion testing actively induces motion. The tests of listening and visualization are employed to assess the pattern, quality, and quantity of the most delicate motions and, in so doing, the potency of the tissues themselves as well as the manifestation of PRM within and surrounding those tissues. The anatomic motion restriction resulting from somatic dysfunction is always associated with local, or distant, impediment of the PRM. Range of motion testing evaluates the availability, amplitude, and ease of motion between adjacent body parts. This includes definition of patterns of soft tissue tension and articular mobility.

It must be stressed here that the terminology 'listening' and 'visualization' is employed figuratively to describe the most passive form of palpation for function. Visualization is employed in association with listening palpation in such a way that the anatomy of the area being palpated is pictured in the mind's eye of the practitioner. These terms are repeatedly used throughout this text, and must not be confused with the sensations obtained from the ears and eyes.

When performing a physical examination, it is most appropriate to start with the least aggressive aspects of examination and continue on to more aggressive procedures. This is because findings obtained by less aggressive procedures can be altered by more aggressive procedures. As such, it is best to employ the test of listening and visualization before palpating for grosser motion restrictions. Ultimately, the identification of changes in subtle motion with the test of listening all but abolishes the need for range of motion testing.

To test for motion, one compares the response of a structure to forces applied in opposite directions, including: flexion versus extension; right versus left rotation; right versus left sidebending; anterior versus posterior translation; right versus left lateral translation; compression versus distraction; abduction versus adduction; lateral (external) rotation versus medial (internal) rotation; and opposing torsions. The specific anatomic relationship being diagnosed will determine which of these opposing motions are assessed and the sequence in which they are assessed.

Between each of the opposing motions there is a neutral point of functional balance. Each motion is defined by physiologic barriers (soft tissue tension) and anatomic barriers (the extreme limit of motion that can be exceeded only by rupture of the structure being tested). Somatic dysfunction between two adjacent anatomic structures is discernible as the presence of a dysfunctional barrier, limiting motion in one direction between the existent physiologic barriers. As such, in the presence of somatic dysfunction, a limitation of motion in one direction as well as a new point of balance, the dysfunctional neutral, will be appreciated.

When testing for any of these paired motions, it is imperative that following the introduction of motion in any given direction, the structure under consideration be allowed to return to the neutral position before proceeding to test for the opposing motion. The quality of motion felt while returning to the neutral position is as important as that of the original motion. If a motion is dysfunctional, the observed motion pattern may reveal restriction of that movement with ease of return to neutral, while the movement in the opposing direction will be free with resistance in the return to neutral.

The hand placement for diagnostic palpation is the same as the hand placement for treatment. For hand placement for all of the following diagnostic procedures the reader is referred to the descriptions of treatment in 'Section 3: Treatment of the patient,' p. 84.

## Tests of listening

The test of listening allows one to effectively assess available motion and the potency of the PRM. When palpated at the head, the PRM is often referred to as the cranial rhythmic impulse (CRI). The PRM is also palpable throughout the body as a biphasic motion consisting of inspiratory and expiratory phases. Somatic dysfunction, as such, can cause the symmetry and potency of this biphasic phenomenon to be impaired. With the test of listening, the area being examined is observed for its motion in association with the PRM. All aspects of motion: quality, asymmetry, and restriction, may be appreciated by listening to the inherent motility of the structure.

When initiating a test of listening one begins with totally passive palpation. This first contact should consist of the lightest possible touch. After establishing palpatory contact, the practitioner must quietly 'listen' to the area being palpated. The practitioner must wait for the perception of inherent motion without doing anything to influence that motion. The perception of the 'tissue breathing' of the PRM may be compared to that of thoracic cage motion during quiet respiration. When unaffected by somatic dysfunction, the tissues give the impression that they are expanding during the inspiratory phase of the PRM, and contracting during the expiratory phase. The amplitude of this motion is about as great as the amplitude observed when palpating a peripheral arterial pulse, but the frequency is roughly one tenth that of the pulse.[6]

The rate of the PRM has been recorded to be between two and 14 cycles per minute with the majority of reported rates, observed by palpation, tending toward the lower half of this range.[7][8][9] This frequency, although distinctly separated from, and usually slower than the rate of pulmonary respiration, occasionally coincides with, and may be entrained with, breathing.

In the absence of somatic dysfunction, the motion of the PRM demonstrates biphasic balance in quality and quantity. In the presence of a somatic dysfunction, the perception of motion within the dysfunctional area is typically modified in such a way that it is unrestricted in one phase of the PRM and restricted in the other phase. The dysfunction is identified in terms of this dysfunctional pattern. A restriction in the inspiratory phase of the PRM is referred to as an expiratory dysfunction, while a restriction in the expiratory phase is an inspiratory dysfunction. It should be recognized that in some dysfunctions, as in sphenobasilar synchondrosis (SBS) compression, the biphasic motion may be generally constrained. In this circumstance, the dysfunction is described in terms of the anatomic condition and not as a restriction of one phase of the PRM.

In cases where the palpable motion of the biphasic PRM (flexion-external rotation during inspiration and extension-internal rotation during expiration) is challenging to perceive, it can be useful to mentally visualize the normal motions of the structure being evaluated. Visualization is accomplished without actively inducing motion. When employing visualization, the practitioner mentally focuses upon, and compares the availability of, the different opposing motions. The mental imaging involved in this process will cause the practitioner to become more aware of subtle palpatory cues from their hands and the direction of unencumbered motion of the PRM will be more readily appreciable, while the dysfunctional direction of motion will not.

If this is still insufficient, the practitioner may proceed to a more active form of visualization, by picturing the structure being diagnosed moving in one direction, then returning to the neutral position, and finally moving in the opposite direction. This process of mentally picturing the motion while palpating it will trigger the subtlest proprioceptive awareness from the practitioner's flexor pollicis longus and flexor digitorum profundus muscles to amplify the perception of the motion. The dysfunction in the direction of the unrestricted motion will prove to be more easily visualized.

The visualization process is greatly enhanced by a thorough knowledge of the anatomy of the area being palpated. Such knowledge will allow the practitioner to more readily appreciate the structure that they are visualizing and the subtle motility that they are listening for. The identification of motion patterns leads to an understanding of areas of functional restriction and subtle variations in the underlying anatomy.

The test of listening requires a very delicate touch. This, however, does not mean that only the superficial layers of tissues are being palpated. By mentally picturing the different structures and the different layers, the practitioner may focus upon deeper structures, with a hand contact that progressively accompanies the progression of the palpation, although without the application of invasive touch.

Once the rhythm has been appreciated, the manifest action of the PRM in a given structure is determined by gently increasing the amount of palpatory contact, until the inherent motion of the specific structure is palpated. The practitioner should mentally visualize the different anatomic layers until the level of the structure being examined is reached. This is accomplished while still applying the lightest touch whereby the inherent motion is appreciated.

The appreciation of the PRM, its rate, potency, and dysfunctional patterns in any given structure, or between structures, requires quiet listening. As such, in order to perceive the PRM, the practitioner must learn to concentrate in a relaxed manner. Time and patience are necessary to obtain the desired information. This conscious touch is not just mechanical touch. It lends itself particularly well to the examination of very ill and fragile individuals.

Somatic dysfunction is often uncomfortable. Procedures that employ palpatory forces greater than those employed in the test of listening and visualization can take the area in the direction of the restricted motion and tend to increase the associated discomfort. Because the test of listening is focused more upon the quality of available motion than it is upon the quantity, the patient is not taken into the position of discomfort associated with the dysfunctional range of motion. By focusing upon the quality of motion, the practitioner knows the position of balance and the direction of restriction from the very beginning of the test of listening. Thus, monitoring the position of functional balance, even in the presence of somatic dysfunction, tends to be soothing to the patient.

When diagnosing with the test of listening the practitioner identifies the inherent forces within the tissues. Having done this, treatment can seamlessly follow through the use of these inherent forces.

## Range of motion testing

If necessary, range of motion testing may be used to strengthen the diagnosis made with the test of listening and visualization. After palpatory listening and visualizing, if the practitioner is hesitant as to what has been observed, it is then appropriate to follow with dynamic motion testing.

Range of motion testing is the assessment of the range of available passive motion between two contiguous anatomic structures. It is most often identified in the context of the pattern of available anatomic motion. These complex motion patterns are defined by breaking them down into their paired components as described above.

Range of motion testing in terms of osteopathic diagnosis should not be confused with that employed for orthopedic diagnosis. The motions evaluated are comparable, but the forces used to assess those motions are very much less forceful. This is of particular importance when diagnosing frail individuals. Typically, the dysfunctional restrictions of greatest significance are found in the minor motions between two adjacent anatomic structures, as exemplified by abduction or adduction restriction in ulnohumeral dysfunction. For these reasons, range of motion testing must be employed using the lightest possible touch that still provides the perception of motion and barrier. The experienced practitioner will soon find that the subtle forces that should be used in range of motion testing, when employed in the gentlest possible manner, point one to the subtle touch employed in the test of listening described above.

# History

With the exception of the most emergent of clinical circumstances, before any treatment is decided upon a thorough understanding of the problem(s) to be addressed must be established. The establishment of a treatable diagnosis begins with the acquisition of the patient's history. The history for the aging patient, as with that for all other patient's, consists of a starting point, the patient's chief complaint, and continues with a sequence of inquiry that becomes progressively broader until a complete picture of the patient's circumstance is obtained. The typical sequence of this process is:

- Chief complaint (CC)
- History of present illness (HPI)
- Review of systems (ROS)
- Past medical history (PMH)
- Social history (SH)
- Past family history (PFH)

The CC establishes the reason for the patient's visit with the healthcare provider. The acquisition of this information is initiated with a simple open-ended question, such as: "What brings you in to see me today?" The patient's response should be recorded in the patient's own words, e.g., "I have a headache and feel like vomiting." The HPI goes on to describe the CC(s) in detail. The ROS, PMH, SH, and PFH provide important additional pertinent information that will help in focusing the physical examination, identifying a diagnosis, and ultimately, determining a treatment protocol.

It is important to recognize that the following areas of information that should be included within the complete history are of particular interest to the osteopathic practitioner. In the context of the patient's CC, HPI, ROS, and PMH, which organ systems are significantly involved and how somatic dysfunction affects the efficient function of these involved systems through its impact upon the following are important to note:

- skeletal, arthrodial, and myofascial mechanics;
- neurophysiology, including sensorimotor, sympathetic, and parasympathetic function;
- tissue perfusion, including arterial, venous, and lymphatic;
- primary respiration.

To delineate the HPI a series of details should be sought out. Particularly, if the CC is a pain complaint, the HPI should include the following information:

- Location: "Where is the pain?" "Does the pain radiate into an adjacent or distant part of the body?" Here it is important to remember that pain complaints may be reflex in origin. What appears to be a primary musculoskeletal complaint may actually be a dermatomally or myotomally-related viscerosomatic reflex. As such, the location of the pain should cause the examiner to look closely at the potentially etiologic visceral organ later in the history when performing the ROS. Conversely what appears to be visceral pain may prove to be a visceral reflection of a somatovisceral reflex, or simply locally suggestive somatic pain.
- Quality: "Describe the pain." "Is it: sharp, dull, aching, throbbing, or burning in nature?"
- Severity: "Describe the pain in terms of a scale of one to ten."
- Timing and frequency: "Is the complaint associated with a specific time of day, week, month, or year?" Musculoskeletal pain from postural imbalance as might be associated with

accommodation for pelvic unleveling from an anatomic short leg frequently occurs at the same time every day, when the patient fatigues. Pain associated with muscle spasm and arthritides is often experienced after periods of immobility when the patient attempts to initiate motion. "Is the pain constant, as is seen with inflammation, or intermittent, as is seen with colic affecting a hollow viscus, and if intermittent, how long does it last?"
- Duration: "How long has the problem persisted?"
- Context: Describe what the patient did to cause the problem, or was doing when the problem occurred.
- Modifying factors: "Describe what makes the problem better or worse," etc.
- Associated signs and symptoms: In the above example the patient's headache is associated with nausea.

The ROS is an extremely important component of the history, in that it provides holistic information that might otherwise be overlooked if the history is limited to the HPI. The ROS should acquire information in each of the ROS body areas and organ systems to be reviewed:

- Allergy/immunologic
- Cardiovascular
- Endocrinology
- Gastrointestinal
- Genitourinary
- Hematologic/lymphatic
- Integumentary
- Musculoskeletal
- Neurological
- Psychiatric
- Pulmonary

- Constitutional: these are a series of generalized symptoms like: quality of sleep, fatigue, fever, and weight loss or gain, that are not necessarily categorizable under any of the body areas or organ systems listed above.
- Head, eyes, ears, nose, mouth, and throat (HEENT) may be inquired about as a separate line of questioning, but they actually involve many of the other body areas or organ systems listed above.

The patient's PMH should be obtained including major illnesses, any current chronic illnesses, and previous surgery. List PMH with diabetes, hypertension, asthma, etc. as it pertains to the patient. This should also include an inventory of any prescription or over-the-counter medications or health supplements that the patient is taking.

The SH and PFH are recorded just like the PMH. The SH should be obtained including living arrangements, occupation, marital status, number of children, drug use (including tobacco, alcohol, or other recreational drug use), recent foreign travel, and exposure to environmental pathogens through recreational activities or pets. The PFH diseases affecting especially, but not necessarily limited to, the patient's immediate family members: grandparents, parents, siblings, and children, should be obtained. This should include whether or not the relative is living or deceased. If living, any specific diseases affecting the relative should be noted, or if deceased, the cause of death obtained.

# Physical examination

The distinctive osteopathic portion of the total physical examination consists of three components: observation, palpation for structure, and palpation for function. Although sequentially prioritized as observation, followed by static palpation, followed by dynamic palpation, with experience the assessment for these components integrates effectively. It is of value to have the patient gowned in such a manner that their back and bare legs may be directly observed and palpated.

Observation, the visual evaluation of the patient, provides the examiner with an appreciation of the patient's tensegral status. This is very important and, when mastered, can provide much of the information necessary to diagnose somatic dysfunction. Observation consists of the acquisition of the information from multiple visible cues that can then be synthesized into a holistic appreciation of the patient's total-body function. As complex as this may initially seem, with experience, it is done quickly. It begins as soon as you first see the patient. You can observe as they walk into the examination room and throughout the acquisition of the history. You can evaluate the patient's posture, and the motion of their head, face, spine, arms, and legs. Observational diagnosis may be substantiated by palpation for structure and function.

Palpation for structure, the tactile evaluation of static anatomy, provides the examiner with an appreciation of the patient's architecture. Palpation for structure provides further delineation of information obtained by observation. This is performed to evaluate for positional asymmetries and structural anomalies that will influence the patient's functional status.

Palpation for function, the tactile evaluation of dynamic capacity, provides the examiner with an appreciation of the patient's ability to perform. This assessment of performance must be considered on the macro and micro levels and should also include the assessment of inherent rhythmicity. The relationship between structure and function is a fundamental principle of somatic function and consequently dysfunction.

Once the practitioner becomes proficient with the examination process, the three steps of observation, palpation for structure, and palpation for function blend seamlessly into one another. When this occurs, all three steps may be performed almost simultaneously.

The distinctive osteopathic assessment should include, to the extent possible, the examination of the patient in the standing, seated, prone, and supine positions. After observation, palpation for structure and palpation for function follow. In the performance of this assessment, it should be noted that although observation and palpation may be performed in each patient position, the actual examination may be edited to avoid unnecessary repetition. The standing examination reveals the most complete picture of the patient's dynamic weight-bearing. The seated position provides a picture of the patient's postural mechanics without the influence of the lower extremities. The prone and supine positions allow for functional assessment independent of the influence of gravity. In each position visual findings may be confirmed with palpation to differentiate between structural and functional influences. Palpation for function, when employed with the patient in each of the positions, provides a slightly different perspective.

## Observation and palpation in the standing position from the front

For psychological reasons it may be appropriate to begin with a cursory examination of the area of the patient's chief complaint. However, whatever the chief complaint is, whenever possible, taking into consideration individual patient limitations, the physical examination should include the assessment of the patient in the standing position. This is because the standing evaluation provides a global overview of the patient's total-body mechanics. The patient's standing posture should first be visually inspected, noting areas of interest. These visual findings may then, as appropriate, be further assessed by palpating for structure and function.

When observed anteriorly, in a patient with good posture, the center of gravity line should lie in the coronal plane, dividing the body into two equal halves. It should pass through the glabella, the middle of the suprasternal notch, the umbilicus, and the pubic symphysis, arriving on the ground equidistant between the patient's feet.

Observe the alignment of the patient's feet. The position of both feet should be such that they form a 30° angle open anteriorly. Weight-bearing should be distributed equally upon both feet. Further observe the feet for pes cavus (high arch) or pes planus (flat foot). These patterns may reflect total foot mechanics where, in pes cavus, the foot is completely positioned in inversion (external rotation), and in pes planus, the foot is completely positioned in eversion (internal rotation). These dysfunctions, when symmetrical, may be the result of a total-body flexion-external rotation pattern with bilateral inversion of the feet or total-body extension-internal rotation with bilateral eversion.

Asymmetrical dysfunction may result from dysfunction of the lower extremity, pelvis, or spine. For instance, a posterior displacement of the distal fibula may result in abduction of the talus and inversion of the foot with a unilateral high medial longitudinal arch, whereas, anterior distal fibular displacement can produce a unilateral flattening of the medial longitudinal arch.

Lateral (external) and medial (internal) rotation articular dysfunctions within the foot (subtalar, talonavicular, and calcaneocuboid) are often the result of sprains and strains. Subtalar dysfunctions between the talus and calcaneus are more commonly encountered with both the talus and calcaneum going into a lateral rotation strain. The talus is displaced anteriorly while the calcaneum is displaced posteriorly. On the contrary, talonavicular and calcaneocuboid articular dysfunctions are more commonly encountered with both the talus and navicular bone, or calcaneus and cuboid, going into a medial rotation strain.

Look at the lower extremities to see if the tibial and femoral diaphyses are aligned straight or are angulated, producing valgus or varus configuration of the knees. Additionally look for torsion between the two bones, and any lateral or medial tibiofemoral strain.

Next, examine the patellae. Look at each patella and the tissues surrounding it for positional asymmetry, possibly indicative of a distant dysfunction. Quite often, deviation of the patella is associated with a dysfunction of the ipsilateral pelvic bone. The tensor fascia lata originates off the anterolateral iliac crest and continues through the iliotibial tract that inserts laterally upon the knee. As such, posterior displacement of the ilium loads the iliotibial tract and consequently the knee with resultant lateral displacement of the patella.

Note any pelvic side shift, the lateral deviation of the pelvis to one side or the other. Subsequently, observe the greater trochanters and the landmarks of the pelvis, particularly the iliac crests, for asymmetry. If the trochanters are level and the iliac crests are asymmetric, pelvic dysfunction, such as a pelvic torsion may be present. It should also be noted that anatomic asymmetry of the pelvic bones, although less commonly encountered, can also result in this finding. If both the trochanters and iliac crests are asymmetric, this is consistent with an anatomic leg length inequity. In this case, a posterior (internal rotation) pelvic bone may be found on the side of the long leg. Such an imbalance can also result from functional leg length inequity from asymmetric foot, ankle, knee, or hip dysfunction.

Then, look at the thoracic cage, observing the ease of respiratory excursion, noting any asymmetric motion of the ribs. Flattening of the thoracic spine will tend to facilitate the inspiration phase of respiration, while increased thoracic kyphosis facilitates the expiratory phase. A thoracic lateral curve will allow a greater degree of rib motion on the side of the convexity of the curve. Posterior rotation of the ribs will be present on the side of the spinal convexity and anterior rotation on the side of the concavity. These findings must be corroborated by posterior observation and palpation for function.

Compare the shoulders. Note the position of the clavicles. Asymmetries of these structures may be the result of sternoclavicular, acromioclavicular, scapulothoracic, thoracic cage, cervical spine, or cranial dysfunction individually, or in any dysfunctional combination that may in turn be the result of articular, muscular, fascial, ligamentous, or membranous dysfunctions.

Observe the carriage of the head and cervical spine. Look for sidebending or rotation that shifts the head to one side. Consider the relationship between the occiput and the atlas. The facial and thoracoabdominal midlines should be in alignment. Shifting of the facial midline to one side may indicate sidebending of the occiput to the opposite side with associated occipital rotation to the same side as the deviation. In the presence of such occipital sidebending and rotation, if the chin is prominent, the side of the anterior occipital condyle is dysfunctional. Conversely, if the chin is retracted, the dysfunction is likely to be on the side of the posterior occipital condyle.

Look closely at the ears, because they tend to mirror the position of the temporal bones. When the ear is flared out, the ipsilateral temporal bone is often found to be in external rotation. If the ear appears pinned against the side of the head, the temporal bone is apt to be in internal rotation.

Next, observe the position of the mandible. Normally, the midline of the chin should be in alignment with the midline of the rest of the face. However, the position of the mandible is influenced by the temporal bones. When somatic dysfunction of the occipital bone upon the atlas is present, the temporal bones tend to follow the rotation of the occiput. If the occiput is rotated to the right, then the right temporal bone will tend to be held in internal rotation, and the left temporal bone will be held in external rotation. If the midline of the chin deviates to the side of the flared ear, it is often the result of the temporal external rotation. If, however, the chin is deviated toward the side of the pinned ear, temporomandibular joint (TMJ) dysfunction is likely present.

As appropriate, one can reinforce visual findings with palpation for structure and function. (See discussion below under the heading: 'Palpation for function in the standing position from the back,' p. 50.)

## Observation and palpation in the standing position from the side

When observed from the side, a vertical line dropped from the external auditory meatus should pass through the humeral head, femoral head, mid knee and lateral malleolus. Deviation of these anatomic landmarks from this alignment should prompt the examiner to look further for postural dysfunction.

Assess the cervical and lumbar lordoses, and thoracic kyphosis for exaggeration of curves or gross and discrete areas of increased or decreased curvature. Weakness of the posterior core musculature, commonly encountered in the older individual, will increase the thoracic kyphosis. Weakness of the anterior core musculature will increase the cervical and lumbar lordoses. A gross pattern, either increased or decreased, that involves all levels of the spine can be the result of cranial dysfunction, pelvic dysfunction, or generalized weakness of the core musculature. Cranial flexion of the SBS and sacrum will tend to decrease

AP curves, while cranial extension will tend to increase curves. The cervical lordosis may also be increased as compensation for increased thoracic kyphosis and the lumbar lordosis may follow sacral extension (sacral anatomic flexion or nutation). In addition, increase of the thoracic and lumbar AP curves are seen as the result of spinal lateral (Fryette type I) curves found in association with pelvic unleveling and scoliosis. (See also 'Spinal motions, Physiologic motion of the spine,' in 'Section 4: Clinical considerations, Chapter 1: Musculoskeletal dysfunctions, Part 1: Axial system,' p. 180.)

Alteration of the normal lumbar lordosis should be noted. Increased lumbar lordosis is seen in individuals with increased anterior pelvic tilt and lumbar lateral curves (see above), often associated with anterior abdominal prominence (see below). Loss of lumbar lordosis, particularly affecting L1–L3, is commonly encountered in association with anterior lumbar (psoas major) muscle spasm.[10]

Locally, alteration in cervical posture, particularly at the level of the upper cervical spine, can occur if the occipital condyles are anterior. This is seen more often with unilateral condylar dysfunction. Under these circumstances an anterior positioning of the head will influence the cervical curvature and the facial profile.

Upper cervical flattening decreases the upper portion of the cervical lordosis. This may result from primary Fryette type II flexion dysfunction (C2–C3 and C3–C4 or in association with a trigeminal (upper respiratory tract) or vagal viscerosomatic reflex.[11] [12] This upper cervical flattening, in turn, will result in compensatory mid to lower cervical hyperlordotic stress that can facilitate instability and degenerative arthritis in the region, with potential compromise of the brachial plexus. Look also at the relationship of the cervical spine with the thoracic kyphosis. A forward displacement of the head may result from flexion dysfunction of the upper cervical spine or from increased upper thoracic kyphosis, a 'dowager's hump'.

Look for protraction or retraction of the pectoral girdle. Protraction of the pectoral girdle is seen with increased thoracic kyphosis, weakened paravertebral musculature, and weakened scapulothoracic, particularly rhomboideus major and minor, muscles. Retraction of the pectoral girdle

is seen in the presence of interscapular thoracic extension dysfunction. Such dysfunction may result from Fryette type II spinal mechanics, or it may represent several spinal segments fixed in extension as can be seen in individuals who have habitually assumed a 'military posture' or exercised extensively lifting free weights or with progressive resistance. This same posture is seen in female patients with large breasts who, of necessity, have been required to shift their center of gravity posteriorly by retracting their scapulae. An area of chronic thoracic extension found slightly lower, from T5 to T9, is encountered in patients with chronic pancreatitis.[13]

Observe the contour of the anterior abdominal wall. Abdominal prominence can result from a myriad of causes including but not limited to increased lumbar lordosis, decreased abdominal wall tone, intra-abdominal masses, ascites, and gastrointestinal distension. Many require definitive medical attention, but several may be addressed with specific musculoskeletal procedures. The former conditions must be thoughtfully ruled out before the use of manipulative procedures. In the presence of these conditions, definitive medical treatment should be initiated before complimentary manipulative procedures are employed.

Abdominal prominence resulting from pathological disruption of structure includes disruption of anterior abdominal wall continuity. This is seen in lateralized inguinal and midline umbilical hernias and midline diastasis recti.

Visceral pathology that must be taken into consideration in patients with abdominal prominence includes:

- Ascites, seen in association with liver failure, renal failure, congestive heart failure, pancreatitis, and a myriad of less common etiologies.
- Visceromegaly (most frequently liver and spleen), and large uterine fibroids.

Gastrointestinal distension is a common cause of abdominal prominence. This can result from constipation and various dietary intolerances. It can also be secondary to pathology affecting the liver and pancreas, gastrointestinal obstruction, and the use of anticholinergic and opiate medications.

Prominence of the abdomen may simply be the result of the accumulation of fat that may be deposited as subcutaneous and omental fat. Although this is most often associated with excessive caloric intake, typically in tandem with decreased physical activity, underlying conditions like hypothyroidism and adrenal insufficiency should be considered. Abdominal obesity must also be taken into consideration as a risk factor in: hyperlipidemias, the development of cardiovascular disease, the presence of increased levels of inflammatory cytokines, insulin resistance, and the development of diabetes.

Simple musculoskeletal etiologies include: the loss of abdominal wall musculoskeletal tone, altered pelvic tilt, and increased lumbar lordosis. It should be noted again here that increased spinal AP curves are found in association with lateral (Fryette type I) curves as seen in the presence of pelvic unleveling and scoliosis.

As appropriate, one can reinforce visual findings with palpation for structure and function. (See discussion below under the heading: 'Palpation for function in the standing position from the back,' p. 50.)

## Observation and palpation in the standing position from the back

The examination of the patient from behind is of particular importance. This position allows the practitioner to most directly assess the structure and function of axial anatomy during weight-bearing.

### Observation

From behind, examine the patient for symmetry of the following anatomic landmarks: ears, mastoid processes, shoulder heights, posterior axillary folds, scapular angles, iliac crests, posterior superior iliac spines (PSISs), gluteal folds, popliteal folds, Achilles tendons, and calcaneus. Look at the patient's inferior hairline at the back of the head. This provides an idea of the position of the occiput and basicranium. Unleveling of the hairline should lead the examiner to consider the possibility of a pattern of occipital sidebending and rotation.

Assess the alignment of midline structures including: the occipital protuberance; the cervical,

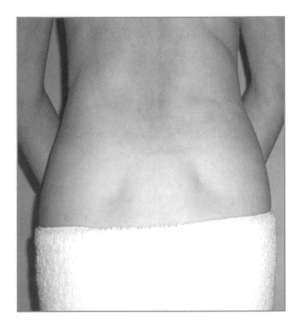

Figure 2.1: Observation from behind

thoracic, and lumbar spinous processes; and the intergluteal fold, often reflecting sacral position. Observe the leveling of the base of the sacrum, the sacral dimples (dimples of Venus) and the rhombus of Michaelis. Spinal sidebending curves result in compensatory positional shifting of these landmarks.

Observe the space between the lateral torso and the arms, the lateral torso contour, as well as the level of contact of the tips of the fingers of the patient when their arms are in a relaxed position at their sides. One side lower than the other may reflect a dysfunction in one of the joints of the arm or pectoral girdle, or vertebral sidebending.

Look for asymmetric paravertebral prominence. This is consistent with the rotational component of a Fryette type I spinal group curve. Such prominence will be located on the side of the convexity of the spinal lateral curve and may be more easily observed with the patient bending forward at the hips. Look for rib humping, seen in association with scoliosis (lateral curvature of the spine greater than 10°), and also the result of the rotational component of the spinal lateral curvature. In the upper thoracic region, the scapula may appear to be more posterior on the side of the paravertebral humping, also caused by vertebral rotation pushing the scapula posteriorly. Fryette type I side-bending curves of the spine may be primary somatic dysfunctions. They are, however, more apt to be secondary to pelvic unleveling affecting the spine from below, or craniocervical dysfunction affecting the spine from above.

Additionally, observe any cutaneous signs: hyperemia, changes in pigmentation, telangiectasia, and acneiform lesions. These findings are commonly seen in the skin over somatic dysfunction affecting the upper thoracic and lumbosacral regions.

### Palpation for structure in the standing position from the back

While observing the patient, it is appropriate to simultaneously palpate the anatomy being evaluated. This provides the practitioner with immediate feedback as to bony architecture and any subtle structural anomalies that may be present, as well as the presence, or absence, of soft tissue tension and texture change.

The palpatory sequence can follow the sequence of visual observation and may be performed simultaneously. The positioning of one's hands bilaterally in contact with the ears, mastoid processes, shoulders, posterior axillary folds, scapular angles, iliac crests, PSISs, gluteal folds, popliteal folds, Achilles tendons, and calcaneus will not only provide tactile cues, but will often allow the practitioner to visually discern subtle asymmetries more easily. Palpation for structure should go on to evaluate, as appropriate to the complaint under consideration, all of the patient's axial and appendicular anatomy. It is during this process that the tissue texture abnormality should be looked for, which is an important finding.

### Palpation for function in the standing position from the back

Although palpation for function in the standing position can, and should, be performed from the front and side, the most effective, and easiest, position for this examination is from behind. This is because it readily allows the examiner to sequentially examine

the sacrum and the pelvic bones, and to therefore get information about pelvic accommodation of forces from above and below. Additionally, during the pelvic bone motion, the posterior superior iliac spine (PSIS) exhibits a greater positional change than the anterior superior iliac spine (ASIS).

When applying the test of listening to the pelvis, different pelvic motions are perceived that are indicative of the dysfunctional area of the body they are responsible for. Appreciation of these differences allows one to identify the dysfunction as either at the level of the sacrum, above in the axial skeletal, or below in the lower extremity. To do this, the practitioner places their thumbs in contact with the PSISs and their hands bilaterally on the iliac crests, and palpates the PRM. (Fig. 2.2)

In the absence of any dysfunction, the pelvic bones should present unrestricted craniosacral external and internal rotation components of

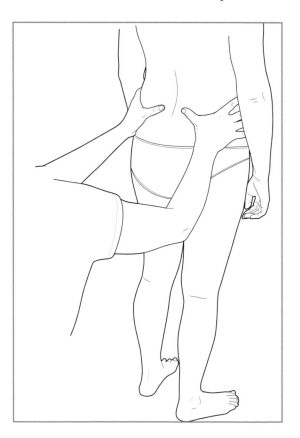

Figure 2.2: Test of listening of the pelvis

motion in each of the three cardinal planes.[14] During craniosacral external rotation, the inspiratory phase of the PRM, the palpable motion is as follows:

- The pelvic bones demonstrate their major component of motion in the sagittal plane, as an anterior rotation that is felt at the iliac crests, with the PSIS moving superiorly.
- In the coronal plane, the minor component of motion is an abduction of the iliac crest, with the PSIS moving laterally.
- In the transverse plane, the minor component of motion is the entire iliac crest moving laterally but to a greater degree at the PSIS than at the ASIS.

As a result of the combination of the three components, during external rotation, the PSIS displays a net upward and lateral movement. During craniosacral internal rotation, the PSIS exhibits a motion in the opposite directions i.e., a net downward and medial movement.

When the two pelvic bones synchronously follow the biphasic PRM, there is a sense of pelvic girdle unity.[15] The biphasic motion is synchronous with the action of the PRM and is associated with craniosacral flexion and extension of the sacrum. With the inspiratory phase of the PRM, as the two pelvic bones externally rotate, the associated lateral movement of the PSISs opens the sacroiliac joints bilaterally, thus allowing the sacral base to move posteriorly into craniosacral flexion. Accordingly, during the expiratory phase of the PRM, when the pelvic bones internally rotate, medial movement of the two PSISs causes the sacroiliac joints to close, following the base of the sacrum as it moves anteriorly into craniosacral extension.

After listening to both pelvic bones as described above, the practitioner can move their thumbs into contact with the PSISs, in a slightly more medial and cephalic position, in such a way that they also contact the base of the sacrum. This position allows a simultaneous test of listening of both pelvic bones and the sacrum, assessing not only their individual motions, but also their relationship, and the freedom of motion of the sacroiliac joints.

**Pelvic torsional pattern**

As described above, in the absence of dysfunction, the pelvic bones follow the sacrum. It should be noted here that because of the intrauterine fetal posture,[16] almost everyone demonstrates a torsional pattern of the pelvis. The structural organization of the body is established early in life. This basic pattern may then undergo modification throughout life from stress-induced somatic dysfunctions.

In addition to the intrauterine origin, a torsional pattern of the pelvis may be associated with the compensatory pattern of the sacrum to a dysfunction of L5 upon S1 or any midline structure above. For instance, when L5 is dysfunctional in a Fryette type II pattern, with either forward bending or backward bending, accompanied by rotation and sidebending to the right, the sacrum accommodates with a left torsion on the right oblique axis. When listening to the sacrum, the left torsion is felt with ease while the right torsion is restricted. The pelvis will also display a torsional pattern on one side to compensate for a dysfunction of rotation on the opposite side of any axial skeletal midline structure above. When listening to the pelvis, as a rule of thumb, the lower the dysfunction in the axial skeleton, the greater the sacral torsional sensation.[17]

Note that there is no sacroiliac joint dysfunction in the case of a sacral torsion. The pattern of pelvic torsion is an accommodation to dysfunction above. This may be as low as L5–S1 or it can be as high as cranial structures. Under these circumstances, both pelvic bones follow the sacrum. These mechanics were demonstrated by Strachan et al. on cadaveric specimens.[18] With a left sacral torsion, the right pelvic bone moves more easily into external rotation and returns to demonstrate a less prominent internal rotation phase. Simultaneously, the left pelvic bone moves easily into internal rotation, with less prominence in the external rotation phase.

During the test of listening, the sense of unity of pelvic girdle motion is constantly present, i.e., the sensation that when one pelvic bone moves, the other one moves in synchrony, although in the opposite direction. It should be recognized that the motions of the pelvic bones described as external or internal rotation, in association with the sacral torsion, are not exactly the same as those which occur with a craniosacral flexion or extension of the sacrum. On the side opposite the rotational component of the sacral torsion, the external rotation of the pelvic bone consists of anterior rotation as the major component of motion, but the two minor components differ with the entire iliac crest moving medially to a greater degree at the PSIS than at the ASIS.

### Pelvic unlinked motion patterns

If during palpation the sense of pelvic girdle unity is absent, with the sensation that both pelvic bones are moving out of synchrony, the dysfunction may be in the lower limbs, the pelvic bones, or the sacroiliac joints. In this case, some restriction of motion is felt under the thumb covering the PSISs and the base of the sacrum.

## Range of motion testing in the standing position

The spinal gross range of motion may be assessed by having the standing patient actively flex, extend, side bend, and rotate each region of the spine, thereby adding to previous observations. As a result of the compensatory response required by the spinal curve that is present, tension between anterior and posterior muscle groups will differ. The patient with a hyperlordotic lumbar spine will demonstrate increased hamstring and hip flexor tension, while their abdominal muscles will have decreased tone. When such individuals forward bend, they typically compensate by flexing their knees.

### Pelvic sideshift test

The practitioner stands behind the standing patient and places one hand on the patient's shoulder, thereby stabilizing it. The practitioner's other hand should be placed in contact with the patient's contralateral hip. A gentle, medially-directed, translatory force is then applied to the hip, against the stabilizing force holding the patient's opposite shoulder. The practitioner's hands are then switched to contact the patient's other shoulder and hip, and the process is repeated in the opposite direction. The symmetry of motion between the two sides is then compared. The pelvic side shift test is defined as positive on the side toward which the patient's pelvis translates most easily.

### Standing flexion test

This procedure is a screening test that is said to determine the side of innominate, iliosacral, somatic dysfunction.[19] It is appropriate to note here that the term iliosacral refers to motion of the ilium, from below upward, upon the sacrum. Although used extensively it must be recognized that there is some question as to the test's validity.[20]

From behind the standing patient, the practitioner's thumbs are placed in contact with the patient's PSISs. The patient is then instructed to slowly bend forward from the hips, moving from below upward. The movement of the practitioner's thumbs with the patient's PSISs is observed. The standing flexion test is said to be positive, indicating the side of the dysfunctional innominate, on the side that the practitioner's thumb moves superiorly, first and furthest, as the patient flexes. It is worth noting that a false positive test can be observed on the side contralateral to asymmetrically tight hamstring muscles.

# Observation and palpation in the seated position

## Observation

Observation and palpation in this position consist, essentially, of examination of the spine, pectoral girdle, and upper extremities. This allows an evaluation to be performed without interference from the lower extremities. This is of particular consequence when there is an inequity of leg length and, as discussed in 'Leg length inequality,' in 'Section 4: Clinical considerations, Chapter 2: Postural imbalance,' p. 237, it is worth noting that over 50% of the population will demonstrate an anatomic leg length inequity of one quarter inch (6 mm) or greater.[21] Ninety per cent of the population has some demonstrable anatomic leg length inequity with an average inequality of 5.2 mm.[22]

Begin by visually inspecting the patient as described above in 'Observation and palpation in the standing position,' from each angle, and note areas of interest such as bilateral asymmetries and cutaneous changes associated with acute or chronic somatic dysfunction. These visual findings may then, as appropriate, be further assessed by palpating for structure and function.

## Palpation for structure in the seated position

Palpate for lumbar, thoracic, and cervical tissue texture changes over the spinous processes and paravertebrally over the transverse processes and, in the thoracic region, also over the rib angles. Using the lightest touch, note skin quality and with slightly more palpatory pressure, subcutaneous tissue texture. In the presence of acute somatic dysfunction, increased sympathetic tone to the skin can result in palpable warmth, an increase in sweating, and palpable subcutaneous fullness. With aging, the elasticity and fullness of the skin normally tends to decrease. Nevertheless, areas where this palpable decrease of cutaneous elasticity and fullness is more prominent may indicate underlying chronic somatic dysfunction. By applying still more palpatory pressure, note any particular alteration in muscular tension.

When palpating the spinous processes, note their alignment and compare interspinous spaces, looking for irregularities. Remember that asymmetry may be due to developmental anatomic variations or pathologic processes such as osteoporosis or osteoarthritis. Approximation of two consecutive spinous processes may be indicative of intersegmental backward bending (anatomic extension), while separation of two spinous processes may indicate forward bending (anatomic flexion). It should be noted that these static observations can also be the result of anatomic variations of the spinous processes and should always be confirmed with tests of listening and, if necessary, range of motion testing of the areas in question.

Next, palpate the pectoral girdle. Patients with shoulder problems usually have protraction of the pectoral girdle. Palpate the myofascial structures of the pectoral girdle. Supraclavicular spaces are usually not as deep in patients with outlet syndrome. Note any asymmetry in the position of the scapulae and clavicles. Palpate the shape of the clavicles that may reflect old traumas with fractures. Compare clavicular obliquity and palpate medial and lateral ends of the clavicles. Prominence may result from sternoclavicular or acromioclavicular joint dysfunction respectively. The sternoclavicular joint is the sole bony articulation between the pectoral girdle and the axial skeleton. As such, sternoclavicular dysfunction can affect the entire pectoral girdle.

The acromioclavicular joint is quite often involved in shoulder dysfunction. Compare the position of the acromion in relation to the lateral part of the clavicle.

Assess the first and second ribs. First rib dysfunction can affect sternoclavicular joint motion.

Palpate and compare the myofascial structures of the upper extremities. Note any differences in quality of the tissues and muscular tone. Assess and compare the two elbows. Note subcutaneous infiltration, evocative of somatic dysfunction. Palpate the hands and wrists. Again note any differences. Local somatic dysfunction is, most often, asymmetrical, whereas, symmetrical findings may reflect an underlying systemic illness, or a prominence of craniosacral flexion or extension in the global body pattern.

## Palpation for function in the seated position

With experience, tests of listening provide precise information as to the functional status of individual segments within the vertebral column. The practitioner places the index and middle fingers of their dominant hand on either side of the spinous process of the vertebra to be assessed. (Fig. 2.3)

With the hand so placed, visualize the vertebra and its articulations with adjacent segments. Listen to the inherent motility of the PRM in that spinal segment and identify whether it moves more freely into flexion or extension, sidebending right or left, and rotation right or left. If necessary proceed to visualization of the motion. To accomplish this, the practitioner successively pictures in their mind's eye each of the motion pairs, looking for asymmetry and restriction. The act of visualization augments the palpatory findings. At this point, if dysfunction is identified, it is appropriate to treat

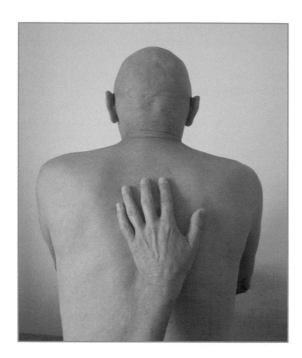

Figure 2.3: Vertebral test of listening

it using indirect principles. (See 'Section 3: Treatment of the patient,' p. 77.) If, however, further clarification of the dysfunctional pattern is necessary, one can proceed to range of motion testing.

Palpation for function of the ribs, sternum, pectoral girdle, and upper extremities follows the same principles. For a description of the hand positions see 'Section 3: Treatment of the patient,' p. 84.

### Range of motion testing in the seated position

If the practitioner has been able to make a diagnosis of somatic dysfunction with tests of listening, and has therefore proceeded to treatment, the range of motion testing in the seated position is not necessary. If, however, there is uncertainty as to the precise dysfunctional pattern present, the observations from the tests of listening should be further delineated by using range of motion testing.

For the different areas of the lumbar, thoracic, and cervical spine, it may be of interest to start with active motion testing before proceeding to segmental motion testing. First this gives the practitioner and the patient an assessment of the patient's overall mobility, and of specific areas of restriction. Secondly it allows the patient to appreciate any improvement when the test is done again after a successful treatment.

To perform active motion testing, the practitioner stands behind the patient and instructs them to bend forward and backward, to side bend to both sides, and to rotate to both sides. Restrictions of motion may then be observed at the different spinal levels.

To test for passive motion of the spine in the seated position, the *active hand-passive hand test* is preferred. It should be stressed again that range of motion testing in terms of osteopathic diagnosis should not be confused with that employed for orthopedic diagnosis. The forces used to assess motions in the osteopathic examination are very gentle. In the active hand-passive hand test, motion is introduced with one hand, the active hand, while the other hand, the passive hand, feels the response at the level being tested. During this test, the practitioner should focus on what the passive hand is feeling. One common mistake is to focus instead on the active hand, and therefore one gets an appreciation of the motion occurring at different, and often multiple, areas. With experience, the practitioner will feel a response under their passive hand to the slightest motion induced with their active hand, and as their skills are developed, direct passive motion testing will blend seamlessly into the indirect procedure of tests of listening.

Start at the level of the lumbar spine. The practitioner stands behind the seated patient and places one forearm over the patient's upper back and shoulders, such that their elbow is over one shoulder and their hand, the active hand, is over the other shoulder. The thumb and index fingers or the index and middle fingers, of the passive hand, are placed on each side of the lumbar vertebra located below the intervertebral space being evaluated as defined with palpation for structure. The tips of the fingers cover the intervertebral space to appreciate the motion occurring at this level. With the active forearm, introduce flexion, extension, sidebending and rotation, and for each of these motions, with the fingers of the passive hand, evaluate the response at the level of the intervertebral space. Note that when doing this test, it is important to introduce every motion from the neutral position. Dysfunction is named in the direction of ease. In this case, the motion to return to the neutral position is qualitatively more difficult. Once a dysfunctional pattern has been diagnosed, it is appropriate to treat it using indirect principles. (See 'Section 3: Treatment of the patient,' p. 77.)

In the same manner as above, test the mid- and inferior thoracic spine. To motion test the upper thoracic spine, the active hand is placed on the patient's head. The fingers of the passive hand are positioned as described for the lumbar spine. Introduction of motion with the active hand must be done very gently, employing the smallest possible amplitude.

Next, evaluate motion at the level of the cervical spine in areas where tissue texture changes have been identified. The hand placement is the same as the one described for the upper thoracic spine, although the proximity of the cervical spine to the top of the head necessitates that the forces employed for the introduction of motion must be smaller than for those used in the upper thoracic spine. As above, somatic dysfunction is present when the motion is easy in the direction of the dysfunction, with returning to the neutral position and motion to the opposite direction more difficult. Always assess quality and quantity of motion. Treat any identified dysfunction using indirect principles. (See 'Section 3: Treatment of the patient,' p. 77.)

Complete range of motion assessment of the cervical spine may be performed with the patient in the seated position. Be aware of the possibility of the occurrence of pain when the patient actively produces the necessary movements. Therefore, insist that the patient moves only through their comfortable range of motion.

Normally, during cervical flexion, the patient must be able to place their chin upon their chest. If this is not possible, measure the distance between their chin and chest with your fingers, and determine what the causative restriction may be. On av-

erage, about 50% of cervical spine flexion occurs at the craniocervical junction with the remaining 50% distributed between C2–C7.

Sidebending of the neck should normally allow the patient to touch their ear to their ipsilateral shoulder, on both sides. Nevertheless, with age, there is a natural decrease in range of motion, and sidebending is the earliest and most often impaired motion in many degenerative diseases.

The seated position is of particular value when testing for range of motion of the pectoral girdle and joints of the upper extremities. For a description of the hand positions for these procedures see 'Section 3: Treatment of the patient,' p. 84.

### Seated flexion test

This procedure is a screening test that is said to determine the side of sacroiliac somatic dysfunction.[23] From behind the seated patient, the practitioner's thumbs are placed in contact with the patient's PSISs. The patient is then instructed to slowly bend forward from the head, moving from above downward. The seated flexion test is positive, indicating the side of the dysfunctional sacroiliac joint, on the side where the thumb moves first and furthest superiorly. There has been some debate as to whether or not the patient's feet should be placed in contact with the floor during the performance of the seated flexion test. Currently this issue seems to have little or no effect upon the outcomes of the test, however the placement of the patient's feet upon the floor tends to reduce the sensation that they might fall forward off the examination table as they forward bend, and is, consequently wherever possible, desirable.

### Adson's test (Fig. 2.4)

Brachial and radial pulses may be evaluated to complete the assessment of the upper extremity. The brachial pulse is on the medial side of the arm, medial to the biceps tendon, just above the elbow, and the radial pulse is usually felt just inside the wrist below the thumb. A difference between the left and right upper extremities is found with impaired circulation typically in association with thoracic outlet syndrome.

Adson's test is employed to demonstrate the reduction or obliteration of the radial artery pulse

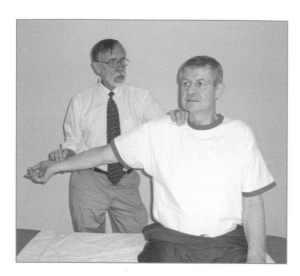

Figure 2.4: Adson's test

with compression of the subclavian artery at the interscalene's triangle. The practitioner palpates the radial pulse while extending and laterally (externally) rotating the patient's arm and shoulder. The patient is then asked to extend and rotate their head in order to look at their hand on the examined side, and next to inspire deeply and hold their breath. A positive sign will result in an absent or diminished pulse, because in this position, the anterior scalene is compressing the subclavian artery.

# Observation and palpation in the prone position

Further observation and palpation for structure and function may be accomplished with the patient in the prone position, if this position is comfortable. However, people with cervical or low back pain or those with shoulder problems may prefer other alternatives. To perform the prone examination, the patient's head should, ideally, be in a neutral position. If there is a preference for the patient to turn their head to one side, it indicates the side of the dysfunction that is usually located in the cervical or upper thoracic area. A pillow placed under the abdomen may provide some comfort if the patient reports that the prone position is stressful to the lumbopelvic area.

## Observation

Begin by visually inspecting the patient, noting areas of interest. Observe for asymmetry in the back, position of the scapulae, position of the pelvic bones, and the dimples of Venus. Record any observed spinal lateral curves and inclination of the sacral base, with the sacral base usually low on the same side as the lateral displacement of the upper end of the intergluteal fold. Observe the paravertebral musculature. Note, if present, the distribution of hair on the patient's back; an asymmetrical pattern is frequently reflective of chronic spinal dysfunction. Observe also any cutaneous pigmentary or trophic changes and the presence of visible capillaries, usually in the lumbosacral or upper thoracic areas, suggestive of underlying dysfunction. Record any scars and inquire as to their etiology.

Observe the lower extremities, noting the symmetry between the two popliteal folds. Also observe the Achilles tendons and the orientation of the posterior aspect of the calcaneus with the distal tibia. Altered calcaneal position may be indicative of dysfunction in the foot. These visual findings may then, as appropriate, be further assessed by palpating for structure and function.

## Palpation for structure in the prone position

Palpate the different layers of tissue from superficial to deep. Start with light palpation of the skin of the back of the patient. Is it soft, smooth, moist, or dry? Note any area with temperature, texture change or both that may indicate underlying somatic dysfunction. Redness that persists after palpation, the 'blush reaction' or 'red reflex,' may also be a sign of dysfunction. When the skin is cool, thin, and dry, with a glossy appearance, the somatic dysfunction is chronic.

Assess subcutaneous tissues for puffiness and edematous areas. Viscerosomatic reflexes are often readily palpable in the subcutaneous tissues, giving a sensation of localized rubbery or puffy quality. For their locations see boxed text 'Viscerosomatic reflexes,' in 'Section 4: Clinical considerations, Chapter 1: Musculoskeletal dysfunctions, Part 1: Axial system,' p. 183.

Next, palpate the muscles of the back. Identify any change in tone such as hypertonicity, hypotonicity, or atonicity. The most superficial spinal muscles are the longest, and the deepest spinal muscles the shortest. Hypertonicity of long and short muscles on the same side may be a response to asymmetrical postural patterns and group curves. In scoliosis, the result of spinal rotation, these muscles create the paravertebral muscular prominence. Hypertonicity of short muscles on one side more closely reflects a segmental dysfunction.

The prone position provides an important opportunity to assess the lower extremities under non-weight-bearing circumstances. Dysfunctional tensions in the hamstrings and calf muscles may otherwise go unappreciated.

## Palpation for function in the prone position

As described above in 'Palpation for function in the seated position,' tests of listening offer precise information about individual segments within the vertebral column. The practitioner places the thumb and index, or the index and middle fingers of their dominant hand on either side of the spinous process of the vertebra to be assessed, and listens to the inherent motion of that vertebra. (For hand placement, see 'Figure 2.3: Vertebral test of listening.')

Tests of listening of the sacrum and pelvic bones may be employed in the prone position. To test the sacrum, while standing at the side of the treatment table at the level of the patient's pelvis, facing cephalically, the practitioner places the palm of their hand on the sacrum, with the tip of the fingers on the sacral base. (Fig. 2.5)

During craniosacral flexion, the sacral base moves posteriorly while the convexity of the sacrum decreases, and during craniosacral extension, the sacral base moves anteriorly while the convexity of the sacrum increases. Palpation of the coccyx may follow. For this, the practitioner places their palm on the sacrum, with the fingers oriented caudally, in such a way that the middle finger lies on the coccyx. In the absence of dysfunction, the coccyx follows the sacrum. During craniosacral flexion, the apex of

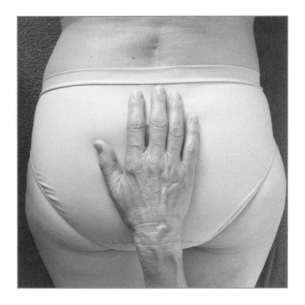

Figure 2.5: Hand placement for test of listening of the sacrum

the coccyx moves posteriorly and during craniosacral extension, it moves anteriorly.

To test the pelvic bones, the practitioner places both hands on the pelvis, in such a way that their thumbs contact the PSISs and their hands lie over the iliac crest on either side. Palpation of the PRM will reveal the inherent motion of the pelvic bones.

## Range of motion testing in the prone position

If necessary, range of motion testing in the prone position may complete the examination. In this position, different finger positions may be described, using short lever principles. To test flexion/extension between two spinal segments, the practitioner stands at the side of the treatment table, with the thumb and index finger of each hand on either side of the spinous processes of the vertebrae. Extension and flexion are successively introduced, by slowly approximating and separating the two spinous processes, allowing them to return to the neutral position after each motion. (Fig. 2.6)

This finger placement may be used to test the lumbar and the thoracic vertebrae. A similar test at the cervical level requires a very delicate touch.

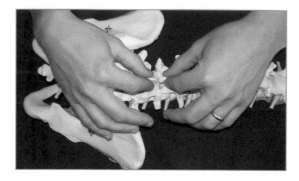

**Figure 2.6:** Hand placement for range of motion testing of flexion/extension

Testing for sidebending may be applied with the same hand position. In order to introduce the sidebending, the practitioner may fix the lower spinous process while sidebending the upper one on one side, returning to the neutral position before introducing the sidebending on the opposite side.

Testing for rotation consists of placing one thumb on the lateral side of the spinous process of the superior vertebra, and the thumb of the other hand on the contralateral side of the spinous process of the inferior vertebra. To introduce rotation on one side, the practitioner pushes the upper spinous process on the opposite side, while applying a counter force on the inferior vertebra. (Fig. 2.7) Next, the practitioner reverses their thumb position in order to test the rotation in the other direction.

Another method for assessing rotation consists of placing the thumb of one hand on the transverse process of the superior vertebra, and the thumb of the other hand on the contralateral transverse process of the inferior vertebra. Rotation is introduced to the left side by pushing gently, anteriorly, upon the right transverse process of the superior vertebra, while applying a counter force on the inferior vertebra. The practitioner then reverses their thumb position to introduce rotation in the opposite direction.

In order to progress with palpation when practicing range of motion testing, whatever the hand position, it is most appropriate to begin with tests of listening before proceeding to range of motion testing.

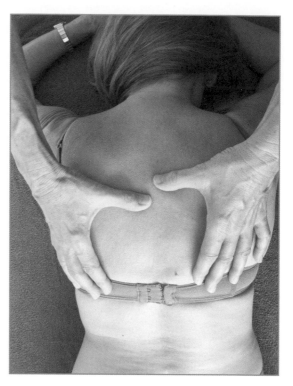

**Figure 2.7:** Hand placement for range of motion testing of rotation

## Observation and palpation in the supine position

During the examination in the supine position, the patient is more able to relax, and can freely see and interact with the practitioner. This gives the patient a sense of control. It is absolutely important that the patient positions themselves in the most comfortable position that they can assume. This assures that the findings from the palpatory examination are not obscured by muscular tension resulting from discomfort. A few adjustments may be necessary to enhance comfort, such as a pillow placed under the head when the patient has significant kyphosis.

Examining the patient in the supine position last in the examination sequence is advantageous in that, when indirect procedures are employed, they may be accomplished with the patient in the supine position for almost all areas of the body. It is thus unnecessary to ask the patient to change position, creating a smooth continuity between examination and treatment.

## Observation

Visually inspect the patient, noting areas of interest. These visual findings may then, as appropriate, be further assessed by palpating for structure and function.

Observe the position that the patient spontaneously assumes, noting any asymmetries, and inquire about any areas of discomfort. Normally, patients position themselves in a release position indicative of their underlying dysfunctional pattern.

Observe the lower extremities. Note the presence of edema, in particular at the level of the ankles and feet. Evaluate the venous status. Record any scars that may be the result of past traumas or surgery.

Look for asymmetry between the two feet. In the resting position, look for the presence of pronation or supination in the feet. Compare the degree of flexion of the ankles. Any asymmetry may be the sign of old ankle injuries. Usually after 50 years of age, feet are more pronated, flatter, and have a decreased range of motion in the ankle and in the first metatarsophalangeal joints. Observe hallux valgus deformities, the phalangeal alignment of the toes, and the presence of mallet toes, hammer toes, and claw toes, calluses or corns.

Note any increase in lateral (external) or medial (internal) rotation in the lower extremity, and determine its origin: pelvis, hip, knee, or foot. Rotational position of the complete lower extremity is frequently associated with an ipsilateral pelvic bone dysfunction, where lateral (external) rotation follows external rotation of the pelvic bone and medial (internal) rotation reveals the same coupled relationship. Symmetrical medially (internally) or laterally (externally) rotated lower extremities may be respectively indicative of craniosacral extension or flexion dysfunctions affecting the sacrum.

Observe the alignment of the tibia and femur, looking for genu valgum or genu varum that persists in the supine position and compare the position and orientation of the two patellae. Notice any deviation. Next look for any lack of extension, either at the level of the hip or the knee. If the hip is slightly flexed and laterally (externally) rotated, suspect a tight ipsilateral psoas muscle.

Examine the pelvis in relation to the treatment table, the lower extremities below, and the torso above. Lateral deviation of the pelvis upon the table from the midline can be indicative of lumbosacral dysfunction. Note any asymmetry of the anatomic landmarks, the ASISs, iliac crests, and greater trochanters.

Assess the thoracic cage and the ease of thoracoabdominal respiration. Observe the symmetry and coordination of respiratory movement between the abdomen and thoracic cage.

Typically, in the upper ribs, during inhalation, the anterior aspect of the ribs moves cephalad resulting in an increase of the anteroposterior thoracic diameter. This is referred to as 'pump handle' motion of the ribs. In the lower ribs, during inhalation, the lateral aspect of the ribs moves cephalad, producing an increase of the transverse diameter of the thorax. This is referred to as 'bucket handle' motion.

All of the ribs demonstrate some degree of both bucket handle and pump handle motion. The upper ribs, however, demonstrate pump handle motion as their major motion with bucket handle motion as a minor motion. Conversely, the lower ribs have bucket handle motion as their major motion with pump handle motion as the minor motion. Articular dysfunctions between the ribs and their respective thoracic spinal segments tend to occur as restrictions of the minor motions. Thus the first and second ribs become restricted in an elevated (inhaled) bucket handle position and the lower ribs become restricted in an inhaled (restricted exhalation) and exhaled (restricted inhalation) pump handle motion.

Diaphragmatic respiration should be unencumbered, with a synchronized alternation between the rise and fall of the abdomen during inspiration and expiration. Note any asymmetry between both sides of the thoracic cage. Rib dysfunction may be painful and the patient may avoid respiratory motion at the level of the dysfunction.

Observe the abdominal contour and its movement during respiration. The contour and movement should be smooth and symmetrical.

Abdominal visceral dysfunction may decrease the abdominal respiratory amplitude.

The sequence of pulmonary respiration should occur as a coordinated action involving all of the above areas. Note any portion of the thoracoabdominal area that does not contribute to the global respiratory motion, indicating an area of dysfunction.

Observe the muscular tone of the abdominal wall, noting areas of poor muscle tone. Look at the location of the umbilicus, which should be centered. If it is not, it may be indicative of intra-abdominal dysfunction or somatic dysfunction at the level of the mid-lumbar spine. In males and some females note the pattern of the hair that is seen extending from the suprapubic area up to the umbilicus or above. This line reflects the functional status of the lumbar spine. Deviation from the midline may be indicative of lumbar somatic dysfunction at the same horizontal level.

Next, observe the position of the head. Note the presence of excessive flexion or extension, sidebending, and rotation. The combination of sidebending and rotation in opposite directions is coherent with occipitoatlantal dysfunction, whereas sidebending and rotation in the same direction is linked with dysfunction in the typical cervical or upper thoracic vertebrae.

## Palpation for structure in the supine position

### Leg length

Start at the level of the feet. With the patient lying straight on the examination table, evaluate leg length. Take both feet within hands, with the patient's heels resting in your palms. Compare the levels of the distal aspects of the medial malleoli. With smaller inequities this method does not effectively differentiate between functional and anatomic leg length differences. To see other methods and find out if and how much heel lift would be appropriate, see the discussion on 'Leg length inequality' in 'Section 4: Clinical considerations, Chapter 2: Postural imbalance,' p. 237.

### Malleoli

On each leg compare the level of the distal medial and lateral malleoli.

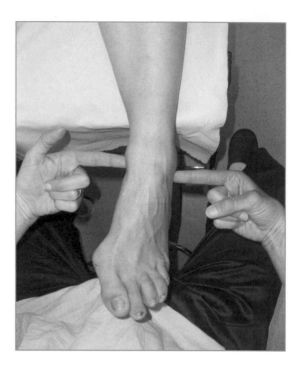

Figure 2.8: Hand placement to compare the level of the distal medial and lateral malleoli

Normally, when the extended index fingers are placed perpendicularly under the malleoli, the superior border of the finger located under the lateral malleolus is at the same level as the inferior border of the finger located under the medial malleolus. (Fig. 2.8) Any difference may be associated with fibular dysfunction.

### Tissue texture changes

Look for tissue texture changes. Circulatory compromise and decreased lymphatic function may affect tissue texture. Edema in the lower extremity can be the result of insufficient venous or lymphatic return, or both. Bilateral lower extremity edema is more likely to result from systemic illness (heart failure, renal failure, hepatic failure, or protein-calorie malnutrition with insufficient serum albumin production), intra-abdominal, or intrathoracic venous or lymphatic obstruction. Asymmetrical lower extremity edema, by contrast, is more apt to represent physical obstruction within the affected extremity. Somatic dysfunction can result in such an obstruction. An elevated dysfunction of the pubic bone places tension upon the ipsilateral adductor magnus with potential compromise of the deep venous and lymphatic vasculature at the adductor hiatus. Note, also, any localized 'puffiness' of the tissues, in particular around the patella, the lateral or medial aspect of the knee, or at the ankle that may indicate a somatic dysfunction.

## Muscular tone

Assess the muscular tone of postural muscles inclined to tightness, in particular the hip adductors, hamstrings, rectus femoris, tensor fascia lata, and piriformis. Evaluate also the peroneus longus, brevis, and tertius; tibialis anterior; vastus medialis and lateralis; transversus; and rectus abdominis muscles, which are inclined to weakness. All these muscles take part in postural balance and their hyper or hypotonicity can be indicative of postural instability.

## Thoracoabdominal area

Palpate the thoracic cage, looking for rib dysfunction in either inspiration or expiration. Assess the sternum and sternocostal joints. Palpate the thoracoabdominal area. Observe temperature changes in the abdominal wall. "Chronic and low vitality conditions will present a cold and clammy skin over the abdomen and cold areas in the skin over the spinal segments involved while just the reverse will be the usual findings in the acute condition."[24]

Look for subcutaneous tissue texture changes. (See boxed text: 'Viscerosomatic reflexes' in 'Section 4: Clinical considerations, Chapter 1: Musculoskeletal dysfunctions, Part 1: Axial system,' p. 184.) Several authors have described a correlation between existing tissue texture changes and dysfunction of the viscera. These palpable findings have been described as "small pearls of tapioca, firm, partially fixed, located under the skin in the deep fascia."[25] They are known as Chapman reflexes: "A system of reflex points that present as predictable anterior and posterior fascial tissue texture abnormalities (plaque-like changes or stringiness of the involved tissues) assumed to be reflections of visceral dysfunction or pathology. Originally used by Frank Chapman, D.O. and described by Charles Owens, D.O."[26]

## Cervical region

Next palpate the cervical region. Note any myofascial tension in the anterior muscles of the neck, posteriorly in the occipital region, and in the paraspinal muscles. Of particular interest in suboccipital headaches is the distribution of the greater occipital nerves (nerves of Arnold). As the medial branch of the dorsal primary ramus of the second cervical spinal nerve, the greater occipital nerve emerges posteriorly from under the inferior oblique muscle, on both sides of the neck, to ascend between the obliquus capitis inferior and semispinalis capitis muscles. It then passes through the trapezius muscle and ascends to innervate the scalp from the occiput to the top of the head.

Cervical vertebra 1 somatic dysfunction, with associated cord level (C2) facilitation, can result in pain referable to the distribution of the greater occipital nerve; upper cervical (vertebral units C1–C2 and C2–C3) somatic dysfunction can result in increased tension of the obliquus capitis inferior with potential entrapment of the greater occipital nerve. The greater occipital nerve is vulnerable, mainly due to its muscular relationship with the inferior oblique capitis. Upper cervical spinal flexion stretches the posterior roots of C2 over the denticulate ligament, while rotation stretches the posterior root of C2 on the side opposite to the rotation.[27] Resultant greater occipital nerve entrapment neuralgia is referred to as C2 neuralgia, or Arnold's neuralgia.

Palpate bony components of the cervical spine. The knowledge of bony and soft tissue anatomic landmarks is of paramount importance for precise palpation. The tips of the transverse processes of C1 are palpable posterior to the mandible, about 1 cm above and in front of the apex of the mastoid process. When dysfunctional, one side is more sensitive than the other, requiring delicacy of touch. Determine the position of these processes, noting if one side is more cephalic, anterior, and prominent.

Cervical vertebra 3 is normally identified at the level of the gonial, or mandibular, angle, the angle formed by the junction of the posterior and lower borders of the mandible. C3 is also normally at the level of the hyoid bone. C4-C5 is at the level of the thyroid cartilage, and C6 is at the level of the cricoid ring. It should be stressed, however, that with the aging patient, postural modification, in particular in the cervical region, or modification of the occlusal pattern, may modify these relationships. The anterior tubercle of the transverse process of C6, the carotid tubercle, also referred to as Chassaignac's tubercle, is a site where the carotid artery may be compressed.

Palpate the spinous processes of the cervical vertebra, to identify any segmental misalignment, depression, or prominence. Evaluation of the spaces between different spinous processes requires a delicate touch. Determine if there is some irregularity. Quite often, the tip of the spinous process of C5, and less often C6, is felt to be anterior to the spinous processes superior and inferior. This can reflect a somatic dysfunction of extension at that level that may be associated with cervical and shoulder pain.

Gently palpate the transverse processes of the cervical vertebrae. Look for posterior prominence that is found associated with ipsilateral rotation of that spinal segment and look for lateral displacement that is associated with contralateral sidebending. Follow the observation of any positional alteration of structure with palpation for function to complete the assessment.

## Palpation for function in the supine position

Complete the examination of suspicious areas with palpation for function, using tests of listening to assess the inherent motility of the PRM in these areas. Start with the lower extremities, paired structures that can be expected to demonstrate biphasic craniosacral external and internal rotation. Start at the level of the feet with both hands over the dorsum of the feet to feel if the motion exists qualitatively and quantitatively in both legs. With experience, the practitioner will have a sense of which leg is dysfunctional, and where.

### Foot
Assess the individual bones of the lower extremities. Apply tests of listening to the calcaneum, talus, cuboid, and navicular bones, as well as the subtalar, calcaneocuboid, cuneocuboid, and

talonavicular articulations. In the absence of any dysfunction, as paired structures, the bones of the feet should demonstrate unrestricted craniosacral external and internal rotation, the result of a combination of the motion in each of the three cardinal planes. One motion is a major component and the two others are minor, although equally important, components.

Craniosacral external rotation demonstrates a pattern resembling inversion of the foot while craniosacral internal rotation resembles eversion. During craniosacral external rotation, the inspiratory phase of the PRM, the palpable motion of each of the bones of the foot is as follows:

- In the sagittal plane, the major component of motion is a plantar flexion.
- In the coronal plane, the minor component of motion is supination, i.e., an elevation of the medial (internal) border of the bone while the lateral (external) border descends.
- In the transverse plane, the minor component of motion is adduction.

Opposite motions occur during craniosacral internal rotation; the expiratory phase of the PRM. Identify dysfunctional restriction in the major and minor components. If necessary, proceed to range of motion testing, and treat any identified dysfunction using indirect principles. (See 'Section 3: Treatment of the patient,' p. 77.)

Subtalar dysfunctions between the talus and calcaneus are very frequently found associated with ankle sprains. Typically the talus and calcaneum both display a lateral (external) rotation dysfunction, but the motion in the sagittal plane between these two bones differs. The talus is displaced anteriorly while the calcaneum is displaced posteriorly. On the contrary, talonavicular, and calcaneocuboid articular dysfunctions are commonly medial (internal) rotation dysfunctions, associated with medial (internal) rotation strain of the talus and navicular bone, or calcaneus and cuboid.

### Fibula
Next, listen to motion between the tibia and fibula, in both the proximal and distal joints. Normally, a posterior or anterior glide of the proximal fibula,

relative to the tibia, should be associated with the opposite motion of the distal tibiofibular joint. Assess the interosseous membrane that may also contribute to tibiofibular dysfunction. Treat any identified dysfunction using indirect principles.

### Knee

Listen to motion at the knee, assessing the motion of the patella, and the tibia relative to the femur in lateral (external)/medial (internal) rotation, abduction/adduction, and lateral/medial translation. If necessary, use range of motion tests to confirm observations obtained from listening. With indirect principles, treat any identified dysfunction. Quite often the fibula is involved in dysfunctions of the knee or foot and it should be considered first. Remember also that physical complaints at the knee can result from dysfunction at the ankle below or hip or pelvis above.

### Hip

Assess the hip joints with tests of listening. Remember that hip dysfunction may be the result of tightened postural muscles associated with postural imbalance. Thus, in the presence of a hip dysfunction visualize these muscles to determine if one of them contributes to the dysfunction; check in particular: hip adductors; hamstrings; the obturator internus and externus muscles; the piriformis; and the iliopsoas group, particularly the psoas major. Treatment of these dysfunctions

using myofascial release will often facilitate a more complete response in the pelvis.

### Pelvis

Additional assessment of the pelvis may be done in the supine position. Start the tests of listening upon the pelvic bones, (Fig. 2.9), and continue with the assessment of the sacrum and lumbar spine.

Note that the non-weight-bearing assessment offers more precise information about the motion of the pelvis than does the standing evaluation. When pelvic dysfunction found during the standing evaluation persists in the supine position, the site of the dysfunction is within the pelvis. On the other hand, if dysfunction observed standing is not present during the non-weight-bearing examination, the pelvic dysfunction is an accommodation to somatic dysfunction somewhere else. Remember that besides musculoskeletal pain dysfunctions, lumbar spine, sacrum, coccyx, and pelvic bones may be responsible for functional abdominal and pelvic visceral complaints. The treatment of identified dysfunctional areas should follow. For a description of the hand positions for treatment procedures see 'Section 3: Treatment of the patient,' p. 84.

### Pelvic floor

Pelvic floor assessment may follow. If the practitioner has appropriate credentials, an internal evaluation may be performed. For a thorough examination, the patient is best positioned in the lithotomy position for vaginal examination, and

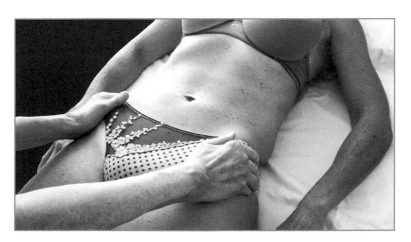

**Figure 2.9:** Hand placement for test of listening of the pelvis

lateral recumbent for anorectal examination. In the lithotomy position, it is best to examine the patient on a table equipped with stirrups for gynecological examination, with the patient positioned such that their perineum is located as close to the edge of the examination table as possible. This position allows for a good evaluation of the levator ani and pelvic wall muscles as well as coccygeal mobility.

Assess the ischial tuberosities. Look for asymmetry of shape and position that may be related to pelvic bone inter- or intraosseous dysfunction. Externally palpate the pelvic floor on the medial side of the ischiatic tuberosities for asymmetry of tonicity and hyper- or hypotonicity.

Introduce a gloved index finger into the vagina, or if the patient is male, the anus. Palpate the vaginal or rectal walls. Note any tenderness, tight muscle fibers, or hypotonicity with palpation. At the level of the ischial spines, palpate the sacrotuberous and sacrospinous ligaments. Asymmetrical ligamentous tension is present when the sacrum is dysfunctionally rotated between the ilia. Assess sacrococcygeal relationship. Hold the coccyx between the intravaginal, or intrarectal, index finger and thumb, externally. Assess the available motion between the sacrum and coccyx.

For the female patient, precise evaluation of the pelvic floor muscles, including the different portions of the levator ani muscle (iliococcygeus, ischiococcygeus, and pubococcygeus) may be further accomplished. In the lithotomy position, the relative position for palpation is described as if the practitioner is facing a clock. About one inch above the vaginal orifice, the pubococcygeus muscle can be palpated from seven to 11 o'clock on the left and from one to five o'clock on the right. Puborectalis muscle evaluation is performed more laterally in the distal vagina. Inserting the finger further into the vagina, the iliococcygeus muscle is palpated from four to eight o'clock while the coccygeus muscle is felt with the finger inserted more deeply into the vagina at five and seven o'clock. Although not described as directly part of the pelvic floor muscle, the obturator internus muscle has a strong relationship with the pubococcygeus muscle. It can be palpated intravaginally with the index finger directed superiorly and laterally on each side at ten and two o'clock. Dysfunction of the obturator internus may contribute to urinary symptoms and dyspareunia.

After palpation, instruct the patient to contract the perineal muscles. To facilitate patient comprehension of what has to be done, tell them to contract their muscles as if they wanted to stop the flow of urine. Ask the patient to contract their vaginal muscles upon the examining finger and assess the different components of the pelvic floor. Note any contractions of other muscles, in particular those of the abdominal wall, hip adductors, and gluteal region, a common pattern in patients with a lack of pelvic floor awareness. Usually, with uterine prolapse, the pubococcygeus muscle is atrophied, and the vagina feels very spacious with freely movable walls.

Follow the examination with treatment. This should include normalization of lumbar spine, pelvic bones, sacrum, and coccyx. Dysfunction of myofascial structures must be addressed, with myofascial techniques and massage. When the treatment is completed the dysfunctional areas should be reassessed. Finally a program to increase awareness and to strengthen the pelvic floor should be considered such as the 'Kegel exercises.' (See 'Section 4: Clinical considerations, Chapter 6: Urogenital dysfunctions,' p. 338.)

**Thoracoabdominal area**

Palpate the thoracic cage, looking for rib dysfunction in either inspiration or expiration. Assess the sternum and sternocostal joints. Apply tests of listening to the diaphragm and try to visualize its different parts to determine where any restriction of mobility may be located; note any difference in tension and freedom of movement between its two halves, as well as its posterior and anterior portions. Release any diaphragmatic dysfunction. If the dysfunction persists, look for primary dysfunction elsewhere that may be a contributing factor, or primarily responsible for it.

Diaphragmatic dysfunction may happen as a primary dysfunction of the diaphragm itself or the consequence of dysfunction of the lower thoracic cage, lumbar spine, or temporal bones. Dysfunction of ribs 6 through 12 can affect the diaphragm at its attachments, while the lower ribs may be dysfunctional because of lower thoracic spinal dysfunction. Diaphragmatic dysfunction is also found associated with motion restriction of the upper lumbar vertebrae. Lumbar vertebral dysfunction impacts the diaphragm through its effect upon the diaphragmatic crura. Dysfunction of the temporal bones that affects the PRM and the cranial diaphragm can, in turn, prevent full excursion of the thoracoabdominal diaphragm.

Palpate the abdominal wall and abdominal contents. Employ tests of listening to evaluate tone and symmetry of the myofascial components of the abdomen. Listen to the inherent motility of the abdomen globally, as well as listening to the abdominal wall and the individual viscera within. Identified areas of dysfunctional tension or restricted motility should be treated.

### Pectoral girdle
Proceed to the assessment of the pectoral girdle. Assess the clavicles and sternoclavicular, acromioclavicular, glenohumeral, and scapulothoracic joints. Also assess associated soft tissues, including myofascial structures and their related vascular, lymphatic, and neural elements.

### Vertebral spine
All the vertebrae may be readily assessed with the patient in the supine position. This position is, however, of particular interest for the examination of the upper thoracic and lumbar vertebrae. This is because it allows evaluation of these areas in association with the examination of the pelvis, cervical, and cephalic regions respectively without requiring that the patient moves. When using indirect procedures, continuity in the treatment of sequential areas is beneficial. Much of the time, multiple areas may be treated. Keeping the same patient position eliminates unnecessary proprioceptive input to the CNS as the result of each positional change, which could interfere with the continuity of the treatment sequence. Areas of identified somatic dysfunction can be treated as necessary. See hand positions in 'Section 3: Treatment of the patient,' p. 84.

### Cervical region
Next palpate the cervical spine for function. With aging, almost every patient experiences neck pain.

Frequently, significant somatic dysfunction is found in the upper cervical region and at the craniocervical junction, where a large percentage of the proprioceptors for the cervical spine are located. Sensorimotor disturbances, such as poor balance, may result from high cervical somatic dysfunction. Because of this extremely sophisticated proprioceptive system and the location of the ascending vertebral arteries, palpation and treatment of this area must be exceptionally gentle. Before articulating the cervical spine, these issues necessitate that a complete medical evaluation of the area be carried out. Indirect procedures are by far the treatment of choice in this delicate area.

With great palpatory precision, assess the cervical vertebrae for function. Tests of listening allow an appreciation of motion without the use of force and amplitude that may be too aggressive for the frail patient. Assess the cervical fasciae and the associated visceral structures. Judicious use of range of motion testing may follow as tolerated by the patient.

### Range of motion testing in the supine position

Each of the tests of listening may be further delineated, if necessary, with gentle passive range of motion testing. All hand positions are the same as those used for treatment. See 'Section 3: Treatment of the patient,' p. 84. Active range of motion testing allows evaluation of available motion and may be necessary to completely assess the extent of the patient's limitations. This is also a good way to have the patient appreciate the amount of improvement after a successful treatment and to let them understand the necessity of measures, such as exercise, to continue to improve their condition and to maintain the improvement.

## Observation and palpation of the neurocranium

For the purpose of clarification the neurocranium and the viscerocranium are discussed separately in this presentation. For the practical purposes of examination of the patient, however, this sequence may be modified according to the needs of the individual. For instance, observation of the viscerocranium may follow observation of the neurocranium, before palpation.

Observation and palpation of the neurocranium is easier in the supine position. It may, however, be done in several different positions, such as the seated position, when a patient may be afraid to lie down because of vertigo. Remember that the more a trustful relationship between patient and practitioner is established, the better the treatment outcome will likely be. The practitioner's body language and touch during palpation and treatment is of paramount importance. A message of trust or distrust is transmitted as soon as the first contact with the patient is made. This is particularly important when touching the skull, because the patient must completely relax for best results.

### Observation of the neurocranium

Although the neurocranium consists of eight bones: the occipital bone, two parietal bones, the frontal bone, two temporal bones, the sphenoid, and ethmoid, they are not all directly accessible, either visually, or by palpation.

Start with general observation of the skull. Ideally, the midline of the skull should be aligned with the midline of the trunk. If this is not the case, dysfunction in the cervical or upper thoracic vertebrae may be present. If possible, any such dysfunction should be addressed before treating dysfunction of the skull. If, for some reason these dysfunctions cannot be immediately addressed, be sure that the patient is able to assume the most comfortable position possible when treating the skull. A common mistake before assessing the skull is to align the patient's head with their trunk, without first treating the spinal dysfunctions. If the patient is inappropriately positioned, the motions felt in the head may not be a reflection of the components of the skull, but rather the result of tractions from the dysfunctional vertebral myofascial structures. As an example, when the head of a patient with a right cervical sidebending is 'aligned', the practitioner will first feel a right sidebending when palpating the occiput or the sphenoid. This represents a reflection of the dysfunction of the cervical spine and not necessarily of the motion of the occiput or sphenoid.

Consider the global pattern of the skull. An increase in the width of the skull may be associated with cranial flexion, whereas a decrease is linked with extension. Remember, however, that only palpation for motion can differentiate a dysfunction with restriction of movement from a morphologically wider, or narrower, skull in which motion is unimpaired.

Look at the superficial tissues of the forehead, around the ears, and wherever else the patient's hair pattern allows observation of the neurocranium. Note any asymmetries in the wrinkles, dermatologic disorders, or stasis. Observe the features of the patient, noting any signs of nervousness, such as tics.

Look for visible asymmetries. Because of the patient's hair, it is easier to observe asymmetries of the viscerocranium structures than those of the neurocranium. Be aware of the fact that the viscerocranium does not necessarily reflect the neurocranium.

Observe the temporal fossae for clues as to the position of the greater wings of the sphenoid. A fossa that is higher, lower, deep, or shallow on one side is indicative of the position of the lateral aspect of the greater wing of the sphenoid on that side. With the patient's eyes closed, note the obliquity of the upper lid margins bilaterally. The lines formed by the lid margins usually mirror the position of the ipsilateral wings of the sphenoid. Information gathered by observation must, of course, be further elucidated. Palpate and employ tests of listening to verify observational findings.

The position of the temporal bones may be extrapolated from observing the position of the auricles, because they mirror the temporal bones. Generally, when the ear is flared out, it is associated with ipsilateral temporal bone external rotation and when it is pinned against the side of the head, it is linked with temporal bone internal rotation. This is, however, not always the case and when observed, should be corroborated with additional assessment.

Observe further the relative positions of upper and lower attachments of the auricle. When the upper attachment is located more anteriorly than the inferior attachment, it is consistent with a component of anterior rotation of the temporal bone.

Conversely, with posterior temporal bone rotation, the upper attachment of the ear will be posterior to the inferior attachment. Anterior or posterior rotation of the temporal bone in the sagittal plane is the major component of external and internal rotation respectively.[28] Although the relative outflare of the ear is easily observed, the relative positions of the upper and lower attachments of the auricle are a more reliable indicator.

Sidebending rotation and torsion of the SBS may be assessed with observation. Imagine a line between the two temporal fossae, the location of the superior temporal surfaces of the greater wings of the sphenoid bone. One side is often lower than the other. When this is on the side of temporal external rotation, it is indicative of a possible pattern of sidebending rotation of the SBS on that side. When the low end of the line is on the side of temporal internal rotation, a pattern of ipsilateral torsion may be present. Palpation for function must be done to confirm these observations.

The frontal bone is also observed without difficulty. Look at the forehead. It will be wider, with receding frontal eminences and longer eyebrows, when associated with a pattern of cranial flexion-external rotation, whereas it will be narrower, with prominent frontal eminences and curved, shorter eyebrows, when associated with a pattern of cranial extension-internal rotation. Observation of the viscerocranium will be discussed below.

## Palpation for structure of the neurocranium

Continue the assessment of the neurocranium with palpation for structure of the different parts of the skull that may be appreciated more readily than with simple observation. Assess the quality of soft tissues, skin, subcutaneous tissues, and muscles. Evaluate in particular the muscles that attach upon the occipital squama and the temporal bone. Hypertonicity in these muscles, either a primary or a secondary dysfunction, may contribute to the decreased sensation of the palpated PRM. Palpation of the viscerocranium will be discussed below.

The occiput and sphenoid are classified as midline bones and, as such, are said to demonstrate flexion and extension during the PRM cycle. This may be true, but it is an over simplification. The basiocciput and body of the sphenoid have their embryologic origin in cartilage and do manifest motion as flexion and extension. The squamous portions of these bones, however, are membranous in origin and move to some degree into external rotation and internal rotation in association with flexion and extension. Consequently, in the presence of SBS dysfunctions like torsions, sidebending rotations, and strains, this relationship can result in lateral asymmetries of the squamous portions of the occiput and, to a lesser extent, the sphenoid bone.

Assess the occipital squama, looking for asymmetry. It will feel caudally displaced (lower) on the side that is in cranial flexion-external rotation, and cephalically displaced (higher) in cranial extension-internal rotation. Be aware of occipitocervical dysfunction with possible sidebending of the head that may produce a difference in the position of the occipital squama. Palpation for function will be necessary to confirm the findings.

Palpation of the sphenoid can be done in the temporal fossa in order to assess the lateral-most aspect of the greater wing of the sphenoid, and in the oral cavity in order to palpate the pterygoid processes. With cranial flexion-external rotation, the temporal fossae are full and the pterygoid processes move laterally and upward, while in cranial extension-internal rotation the temporal fossae are deep and the pterygoid processes move medially and downward.

The temporal bones can be palpated at the level of the temporal squama, including the zygomatic process, and also at the mastoid process. On each side, with cranial flexion-external rotation, the temporal squama is full. This normally follows the lateral displacement of the greater wing of the sphenoid. The tip of the mastoid process is posterior, medial, and high with cranial flexion-external rotation. With cranial extension-internal rotation, the temporal squama is flatter, and the tip of the mastoid process is anterior, lateral, and low.

Palpation of the frontal bone gives information that can be analyzed using the same principles as described above in 'observation.' It will feel wider, with receding frontal eminences in cranial flexion-external rotation, and narrower, with prominent frontal eminences in cranial extension-internal rotation.

Finally, palpate the parietal bones, which are sometimes not easy to evaluate visually if the patient has hair. The medial edge of the parietal is flattened in cranial flexion-external rotation, and prominent in extension-internal rotation.

## Palpation for function of the neurocranium

### Vault hold and cradling the skull (Figs. 2.10 & 2.11)

Start the palpation for function with a global assessment of the skull. The 'vault hold' is a standard procedure to accomplish this assessment. With the patient supine, the practitioner, seated at the patient's head, contacts the skull in such a way that the hands gently cradle the lateral parts of the skull. The tips of the index fingers are on the top of the greater wings of the sphenoid; the middle fingers are on the temporal squamae of the temporal bones, anterior to the external auditory meatus; the ring fingers are on the temporal bones, behind the external auditory meatus, on the mastoid portions of the temporal bones; and the little fingers are on the occipital squama. The thumbs are interlocked over the sagittal suture without contacting the suture if possible.

A slightly different hand position has been described in the 1951 Sutherland-approved edition of 'Osteopathy in the Cranial Field': "Index fingers at the frontosphenoidal area or on the lateral surface of the great wings, the middle or proximal phalanges of the middle fingers on the anterior inferior angles of the parietals, the ring fingers on the mastoid angles of the parietals and the little fingers on the occipital squama."[29] This alternative allows for a particularly good appreciation of the PRM and the cranial membranes.

We propose a third position that may seem more ergonomically satisfactory for some practitioners. We named this hold 'cradling the skull.'[30] With the patient supine, the practitioner, seated at the patient's head, places their hands under the occiput in such a way that the distal pads of the index, middle, and ring fingers are in contact with the occiput along and inferior to the superior nuchal line. The lateral aspects of the distal phalanges of the thumbs contact the greater wings of the sphenoid bilaterally.

As soon as you properly apply one of these holds, the patient should immediately feel a sensation of confidence and relaxation. Under these circumstances, you will acquire a good appreciation of the dynamics of the cranium, and the cranial rhythmic impulse (CRI) may be optimally palpated.

### Listening

Place your hands as described above, with either of the vault holds, or cradling the skull, and as

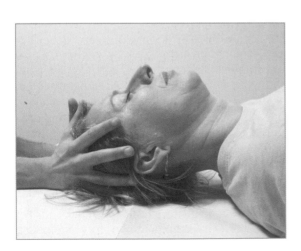

Figure 2.10: Hand placement for vault hold

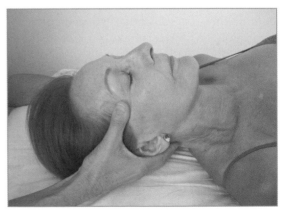

Figure 2.11: Hand placement for cradling the skull

stated by Sutherland, "allowing the physiological function within to manifest its own unerring potency rather than the use of blind force from without."[31]

Note the different sensations that you are feeling. Does the skull feel hard, heavy, compact, tight, restricted, compressed, or do the tissues give you a sense of vitality? Quietly 'listen' and wait for the perception of inherent motion that can be described as the perception of 'tissue breathing.' The PRM may be compared to that of thoracic cage motion during quiet respiration with the sensation of an expansion during the inspiratory phase (cranial flexion-external rotation), and of a contraction during the expiratory phase (cranial extension-internal rotation). Normally, its amplitude is as detectable as the amplitude palpated upon a peripheral arterial pulse, but its frequency is much lower, approximately one tenth that of the pulse, or lower.[32][33][34][35]

Observe the CRI, the palpated sensation of the PRM. Do you feel expansion and contraction? How would you describe this inherent motility? Do you perceive a strong, powerful, vigorous dynamic, or weak, frail, anemic phenomena? Do you feel balance in power and amplitude of the CRI? Do you feel resilience and potency, or irregularities with immobility or agitation? Do you experience stillness during this process of listening?

From this first assessment you get a sense of the status of your patient. We have shown that the palpable CRI is congruous with the low-frequency Traube-Hering oscillations in blood flow velocity.[36] Further, these low-frequency Traube-Hering oscillations are mediated through sympathetic activity.[37][38] With aging, alteration in autonomic function modifies the low frequency recorded in young adults.[39] This may contribute to the difference felt between young and older subjects. Usually, a potent PRM is found in healthy, young individuals, whereas power of the CRI may decrease in older individuals. It should be noted, however, that the potency of the PRM may be maintained at any age when individuals stay healthy, while somatic dysfunction or other health issues will affect it. Assessment of the PRM is a good tool to evaluate the patient, to diagnose any dysfunction, and then to use

its potency in the therapeutic phase, as described in 'Section 3: Treatment of the patient,' p. 77.

Ideally the skull should demonstrate symmetrical unrestricted motility. With your hands still in one of the positions described above, compare the sensations perceived on the right and left sides of the head. In the presence of dysfunction, restriction of motility may affect the complete skull or be limited to one side. Dysfunction may be located in the structures of the skull or in its content. Somatic dysfunction affecting the motion of the skull may be found in the vault, the cranial base, the cervical area, or even somewhere lower in the body. The dysfunction acts as an anchor towards which all tissues seem to be attracted and the restriction of motility is indicative of the location of the dysfunction.

### Cranial and spinal membranes

As stated by Becker, "The greatest and most direct conditioner of stress reactions are membranous articular strains in the craniosacral mechanism that lead to a disturbance of mobility and motility of the cranial articular mechanism, abnormal patterns of mobility of the reciprocal tension membrane, venous retardation, loss of mobility and motility of the pituitary gland within the sella tursica (*sic*), disturbances of the hypothalamic areas, hyper- and hypo-irritability of the central innervation of the sympathetic and parasympathetic nervous systems, and hormonal changes that accompany all of this reaction to strain and stress."[40]

When listening to the skull, focus attention to distinguish between the bony layer of the skull and the membranous layer of the dural membranes. The external layer of the dura mater is contiguous with the inner cranial periosteum, thereby functionally uniting all of the cranial bones. The internal layer of the dura mater folds upon itself to form the falx cerebri, the tentorium cerebelli, the falx cerebelli, and the diaphragma sellae.

These portions also play a significant role in uniting the cranial bones. In the sagittal plane, the falx cerebri links the frontal and ethmoid bones in the anterior portion of the skull with the occiput in the posterior portion of the skull. Transversally, the tentorium cerebelli unites the occiput, the parietomastoid sutures, and the two temporal bones with the clinoid processes of the sphenoid bone. Additionally, the cranial dural membranes contribute to the fluid exchanges between the cerebrospinal fluid and the blood and establish close relationships with the cranial nerves.

Using layer palpation, learn to distinguish the palpatory sensation of the cranial bones compared to the dural membranes. The cranial bones of the older patient normally demonstrate a sensation of density with compliance, whereas the dural membranes exhibit less density with greater compliance. Assess for restriction of mobility and asymmetry of tension of the dural membranes. Listen to the 'Sutherland fulcrum,' at the level of the straight sinus, where the three sickle-shaped folds formed by the two sides of the tentorium cerebelli and the falx cerebelli come together.[41] This area constitutes a suspended area of reciprocal tension between the three folds. Next, evaluate the sense of continuity of the core link: the connection of the spinal dura mater from the occiput at the foramen magnum to the sacrum.[42]

**Sphenobasilar synchondrosis**

Use one of the handhold positions described above, either one of the vault hold positions or cradling the skull. Additional hand placements are described in 'Section 3: Treatment of the patient,' p. 145. When restriction of motility involves the complete skull with global restriction of motility manifesting on both sides of the skull, a SBS dysfunction may be present. When restriction is limited to one side, a unilateral dysfunction, such as occipitomastoid (OM) or sphenosquamous compression may be found. To further localize such a unilateral dysfunction, compare the sensation in the anterior and posterior halves of the skull on the dysfunctional side.

Sphenobasilar synchondrosis dysfunctions are described as: compression; cranial flexion or extension; torsion; sidebending-rotation; and vertical or lateral strains:

- Compression: Usually the result of serious traumas applied to the head, such as a difficult birth or a severe fall on the head. No motility persists at the level of the SBS.
- Cranial flexion dysfunction: When the SBS moves freely into cranial flexion and cannot move into cranial extension. The whole skull may be in a state of cranial flexion-external rotation and the PRM is facilitated in the inspiratory phase. Conversely, a cranial extension dysfunction is found when the SBS moves freely into cranial extension and cannot move into cranial flexion. The whole skull may be in a state of cranial extension-internal rotation and the PRM is facilitated in the expiratory phase.
- Torsion: When the greater wing of the sphenoid moves superiorly on one side and the other inferiorly, while the occipital squama moves inferiorly on the side of the superior greater wing and superiorly on the other side.
- Sidebending-rotation: When the greater wing of the sphenoid and the occipital squama move inferiorly on the same side and separate from one another on that side, while they both move superiorly and toward one another on the opposite side. Most of the time they separate from one another on the lower side; there are, however, infrequent exceptions where they are found to be separated on the higher side.
- Vertical strain: When a vertical shift between the occiput and the sphenoid takes place at the level of the SBS. It follows an upward or downward force, applied either anterior or posterior to the SBS. An inferior vertical strain is present when the posterior articular surface of the sphenoidal body moves inferiorly and the anterior articular surface of the basiocciput moves superiorly. Similarly, a superior vertical strain is present when the posterior sphenoidal body is elevated and the anterior articular surface of the basiocciput is low.
- Lateral strain: When a lateral force is applied anterior or posterior to the SBS causing a shift between the occiput and the sphenoid. A right lateral strain is present when the posterior articular surface of the sphenoidal body is moved to the right and the anterior articular surface of the basiocciput is moved to the left. Likewise, with a left lateral strain, the posterior sphenoidal body is moved to the left, and the anterior articular surface of the basiocciput is moved to the right.

Although some authors report that the SBS begins to ossify at the age of eight,[43] the majority affirm that the SBS does not start fusion until shortly after puberty, and that the process lasts approximately until 25 years of age.[44] [45] [46] [47] [48] In the aging adult, because of the degree of ossification of the SBS, any cranial flexion or extension that is felt is more likely the result of bony compliance than real articulatory motion. Further, the motions palpated are also the product of membranous patterns. These patterns may be established as early as during fetal life, and during their development, consequently palpated cranial bone motions often mirror these early patterns.[49]

A thorough knowledge of anatomy is necessary to visualize aspects of the SBS that cannot be palpated directly. Visualization must be employed in association with listening palpation. When assessing the SBS, the location and orientation of the articular surfaces, as well as surrounding structures must be pictured in the mind's eye of the practitioner. Remember that the contact points of your hands upon the sphenoid and occiput are on portions of the bones that are of membranous origin, while the SBS is part of the less flexible cartilaginous base. Thus, when assessing the movement of the sphenoid's body at the level of the SBS, the first sensation is through the greater wings and what is felt could be the result of the greater wings' flexibility and not necessarily the motion of the sphenoidal body at the level of the SBS. Without precise visualization of the SBS, it is easy to commit the error of palpating the superficial motion and assuming that what is being perceived is the motion of the SBS, even in the presence of SBS compression or complete ossification.

After listening to the SBS, determine the dysfunctional pattern and use indirect principles in conjunction with the inherent forces of the PRM to treat what has been found.

**Cranial base**
After the SBS, assess the remaining articulations of the cranial base, including the articulations of the two temporal bones, with the basilar area of the occiput (the OM and petro-occipital sutures) and the sphenoid (the sphenopetrosal synchondroses). Each of these articulations involves the

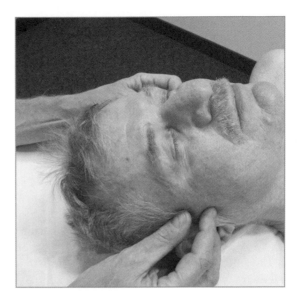

Figure 2.12: Hand placement for global hold of the temporal bones

temporal bone. Thus, start with a global hold of the temporal bone. (Fig. 2.12)

With the patient in a supine position, the practitioner, seated at the head of the table, places their thumbs and index fingers superior and inferior to the zygomatic processes, the middle fingers at the external auditory meatus, the ring fingers on the tip of the mastoid processes, and the little fingers on the superior part of the mastoid portions. Listen to the motion of the temporal bones that should be free in both external and internal rotation. During craniosacral external rotation, the inspiratory phase of the PRM, the palpable motion is as follows:[50]

- The temporal bones demonstrate the major component of their motion in the sagittal plane, as an anterior rotation that is felt at the level of the zygomatic processes, moving inferiorly, and at the level of the tip of the mastoid processes, moving superiorly.
- In the coronal plane, the minor component of motion produces an abduction of the temporal squamae, moving laterally, and an adduction of the tip of the mastoid processes, moving medially.

- In the transverse plane, the minor component of motion is that of the whole temporal bone moving laterally but to a greater degree at the posterior portion than at the anterior portion.

In case of a restriction of motility, visualize the whole temporal bone and picture which part of the bone is restricted. Visualization of the different joints helps to determine the site of dysfunction. If necessary, confirm the palpation with a study of each of the articulations as described in 'Section 3: Treatment of the patient,' p. 148.

Dysfunction involving the OM suture is frequent. It is often the result of the individual falling backward, or of chronic postural dysfunction from excessive tension through the sternocleidomastoid muscle. OM sutures between the occipital squama and the two mastoid parts of the temporal bones demonstrate variable patterns of ossification and individual asymmetries.[51] Ossification occurs between 30 and 70 years of age and typically the suture does not completely ossify.[52] [53]

The complaints most often associated with OM dysfunction are headache, cervical pain, motion restriction, and dizziness, or occasionally vagal dysfunction because of vagus nerve entrapment in the jugular foramen.

Dysfunction involving the petro-occipital sutures is often associated with OM dysfunction. The petro-occipital suture, also named petro-occipital fissure or petro-occipital synchondrosis remains somewhat unossified in the non-pathological state until late in adulthood. The soft tissues of the unfused petro-occipital suture may act to dampen the transmission of postural forces, protecting the content of the temporal petrous portion in so doing, in particular the vestibular apparatus and the cochlear apparatus.[54] With aging, however, the petro-occipital suture goes through distinctive changes in ossification, although this ossification begins much later than in other synchondroses of the cranial base. Usually, a greater degree of ossification occurs in male crania, with individual asymmetries. It is hypothesized that epigenetic factors influence its ossification, such as basic biomechanical factors altering the cellular

environment and gene expression.[55] It is also suggested that the ossification of the suture results in a loss of its dampening effect, a possible factor in age-related conductive hearing loss, upper respiratory dysfunction, and apnea.

Sphenopetrosal synchondrosis dysfunction is frequently associated with other dysfunctions of the cranial base. Ossification of this synchondrosis starts at around 40 years of age, but it never ossifies completely.[56] [57] Because of its close relationship with the pharyngotympanic tube (Eustachian or auditory tube) partially fixed to the external cranial base under it, sphenopetrosal synchondrosis dysfunction may contribute to catarrhal inflammation of the Eustachian tube. Its assessment and treatment is also of particular interest in patients with postural and orofacial dysfunctions.

### Vault

The cranial vault or calvaria is easily accessible and its components are derived from a membranous origin. Palpation of the parietal bones allows for a good appreciation of the sutures of the vault, i.e., the coronal, lambdoid, sagittal, sphenoparietal, and parietomastoid sutures. With both hands on the parietal bones, listen to their motion. If a restriction is sensed, visualize the parietal bones and see in your mind's eye what part is restricted. Visualization of the different sutures helps to determine the site of dysfunction. If necessary, confirm the palpation with a study of each of the articulations as described in 'Section 3: Treatment of the patient,' p. 153.

Palpation of the parietal bones also allows for a good appreciation of intracranial fluids. The venous sinuses have a close relationship with the sutures of the cranial vault, in particular the superior sagittal sinus along the sagittal suture, and the lateral sinuses with the parietomastoid sutures.

Evaluate the relationship between the frontal, sphenoid, and parietal bones. Next, consider the relationship between the frontal bone and the viscerocranium. Frontal dysfunctions are of significance when problem-solving complaints involving the viscerocranium, such as ocular or upper respiratory disorders.

After you have completed your assessment, a possible sequence for the treatment of somatic dysfunction of the neurocranium is to begin by addressing membranous strain patterns. Next, if possible, the SBS may be treated, followed by other dysfunctions of the base and vault.

# Observation and palpation of the viscerocranium
## Observation of the viscerocranium

From the 13 bones that form the viscerocranium or facial skeleton, only eight are easily observed and palpated. They are the two zygomatic bones, the two maxillae, the two nasal bones, and the two lacrimal bones. The two palatine bones can be partially observed and palpated intra-orally where they form the posterior part of the hard palate. The two inferior nasal conchae and the vomer cannot be directly observed or palpated. The mandible will be considered here for functional reasons, although it is not actually part of the viscerocranium, nor is it part of the neurocranium.

Like the cranial base, the face is shaped by genetic factors. Nevertheless, the facial characteristics of the aging individual result also from the influence of strong epigenetic factors, such as the action of the facial musculature and surrounding fasciae. As the individual matures, the facial soft tissues reveal that person's habits of facial expression or usage of other oral functions, such as respiration, mastication, language, and visual functions. Negative emotions and the stresses of life will create a pattern of internal rotation in the soft tissues, whereas positive emotional events and a comfortable environment contribute to produce external rotation. The face allows us to communicate with the world. The status of this communication may be seen in the creases surrounding sensory structures, such as the eyes, mouth, and nose that are interfaces between the outside world and the inner individual. Additionally, some areas of the facial skeleton experience resorption with aging, in particular the midface skeleton.[58]

Observe the overall aspect of the viscerocranium. Note the quality of the skin—look for ruddiness, pallor, dryness, scaliness, eruptions, and excoriations. Spot any asymmetry of the forehead, eyebrows, eyes, nares, cheeks, lips, and jaw line. Study the midline of the face, from the metopic suture and nose to the symphysis menti. These structures should be in straight alignment. Curvature of this alignment, with facial asymmetry, such that one side of the face is relatively smaller on the side of the concavity, is consistent with SBS dysfunction. Angular disruption of the midline is typically consistent with local dysfunction affecting the individual viscerocranial bones.

Look at the zygomatic bones. They form an important link between the viscerocranium and the neurocranium. They also absorb some of the stress applied to the viscerocranium, as occurs during mastication, so that forces are not completely transmitted to the neurocranium. With cranial flexion-external rotation, the anterosuperior, or orbital, border of the zygoma is everted, whereas the posteroinferior or zygomatic border is inverted. With cranial extension-internal rotation, the opposite occurs with the anterosuperior border inverted, and the posteroinferior border everted. Note that the prominence of the cheekbone corresponds to the posteroinferior border. Therefore, a patient who has a prominent cheekbone may have an extension-internal rotation dysfunction of the zygoma on that side.

Observe the bony orbit for size and symmetry. Consider the orbital diameter that connects the superomedial angle of the orbit to the inferolateral angle. Usually, a wider diameter reflects a pattern of cranial flexion-external rotation, whereas a narrower diameter reflects a pattern of cranial extension-internal rotation. Cranial flexion-external rotation is also associated with a decrease of the orbital depth, and hyperopia, while extension-internal rotation is associated with increased orbital depth, and myopia.

Look at the eyes, noting any alteration in size, shape, and position. Observe for symmetry and quality of ocular movement. Note the neutral resting position of each eye and any tendency for deviation from bilateral ocular alignment. Try to see if asymmetry of ocular movement is associated with vertebral or cranial dysfunction. For instance, a patient with occipitoatlantal dysfunction with sidebending left and rotation right may demonstrate a subtle exotropia of the left eye and esotropia on the right eye. Record any nystagmus, and if identified, a thorough neurological examination is indicated for potential neuropathology.

Examine the nose, its size, shape, and position. Observe the alignment of the various portions of the nose—the nasal bones, the nasal lateral cartilages, and the tip of the nose. If asymmetry is noted, identify the dysfunctional portion. Assess the two nares for symmetry of size, shape, and position. Asymmetries are common. They may follow trauma to the nose, with resulting dysfunction often involving: the frontoethmoidal suture; the frontonasal suture; the relationship between the nasal bones and lateral cartilages; and the septal cartilage with associated septal deviation. Note if the patient is breathing through the nose, and equally through both nares, without any difficulty or noise. Ask the patient if one side is chronically obstructed that may be the side of dysfunction. Osteopathic procedures may not change the structural alignment, but they may improve respiratory function.

Check the lower part of the viscerocranium. Look at the maxillae and note any asymmetry. Usually, the upper lip is a good indication of the maxillae, and it mirrors any asymmetry, while the lower lip reflects the mandible. In the male patient, the distribution of facial hair, in particular at the level of the moustache, is a good indication of the position of the maxillae.

Assess the nasolabial sulci for depth and obliquity. Increased depth of the nasolabial sulcus on one side is indicative of external rotation of the ipsilateral maxilla or the zygoma, or both, whereas decreased depth is consistent with internal rotation. Observe the philtrum (the groove above the upper lip) and the philtral ridges. The orientation of both the nasolabial sulci and the philtral ridges reflects the maxillae. The more horizontal these landmarks are the more external rotation is present in the maxilla; the more vertical, the more internal rotation.

Note the alignment of the lips and their relationship to one another. When they are in contact, there should normally be no protrusion of the lips or tension of perioral muscles, which when present may indicate occlusal disorder or nervousness. Ask the patient to clench their teeth and look at the masticatory musculature for asymmetry.

Look for evidence of scars on the chin, which may be the result of a fall with possible associated TMJ joint or occipitocervical dysfunction. Examine the mandible for position and symmetry. Note the alignment of the symphysis menti with the midline of the face above and the suprasternal notch below. Inspect the preauricular area for swelling or erythema, a sign of TMJ dysfunction. The condyles of the mandible articulate in the mandibular fossae of the temporal bones, and when a temporal bone is externally rotated, the mandibular fossa on that side is displaced posteriorly, whereas it is displaced anteriorly during internal rotation of the temporal bone. As a result, the chin will be displaced toward the side of temporal external rotation and away from the side of internal rotation. Thus, when the midline of the chin deviates to the side of the flared ear, a temporal dysfunction in external rotation may be suspected. On the other hand, when the chin deviates toward the side of the pinned ear, a TMJ joint dysfunction may be present.

Ask the patient to slowly open their mouth while observing for displacement of the symphysis menti. Note any distorted pattern, a sign of TMJ dysfunction, with usually a deviation of the mandible toward the affected side. Have the patient move their mandible laterally to the right and left and evaluate the ease of movement and amplitude of displacement bilaterally. Observe and note the presence of a dominant side to the masticatory pattern.

Have the patient open their mouth. Observe their teeth and note any dental malalignment, crowding, crowns, and bridges. Look for the presence of dental imprints on the lateral portions of the tongue, a sign of lingual malposition, or dysfunctional occlusion, or both. Have the patient clench their teeth and observe the occlusal pattern. Normally, the midline between the upper and lower incisors should be aligned. Additionally, the upper incisors should slightly override the lower incisors and the upper molars should rest on the lower molars. See 'Stomatognathic system,' in 'Section 4: Clinical considerations, Chapter 2: Postural imbalance,' p. 235.

## Palpation for structure of the viscerocranium

Palpation for structure substantiates the findings of visual observation. Start with palpation of the zygomatic bones. They are almost completely palpable. Look for asymmetry. On each side palpate the anterosuperior and posteroinferior borders, to determine difference between cranial flexion-external rotation and extension-internal rotation as described in the paragraph above: 'Observation of the viscerocranium.'

Palpate the nasal bones to differentiate between external rotation, where the posterior border of the nasal bone seems displaced laterally, and internal rotation, where it seems displaced medially. In the same way palpate the frontal processes, the body, and the alveolar processes of the maxillae to look for asymmetry. Palpation of the palate may be done intraorally. On the side of external rotation, the maxilla will appear to be wider, and the palate lower and flattened, while with internal rotation, the maxilla appears narrow, and the palate high and arched.

On each side of the face, palpate the condyles of the mandible. Ask the patient to slowly open and close their mouth to facilitate this process. Note any asymmetry in size and position of the condyles, any subcutaneous tissue texture abnormality and tenderness, and the extent of mandibular condylar movement. Normally, the TMJ is quiet during the opening of the mouth. Crepitus (clicking or popping sounds) are indicative of a dysfunction. Assess the degree of mandibular opening by measuring the distance between the incisal edges of the upper and lower anterior teeth. In the adult patient, an opening of less than 35 mm is considered abnormal.

Examine the masticatory musculature. On each side, the masseter can be palpated at their attachments to the zygomatic arch and angle of the mandible. The temporalis muscles are found externally in the temporal fossae. They can also be palpated intraorally along the anterior aspect of the ramus of the mandible. The medial pterygoid is felt intraorally in the lingual vestibule in the retromolar region and the lateral pterygoid palpation, although difficult, is possible intraorally posterior to the maxillary tuberosity.[59]

Discuss masticatory patterns with the patient. Explain the necessity to masticate on both sides as much as possible.

## Palpation for function of the viscerocranium

Although the frontal and sphenoid bones are parts of the neurocranium, remember that they have an important influence on the ocular and respiratory functions of the viscerocranium. Dysfunction of these bones must be addressed as much as possible before treating the viscerocranium.

Employ tests of listening to confirm observational findings. Listen to the components of the orbit, and to the ocular globe. Listen to the components of the nose, often in dysfunction, with complaints such as rhinitis and sinusitis. Check the TMJs with tests of listening and if somatic dysfunction is identified, treat it using indirect principles. Osteopathic treatment may be employed to address pain, function, and structure. See hand placement in 'Section 3: Treatment of the patient,' p. 84.

# References

1. Willard A. The application of the principles of osteopathy. Year Book of the Academy of Applied Osteopathy. American Academy of Osteopathy. Indianapolis, IN. 1940:3–13.
2. Glossary of Osteopathic Terminology. In: Chila AG. ed. Foundations of Osteopathic Medicine. 3rd ed. Philadelphia: Wolters Kluwer/Lippincott Williams and Wilkins; 2011:1106.
3. Simpson GG. Biology and the nature of science. Science. 1963 Jan 11;139(3550):81–8.
4. Nelson K, Mnabhi A, Glonek T. The Accuracy of Diagnostic Palpation: The Comparison of Soft Tissue Findings with Random Blood Sugar in Diabetic Patients. Osteopathic Family Physician Nov-Dec 2010 2(6):165–9.
5. Tarr R, Nelson K, Vatt R, Richardson D. Palpatory findings associated with the diabetic state. J Am Osteopath Assoc. 1985:604–5.
6. Nelson K, Sergueef N, Lipinski C, Chapman A, Glonek T. The cranial rhythmic impulse related to the Traube-Hering-Mayer oscillation: Comparing laser-Doppler flowmetry and palpation. J Am Osteopath Assoc. March; 2001:163–73.
7. Woods JM, Woods RH. A physical finding relating to psychiatric disorders. J Am Osteopath Assoc. 1961 Aug;60:988–93.
8. Glonek T, Sergueef N, Nelson K. Physiological Rhythms/ Oscillations. Chapt. 11. In: Chila AG. ed. Foundations of Osteopathic Medicine. Wolters Kluwer/Lippincott Williams and Wilkins; 2011:162–90.

9. Sergueef N, Greer MA, Nelson KE, Glonek T. The palpated cranial rhythmic impulse (CRI): Its normative rate and examiner experience. International Journal of Osteopathic Medicine. 2011;14:10–16.

10. Nelson KE, Rottmen J. The female patient, Chapt. 9. in: Somatic Dysfunction in Osteopathic Family Medicine. Nelson KE, Glonek T, eds. Baltimore, MD: Lippincott, Williams & Wilkins; 2007:111.

11. Nelson KE. Viscerosomatic and somatovisceral reflexes Chapt. 5, in: Somatic Dysfunction in Osteopathic Family Medicine. Nelson KE, Glonek T, eds. Baltimore, MD: Lippincott, Williams & Wilkins; 2007:37–45.

12. Nelson KE. The patient with an upper respiratory infection. Chapt. 16. in: Somatic Dysfunction in Osteopathic Family Medicine. Nelson KE, Glonek T, eds. Baltimore, MD: Lippincott, Williams & Wilkins; 2007:222.

13. Nelson KE. Viscerosomatic and somatovisceral reflexes Chapt. 5, in: Somatic Dysfunction in Osteopathic Family Medicine. Nelson KE, Glonek T, eds. Baltimore, MD: Lippincott, Williams & Wilkins; 2007:44.

14. Sergueef N. L'odyssée de l'iliaque. Paris: Spek; 1985.

15. Sergueef N. L'Odyssée de l'iliaque. Paris: Spek; 1985.

16. Sergueef N. Cranial Osteopathy for Infants, Children and Adolescents. Edinburg, UK. Churchill Livingstone, Elsevier; 2007.

17. Sergueef N. Normaliser la colonne sans 'manipulation vertébrale'. Paris: Spek; 1994.

18. Strachan WF, Beckwith CG, Larson NJ, Grant JH. A study of the mechanics of the sacroiliac joint. J Am Osteopath Assoc. 1938;37(2): 575–8.

19. Glossary of Osteopathic Terminology. In: Chila AG. ed. Foundations of Osteopathic Medicine. 3rd ed. Philadelphia: Wolters Kluwer/Lippincott Williams and Wilkins; 2011:1092.

20. Vincent-Smith B, Gibbons P. Inter-examiner and intra-examiner reliability of the standing flexion test. Man Ther. 1999 May;4(2):87–93.

21. Nelson KE, Mnabhi A. The patient with back pain: Short leg syndrome and postural balance, Chapt. 26. In: Nelson, Glonek, eds., Somatic Dysfunction in Osteopathic Family Medicine. Baltimore, MD: Lippincott, Williams & Wilkins; 2007:408–33.

22. Knutson GA. Anatomic and functional leg-length inequality: a review and recommendation for clinical decision-making. Part I, anatomic leg-length inequality: prevalence, magnitude, effects and clinical significance. Chiropr Osteopat. 2005 Jul 20:13:11.

23. Glossary of Osteopathic Terminology. In: Chila AG. ed. Foundations of Osteopathic Medicine. 3rd ed. Philadelphia: Wolters Kluwer/Lippincott Williams and Wilkins; 2011:1092.

24. Northup T. L. Manipulative treatment of mucous colitis. Year Book of the Academy of Applied Osteopathy. American Academy of Osteopathy. Indianapolis, IN. 1940;3:110.

25. Washington K, Mosiello R, Venditto M, Simelaro J, Coughlin P, Crow WT, Nicholas A. Presence of Chapman reflex points in hospitalized patients with pneumonia. J Am Osteopath Assoc. 2003 Oct;103(10):479–83.

26. Glossary of Osteopathic Terminology. In: Chila AG. ed. Foundations of Osteopathic Medicine. 3rd ed. Philadelphia: Wolters Kluwer/Lippincott Williams and Wilkins; 2011:1090.

27. Vital JM, Grenier F, Dautheribes M, Baspeyre H, Lavignolle B, Senegas J. An anatomic and dynamic study of the greater occipital nerve (n. of Arnold). Applications to the treatment of Arnold's neuralgia. Surg Radiol Anat 1989;11(3):205–10.

28. Sergueef N. Le B.A.BA du crânien. Paris, France: Spek; 1986.

29. Magoun HI. Osteopathy in the cranial field. Kirksville, MO: The Journal Printing Company; 1951:97.

30. Sergueef N. Cranial Osteopathy for Infants, Children and Adolescents. Edinburg, UK. Churchill Livingstone, Elsevier; 2007.

31. Sutherland WG. The cranial bowl. Mankato, MN: Free Press Company; 1939. Reprinted : Indianapolis, IN: American Academy of Osteopathy; 1986:8.

32. Nelson K, Sergueef N, Lipinski C, Chapman A, Glonek T. The cranial rhythmic impulse related to the Traube-Hering-Mayer oscillation: Comparing laser-Doppler flowmetry and palpation. J Am Osteopath Assoc. March 2001:163–73.

33. Nelson KE, Sergueef N, Glonek T. Recording the Rate of the Cranial Rhythmic Impulse. J Am Osteopath Assoc. 2006; 106(6):337–41.

34. Glonek T, Sergueef N, Nelson KE. Physiological Rhythms/Oscillations. Chapt. 11. In: Foundations for Osteopathic Medicine. Chila AG. ed. 3rd ed. Philadelphia: Wolters Kluwer/Lippincott Williams and Wilkins; 2011:162–190.

35. Sergueef N, Greer MA, Nelson KE, Glonek T. The palpated cranial rhythmic impulse (CRI): Its normative rate and examiner experience Int J Osteopathic Med. 2011; 14(1):10–16. Online publication: 31-DEC-2010.

36. Nelson KE, Sergueef N, Lipinski CL, Chapman A, Glonek T. The cranial rhythmic impulse related to the Traube-Hering-Mayer oscillation: comparing laser-Doppler flowmetry and palpation. J Am Osteopath Assoc 2001;101:163–73.

37. Akselrod S, Gordon D, Madwed JB, Snidman NC, Shannon DC, Cohen RJ. Hemodynamic regulation: investigation by spectral analysis. Am J Physiol Heart Circ Physiol 1985;249:H867–75.

38. Saul PJ, Rea RF, Eckberg DL, Berger RD, Cohen RJ. Heart rate and muscle sympathetic nerve variability during reflex changes of autonomic activity. Am J Physiol 1990; 258:H713–21.

39. Jarisch WR, Ferguson JJ, Shannon RP, Wei JY, Goldberger AL. Age-related disappearance of Mayer-like heart rate waves. Experientia. 1987 Dec 1;43(11–12):1207–9.

40. Becker RE. Diagnostic touch: its principles and application. Part IV. Trauma and stress. Year Book of the Academy of Applied Osteopathy. American Academy of Osteopathy. Indianapolis, IN. 1965;2:174.

41. Sutherland WG. Teachings in the science of Osteopathy. Fort Worth, TX: Sutherland Cranial Teaching Foundation, Inc.; 1991:45.

42. Glossary of Osteopathic Terminology. In: Chila AG. editor. Foundations of Osteopathic Medicine. 3nd edition. Philadelphia: Wolters

Kluwer/Lippincott Williams and Wilkins; 2011:1090.

43. Madeline LA, Elster AD. Suture closure in the human chondrocranium: CT assessment. Radiology. 1995 Sep;196(3):747–56.

44. Irwin GL. Roentgen determination of the time of closure of the spheno-occipital synchondrosis. Radiology, 1960; 75:450–453.

45. Mann SS, Naidich TP, Towbin RB, Doundoulakis SH. Imaging of postnatal maturation of the skull base. Neuroimaging Clin N Am 2000 Feb;10(1):1–21,vii.

46. Melsen B. Time of closure of the spheno-occipital synchondrosis determined on dry skulls. A radiographic craniometric study. Acta Odontol Scand 1969;27(1): 73–90.

47. Okamoto K, Ito J, Tokiguchi S, Furusawa T. High-resolution CT findings in the development of spheno-occipital synchondrosis. Am J Neuroradiol. 1996;17(1):117–20.

48. Williams PL, editor. Gray's anatomy. 38th ed. Edinburgh: Churchill Livingstone; 1995.

49. Sergueef N. Cranial Osteopathy for Infants, Children and Adolescents. Edinburgh: Churchill Livingstone Elsevier; 2007.

50. Sergueef N. Le B.A.BA du crânien. Paris, France: Spek; 1986.

51. Mann SS, Naidich TP, Towbin RB, Doundoulakis SH. Imaging of postnatal maturation of the skull base. Neuroimaging Clin N Am 2000 Feb; 10(1):1–21,vii.

52. Todd TW, Lyon DW. Endocranial suture closure. Its progress and age relationship. Part I. Adult males and white stock. Am J Phys Anthropol 1924;7:325–84.

53. Todd TW, Lyon DW. Cranial suture closure. Its progress and age relationship. Part II. Ectocranial closure in adult males of white stock. Am J Phys Anthropol 1925;8: 23–45.

54. Balboni AL, Estenson TL, Reidenberg JS, Bergemann AD, Laitman JT. Assessing age-related ossification of the petro-occipital fissure: laying the foundation for understanding the clinicopathologies of the cranial base. Anat Rec A Discov Mol Cell Evol Biol 2005;282: 38– 48.

55. Balboni AL, Estenson TL, Reidenberg JS, Bergemann AD, Laitman JT. Assessing age-related ossification of the petro-occipital fissure: laying the foundation for understanding the clinicopathologies of the cranial base. Anat Rec A Discov Mol Cell Evol Biol 2005;282:38– 48.

56. Todd TW, Lyon DW. Endocranial suture closure. Its progress and age relationship. Part I. Adult males and white stock. Am J Phys Anthropol 1924;7:325–84.

57. Magoun HI. Osteopathy in the cranial field. 2nd ed. The Journal Printing Company: Kirksville, MO; 1966:147.

58. Mendelson B, Wong CH. Changes in the Facial Skeleton With Aging: Implications and Clinical Applications in Facial Rejuvenation. Aesthetic Plast Surg. 2012; May 12.

59. Barriere P, Lutz JC, Zamanian A, Wilk A, Rhiem S, Veillon F, Kahn JL. MRI evidence of lateral pterygoïd muscle palpation. Int J Oral Maxillofac Surg. 2009 Oct;38(10):1094–5.

# SECTION 3

# Treatment of the patient

*To find health should be the object of the doctor. Anyone can find disease.*

—A. T. Still[1]

*There is a very great art in the application of the science of osteopathy. No one has ever attained perfection in it. There is no other art or skill similar to it. We all begin at zero and we learn only by practice. We may be taught how to proceed but everyone must acquire his own skill.*

—H. H. Fryette[2]

## Osteopathic treatment

Osteopathy, throughout the world, exists through a diverse group of healthcare practitioners. This community of osteopaths (Diplomat of Osteopathy, or Doctor of Osteopathic Medicine) shares the fundamental philosophy of osteopathy, and the recognition of the contribution of function, and dysfunction, of the structure of the body upon the establishment and maintenance of the health of their patients.

Originally, Still proposed that his philosophy and principles of healthcare be taught at Baker University in Baldwin City, Kansas, instead of the medical curriculum for a MD degree, similar to the practice, at the time, for the granting of medical degrees in homeopathy. When his offer was rejected, he elected to establish his own school and coined the name 'osteopathy' for the course of study. This evolved into the integrative form of medical practice, osteopathic medicine, as practiced in the United States and elsewhere. As the awareness of osteopathic philosophy and principles spread throughout the world, because of the resistance demonstrated by mainstream medicine, many practitioners have chosen to limit the scope of osteopathic practice to that originally proposed by Still.

A strong argument can be made for keeping the purity of the original nineteenth-century osteopathic concept. An equally strong argument can be made in support of integrating the advances of twenty-first-century medicine into osteopathic practice. However one chooses to approach this issue, advances of modern medicine must be recognized. If modern infectious disease practices had been available in 1864, when Still lost three of his children to spinal meningitis, it is entirely possible that he may not have lost his faith in his medical training, and osteopathy might never have been born. Whether one chooses to follow the practice of pure osteopathy, or the practice of integrative osteopathic medicine, it must be accepted that complete modern healthcare necessitates that, if the practice of osteopathic medicine is not chosen, the practitioner of osteopathy must be fully aware of the limitations of their area of practice, and know how to work as a member of an inclusive twenty-first-century healthcare team.

The philosophy of osteopathy is firmly grounded upon the concept of the triune body, mind, and spirit, the nature of humanity.[3] This concept, as embraced by Still and later by Sutherland, was thoroughly developed in the eighteenth century by Emanuel Swedenborg, a Swedish scientist and theologian.[4] It recognizes the reciprocal influence of the body and spirit upon one another, and the importance of the mind as the bridge between the two. Thus the therapeutic approach of osteopathy employs the body as a source of physical, as well as emotional and spiritual healing, health promotion, and maintenance, and at the same time recognizes the impact that mental and spiritual influences have upon the body.

The osteopathic philosophy, in the context of the corporeal component of the triune nature of humanity, may be summarized by the following four principles:[5]

1. *The human being is a dynamic unit of function.* As such, the level of efficiency of function of any area of the body will impact all other body areas through membranous, myofascial, bony articular, neurological, and vascular interactions, and through the primary respiratory mechanism (PRM).
2. *The body possesses self-regulatory mechanisms that are self-healing in nature.* Its function is directed toward homeostasis, the maintenance of physiological balance as a result of the dynamic state of equilibrium between interdependent body functions and consequently optimal health status.
3. *Structure and function are interrelated at all levels.* Structure determines function and is, in turn, influenced by function and dysfunction.
4. *Rational treatment is based upon these principles.* Optimal structure and structural interrelationships result in optimal function. Somatic dysfunction, the impediment of normal function, will, over time, result in abnormal structure. The modification of structure becomes progressively greater as the individual ages. The body's self-healing capacity can be impaired by the inability to compensate for age, illness, and somatic dysfunction. The progression of time (aging) is permanent, while illness may be treated to a greater or lesser extent by standard medical means and somatic dysfunction addressed by osteopathic manipulative treatment (OMT). The alleviation of somatic dysfunction in any anatomic area affects the entire body. The objective of distinctive osteopathic practice is, therefore, to diagnose and treat somatic dysfunction at the various levels of fluid, membranous, myofascial, ligamentous, intra-, and interosseous dysfunction, thereby enhancing the whole-body capacity for repair and maintenance of health. The treatment of somatic dysfunction, through the body's self-healing capacity, will act to maintain health, and in the presence of disease, enhance the body's self-healing capacity and consequently the effectiveness of standard medical treatment.

## Determining the application of osteopathic manipulative treatment

Treatment is specifically determined by the diagnosis of the condition to be treated. Osteopathic manipulative treatment is employed to treat one thing only: somatic dysfunction. As in any other area in healthcare, before a specific treatment intervention can be applied, a specific diagnosis must be made. (See 'Section 2: Osteopathic assessment,' p. 39.)

The diagnosis of somatic dysfunction is based upon the identification of palpably *abnormal soft tissue texture* (T). It is defined by *positional asymmetry* of anatomic structure (A), and *restriction of motion* (R), within the normal limits of physiologic motion of the anatomy being examined. *Tenderness to palpation* (T), an involuntary response on the part of the patient, is the final component that is in actuality linked closely to tissue texture abnormality. The resultant mnemonic TART describes the criteria, the presence of any one of which is sufficient, for the diagnosis of somatic dysfunction. Whatever the dysfunctional pattern, positional asymmetry and restriction of motion is of primary importance when deciding how to apply the most appropriate OMT intervention.

Once the pattern exhibited by the anatomic area of dysfunction has been identified, it is appropriate to decide what is maintaining it. Determining if it is articular, muscular, or fascial will assist in the selection of a manipulative procedure that will be the most effective.

When diagnosing with the test of listening (see 'Section 2: Osteopathic assessment,' p. 41.) the tensegral balance of inherent forces within the tissues is evaluated. Through discerning touch, the practitioner establishes an awareness of forces that have been, and are currently being, applied to the tissues, as well as the state of fascial, ligamentous, and articular relationships. Through their touch, the practitioner feels also the biodynamic intrinsic force within the tissue manifesting its own unerring potency. Becker defined this appreciation of biodynamic potency as: "...a functioning point of stillness, a fulcrum point, within the bioenergy field in body physiology over, around, and through which these patterns of activity are manifesting themselves."[6]

The absence of a clearly identifiable dysfunctional pattern in the presence of tissue texture abnormality and tenderness to palpation should lead one to consider a reflexly-mediated, viscerosomatic or somatosomatic, etiology. Under these circumstances the source of the reflex should be sought out and specifically treated, as appropriate, using accepted medical treatments. Osteopathic manipulative treatment may be integrated into the complete treatment protocol, but failure to diagnose the underlying pathology is medical malpractice.

An additional criterion for an OMT procedural selection is the level of tolerance of the individual patient. Young, healthy adults are physiologically most tolerant to OMT. As an individual ages, their tolerance for manipulative procedures decreases. The existence of concomitant medical illness further decreases patient tolerance. The presence of acute or chronic inflammatory states is particularly tolerance limiting. If an otherwise healthy-appearing patient reacts with unexpected intensity to what should have been appropriately selected OMT, the presence of an undiagnosed illness, particularly, but not limited to, collagen vascular disease, should be actively sought out.

## Osteopathic forms of treatment

Over the years a plethora of types of OMT have been described. These are fundamentally based upon traditional manual therapies, some of which, tui na for example, go back in time for thousands of years. In fact, all variations of OMT are based upon two fundamental classes of treatment procedures: direct and indirect techniques and these two forms of OMT have one very important aspect that they share. They are predicated upon the precise diagnosis of somatic dysfunction in the context of physical motion and the restriction of that motion within its normal range. (See 'Section 2: Osteopathic assessment,' p. 39.) The restriction of motion is described as being the result of a dysfunctional, or restrictive, barrier. Osteopathic manipulative treatment is, for the most part, focused upon the re-establishment of normal function by the elimination of the dysfunctional, or restrictive, barrier. Manipulative procedures that move against the barrier (said to be engaging the barrier) are referred to as *direct* procedures. Those procedures that position the patient away from the barrier are *indirect* procedures. Additionally, *combined* procedures sequentially employ both indirect and direct treatment methods. This is most typically done by starting with the patient in the indirect position, allowing a release of dysfunctional tension to occur, and then moving in the direction of the restrictive barrier, often taking the dysfunctional area through a full range of motion.

OMT procedures are further delineated by identifying the final corrective force employed. In the case of indirect procedures this is often force that is inherent within the tensegral structure of the body that may be further augmented by employing practitioner-induced compressive, distractive, or vibratory forces and, or, the dynamic presence of the PRM. (See 'Section 1: Osteopathy, fascia, fluid, and the primary respiratory mechanism,' p. 18.) Direct procedures take into consideration the origin of the final corrective force that is applied against the barrier, be it a patient applied force, as occurs in muscle energy procedures, or physician applied. The method of application of the final corrective force may then be further subdivided according to the velocity with which the force is applied and the amplitude of the resultant induced motion directed against the barrier.

Finally, the various OMT categories may be considered in the relative context of how aggressive they are. The more aggressive a procedure type, the more rapidly the limit of patient tolerance may be reached. For the purposes of discussion, a continuum listing the types of OMT from the most to least aggressive can be developed. This is certainly not absolute, but it can serve as an aide in the selection of OMT for any given patient. As stated, this is a very arbitrary listing, in that indirect procedures can occasionally be quite aggressive and, an additional aspect, the duration of time required accomplishing the desired therapeutic effect, also impacts patient tolerance and consequently OMT dosage.

In general, the longer it takes to apply a given intervention, the greater its dosage. It could therefore be argued that five to ten minutes of indirect myofascial release could expose a patient to a greater dose of OMT, and consequently be more aggressive, than a single precisely applied high velocity, low amplitude (HVLA) procedure lasting only a few seconds. Certainly an accomplished osteopathic practitioner should possess the skills to intelligently employ the entire procedural spectrum. "One must not be a blacksmith only, and only able to hit large bones and muscles with a heavy hammer, but one must be able to use the most delicate instruments of the silversmith in adjusting the deranged, displaced bones, nerves, muscles and remove all obstructions, and thereby set the machinery of life moving. To do this is to be an osteopath."[7]

## Osteopathic manipulative treatment categories from most to least aggressive

Essentially, all of the procedural categories listed below require that the dysfunctional barrier be specifically defined and precisely addressed. Some of them, like inhibitory pressure, are employed to treat acute, reflex-mediated myofascial tissue texture change; the 'barrier' associated with increased soft tissue tension must still be appreciated. Additionally, although many of the procedures listed, for example: range of motion; articulation; soft tissue; direct and indirect myofascial release; and cranial osteopathic procedures should be specifically applied, they may also be employed for the general effect they have upon the patient.

*Direct procedures*, wherein the restrictive barrier is engaged and an exogenous, or in the case of muscle energy, patient-generated, final corrective force is employed, are among the more aggressive forms of OMT.

1. *High velocity, low amplitude*, also known as thrust or impulse technique, employs a rapid, practitioner-generated, therapeutic force of brief duration (high velocity) applied over a very short distance (low amplitude) within the anatomic range of motion of a joint.

2. *Articulation* applies a low velocity, moderate to high amplitude practitioner-generated force against the restrictive barrier such that a joint is carried through its full motion.

3. *Springing* applies low velocity, moderate amplitude practitioner-generated forces through which the restrictive barrier is repeatedly engaged to increase freedom of motion. It is a form of articulation.

4. *Positional technique* applies a combination of practitioner-generated leverage and patient-generated respiratory movement, using a fulcrum to localize forces against the dysfunctional barrier to achieve mobilization. This process may be incorporated into springing or thrust procedures.

5. *Range of motion* (ROM), similar to articulation, applies active (patient-generated) or passive (practitioner-generated) movement of a body part to its physiologic or anatomic limit in any or all planes of motion.

6. *Traction* applies continuous or intermittent, high or low amplitude, practitioner- (or device-) generated force to stretch or separate dysfunctional tissues along a longitudinal axis.

7. *Soft tissue* (ST), also called myofascial treatment, usually involves any combination of lateral stretching, linear stretching, deep pressure, traction, or separation of muscle origin and insertion and associated myofascial elements, while monitoring tissue response and motion changes by palpation.

8. *Facilitated oscillatory release technique* (FOR) is the application of a manual oscillatory force that is employed to augment the final corrective force of any other articulatory, ligamentous or myofascial procedure. As such, it may be used with direct, indirect, and combined procedures.

9. *Muscle energy* (ME) applies a patient-generated force as the patient, upon request, actively contracts their muscles from a

precisely controlled position in a specific direction, against an accurately executed, practitioner-generated counterforce. This procedural category is somewhat arbitrarily placed at this point in the aggressiveness continuum, because the final corrective force is patient-generated, thereby providing the patient with control over the intensity of the intervention.

10. *Myotension* applies a patient-generated force of alternating muscle contraction and relaxations against a distinctly executed practitioner-generated counterforce to relax, strengthen, or stretch muscles, or mobilize joints.

11. *Progressive inhibition of neuromuscular structures* (PINS) applies inhibitory pressure sequentially along a series of points between two related tender points. Because this consists of the methodical application of a series of inhibitory pressure procedures, it may be considered to be more aggressive than inhibitory pressure applied to a single point.

12. *Inhibitory pressure* is an extremely low velocity, essentially no amplitude technique form wherein very slowly increasing pressure is applied to and held to reduce reflex activity and produce relaxation in soft tissues with acute, often reflex-mediated, tissue texture change. This may be employed to treat the somatic component of acute viscerosomatic, and somatosomatic reflexes, while providing a somatovisceral influence.

13. *Direct myofascial release* (MFR) is a category of procedures wherein the dysfunctional myofascial barrier is engaged and the tissues are loaded with a constant force, similar to that of inhibitory pressure, until tissue release occurs.

*Combined procedures* consist of the sequential application of indirect and direct principles. The initial positioning is typically indirect, away from the dysfunctional barrier. After a therapeutic release is obtained, direct forces are applied in the direction of the previously identified dysfunctional barrier.

14. *Facilitated positional release* (FPR) is a form of myofascial release wherein the dysfunctional region of the body is placed into a neutral position, reducing tissue and articular tensions in all planes, and an activating force of compression, distraction, or torsion is applied to facilitate the therapeutic release.

15. *Still technique* is a specific, non-repetitive articulatory method that is initially indirect, and is followed by taking the dysfunctional area through a direct range of motion. Attributed to Andrew Taylor Still.

16. *Percussion vibrator technique* is a manipulative technique involving the specific application of mechanical vibratory force to treat somatic dysfunction. This osteopathic manipulative technique was developed by Robert Fulford, DO.

17. *Integrated neuromusculoskeletal release* (INR) is a form of myofascial release that is intended to stretch and reflexly release patterned soft tissue and articular restrictions in which both direct and indirect forces are applied in combination.

*Indirect procedures*, wherein the restrictive barrier is disengaged and the dysfunctional body part is moved away from the restrictive barrier, for the most part constitute the gentlest, and when time required for application is not taken into consideration, least aggressive, low dosage forms of OMT. The patient may be positioned such that forces accumulate in the direction away from the dysfunctional barrier or until tissue tension is equal in one or all planes and directions.

18. *Counterstrain* (CS) (originally *spontaneous release by positioning*, later termed *Strain-Counterstrain®*) is potentially more aggressive than other forms of indirect procedures because the final corrective force is an applied, indirect counterstrain. That is, the dysfunctional tissues are loaded in the direction opposite that of the original strain that resulted in dysfunction. As originally described Jones,[8] the patient is precisely positioned, and that position is held for 90 seconds in order to obtain a release. Counterstrain is placed here because it employs indirect positioning. When time of procedural application is taken into account, combined procedures like facilitated positional release may be less aggressive because they typically require significantly less time to accomplish.

19. *Functional technique*, guided by the tensegrital sensations of ease and bind within the dysfunctional area, is when the tissues are taken in the direction of ease to a neutral position, resulting in reduction of tissue tension in all planes, and the area is held in position or sequentially moved, tracking the sensation of decreasing tissue resistance. Compression to exaggerate the position may be added and held until a total release of tissue tension occurs.

20. *Fascial unwinding* is an extensive form of fascial release (see below), involving constant feedback from myofascial tensions within the patient's body that allows the practitioner, using the sensations of ease and bind, to move the patient's body, or a portion thereof through a series of sequential releases. This is placed above fascial release in the continuum because it consists of a series of releases one after another.

21. *Fascial release* or *myofascial release* (MFR) is guided by the tensegrital sensations of ease and bind. Within the dysfunctional area the tissues are taken in the direction of ease to a neutral position, resulting in reduction of tissue tension in all planes. The area is then held in the position of functional balance until a release occurs and freedom of movement is achieved.

22. *Osteopathy in the cranial field* (OCF)*, or cranial treatment (CR), is a method of treatment that employs forces that are inherent within the tensegrital structure of the body, particularly the dural reciprocal tension membrane, and augments those forces using the inherent rhythmicity of the PRM to induce functional balance and enhance the power of the PRM.

23. *Balanced ligamentous tension* (BLT)* or *ligamentous articular strain technique* (LAS), is a form of articular manipulation that employs the principles of cranial osteopathy, using the tensegrital structure of the body and the inherent rhythmicity of the PRM, to induce functional balance and enhance the power of the PRM.

24. *Visceral manipulation* (VIS)* or *ventral technique*, is a form of treatment intended to improve physiological function of the viscera.

Following tensegrital sensations of ease and bind within, the viscus to be treated is taken, often toward the fascial attachments of the organ being treated, to a point of fascial balance. Inherent visceral rhythmicity, closely related to, if not the PRM itself, may be employed to establish freedom of visceral motion, and consequently function.

*Although listed separately the above manipulative procedural descriptions are quite certainly addressing the same thing: the holistic anatomy and physiology of the human body. As such, they have far more in common than any differences that separate them. It is the author's opinion that the greatest difference between all of the above variations of OMT, aside from the anatomy of the dysfunctional areas being specifically addressed, is whether the treatment procedure follows direct or indirect principles. Procedures as apparently different as HVLA and cranial osteopathy actually are all directed at the same endpoint: the alleviation of somatic dysfunction and the optimization of human physiology; the inherent ability of the body for self healing. Consequently all of these procedural types have a place in the complete osteopathic armamentarium.

The consideration of the diagnosis of the mechanical pattern of the dysfunction, the anatomic component (articular, muscular, fascial, and membranous), or the physiological component (neuroreflex and inherent rhythm) responsible for the dysfunction, and the patient's tolerance may then be employed, allowing the practitioner to identify the most appropriate choice of OMT procedure for the individual patient.

## Response to treatment

Having diagnosed the dysfunction to be treated and decided upon the most appropriate procedure to employ therapeutically it is now appropriate to determine the amount of OMT (dosage) to apply. How much OMT is enough? A very simple rule of thumb is to treat the patient until a response occurs. What kind of response should one look for? Relaxation of the soft tissues in the area being treated is a good response, often referred to as a release. Increased muscular tension during the application of OMT is an indication that the patient's tolerance has already been exceeded. At this point treatment should be stopped and reattempted later, after the patient has rested. At that time a less aggressive procedure should be selected. Alteration in autonomic tone is also indicative of a response. The establishment of a still point followed by increased amplitude of the PRM is favorable. Cutaneous vasodilatation (redness and increased skin temperature) or increased perspiration indicates that it is time to stop. Increased heart or respiratory rate also indicates that one has reached the patient's level of tolerance. If the patient expresses the feeling that the intervention is too uncomfortable, the practitioner should stop and choose a less aggressive approach, or wait and try again at a later time.

As mentioned earlier, the patient's overall health status exerts a significant effect upon their tolerance to whatever procedure is applied. The sicker the individual is, the lower one can expect their tolerance to be. As such, smaller doses of less aggressive OMT will provide optimal therapeutic response without exceeding the patient's level of tolerance. When uncertain as to how much a particularly ill individual will safely tolerate, it is always best to err on the side of caution. One can always slowly increase the dosage of OMT with each successive treatment, but once a patient has been overdosed one must wait for them to recuperate and valuable time is lost.

How often should the individual be treated? This question is not an easy one to answer. Certainly if the patient has an excellent response to the first treatment, if the somatic dysfunction being treated completely resolves and the patient's PRM demonstrates strong amplitude post-intervention, one treatment may well be sufficient. If, however, one is treating a particularly severe problem, or if the condition is a chronic one, multiple interventions may be necessary. This having been said, there should be no reason to treat a patient more than three to five times before releasing them to return for any future treatment on their own, as necessary.

Patients with chronic established conditions may require maintenance treatment, but under these circumstances they should be shown what to expect from effective treatment and then given the opportunity to determine their own maintenance

schedule. Such a schedule should rarely include revisits more frequent than once a month, unless addressing an acute exacerbation of the chronic condition. In the event of such an exacerbation, the three to five treatment schedule described above should apply.

The appropriate follow-up treatment schedule and subsequent OMT dosage may be determined by observing the patient's response to the initial treatment. After the patient has been effectively treated the first time, they may need to be seen for a second visit re-evaluation and further treatment. If appropriate, this is best done in 48–72 hours. The patient response sequence after a successful intervention often proceeds as follows:

- Immediately post-treatment the patient should experience symptomatic relief. This period of relief may be transient, lasting a few hours, or it may be permanent. Failure of the patient to experience this initial period of relief is indicative that the initial diagnosis was incorrect, or that the treatment applied was ineffective. This creates a therapeutic dilemma, in that further treatment, at this time, significantly increases the probability of exceeding the limits of patient tolerance. Under these circumstances, the diagnosis should be thoroughly reconsidered and, if still deemed correct, only the least aggressive forms of OMT should be employed. At the end of this first visit the patient should be cautioned to refrain from overactivity until they are re-evaluated, because, human nature is such that when the individual feels relief they assume that they are completely recovered, and this is all too often not the case.
- Following the period of symptomatic relief the patient may experience a rebound reaction with an exacerbation of their original symptoms. They should be cautioned about this possibility, to avoid unnecessary concern. The rebound reaction should last no more than 24 hours, but 48 hours is acceptable for aged individuals who demonstrate a slower physiological response. If the patient experiences the initial period of relief but the rebound reaction is protracted beyond the acceptable 24-48 hours it is probable that the diagnosis was correct, but that the

treatment was too aggressive, resulting in an excessive reaction. As such the aggressiveness of the second OMT intervention should be appropriately reduced. As mentioned above, if an otherwise healthy-appearing patient reacts with an unexpectedly intense rebound reaction to what should have been appropriately selected OMT, the presence of an undiagnosed illness, particularly, but not limited to, collagen vascular disease, should be actively sought out.

- The rebound reaction is followed by a period of functional recovery and symptom relief that can last from days to indefinitely. It is during this period of functional recovery that it is appropriate to see the patient for follow-up to reassess them for residual dysfunction.
- The second visit is consequently appropriately scheduled in 48 hours (72 hours for elderly slow reactors) following the initial treatment so that the patient may be reassessed during the period of functional recovery and symptom relief, but before they have had opportunity to reinjure themselves. It is at this time that the best idea of the impact of the initial treatment upon the patient's dysfunction may be appreciated.
- Following the second, and any subsequent revisits, if residual somatic dysfunction is still present, revisits should be scheduled by approximately doubling the length of time between them. If the treatment regimen is effective, the patient should continue to demonstrate functional recovery and remain symptom-free as the duration between treatments is increased. At any point during this treatment sequence, if it is felt that the problem has been resolved, the patient should be released to return on an 'as necessary' schedule. If, however, during this time, the patient shows the appropriate response sequence but fails to remain symptom free for the progressively increasing interval between treatments, it is indicative that contributing circumstances are present that should be sought out and addressed. These can be: viscerosomatic and somatosomatic reflexes; dysfunctional accommodation to asymmetrical postural mechanics; overuse syndromes; and somatoemotional issues.

## The treatment of trauma patients

Osteopathic manipulative treatment is used specifically to treat somatic dysfunction, and in most instances it is intended to increase available motion. It is, therefore, inappropriate to manipulate structurally unstable areas of the musculoskeletal system. Bearing this caution in mind, the practitioner should recognize that physical trauma patients can still benefit greatly from correctly applied OMT.

Recognizing that trauma frequently results in torn soft tissue and fractures, extreme caution must be taken not to apply force through such areas. Having recognized this, areas adjacent to traumatized unstable tissues often demonstrate somatic dysfunction. Appropriate treatment of these areas results in decreased patient discomfort and augmentation of healing because of decreased tensegrital stress and increased tissue perfusion in the traumatized area.

Nevertheless, because physical trauma results from exogenous force, initially it is very difficult to estimate the patient's tolerance. A simple approach to this dilemma is to determine, as above, the patient's estimated level of tolerance and then to apply about one-half of that dose. Subsequent treatments then may be adjusted as outlined above. It is particularly under these circumstances that the use of indirect procedures (counterstrain, facilitated positional release, myofascial release, and osteopathy in the cranial field) can produce impressive results. Furthermore, the diagnostic palpatory skill required to employ these indirect procedures is particularly useful when initially diagnosing acute trauma that presents without immediately apparent tissue disruption.

# Procedures

The individuals who employ the procedures described below should be trained, qualified health-care providers and must recognize that when any intervention is applied to another human being, it is not without risk. The practitioner is urged to realise that the procedures described below, when employed to treat patients with concomitant organic pathology, must be used in an adjunctive or integrative fashion. Underlying systemic dysfunctions and diseases must first be diagnosed and treated, with appropriate recognized medical management. The possibility of somatic dysfunction as the result of viscerosomatic reflexes must always be borne in mind.

Although, as above in this chapter, a continuum of OMT procedural categories from most to least aggressive has been described, it cannot be stressed enough that the selection of the lowest dose of the least aggressive procedure that will effectively get the job done is always the best choice. It is, at all times, better to underdose than to have to deal with the results of over-treatment. Because this text addresses the care of aged and often fragile individuals, the discussion of treatment procedures that follows focuses upon indirect procedures that lie firmly at the least aggressive end of the treatment continuum. As Anne L. Wales observed: "The fact that the active force, operating in these procedures upon the area of stress, comes from within the body minimizes the risk of trauma."[9]

With the above in mind, one must recognize that, particularly when treating aged patients, chronic and, often reticent, somatic dysfunction is frequently encountered. An effective method for augmenting the power of indirect OMT procedures is the addition of pumping. This consists of following the freedom of the major and minor movements of the dysfunctional area in association with the movement of the PRM. The movement of the PRM within the dysfunctional pattern may be enhanced to gently encourage the area being treated in the direction of the restriction. This is not, in the purist sense, a direct procedure because, although working in the direction of the restriction, the dysfunctional barrier of the dysfunction is, in itself, never engaged. The pumping process is introduced from the position of ease and employs the rhythm and potency of the PRM to remove the dysfunctional restriction. The operator continues this pumping action up to the point of

release. This procedure is very effective when the minor movements and PRM are employed specifically along with the more easily discernible major movements.

When treating the patient the practitioner must not only make the correct diagnosis and apply the most appropriate intervention; they must do so in such a manner that avoids pain, creates an environment of trust and instills confidence. In this sense it is important to remain constantly sensitive to cues from the patient, to remember the importance of body language and the messages transmitted from the time the patient is first touched through to the conclusion of the treatment. These actions demonstrate to the patient that the practitioner is mastering the problem which, in turn, allows the patient to respond more effectively to the treatment by avoiding the sympathetic response of fight, flight, or freeze.

Because of the complexity of the dysfunctional pattern present, the older patient may, at first, appear to the novice practitioner, to be an overwhelming treatment challenge. All too often the beginner feels that they must treat everything. They have a tendency to focus upon structures that should be symmetrically balanced.

The goal of treatment is, however, to enhance the patient's level of function, and not necessarily to bring back symmetry, particularly if the patient is over 50 years of age. Ideally the treatment should focus upon what is thought to be the most important place to treat: the biodynamic center of the dysfunction: the area or focal point that is responsible for the greatest amount of compensation.

Tests of listening allow one to define the primary dysfunctional areas, versus areas of compensation. When listening to the biodynamic center of the dysfunction, the restriction of motion is felt to be greatest, demonstrating a pattern wherein motion is present in one direction only. This is the direction of dysfunction. When listening to areas of compensation, the motion pattern felt is diminished in quantity and quality in one direction as compared to normal, but motion is still present to some extent in all of its aspects.

# Lower extremity procedures

## Foot global myofascial procedure

### Indications

Pes planus; plantar fasciitis; hallux valgus; toe deformities.

### Procedure

(Example: globally balancing the myofascial components of the left foot. (Fig. 3.1))

**Patient supine.**
Practitioner seated at the foot of the patient on the side of the dysfunction.

With your right hand, hold the distal foot between your thumb and fingers while cradling the left heel with your left hand. While paying attention to the PRM, allow the myofascial structures of the foot to move into the position of ease. Most often this will involve a torsional pattern with the distal foot moving into internal rotation. Identify the position of equally diminished tension in all directions within the dysfunctional pattern, while allowing the motion of the PRM to remain unencumbered. Balance the foot in this position and await a release. For acute dysfunctions this should prove sufficient. For chronic conditions it can

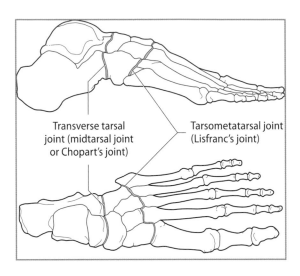

Figure 3.2: The transverse tarsal and tarsometatarsal joints

Transverse tarsal joint (midtarsal joint or Chopart's joint)

Tarsometatarsal joint (Lisfranc's joint)

prove beneficial to very gently encourage the PRM in its more prominent phase.

### Remarks

With the same hand positions, it may be possible to focus more specifically, as necessary, either at the level of the transverse tarsal joint (midtarsal joint or Chopart's joint) or the tarsometatarsal joint (Lisfranc's joint). (Fig. 3.2)

By focusing on the medial plantar surface of the foot, the myofascial dysfunctions contributing to plantar fasciitis may be addressed.

## Achilles tendonitis

### Indications

**Achilles tendinitis.**

### Procedure

(Example: left Achilles tendinitis. (Fig. 3.3))
Patient prone, lying upon the table in such a way that the left foot extends beyond the foot of the table.

Practitioner seated beside the table, to the patient's left, facing the leg.

With your right hand, hold the calcaneus in such a way that your index finger and thumb hold

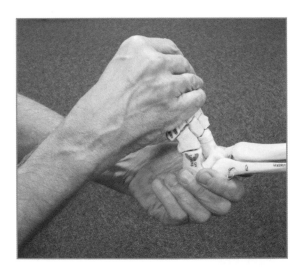

Figure 3.1: Hand placement for global myofascial procedure of the left foot

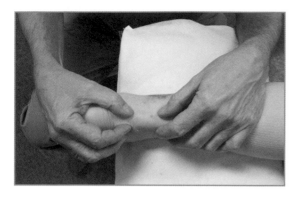

Figure 3.3: Hand placement for diagnosis and treatment of left Achilles tendinitis

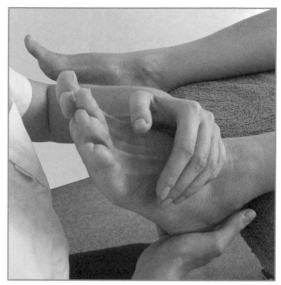

Figure 3.4: Hand placement for diagnosis and treatment of left subtalar dysfunction

the Achilles tendon on either side, at the level of its insertion. Your left hand rests upon the distal calf in such a way that your left index finger and thumb hold the tendon on either side, at approximately the level of the musculotendinous junction. Listen to motion in the fibers of the Achilles tendon between your two hands. Sensing the motion pattern demonstrated by the tendon, follow it until a point of myofascial and ligamentous balance is obtained. At this point any dysfunctional pattern should begin to release. Maintaining the position of balance, and while following the PRM, await a complete release.

### Remarks

At any point during this procedure, you may become aware of a focal point of tension somewhere within the Achilles tendon. At this time, it is appropriated, while maintaining the finger-thumb hold upon the tendon, to move your hands so that the tendon is held immediately proximal and distal to the focal point of tension.

This procedure will be more effective if concomitant calcaneal dysfunction and global postural mechanics are also addressed.

## Subtalar procedure

### Indications

Ankle sprain with motion restriction affecting the subtalar joint with decreased dorsiflexion.

### Procedure
(Example: left subtalar dysfunction. (Fig. 3.4))

**Patient supine.**
Practitioner seated at the foot of the treatment table, on the side of the dysfunction.

With your right hand, cradle the calcaneus of the patient's left foot, and with your left hand, hold the medial aspect of the foot in such a manner that the radial aspect of your hand contacts the dorsum of the patient's foot over the neck of the talus. Listening to the talocalcaneal relationship, follow the tissues in the direction of unrestricted motion (inversion/eversion). Freedom of calcaneal inversion and plantar flexion is most often (but not always) encountered. Follow in the direction of unrestricted motion until a point of myofascial and ligamentous balance is obtained. Hold in this position, while maintaining synchronicity with the PRM, and await release.

## Cuboid procedures

### Indications

Cuboid dysfunction relative to the calcaneus or the navicular bone and occasionally involving the

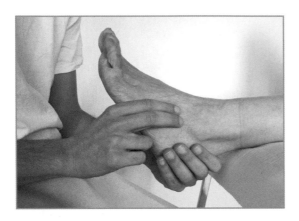

Figure 3.5: Hand placement for diagnosis and treatment of left cuboid dysfunction

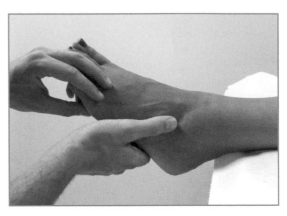

Figure 3.6: Alternative hand placement for diagnosis and treatment of left cuboid dysfunction

third cuneiform or the fourth and fifth metatarsal bones. Often referred to as 'dropped,' because the cuboid is found in internal rotation and the lateral longitudinal arch is decreased.

### Procedure

(Example: left cuboid dysfunction. (Fig. 3.5))

**Patient supine.**
Practitioner seated at the foot of the treatment table, on the side of the dysfunction.

With your right hand, hold the lateral aspect of the patient's left foot in such a manner that your thumb contacts the proximal and medial aspects of the plantar surface of the cuboid, and your middle finger (or index finger) contacts the dorsum of the cuboid in the same proximal and medial location. With your left hand, cradle the left calcaneus. With your hands thus positioned, listen to the cuboid and follow its motion in the direction of freedom until a point of balance is obtained. Hold in this position of myofascial and ligamentous balance, and while maintaining synchronicity with the PRM, await release.

### Alternative procedure

(Example: left cuboid dysfunction. (Fig. 3.6))

With the patient and practitioner in the same position as described above, with your right hand, hold the lateral aspect of the patient's left foot in such a manner that your thumb contacts the dorsum

of the proximal and medial aspects of the cuboid, and your index finger contacts the plantar surface of the cuboid in the same proximal and medial location. Then, hold the distal fourth and fifth left metatarsal heads between your index and middle fingers (dorsum) and the thumb (plantar). With your hands so positioned, listen to the motion between the cuboid and metatarsals, find the point of optimal balance, and await a release.

## Navicular procedure

### Indications

Navicular dysfunction relative to the talus or the three cuneiforms. Also referred to as 'dropped,' because the navicular is found in internal rotation. This dysfunction is associated with pes planus affecting the medial longitudinal arch of the foot.

### Procedure

(Example: left navicular dysfunction. (Fig. 3.7))

Patient supine with their right hip and knee flexed so that they can position their left foot beyond the end of the treatment table.

Practitioner is seated at the foot of the table, to the patient's right, facing the medial aspect of the patient's left foot.

With the thumb and index finger of your left hand, hold the dorsum of the patient's left foot over the neck of the talus. With your right hand,

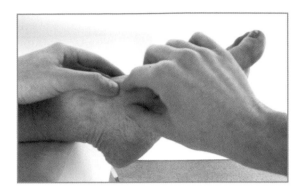

Figure 3.7: Hand placement for diagnosis and treatment of left navicular dysfunction

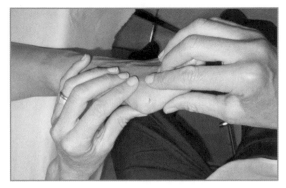

Figure 3.8: Hand placement for diagnosis and treatment of left hallux valgus

hold the navicular bone in such a way that your thumb contacts the plantar surface and your index finger the dorsal surface. Follow in the direction of unrestricted talonavicular motion until a point of myofascial and ligamentous balance is obtained. Hold in this position, and while maintaining synchronicity with the PRM, await release.

Note: While still using a left-sided dysfunction as an example, the above procedure may be modified to treat dysfunction between the navicular and cuneiforms by holding the navicular bone between the thumb and index finger of your left hand and the cuneiforms with the thumb and index finger of your right hand.

## Hallux valgus procedure

### Indications

Treatment of the myofascial and ligamentous tensions that lead to the development and maintenance of hallux valgus deformity.

### Procedure

(Example: left hallux valgus. (Fig. 3.8))

Patient supine with their right hip and knee flexed so that they can position their left foot beyond the end of the treatment table.

Practitioner seated at the foot of the table, to the patient's right, facing the medial aspect of the patient's left foot.

With the thumb and index finger of your left hand, hold the distal aspect of the patient's first

metatarsal in such a manner that your thumb contacts the plantar surface and your index finger the dorsal surface. With the thumb and index finger of your right hand, hold the metatarsal phalangeal end of the patient's first proximal phalange. Follow metatarsal phalangeal motion in the direction of freedom, most often with the toe in internal rotation, abduction, and plantar flexion, until a point of myofascial and ligamentous balance is obtained. Hold this position, and while maintaining synchronicity with the PRM, await release.

### Remarks

This procedure augments the body's self healing mechanism, but in itself will not immediately reverse the bony changes seen in hallux deformity. To maximize the efficacy of this procedure, talo-navicular-tarsal dysfunctional relationships and global postural mechanics that shift weight-bearing in the foot into an extension-internal rotation pattern must also be addressed.

The principles of this procedure may be applied to all of the metatarsal, phalangeal, and inter-phalangeal joints of all of the toes, including conditions like hammer toes.

## Tibiofibular procedures

### Indications

Proximal or distal tibiofibular dysfunction, or both, often presenting as knee or ankle complaints and potentially affecting the foot's mechanics. Achilles tendonitis. Leg cramps.

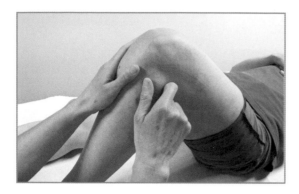

Figure 3.9: Hand placement for diagnosis and treatment of left proximal tibiofibular dysfunction

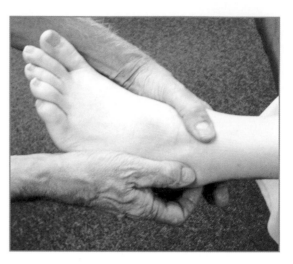

Figure 3.10: Hand placement for diagnosis and treatment of left distal tibiofibular dysfunction

### Proximal tibiofibular procedure

(Example: left proximal tibiofibular dysfunction. (Fig. 3.9))

Patient supine with their left hip and knee flexed sufficiently so that the left foot rests flat upon the table top.

Practitioner seated on the treatment table, on the left side, at the level of or just distal to, the patient's foot, facing toward the patient's head.

With your right hand, hold the left proximal fibula in such a manner that your thumb contacts the anterior aspect and your index finger the posterior aspect of the fibular head. Your left hand holds the anteromedial aspect of the tibia in such a manner that your thumb contacts the lateral aspect of the proximal tibia just anterior to the proximal tibiofibular joint, with your fingers contacting the anteromedial aspect of the tibia. Follow in the direction of unrestricted fibular motion (anteroinferior/posterosuperior glide) until a point of myofascial and ligamentous balance is obtained, and while maintaining synchronicity with the PRM, await release.

### Distal tibiofibular procedure

(Example: left distal tibiofibular dysfunction. (Fig. 3.10))

Patient supine with their right hip and knee flexed so that they can position their left foot beyond the end of the treatment table.

Practitioner seated or standing at the foot of the table.

Hold the left lateral malleolus with your right hand in such a manner that your thumb contacts the anterior aspect and your index finger the posterior aspect. Your left hand then holds the medial aspect of the tibia in such a manner that your thumb contacts the anterior tibial surface and your fingers the posterior surface. Follow in the direction of unrestricted fibular motion (predominantly anterior/posterior motion) until a point of myofascial and ligamentous balance is obtained and await release.

### Combined proximal/distal tibiofibular procedure

(Example: combined proximal/distal left tibiofibular dysfunction. (Fig. 3.11))

**Patient supine.**
Practitioner seated on the left side of the table, facing the patient at the level of the calf.

With your right hand, hold the left proximal fibula so that your thumb contacts the anterior aspect and your index finger the posterior aspect of the fibular head. Next, your left hand holds the left lateral malleolus such that your thumb contacts the anterior aspect and your index finger the posterior aspect. Follow in the direction of unrestricted fibular motion until a

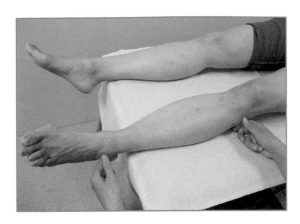

Figure 3.11: Hand placement for diagnosis and treatment of combined proximal/distal left tibiofibular procedure

point of myofascial and ligamentous balance is obtained. Maintain synchronicity with the PRM and await a release.

## Remarks

When treating tibiofibular dysfunction, the process of visualization of the dysfunctional tensions within the interosseous membrane enhances diagnostic understanding. Incorporating this information into the treatment procedure, when searching for balance of tension, will often facilitate the release of otherwise resistant dysfunctions.

In cases of physiologic dysfunction, the motions of the proximal and distal tibiofibular joints are coupled in opposite directions (anterior proximal/posterior distal or posterior proximal/anterior distal), thus resulting in a scissor-like action between the tibia and the fibula. In traumatic non-physiologic dysfunction, tibiofibular mechanics are determined by the direction of the exogenous forces that were responsible for the trauma. Most commonly encountered under these circumstances is a superior subluxation of both the proximal and distal tibiofibular joints.

In each of the procedures above, for chronic cases, the release of the dysfunction may be facilitated by a pumping action. Following the rhythm of the PRM augments this process.

## Knee procedures

### Indications

Knee dysfunctions, sprains, strains, pain, and functional complaints like clicking and popping within the joint.

Note: Because of the complexity of the internal anatomy of the knee, when addressing knee complaints, ligamentous instability and internal structural disruption must be thoroughly ruled out or, if diagnosed, appropriate treatment initiated before the treatment of somatic dysfunction is started. Manipulative treatment without effective stabilization is inappropriate for patients with structural instability. This having been said, once appropriate treatment of orthopedic conditions has been initiated, the integrative treatment of concomitant somatic dysfunction, applied while avoiding stress to unstable anatomy, can enhance the patient's recuperative capacity. It is under these circumstances that the gentlest of indirect functional procedures are appropriate.

It must also be recognized that knee pain is often a symptom that is the result of distal tibiofibular or pelvic somatic dysfunction, and it should be treated accordingly. Proximal tibiofibular pain as a result of compensatory stress induced by distal tibiofibular dysfunction can be misinterpreted as knee pain, while internal rotation (posterior) dysfunction of the innominate results in anterior knee pain, with anteromedial pain associated with sartorius tension and anterolateral pain with tensor fascia lata

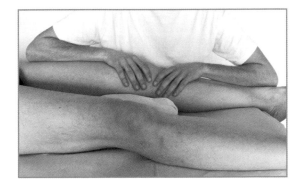

Figure 3.12: Hand placement for diagnosis and treatment of left knee dysfunction

tension. Posterior knee (popliteal) pain is found in association with external rotation (anterior) dysfunction of the innominate through increased hamstring tension.

If the patient presents with a unilateral knee complaint, a local, tibiofibular, knee or pelvic etiology should be sought out. If the complaint is bilateral, a more global postural etiology, an extension pattern (sacral, spinal, or sphenobasilar) with genu valgus, or a flexion pattern with genu varum, is more likely.

### Procedure

(Example: left knee dysfunction. (Fig. 3.12))

Patient supine with a small pillow under the left knee to introduce slight flexion.

Practitioner seated beside the treatment table, on the left side of the patient, at the level of the knee.

With your right hand, hold the anterior surface of the distal thigh such that your fingers contact the medial femoral epicondyle, with your index finger palpating the tibiofemoral joint line. Your thumb should be positioned inferior to the lateral femoral epicondyle to palpate the lateral joint line. Your left hand holds the anterior surface of the proximal tibia over the tibial tuberosity, with your thumb and index finger respectively palpating the lateral and medial joint lines. Listen to the motions between the tibia and femur (flexion/extension, external/internal rotation, abduction/adduction, medial/lateral glide, anterior/posterior glide, and compression/distraction). For each of the above coupled motions, follow them in the direction of unrestricted motion, stacking them, until the final position of ligamentous and myofascial balance is obtained. At this point, while maintaining the position of balance, listen to and follow the PRM. Wait for a release.

### Remarks

With the supine patient position described above, patellar myofascial dysfunction may be addressed by moving your hands so that they surround the patella.

### Alternative procedure

(Example: left knee dysfunction. (Fig. 3.13))

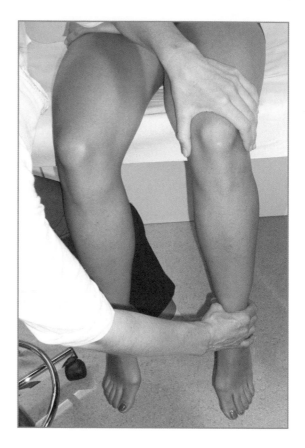

Figure 3.13: Alternative hand placement for diagnosis and treatment of left knee dysfunction

Patient comfortably seated, on the side of the treatment table.

Practitioner seated in front of the patient, to the side opposite the dysfunction.

Your left hand should hold the medial and lateral epicondyles of the femur such that your index finger palpates the lateral tibiofemoral joint line and your thumb the medial joint line. With your right hand, hold the distal tibia. Listen to and visualize, as above, the pattern of motion present. Employ indirect principles and follow the pattern into the position of ligamentous and myofascial balance. Employ the pumping action of the PRM to facilitate a release.

### Remarks

Performing this procedure with the knee in varying degrees of flexion will allow you to position the knee in a manner that most closely approximates the position in which the dysfunction has occurred.

In the hand placement described above (see 'Figure 3.13: Alternative hand placement for diagnosis and treatment of left knee dysfunction'), slightly moving your right hand distally will allow you to treat not only the knee but also, with experience, the ankle, as well as tibiofibular and myofascial dysfunction of the leg.

## Popliteal release

### Indications

Compromise of venous and lymphatic return due to dysfunctional myofascial tension of the popliteal space.

### Procedure

(Example: right popliteal space dysfunction. (Fig. 3.14))

Patient supine with right hip and knee flexed and right foot flat upon the treatment table.

Practitioner standing, facing the patient's head, on the side of the dysfunction, at the level of the patient's foot.

Hold the medial aspect of the patient's popliteal space (semimembranosus, semitendinosus, and medial head of gastrocnemius tendons) with the pads of the fingers of your right hand, and the lateral aspect (biceps femoris and lateral head of gastrocnemius tendons) in a similar fashion with your left hand. Your thumbs rest

anteriorly upon the medial and lateral aspects of the proximal tibia.

Employing indirect principles, assess tension in the soft tissues of the medial and lateral popliteal space. Follow the tissues into the position of ligamentous and myofascial balance. Employing pumping action of the PRM will facilitate a release.

### Remarks

Prior to the application of any central venous and lymphatic procedures to address peripheral congestion, local myofascial obstruction of venous and lymphatic drainage should be addressed.

## Hamstring release

### Indications

Lumbopelvic dysfunctions; limited hip flexion and posterior thigh pain; knee dysfunction.

### Procedure

(Example: dysfunctional left hamstring tension. (Fig. 3.15))

Patient supine with left hip and knee flexed. Practitioner standing, facing the patient's head, on the side of the dysfunction, at the level of the patient's knee.

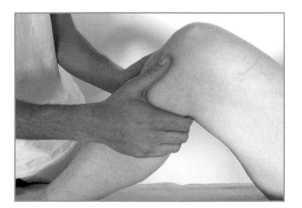

Figure 3.14: Hand placement for popliteal release

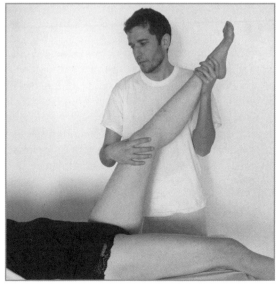

Figure 3.15: Hamstring release

With your left hand, hold the posterior aspect of the ankle. Your right hand rests upon the anterior knee. The patient is instructed to slowly extend their left knee, while you monitor the ease of motion. At the first sense of resistance to extension, using indirect principles, assess the ease of external/internal rotation and abduction/adduction of the hip and knee. Follow the pattern of hip and knee ease of tension into the position of ligamentous and myofascial balance. From this position, employ the pumping action of the PRM to facilitate a release.

### Remarks

If release does not readily occur, it is useful to observe patient pulmonary respiratory motion to identify the phase (inspiratory or expiratory) in which further ease of tension occurs. During normal respiration, ask the patient to breathe more slowly, prolonging the respiratory phase that provides the greatest ease of tension.

## Hip joint procedure

### Indications

Hip pain, dysfunction, and arthritis, psoas dysfunction, piriformis dysfunction and associated knee and lumbopelvic pain and dysfunction.

### Procedure

(Example: left hip dysfunction. (Fig. 3.16))

Patient supine with their left hip and knee flexed.

Practitioner standing beside the treatment table on the side of the dysfunctional hip, at the level of the pelvis.

With your right hand, contact the left pelvic bone in such a way that your thumb rests upon the anterosuperior iliac spine (ASIS) with your index finger extended, pointing posteriorly, along the iliac crest. Your left hand holds the patient's anterior thigh in such a way as to hold the knee against the anterior aspect of your left shoulder. Hip flexion should be gently increased, or decreased, to obtain a position of opti-

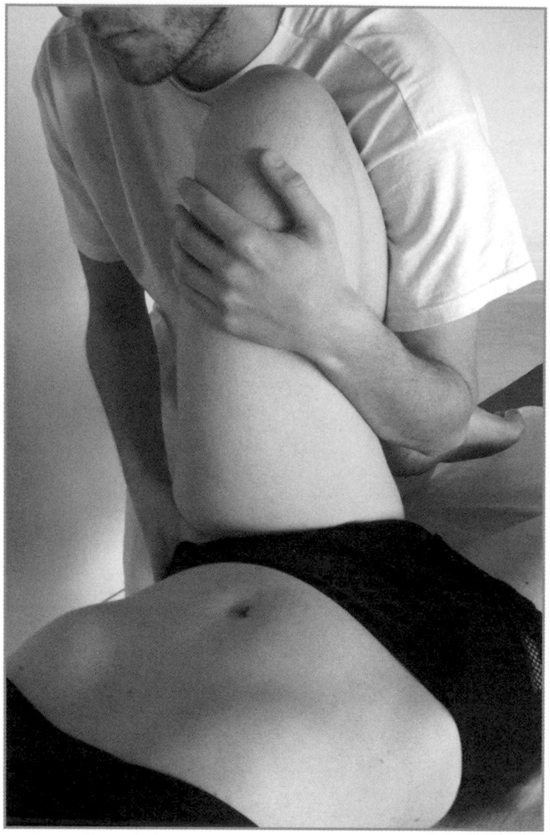

Figure 3.16: Hand placement for diagnosis and treatment of left hip dysfunction

mal functional balance. From this position, listen to the motions at the hip (flexion/extension, abduction/adduction, external/internal rotation, and the minor motions of medial/lateral glide, cephalocaudal glide, and compression/distraction). Because the hip is not being directly palpated, it is particularly useful to visualize the relationship between the femoral head and the acetabulum during this process. Follow each of the coupled motions in the direction of unrestricted motion, stacking them until the final position of ligamentous and myofascial balance is obtained. At this point, while maintaining the position of balance, listen to and follow the PRM, and wait for a release.

## Pelvic procedures

Because dysfunctions in the pelvic and lumbosacral areas can be the result of pelvic splanchnic viscerosomatic reflexes, they should prompt the practitioner to seriously look for, and rule out, underlying visceral pathology. See further: 'Vertebral somatic dysfunction' in 'Section 4: Clinical considerations, Chapter 1: Musculoskeletal dysfunctions, Part 1: Axial system,' p. 183.

## Global pelvic balancing

### Indications

Pelvic somatic dysfunction; pelvic visceral dysfunctions, including constipation and urinary tract complaints; pelvic floor dysfunctions; knee dysfunction; functional leg length inequity.

### Procedure (Fig. 3.17)

Patient supine with their hips flexed or extended according to comfort.

Practitioner standing on either side of the table, at the level of the pelvis.

Place your hands bilaterally upon the patient's pelvis in such a way that your thumbs or thenar eminences contact the ASISs, with your index fingers extended posteriorly curling laterally around the iliac crests. Listen to the position and inherent motion of the pelvic bones, feeling for internal or external rotation in the context of the major and minor motions. Follow the motion pattern in the direction of ease until a point of myofascial and ligamentous balance is obtained. Maintaining synchronicity with the PRM, await a release.

### Alternative procedure (Fig. 3.18)

Patient supine with their legs straight.

Practitioner standing on either side of the table, caudal to the level of the pelvis.

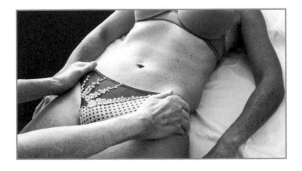

Figure 3.17: Hand placement for global pelvic balancing

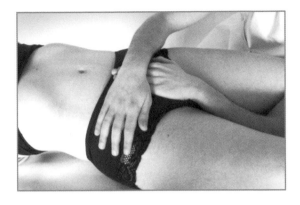

Figure 3.18: Alternative hand placement for global pelvic balancing

Place your caudal hand palm down upon the lower abdomen, with your fingers extended cephalically. The proximal-most aspect of the palm should rest just inferior to the pubic symphysis. Your cephalic forearm and hand should rest transversally across the lower abdomen, in such a manner to contact the ASISs bilaterally. Listen to the position and inherent motion of the pelvic bones and visualize the pelvic bowl and floor. Look for pelvic anteversion, where the pelvis is tilted forward, and retroversion, tilted backwards. Both of these misalignments affect the load on the pelvic floor. See further discussion of pelvic bones in 'Section 4: Clinical considerations, Chapter 6: Urogenital dysfunctions,' p. 324. With your cephalic forearm and hand, listen to the position and inherent motion of the pelvic bones, feeling for internal or external rotation. Follow the motion pattern in the direction of ease until a point of myofascial and ligamentous balance is obtained. Maintain synchronicity with the PRM and await a release.

### Remarks

The objective of treatment is to have both sides of the pelvis moving freely, with external and internal rotation in synchrony with the PRM. Pelvic dysfunctions often demonstrate asymmetric motion patterns with a more significant degree of motion restriction on one side. The release of the side of greater restriction may be augmented through the use of a pumping procedure that employs the inherent forces of the PRM.

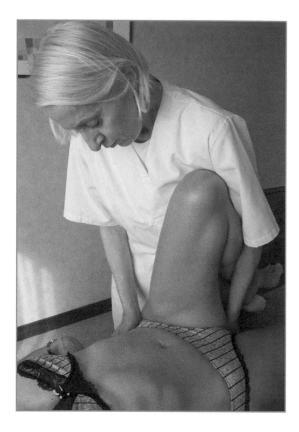

Figure 3.19: Hand placement for diagnosis and treatment of left pelvic bone

## Pelvic bone procedure

### *Indications*

Sacroiliac (SI) dysfunction; pelvic visceral dysfunction, including constipation and urinary tract complaints; pelvic autonomic dysfunction; pelvic floor dysfunction; compensatory knee dysfunction; functional leg length inequity.

### *Procedure*

(Example: left pelvic bone.)

In a position similar to that of the hip joint procedure described above, the patient is supine with their left hip and knee flexed. (See 'Figure 3.16: Hand placement for diagnosis and treatment of left hip dysfunction,' p. 94.)

The practitioner stands beside the treatment table on the patient's left side, at the level of the pelvis.

With your right hand, contact the dysfunctional left pelvic bone in such a way that your thumb rests upon the ASIS, with your index finger extended, pointing posteriorly, along the iliac crest. Alternatively, your right hand may be placed more posteriorly along the iliac crest, thereby allowing you to monitor the left SI joint with the pad of your middle finger. With the patient's hip and knee flexed, your left hand should hold the patient's anterior thigh in such a way as to hold the knee against the anterior aspect of your left shoulder. Alternatively, you can hold the patient's left ischial tuberosity with your left hand, providing greater control of the pelvic bone and an increased sense of the soft tissues attached there. (Fig. 3.19)

Listen to the left pelvic bone and SI joint and, by gently shifting the position of your torso, introducing internal or external rotation in the context of the major and minor motions of the pelvic bone, follow the motion pattern in the direction of ease until a point of pelvic and SI myofascial and ligamentous balance is obtained. Maintaining synchronicity with the PRM, await a release.

## Pubic symphysis procedure

### *Indications*

Pelvic somatic dysfunction; pelvic visceral dysfunctions, including constipation and urinary tract complaints; pelvic floor dysfunctions; functional leg length inequity; unilateral lower extremity edema.

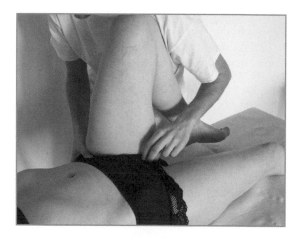

Figure 3.20: Hand placement for diagnosis and treatment of pubic symphysis dysfunction

## Procedure

(Example: superior left pubic bone. (Fig. 3.20))

Patient supine with their left hip and knee flexed.

Practitioner stands beside the treatment table on the patient's left side, at the level of the pelvis.

With your right hand, contact the left pelvic bone in such a way that your thumb lies upon the ASIS, with your fingers resting along the iliac crest. With the patient's hip and knee flexed, hold the knee against the anterior aspect of your left shoulder. With the index and middle fingers, and thumb of your left hand, contact the superior and inferior borders respectively of the left pubic bone, just lateral to the symphysis. From this position, listen to the left pelvic bone and pubis, and by gently shifting the position of your torso, introduce internal rotation (consistent with superior movement of the pubis) in the context of the major and minor motions of the pelvic bone. Follow the motion pattern in the direction of ease until a point of pelvic and pubic myofascial and ligamentous balance is obtained. Maintaining synchronicity with the PRM, await a release. This release may be augmented through the use of a pumping procedure that employs the inherent forces of the PRM.

## Remarks

Unilateral lower extremity edema can be the result of an ipsilateral superior pubic bone dysfunction that places tension upon the adductor magnus, with potential compromise of the deep venous and lymphatic vasculature at the adductor hiatus.

When treating an inferior pubic bone dysfunction, the practitioner introduces external rotation of the pelvic bone, consistent with inferior movement of the pubis.

# Sacroiliac procedures

## Indications

Sacroiliac dysfunction; pelvic somatic dysfunction; pelvic visceral dysfunction; pelvic autonomic dysfunction; pelvic floor dysfunction; compensatory knee dysfunction; functional leg length inequity.

## Supine procedure

(Example: left SI dysfunction. (Fig. 3.21))

Patient supine, lying close to the edge of the table with the left hip and knee flexed.

Practitioner seated on the patient's left side, at the level of the pelvis.

Place the patient's left foot on the anterior surface of your left thigh, and hold their left knee with your left hand. From this stance you can modify the position of the patient's lower extremity by moving your thigh and left hand, thereby influencing the pelvic bone and SI joint. Next, place your right hand palm up beneath the patient's left pelvic bone in such a way that your index and middle fingers palpate the left SI joint. While listening to the SI joint, adjust the positioning of the patient's lower extremity through flexion/extension, internal/external rotation, and abduction/adduction of their hip until the final position of SI and pelvicligamentous and

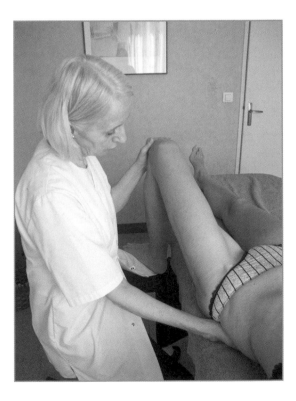

Figure 3.21: Hand placement for diagnosis and treatment of left SI dysfunction in the supine position

myofascial balance is obtained. Hip flexion induces pelvic bone internal rotation (posterior pelvic bone), while extension induces pelvic bone external rotation (anterior pelvic bone). Hip extension may be obtained by lowering your left thigh or elevating the table. While maintaining the position of SI and pelvic ligamentous and myofascial balance, follow the PRM, and wait for a release.

### Remarks

This procedure allows for the balancing of tension in the myofascial components surrounding the pelvic bone, particularly the iliolumbar, sacrospinous, and sacrotuberous ligaments, and the piriformis and gluteal muscles. To accomplish this, a thorough knowledge of and ability to visualize the anatomy of the region is imperative.

Because the patient is supine, it allows increased precision when treating pelvic bone internal rotation (posterior pelvic bone).

### Prone procedure

(Example: left SI dysfunction. (Fig. 3.22))

**Patient prone.**
Practitioner standing on the patient's left side, at the level of the pelvis.

Place your left hand palm down upon the patient's pelvis in such a way that the pads of your fingers are over the left SI joint. With your right hand, hold the patient's left ankle, and ask the patient to flex their knee. While listening to the relationship between the sacrum and pelvic bones, adjust the positioning of the patient's lower extremity through flexion/extension of the knee, and internal/external rotation, abduc-

tion/adduction of the hip until the final position of SI and pelvic ligamentous and myofascial balance is obtained. At this point, while maintaining the position of balance, follow the PRM, and wait for a release.

### Remarks

The positioning of your left monitoring hand may be varied by placing it transversely with the pads of your fingers upon the SI or sacrospinous and sacrotuberous ligaments, thereby allowing you to focus attention specifically on those areas. (Fig. 3.23)

### Alternative prone procedure

(Example: left SI dysfunction. (Fig. 3.24))

Patient prone, lying close to the edge of the table with the left hip and knee flexed in such a way that the thigh and leg hang over the side of the table.

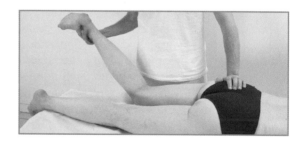

Figure 3.23: Hand placement for SI ligaments release

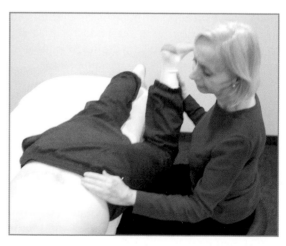

Figure 3.24: Hand placement for diagnosis and treatment of left SI dysfunction in the prone position

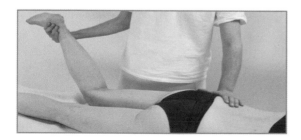

Figure 3.22: Hand placement for diagnosis and treatment of left SI dysfunction in the prone position

Practitioner seated on the patient's left side, at the level of the pelvis.

Place the patient's left leg on the anterior surface of your right thigh, and hold the proximal left leg with your right hand. Next, place your left hand transversely, with the pads of your fingers over the SI joint. From this position, by moving your thigh and right hand, you can modify the positioning of the patient's lower extremity and thereby influence the pelvic bone and SI joint. While listening to the SI joint, adjust the positioning of the patient's lower extremity through flexion/extension, internal/external rotation, and abduction/adduction of the hip until the final position of SI and pelvic ligamentous and myofascial balance is obtained. Hip flexion induces pelvic bone internal rotation (posterior pelvic bone), while extension induces pelvic bone external rotation (anterior pelvic bone). Maintain the position of SI and pelvic ligamentous and myofascial balance, follow the PRM, and wait for a release.

### Remarks

This procedure may be further modified to allow you to balance dysfunction in the pelvic floor. Place your left hand in contact with the patient's ischial tuberosity, with your fingers directed medially to palpate the pelvic floor, and position the patient's lower extremity as described above to obtain ligamentous and myofascial balance, and release.

### Seated procedure

(Example: right SI dysfunction. (Fig. 3.25))

Patient seated on the side of the table, with their right foot resting upon an adjustable height stool in such a manner that their posterior thigh barely contacts the table top.

Practitioner seated, facing the patient from behind.

With the pads of the index, middle, and ring fingers of your left hand, contact the base of the patient's sacrum. Your right hand then contacts the right pelvic bone in such a way that your thumb rests upon the posterior superior iliac spine (PSIS), with your fingers directed anteriorly along and below the iliac crest. While listening to the SI joint, employing indirect principles, the position of the pelvic bone may be taken in the direction of ease, by instructing the patient to abduct or adduct, and externally or

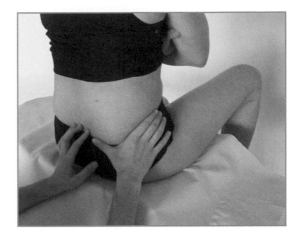

Figure 3.25: Hand placement for diagnosis and treatment of right SI dysfunction in the seated position

internally rotate their right thigh. If necessary, flexion can be introduced by increasing the height of the stool, or by lowering the height of the table. If this is not possible, placing a small pillow under the patient's right thigh will also introduce hip flexion. The position of the sacrum may be similarly modified by instructing the patient to slightly flex or extend, rotate, side bend, or rotate and side bend their head and neck, and if necessary upper torso, until a position of sacral balance is obtained. Follow the motion pattern between the sacrum and pelvic bone in the direction of ease until a point of myofascial and ligamentous balance is obtained. Maintaining synchronicity with the PRM, await a release.

## Global sacral release

### Indications

Sacroiliac dysfunction; pelvic somatic dysfunction; pelvic visceral dysfunction; pelvic autonomic dysfunction; pelvic floor dysfunction.

### Procedure (Fig. 3.26)

Patient prone, lying with their feet beyond the foot end of the table. The patient's head, if possible, should rest in the midline without cervical rotation. This may be accomplished by having the patient lace their fingers together, place their hands palm down on the table, and rest their forehead upon the dorsa of their hands.

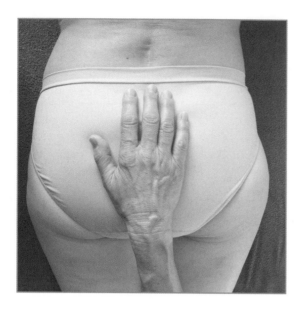

Figure 3.26: Hand placement for global sacral release

Practitioner standing on either side of the patient, at the level of the pelvis.

Place your dominant hand palm down upon the sacrum, in such a way that your thenar and hypothenar eminences rest upon the sacral inferolateral angles, and your fingers point cephalad to rest upon the sacral base. While listening to the sacrum, observe flexion, extension, sidebending, rotation, and the inherent sacral intraosseous motility (craniosacral inspiration/expiration). Follow the sacrum into the position of balance. Follow the PRM and wait for a release, often in association with a still point.

### Remarks

The above hand position allows you to assess the motion of the sacrum. If resistance is felt, you should visualize the site of the restriction (SI joint, L5–S1, coccyx or myofascial structures, or both) and if necessary employ another procedure to treat the dysfunction.

By following the PRM to a still point, this procedure modifies parasympathetic tone. This may be useful for visceral dysfunction resulting from sacral parasympathetic dysfunction.

This procedure may also be employed to enhance the drainage of the cerebrospinal fluid (CSF) surrounding the sacral nerves as they exit the sacral foramina.

## Pelvic floor procedures

### Indications

Pelvic floor dysfunction; pudendal nerve entrapment; pelvic visceral dysfunction; pelvic congestion; pelvic autonomic dysfunction; SI dysfunction; lower extremity vascular disorders.

### Global pelvic floor procedure (Fig. 3.27)

Patient prone, lying with their feet beyond the foot end of the table. The patient's head, if possible, should rest in the midline without cervical rotation. This may be accomplished by having the patient lace their fingers together, place their hands palm down on the table, and rest their forehead upon the dorsa of their hands.

Practitioner standing on either side of the patient, at the level of the pelvis.

Place the pads of your thumbs bilaterally in contact with the medial aspect of the patient's ischial tuberosities. In this position, palpate for asymmetrical myofascial and ligamentous (sacrotuberous ligaments) tension within the pelvic floor. Address identified tension by instructing the patient to, as appropriate, abduct or adduct

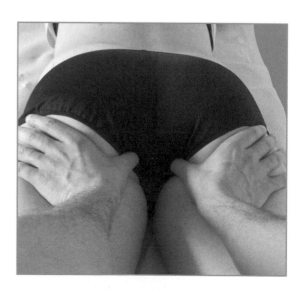

Figure 3.27: Hand placement for global pelvic floor release

and externally or internally rotate their thighs until optimal relaxation of the pelvic floor is obtained. It is useful to observe patient pulmonary respiratory motion to identify the phase (inspiratory or expiratory) in which further ease of tension occurs. During normal respiration, ask the patient to breathe more slowly, prolonging the respiratory phase that provides the greatest ease of tension. With your thumbs directed superiorly and laterally, follow the motion pattern of the pelvic floor in the direction of ease until a point of myofascial and ligamentous balance is obtained. Maintaining synchronicity with the PRM, await a release.

### Remarks

For additional procedures useful for addressing pelvic floor dysfunction, the reader is referred to the pelvic bone and SI procedures described above.

### Unilateral pelvic floor procedure

(Example: left pelvic floor dysfunction. (Fig. 3.28)

**Patient prone.**
Practitioner standing on the patient's right side, at the level of the pelvis.

Place your right hand palm down upon the patient's left buttock in such a way that your thumb is in contact with the medial aspect of the left ischial tuberosity, and your fingers extend laterally. Ask the patient to flex their left knee and hold the patient's left ankle with your left hand. While lis-

tening to the pelvic floor with your right thumb, adjust the positioning of the patient's lower extremity through flexion/extension of the knee, and internal/external rotation, and abduction/adduction of the hip until optimal relaxation of the pelvic ligamentous and myofascial structures is obtained. At this point, while maintaining the position of balance, follow the PRM, and wait for a release.

### Remarks

Exercise caution when introducing internal/external rotation, and abduction/adduction of the hip in patients with knee pathology.

This procedure is of value when addressing entrapment of the pudendal nerve as it passes through the Alcock's canal, and also, for the alleviation of pelvic congestion.

By moving your right thumb superiorly to contact the medial aspect of the ischial spine, the above procedure can be modified to work upon the sacrospinous ligament. This modification is particularly useful when treating entrapment of the pudendal nerve that lies in close contact with the sacrospinous ligament before entering the Alcock's canal.

## Coccygeal procedure

### Indications

Coccygeal dysfunction; sacrotuberous and sacrospinous ligament dysfunction.

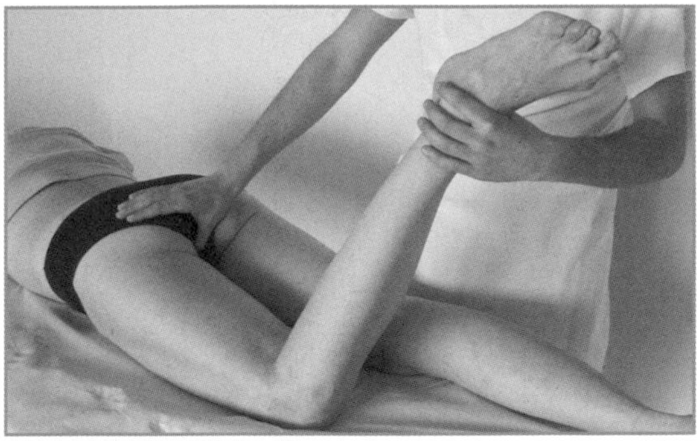

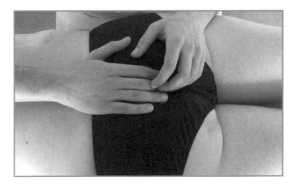

Figure 3.28: Hand placement for unilateral pelvic floor release

Figure 3.29: Hand placement for diagnosis and treatment of coccygeal dysfunction

### Procedure (Fig. 3.29)

Patient lying prone, with their feet positioned off the end of the treatment table. The patient's head should, if possible, rest in the midline without cervical rotation. This may be accomplished by having the patient place their hands, with interlaced fingers, palms down on the table, and rest their forehead upon the dorsa of their hands.

Practitioner seated on either side of the table, facing the patient's pelvis.

Place your cephalic hand upon the patient's sacrum in such a way that your thenar and hypothenar eminences contact the base of the sacrum and your middle finger rests upon the coccyx. The tips of the index and middle fingers of your caudal hand should then be placed in contact with the middle finger of your cephalic hand over the coccyx. Listen to the coccygeal motion and follow the coccyx in the direction of freedom of motion. This is most frequently flexion, with some degree of sidebending and rotation (usually in the same direction). In this procedure, because the coccyx is an extension of the sacrum, it is of particular importance that you follow the craniosacral flexion/extension motion of the sacrum with the cephalic hand. With the coccyx in the position of balanced myofascial and ligamentous tension, while following the PRM, await a release.

### Remarks

Follow the craniosacral motion of the sacrum in a pumping fashion to augment the release of the coccyx.

Before applying the coccygeal procedure, it is appropriate to identify and treat any concomitant sacral, sacrotuberous, and sacrospinous ligament dysfunctions.

It is possible to perform the coccygeal procedure by holding the coccyx between a gloved finger of one hand inserted into the patient's rectum and the middle finger of the other hand placed externally upon the coccyx. This procedure, however, should be performed only by practitioners who are legally qualified to do so.

# Global sacroiliac and lumbosacral release

### Indications

Sacroiliac dysfunction; lumbosacral dysfunction; pelvic visceral dysfunction; pelvic autonomic dysfunction; pelvic floor dysfunction; functional leg length inequity.

### Procedure

(Example: general sacral motion restriction. (Fig. 3. 30))

Patient prone, lying with their feet beyond the foot end of the table. The patient's head, if possible, should rest in the midline without cervical rotation. This may be accomplished by having the patient lace their fingers together, place their hands palm down on the table, and rest their forehead upon the dorsa of their hands.

Practitioner standing on either side of the patient, at the level of the pelvis.

Your caudal hand should be placed in such a manner that your index finger and thumb contact the inferolateral angles (ILA) of the patient's sacrum, while the index finger and thumb of your cephalic hand contact the lateral aspects of the sacral base. While listening to the sacrum, observe flexion, extension, sidebending, and rotation. Em-

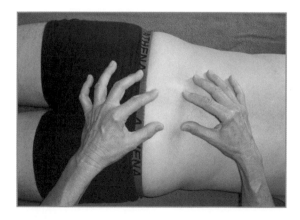

Figure 3.30: Hand placement for global sacroiliac and lumbosacral release

ploy indirect principles and follow the sacrum in the direction of ease. While maintaining the position of sacral ligamentous and myofascial balance, follow the PRM, and wait for a release.

### Remarks

The establishment of a position of sacral ligamentous and myofascial balance may be facilitated by instructing the patient to rotate their head and cervical spine to the left or right, and by dorsiflexing or plantarflexing one or both feet. Dorsiflexion of the foot enhances craniosacral flexion of the sacrum, while plantar flexion enhances craniosacral extension.

Alternatively, the sacrum may be monitored by placing your index fingers bilaterally in contact with the base, while your thumbs bilaterally palpate the ILAs.

## Lumbosacral procedures

### Indications

Lumbosacral dysfunction; low back pain.

### Prone procedure

(Example: lumbosacral torsions and Fryette type I and type II lumbosacral dysfunctions; (Fig. 3.31) see further discussion of 'The pelvis and the lumbar spine' in 'Section 4: Clinical considerations, Chapter 1: Musculoskeletal dysfunctions, Part 1: Axial system,' p. 180.)

Patient prone, lying with their feet beyond the foot end of the table to reduce lumbosacral anatomic extension stress. The patient's head, if possible, should rest in the midline without cervical rotation. This may be accomplished by having the patient lace their fingers together, place their hands palm down on the table, and rest their forehead upon the dorsa of their hands.

Practitioner stands on either side of the patient, at the level of the pelvis.

Your caudal hand is placed in such a manner that your index finger and thumb contact the sacral sulci at the base of the sacrum. The index finger and thumb of your cephalic hand contact either side of the spinous process of L5. Listen, and employing indirect

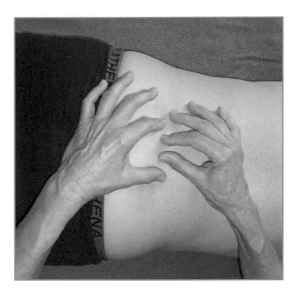

Figure 3.31: Hand placement for diagnosis and treatment of lumbosacral dysfunction in the prone position

principles, follow the motion of the sacrum and L5 in the direction of ease (flexion, extension, sidebending, and rotation). While maintaining the position of sacral and lumbar ligamentous and myofascial balance, follow the PRM, and wait for a release.

### Remarks

The acquisition of the optimal lumbosacral position of ease may be facilitated by instructing the patient to rotate their head and cervical spine to the left or right, and by dorsiflexing or plantarflexing one or both feet. Dorsiflexion of the foot enhances craniosacral flexion of the sacrum, while plantarflexion enhances craniosacral extension.

### Supine procedure

(Example: L5 rotated right, sacrum rotated left. (Fig. 3.32))

**Patient supine.**

Practitioner stands on the right side of the patient, at the level of the pelvis.

Flex your right hip and knee and place your right foot transversely upon the table top about 6–10 inches caudal to the patient's pelvis.

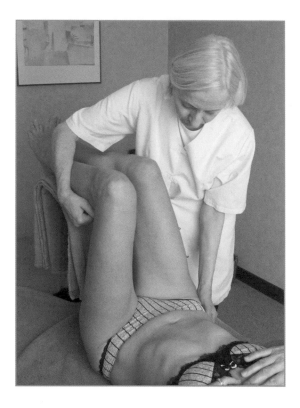

Figure 3.32: Hand placement for diagnosis and treatment of lumbosacral dysfunction in the supine position

Instruct the patient to flex both hips and knees and to place their calves upon your right thigh. Then place your left hand upon the patient's right iliac crest, and with your right forearm and hand hold the patient's legs against your torso. Next, visualize and listen to the motion of the pelvis. Using the patient's legs as levers, follow the motion of each pelvic bone into external or internal rotation, with flexion/extension and abduction/adduction. Deviation of the patient's legs and ankles to the left of the midline of their pelvis introduces left pelvic torsion, while deviation to the right introduces right pelvic torsion. Increasing flexion of one hip increases internal rotation of the ipsilateral pelvic bone, while extension increases external rotation. In the above example there is an internal rotation of the pelvic bone on the left and external rotation on the right, as a result of the left rotation of the sacrum. After following the motion

of the pelvic bones into the position of myofascial and ligamentous balance, you should concentrate upon the intersegmental relationship between the sacrum and L5, following flexion, extension, sidebending left/right, and rotation left/right to the position of optimal balance. While maintaining this position of pelvic and lumbosacral intersegmental balanced ligamentous tension, follow the PRM, and wait for a release.

### Remarks

This procedure is particularly useful in that it allows one to work globally on the pelvis, while also focusing attention more locally on either or both SI joints and L5–S1, or segmentally even higher in the lumbar spine. With the use of precise listening, it can also be useful to release all ligamentous and myofascial tensions involving the sacrotuberous and sacrospinous ligaments and the piriformis, psoas, and internus obturator muscles.

### Seated procedure (Fig. 3.33)

(Example: L5 sidebend right, rotated left, as the lowest articulation in a Fryette type I group curve. This is also consistent with a sacral forward torsion, rotated right on the right oblique axis. See further discussion of 'The pelvis and the lumbar spine' in 'Section 4: Clinical considerations, Chapter 1: Musculoskeletal dysfunctions, Part 1: Axial system,' p. 182.)

With the tips of the thumb and index finger of your left hand, contact the spinous process of L5 in such a way that the interspinous tissues between L5 and S1 are also contacted. Next place your right hand upon the patient's right shoulder. With your left hand, listen to the intersegmental relationship between L5 and S1. Employ indirect principles and take L5 upon S1 in the direction of ease, by introducing sidebending right and rotation left from above, through the patient's right shoulder, with your right hand. Using indirect principles, follow the motion pattern between L5 and S1 until a point of myofascial and ligamentous balance is obtained. Await a release.

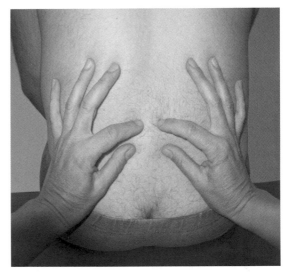

Figure 3.34: Hand placement for diagnosis and treatment of lumbosacral dysfunction in the seated position

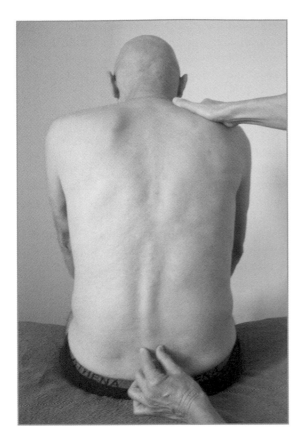

Figure 3.33: Hand placement for diagnosis and treatment of lumbosacral dysfunction in the seated position

### Alternative seated procedure (Fig. 3.34)

(Example: lumbosacral torsions and Fryette type I and type II lumbosacral dysfunctions. See further discussion of 'The pelvis and the lumbar spine' in 'Section 4: Clinical considerations, Chapter 1: Musculoskeletal dysfunctions, Part 1: Axial system,' p. 182.)

Patient seated with their legs hanging off the side of the treatment table.

Practitioner seated, facing the patient from behind.

Contact the base of the patient's sacrum bilaterally with the pads of your thumbs, while your index fingers contact either side of the spinous process of L5. Listen to the lumbosacral junction, and employ indirect principles to follow L5 and the sacrum in the direction of ease. This may be enhanced by instructing the patient to slightly flex or extend, rotate, and side bend their head and neck, and if necessary upper torso until a position of lumbosacral myofascial and ligamentous balance is obtained. Even greater fine tuning may be obtained by monitoring the lumbosacral junction with one hand and introducing flexion, extension, rotation, and sidebending from above with the other hand. Maintaining synchronicity with the PRM, await a release.

### Remarks

The practitioner should be cautious in that, if the dosage tolerance of the patient is exceeded, this seated lumbosacral procedure occasionally results in a presyncopal patient response.

## Lumbar procedures

Because dysfunction in the upper lumbar area can be the result of viscerosomatic reflexes, it should prompt the practitioner to seriously look for, and rule out, underlying visceral pathology. See further: 'Vertebral somatic dysfunction' in 'Section 4: Clinical considerations, Chapter 1: Musculo-skeletal dysfunctions, Part 1: Axial system,' p. 183. Treatment procedures should never be applied to or through areas of spinal instability, hypermobility, or spinal levels with neurological compression.

# Global lumbar spine procedures

## Indications

Lumbosacral and lumbar dysfunctions; low back pain.

## Prone procedure

(Example: lumbar paravertebral muscular tension. (Fig. 3.35))

Patient prone, lying with their feet beyond the foot end of the table to reduce lumbosacral anatomic extension stress. The patient's head, if pos-

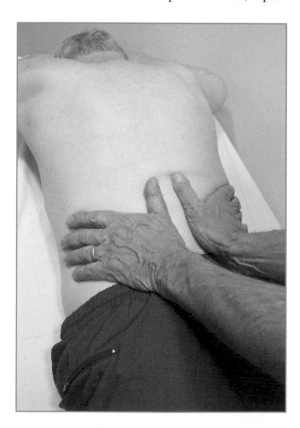

Figure 3.35: Hand placement for global lumbar release

sible, should rest in the midline without cervical rotation. This may be accomplished by having the patient lace their fingers together, place their hands palm down on the table, and rest their forehead upon the dorsa of their hands.

Practitioner stands on either side of the patient, at the level of the pelvis, facing toward the patient's head.

Place your thenar eminences bilaterally contacting the medial aspects of the patient's lumbar paravertebral muscles, in such a way that your fingers extend obliquely, laterally, and cephalically. Listen to the lumbar spine and its myofascial and ligamentous elements for rotational and lateral translatory asymmetry. Using indirect principles follow the tissues in the direction of ease. Employ the PRM in a pumping fashion until the dysfunctional tissues demonstrate a quality of motion allowing them to return to neutral without resistance. The above process should be repeated in the direction opposite the initial asymmetry, if necessary, until both sides demonstrate equal quality of motion.

## Remarks

If the patient is tense, muscular, or obese, it may prove difficult to identify any apparent asymmetry of the lumbar spine and its myofascial and ligamentous elements. Under these circumstances, you can introduce a rotational and lateral translatory motion gently to the left through your right hand. After allowing the tissues to return to neutral, repeat the process by introducing rotation and lateral translation to the right through your left hand. Compliance with, versus resistance to, these opposing motion patterns is then compared, and the indirect procedure described above applied.

## Alternative hand placement

(Example: rotation and lateral translation to the left. (Fig. 3.36))

Once the dysfunctional asymmetry has been identified, using the method described above, stand on the patient's left side, at the level of the lumbosacral junction. The fingers of your right hand should hold the ASIS of the patient's right pelvic bone. With the fingers of your left hand extended laterally, the proximal aspect of your the-

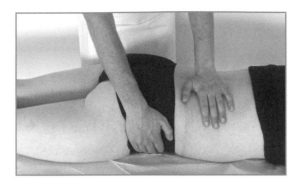

Figure 3.36: Alternative hand placement for global lumbar release

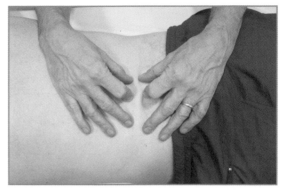

Figure 3.37: Hand placement for diagnosis and treatment of segmental lumbar dysfunction in the prone position

nar and hypothenar eminences should contact the right lumbar paravertebral muscles. Follow the lumbar ligamentous and myofascial motion with your left hand, while gently lifting and rotating the patient's pelvis in the direction of ease with your right hand. Return to neutral and repeat in a pumping fashion until the dysfunctional tissues return to neutral without resistance. This process should be repeated in the direction opposite the initial asymmetry, until both sides demonstrate equal quality of motion.

### Remarks

Osteopathic manipulative treatment procedures are intended to enhance function by reducing motion restriction associated with dysfunction. As such, it is potentially injurious to increase available motion under circumstances of anatomic instability with potential for hypermobility. Consequently, these procedures should not be applied to areas of lumbar or lumbosacral instability in clinical conditions like spondylolisthesis and intervertebral disc herniation.

## Segmental lumbar spine procedures

### Indications

Lumbosacral and lumbar single segment dysfunctions; low back pain; psoas and thoracoabdominal diaphragm dysfunctions.

### Prone procedure

(Example: L3–L4 dysfunction. (Fig. 3.37))

Patient prone, lying with their feet beyond the foot end of the table to reduce lumbosacral anatomic extension stress. To further reduce the lumbar lordosis, it may be desirable to place a small pillow under the patient's abdomen. If possible, the patient's head should rest in the midline without cervical rotation. This may be accomplished by having the patient rest their forehead upon the dorsa of their hands, with their fingers laced together.

Practitioner sits on either side of the patient, at the level of the lumbar spine.

Place your caudal hand in such a manner that your index finger and thumb contact either side of the spinous process of L4. With the index finger and thumb of your cephalic hand, contact either side of the spinous process of L3. Listen, and employing indirect principles, follow the motion of L3 in the direction of ease (flexion, extension, sidebending, and rotation). While maintaining the position of intersegmental lumbar balanced ligamentous tension, follow the PRM in a pumping fashion, and wait for a release.

### Supine procedure

(Example: L1–L2 dysfunction. (Fig. 3.38))

**Patient supine.**
Practitioner standing on either side of the patient, at the level of the pelvis.

Hold the patient around their waist with both hands in such a manner that your index fingers

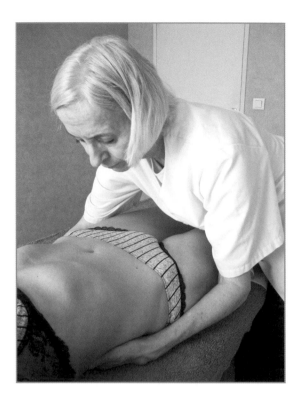

Figure 3.38: Hand placement for diagnosis and treatment of segmental lumbar dysfunction in the supine position

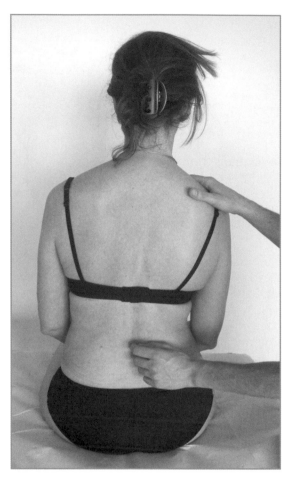

Figure 3.39: Hand placement for diagnosis and treatment of segmental lumbar dysfunction in the seated position

contact the transverse processes of L1 bilaterally, and your middle fingers contact the transverse processes of L2. Listen, and employing indirect principles, follow the motion between L1 and L2 in the direction of ease (flexion, extension, sidebending, and rotation). While maintaining the position of intersegmental lumbar balanced ligamentous tension, follow the PRM, and wait for a release.

### Seated procedure

(Example: L2–L3 flexed, side bent right, rotated right dysfunction. (Fig. 3.39))

Patient seated on the side of the table.

Practitioner standing facing the patient from behind.

With the tips of the index finger and thumb of your left hand, bilaterally contact the spinous process of L2 in such a way that the interspinous tissues between L2 and L3 are also contacted. Next, place your right hand so that it rests upon the patient's right shoulder. With your left hand, listen to the intersegmental relationship between L2 and L3. Employ indirect principles and take L2 upon L3 in the direction of ease, by introducing flexion, sidebending right, and rotation right from above, through the patient's right shoulder, with your right hand. Follow the motion pattern between L2 and L3 until a point of myofascial and ligamentous balance is obtained. Maintaining synchronicity with the PRM, await a release.

### Remarks

This procedure is applicable for treating intersegmental dysfunctions from the mid- to low thoracic spine to the lumbosacral junction.

When introducing motion from above through the patient's shoulder, it is extremely important that you focus upon the listening hand (left hand in the above example) that is monitoring the lumbar dysfunction, and not upon the active hand (right hand). Failure to do this can potentially provide confusing information from asymmetrical mechanics affecting the body between the active hand and the listening hand.

# Lumbopelvic muscular procedures

## Piriformis release

### Indications

Piriformis dysfunction resulting in buttock pain, external rotation of the hip, functional inequity of leg length, and either sciatic nerve compression with sciatica, or pudendal nerve compression with pelvic floor pain.

### Procedure

(Example: left piriformis dysfunction. (Fig. 3.40))

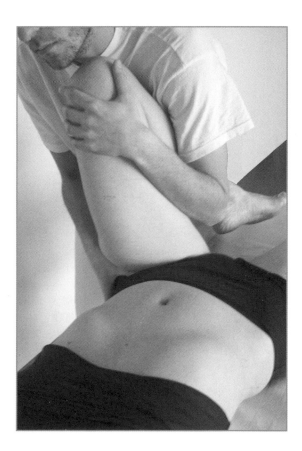

Figure 3.40: Hand placement for piriformis release

Patient supine with their left hip and knee flexed.

Practitioner standing beside the treatment table on the side of the dysfunctional piriformis, at the level of the pelvis.

With your right hand, contact the left pelvic bone so that your fingers extend posteriorly to palpate the left greater trochanter at the point of insertion of the piriformis muscle. Your left hand holds the patient's anterior thigh, holding the knee against the anterior aspect of your left shoulder. By adjusting hip flexion, abduction, and external rotation, place the hip in the position of ease. Visualize and listen to the dysfunctional piriformis muscle, following it into the final position of myofascial balance. At this point, while maintaining the position of balance, wait for a release.

### Remarks

An isometric modification may be added in the case of chronic conditions where the release of dysfunctional piriformis tension does not readily occur. Ask the patient to very gently and briefly (about two seconds) contract the piriformis, pushing their knee in the direction of the holding force of your left hand (a combination of hip external rotation and abduction). When the patient is instructed to relax, listen carefully to the dysfunctional piriformis muscle, noting the ease and degree that relaxation occurs. This process may be repeated several times, as necessary, to obtain optimal muscular relaxation. For best results, each sequential contraction should employ slightly different amounts of hip external rotation and abduction, dependent upon the sensation of the ease and degree of relaxation, as observed by listening.

Note: This is not a traditional muscle energy procedure in that, following the therapeutic contraction, the muscle is not stretched to directly take it to a new barrier. Rather, the improvement of the quality of piriformis relaxation is the desired goal of the procedure.

## Obturator internus release

### Indications

Obturator internus dysfunction resulting in hip pain, external rotation of the hip, pelvic bone, and pelvic floor dysfunction.

### Procedure

This procedure is essentially the same as the piriformis muscle procedure described above. It differs in that the monitoring hand should be placed so that the fingers contact the point of insertion of the obturator internus, located more posteriorly upon the greater trochanter, and the position of ease is obtained with hip flexion of approximately 90°.

## Iliopsoas release

### Indications

Psoas major spasm resulting in lumbosacral, SI, inguinal pain, or pain involving any combination of these structures; restricted hip extension; pelvic sideshift opposite the side of dysfunction; iliacus spasm; SI, inguinal, or intrapelvic pain, or pain in these areas in any combination.

### Procedure

(Example: left iliopsoas dysfunction. (Fig. 3.41))

Patient supine with their left hip and knee flexed.

Practitioner standing beside the treatment table on the side of the dysfunctional iliopsoas, at the level of the pelvis, facing toward the patient's head.

Place the pads of the fingers of your right hand over the left lower quadrant of the patient's abdomen, just above the lateral half of the inguinal ligament, to contact the distal aspect of the left iliopsoas muscle group.

Your left hand holds the patient's anterior thigh, holding the knee against the left side of your anterior chest. By adjusting hip flexion, abduction, and external rotation, place the hip in the position of ease. Visualize and listen to the dysfunctional iliopsoas muscle group, and determine the component (psoas major, psoas minor, or iliacus) demonstrating greatest tension. Follow it into the position of myofascial balance and wait for a release.

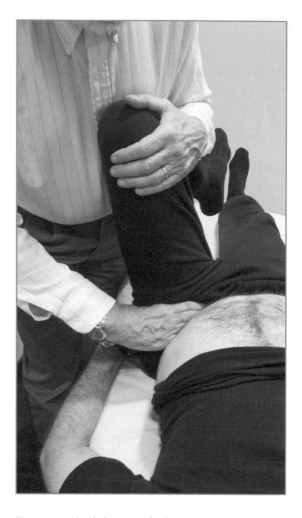

Figure 3.41: Hand placement for iliopsoas release

### Remarks

Psoas major dysfunction is typically associated with an ipsilateral flexed upper lumbar somatic dysfunction. This flexed upper lumbar dysfunction should be treated before addressing the dysfunctional psoas.

The psoas major consists of five digitations, each originating from the bodies of two adjacent vertebrae and their intervertebral disc from T12–L5. It consequently can be considered to function as a series of individual smaller muscles, each with a slightly different dysfunctional potential. Visualization can be employed to identify which component within the greater psoas major is dysfunctional. As such, during the treatment procedure, one can more precisely address the dysfunction by varying the amount of hip flexion in conjunction with external/internal rotation and abduction/adduction, thereby giving the greatest degree of myofascial ease and relaxation.

The iliacus portion of the iliopsoas group does not traverse the lumbosacral junction, but rather originates from the inner aspect of the pelvic bone. To specifically address dysfunction of the left iliacus using the above psoas major procedure, the right hand that is placed over the left lower quadrant of the patient's abdomen should be moved in such a way that the fingers, directed medially, curl over the ASIS so that the tips of the fingers are directed toward the iliac fossa of the pelvic bone to palpate the iliacus muscle. (Fig. 3.42) The left hand and anterior chest are employed as described

above and the patient is positioned in such a manner as to obtain myofascial balance and release.

An isometric modification may be added in the case of chronic conditions where the release of dysfunctional iliopsoas tension does not readily occur. Ask the patient to very gently and briefly (about two seconds) contract the iliopsoas group flexing their hip against the holding force of your left hand. When the patient is instructed to relax, listen carefully to the dysfunctional muscle group, noting the ease and degree that relaxation occurs. This process may be repeated several times, as necessary, to obtain optimal muscular relaxation. For best results, each sequential contraction should employ slightly different amounts of hip flexion and external/internal rotation and abduction/adduction, dependent upon the sensation of the ease and degree of relaxation, as observed by listening.

Note: This is not a traditional muscle energy procedure in that, it is indirect, and following the therapeutic contraction, the muscle is not stretched to directly take it to a new barrier. Rather, the improvement of the quality of iliopsoas relaxation is the desired goal of the procedure.

## Quadratus lumborum release
### Indications

Flank pain; lumbosacral dysfunction, SI dysfunction or both; pelvic unleveling with functional shortening of the ipsilateral lower extremity; ipsilateral lower rib dysfunctions.

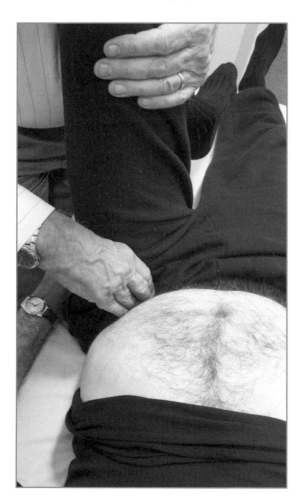

Figure 3.42: Hand placement for iliacus release

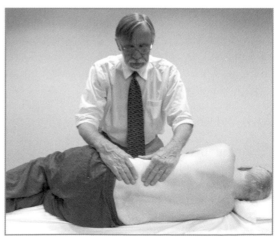

Figure 3.43: Hand placement for quadratus lumborum release

### Procedure

(Example: left quadratus lumborum dysfunction. (Fig. 3.43))

Patient lying on their right side with their hips and knees flexed for comfort and positional stability.

Practitioner standing beside the treatment table in front of the patient, at the level of the lumbar spine.

Place the right hand palm down upon the iliac crest, with the fingers directed posteriorly and cephalically toward the lumbar spine. Place the left hand palm down upon the lower rib cage, with the fingers directed posteriorly and caudally. This hand placement allows you to simultaneously listen to the quadratus lumborum, pelvic bone, and lower ribs. Follow the motion felt at the level of the pelvic bone and lower ribs into the position of ligamentous and myofascial balance, most of the time in a torsional pattern between your two hands. Wait for a release. If necessary, the release may be facilitated by a pumping action between your two hands.

# Thoracic procedures

Because dysfunction in the thoracic area can be the result of sympathetically-mediated viscerosomatic reflexes, it should prompt the practitioner to seriously look for, and rule out, underlying visceral pathology. See further: 'Vertebral somatic dysfunction' in 'Section 4: Clinical considerations, Chapter 1: Musculoskeletal dysfunctions, Part 1: Axial system,' p. 183.

## Global thoracic cage procedures

### Indications

Thoracic cage somatic dysfunction with decreased compliance; pulmonary dysfunction; cardiac dysfunction; venous and lymphatic congestion.

Note: The practitioner is urged to recognize that this procedure, and any other procedure, when employed to address pulmonary and cardiac dysfunctions must be used in an adjunctive or integrative fashion. Underlying pulmonary and cardiac dysfunction and disease must first be diagnosed and treated with appropriate recognized medical management.

### Sternocostal procedure (Fig. 3.44)

**Patient supine.**
Practitioner standing beside the treatment table on either side, at the level of the thorax, facing toward the patient's head.

Place your thenar eminences bilaterally in contact with the medial aspects of the patient's chest, in such a way that your thumbs are directed superiorly, and your fingers laterally. Listen to the thoracic cage and its myofascial and ligamentous elements for rotational, lateral translatory, and inspiratory or expiratory asymmetry. Employ indirect principles and follow the tissues in the direction of ease. Observe patient pulmonary respiratory motion to identify the phase (inspiratory or expiratory) in which further ease of tension occurs. Ask the patient to breathe more slowly, prolonging the respiratory phase that provides the greatest ease of tension, until the dysfunctional tissues demonstrate a quality of motion allowing them to return to neutral without resistance. The above process should be repeated in the direction opposite the initial asymmetry, if necessary, until both sides demonstrate equal quality of motion.

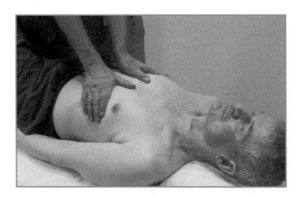

Figure 3.44: Hand placement for sternocostal release

### Alternative procedure (Fig. 3.45)

Place one hand upon the sternum, in such a way that the fingers point cephalically and the little finger and index finger, or thumb, bilaterally contact the medial aspects of the costal cartilages on either side of the sternum. Place your other hand, so that your thenar eminence contacts the rib(s) to be examined and treated, over the costal cartilage(s), with your fingers extended laterally around the patient's thoracic cage.

### Sterno-occipital procedure (Fig. 3.46)

**Patient supine.**
Practitioner seated at the head of the table.

With one hand cradling the occiput, place the other hand upon the sternum with the palm over the sternal body and the fingers directed inferiorly. Listen and follow the sternum and occiput, allowing them both to move into the position of ease. This is often accompanied by spontaneous respiratory cooperation by the patient, in the form of a deep breath. If this does not occur, or if the release is incomplete, it is useful to observe the patient's pulmonary respiratory motion to identify the phase (inspiratory or expiratory) in which further ease of tension occurs. Ask the patient to breathe more slowly, prolonging the respiratory phase that provides the greatest ease of tension.

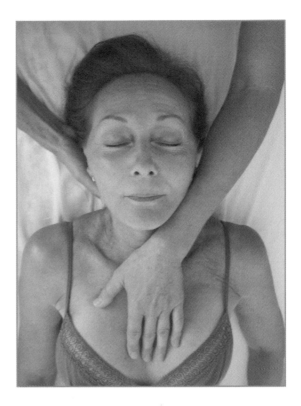

Figure 3.46: Hand placement for sterno-occipital release

### Remarks

In female patients, the hand placement should be adjacent, medial, and inferior, or superior, to the breast tissue. Direct contact with the breast is not appropriate; it is often uncomfortable for the patient, and provides no therapeutic advantage.

These procedures may be started by listening to the chest cage using the hand placed upon the sternum. This will allow a global sense of chest cage motility and assist in the identification of areas of restriction requiring further evaluation and treatment, such as the sternomanubrial junction.

During the procedure application, the depth of the tissue being treated may be adjusted for by increasing or decreasing the pressure applied through the hands. This pressure should be determined by listening and visualization using the lightest touch and should never begin to introduce deformation of the structures being palpated.

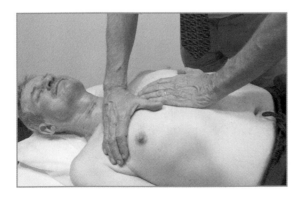

Figure 3.45: Alternative hand placement for sternocostal release

## Global thoracic spine procedure

### Indications

Back pain and chest wall pain with thoracic spinal and rib dysfunctions; paraspinal myofascial dysfunction; pectoral girdle dysfunction; decreased thoracic cage compliance complicating cardiopulmonary diseases; venous and lymphatic congestion; sympathetic dysautonomia.

### Procedure

(Example: decreased thoracic cage mobility, patient initially positioned on the side of greatest comfort, in this instance, their right side. (Fig. 3.47))

Patient lying on their side with their hips and knees flexed for comfort and positional stability, and with one or several pillows, as necessary, supporting their head and cervical spine.

Practitioner standing beside the treatment table in front of the patient, at the level of the thoracic spine.

Place your right hand between the patient's left arm and thoracic cage, in such a way that the pads of your fingers contact the left paravertebral region of lower thoracic vertebrae. Your left hand should rest palm down upon the left scapula, with the fingers directed medially and caudally toward the mid-thoracic spine. This hand placement allows you to listen to the thoracic spine, ribs, and myofascial structures of the left hemithorax. Follow the motion felt into the position of ligamentous and myofascial balance, most of the time in a

torsional pattern, between your two hands. Wait for a release. If necessary, the release may be enhanced by employing a pumping action between your two hands. Upon completion, repeat the procedure with the patient lying on their left side.

## Segmental thoracic spine procedures

### Indications

Thoracic somatic dysfunction and segmentally related sympathetic somatovisceral influences.

### Lateral decubitus procedure

(Example: T6–T7 extended, side bent left, rotated left dysfunction. (Fig. 3.48))

Patient lying on their right side with their hips and knees flexed for comfort and positional stability, and with one or several pillows, as necessary, supporting their head and cervical spine.

Practitioner standing beside the treatment table in front of the patient, at the level of the thoracic spine.

Place your right hand between the patient's left arm and thoracic cage, in such a way that your index and middle fingers contact either side of the spinous process of T7. Place your left hand with your fingers directed caudally, such that the index and middle fingers contact either side of the spinous process of T6. Listen to the motion between T6 and T7, and employ indirect principles to take T6 upon T7 in the direction of ease, by introducing extension, rotation

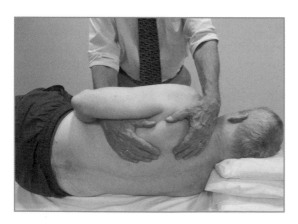

Figure 3.47: Hand placement for global thoracic release

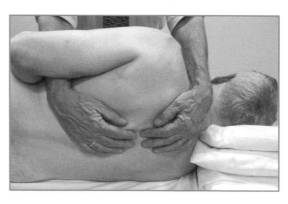

Figure 3.48: Hand placement for diagnosis and treatment of segmental thoracic dysfunction in the lateral decubitus position

left, and sidebending left with your left hand until a point of myofascial and ligamentous balance is obtained. Maintaining synchronicity with the PRM, await a release.

## Remarks

Alternative hand placement: In the above procedure, the use of the thumb and index finger for spinous process contact may be employed as an alternative to the use of the index and middle fingers.

## Seated procedure

(Example: T5–T6 extended, side bent right, rotated right dysfunction. (Fig. 3.49))

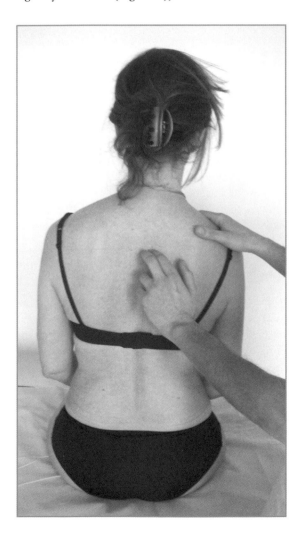

Figure 3.49: Hand placement for diagnosis and treatment of segmental thoracic dysfunction in the seated position

**Patient seated on the side of the table.**
Practitioner standing facing the patient from behind.

With the tips of the index and middle fingers of your left hand contact the spinous process of T5, in such a way that the interspinous tissues between T5 and T6 are also contacted. Next place your right hand upon the patient's right shoulder. With your left hand, listen to the intersegmental relationship between T5 and T6. Employ indirect principles and take T5 upon T6 in the direction of ease, by introducing extension, sidebending right, and rotation right from above, through the patient's right shoulder, with your right hand. Using indirect principles, follow the motion pattern between T5 and T6 until a point of myofascial and ligamentous balance is obtained. Maintaining synchronicity with the PRM, await a release. The release of the dysfunction may be facilitated by a pumping action that follows the rhythm of the PRM.

## Remarks

As compared to the lateral decubitus procedure, this procedure lends itself more readily to the treatment of dysfunctions in the upper-middle thoracic region.

To treat the upper thoracic region, the active hand that is placed upon the shoulder can be moved to contact the top of the patient's head. (Fig. 3.50) It must be stressed that at no time during this procedure should any compression be applied to the head or through the cervical spine. Further, when introducing motion from above through the patient's head and neck, it is extremely important that you focus upon the listening hand (left hand in the above example) that is monitoring the thoracic dysfunction, and not upon the active hand (right hand). Failure to do this can potentially provide confusing information from asymmetrical mechanics affecting the body between the active and listening hands.

## Sutherland's procedure[10]

(Example: T5–T6 extended, side bent left, rotated left dysfunction. (Fig. 3.51))

"One of the frequent fascial drags occurs at the upper dorsal region, an area that became designated as 'the old-age center' during the early presentation of the science of osteopathy."[11]

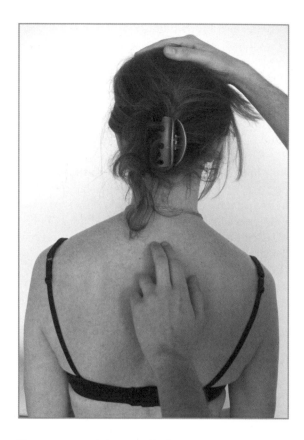

Figure 3.50: Hand placement for diagnosis and treatment of segmental upper thoracic dysfunction in the seated position

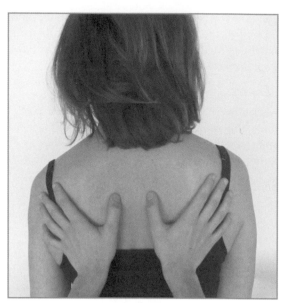

Figure 3.51: Hand placement for Sutherland's procedure; initial phase

Patient seated on the side of the table.

Practitioner standing, facing the patient from behind.

Place a finger upon each transverse process of T5. Instruct the patient to alternately raise one shoulder, and lower the other while you palpate for freedom of motion. In this example, you will feel restriction of movement of the left transverse process of T5 when the patient elevates their left shoulder, and freedom when they lower it, whereas the right transverse process will demonstrate relative freedom of motion during elevation and depression of the right shoulder. Once the dysfunction has been identified, shift your fingers so that they contact the right transverse process of T5 and the left transverse process of T6. Using indirect principles, follow the transverse processes anteriorly (T5 right and T6 left) in the plane of the articular facets, to exaggerate the dysfunction.

The patient should then be instructed to elevate their right shoulder while lowering their left shoulder and carrying it slightly posteriorly. When the point of myofascial and ligamentous balance is found, respiratory cooperation may be employed. Instruct the patient to inhale and hold their breath. Hold this position and await a release.

## Remarks

If the dysfunction is T5, flexed, rotated, and side bent to the left, there will be freedom of motion of the right transverse process of T5 when the patient elevates their right shoulder and restriction when they lower it. The ligamentous imbalance of the dysfunction will be felt to be mainly on the side of convexity and respiratory cooperation using exhalation may be employed.

### Costovertebral procedure

(Example: T5–T6 extended, side bent left, rotated left dysfunction. (Fig. 3.52))

This procedure uses the ribs as levers to address thoracic vertebra dysfunction.

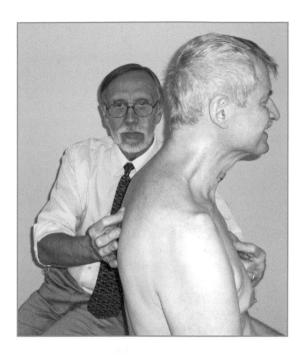

Figure 3.52: Hand placement for costovertebral procedure

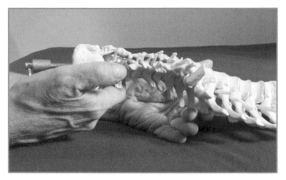

Figure 3.53: Hand placement for cervicothoracic procedure

head, neck, upper back, upper extremity, or any combination of these structures. The presence of upper thoracic sympathetic and upper cervical parasympathetic reflexes can result in multiple somatovisceral complaints.

Patient seated on the side of the table.

Practitioner seated on the table, on the patient's left side.

Place the thumb and index finger of your right hand on either side of the spinous process of T5. The thumb and index finger of your left hand should respectively contact the left and right costal cartilages of the fifth ribs. Listen to the vertebra and ribs. In this example, with left rotation and sidebending of T5, the left fifth rib will be felt to move posteriorly and inferiorly, while the right fifth rib will be felt to move anteriorly and superiorly. Follow the motion into the position of ligamentous and myofascial balance, and following the PRM, wait for a release. When necessary, the release may be enhanced by employing a pumping action between your two hands.

# Cervicothoracic procedure

## Indications

Upper thoracic and cervical somatic dysfunction with pain, or functional complaints, involving the

## Procedure (Fig. 3.53)

**Patient supine.**

Practitioner seated at the head of the table.

With one hand cradle the patient's occiput, while the pads of the index and middle fingers of your other hand contact the spinous process(es) of the dysfunctional area. Listen to the myofascial and ligamentous elements of the region for flexion, extension, rotation, lateral translation, and sidebending asymmetries. If necessary, upper thoracic or cervical dysfunction may be further assessed by introducing motion from above. With your occipital hand, gently increase and decrease occipital flexion to produce cervical or upper thoracic flexion and extension, and introduce rotation and sidebending as necessary. Sidebending is associated with translation to the opposite side. The introduction of motions that are too gross will result in loss of localization. Using indirect principles, follow the tissues in the direction of ligamentous and myofascial balance. Employ the PRM in a pumping fashion, and await a release.

## Remarks

If resistance to release is encountered during treatment, assess the spinal segments above and below the dysfunctional area for contributory dysfunction and, if found, treat it and return to the initial area.

Because dysfunction in this area can be the result of viscerosomatic reflexes, it should prompt the practitioner to seriously look for, and rule out, underlying visceral pathology. See further: 'Vertebral somatic dysfunction' in 'Section 4: Clinical considerations, Chapter 1: Musculoskeletal dysfunction, Part 1: Axial system,' p. 183.

## Rib procedures for the fourth to tenth ribs

### Indications

Back pain, intercostal pain, and chest wall pain with thoracic rib dysfunctions; scapulothoracic dysfunctions; decreased thoracic cage compliance complicating cardiopulmonary diseases; venous and lymphatic congestion; sympathetic dysautonomia.

### Sutherland's procedure[12] (Fig. 3.54)

Patient seated on the side of the table.

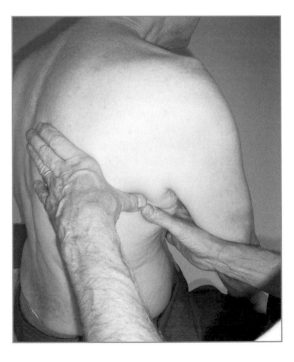

Figure 3.54: Hand placement for diagnosis and treatment of rib dysfunction; Sutherland's procedure

Practitioner seated, facing the patient on the side of the dysfunction.

Place your hands so that your index fingers and thumbs follow the course of the dysfunctional rib. Your thumbs should contact the dysfunctional rib laterally near the posterior axillary line. Posteriorly, the pad of your index finger should rest approximately upon the angle of the rib and anteriorly your index finger should extend toward the costochondral junction. Hold the rib to keep it from moving anteriorly and ask the patient to slowly rotate their pectoral girdle in order to bring the opposite shoulder posteriorly, until a point of balance is obtained. Listen and follow the rib in the direction of freedom of motion (anterior/posterior, cephalad/caudal, lateral translation, and rotation) until a point of balanced ligamentous and myofascial tension is obtained. Observe the patient's breathing to identify the phase (inspiratory or expiratory) in which further ease of tension occurs. Ask the patient to breathe slowly, prolonging the respiratory phase that provides the greatest decrease of tension. Await a complete release.

### Alternative procedure

Patient and practitioner seated as above. Place the index and middle fingers of your hands so that they contact the rib posteriorly, just lateral to the costotransverse articulation, and anteriorly, lateral to the sternocostal articulation. Listen and follow the rib in the direction of freedom of motion until a point of balanced ligamentous and myofascial tension is obtained. Employ the patient's respiration as above to obtain the greatest decrease of tension and await a complete release.

## First rib procedures

### Indications

First rib dysfunction; thoracic outlet syndrome associated with anterior and middle scalene dysfunction; overuse syndrome of the scalene muscles seen in association with chronic obstructive pulmonary disease.

### First rib procedure seated

(Example: left first rib dysfunction. (Fig. 3.55))

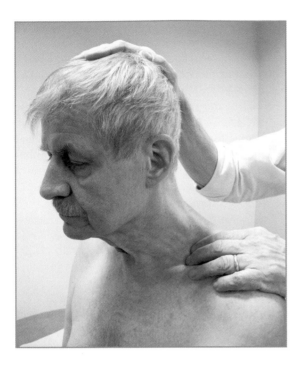

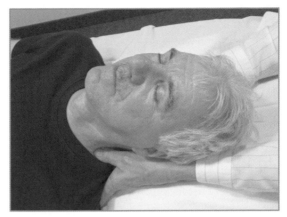

Figure 3.56: Hand placement for diagnosis and treatment of first rib dysfunction in the supine position

Figure 3.55: Hand placement for diagnosis and treatment of first rib dysfunction in the seated position

**Patient supine.**

Practitioner seated at the head of the treatment table.

Place your left hand in such a way that the pad of your thumb rests between the sternocleidomastoid and trapezius muscles contacting the superolateral aspect of the first rib. Your right hand cradles the patient's occiput. Listen to the motion of the rib, and adjust the position of the patient's head and neck using flexion, extension, rotation, and sidebending right/left until a point of balanced ligamentous and myofascial tension is obtained. Monitor the patient's breathing and identify the respiratory phase that decreases tension. Instruct the patient to slowly breathe, prolonging the respiratory phase that provides the greatest decrease of tension. Await a complete release.

### Remarks

Most of the time, the fist rib will display an inspiratory or elevated dysfunction. In this case, the respiratory phase that provides the greatest decrease of tension will be inspiration. Because of the insertion of the anterior and middle scalene muscles upon the first rib, decrease of tension can frequently be obtained by sidebending the head and neck to the side of the dysfunctional rib, with variable amounts of rotation to the opposite side, and flexion.

Patient seated on the side of the table.

Practitioner standing behind the patient.

Place your left hand in such a way that the pad of your index or middle finger contacts the superolateral aspect of the first rib. Your right hand rests on the top of the patient's head. Listen to the motion of the rib, and adjust the position of the patient's head and neck using flexion, extension, rotation, and sidebending right/left until a point of balanced ligamentous and myofascial tension is obtained. Monitor the patient's breathing and identify the phase (inspiratory or expiratory) in which further ease of tension occurs. Instruct the patient to slowly breathe, prolonging the respiratory phase that provides the greatest decrease of tension. Await a complete release.

### First rib procedure supine

(Example: left first rib dysfunction. (Fig. 3.56))

## Second rib procedure

### Indications

Second rib dysfunction; overuse syndrome of the scalene muscles seen in association with chronic obstructive pulmonary disease.

### Second rib procedure

(Example: left second rib dysfunction. (Fig. 3.57))

Patient seated on the side of the table.

Practitioner standing behind the patient.

Place your left hand in such a way that the pad of your thumb contacts the angle of the second rib just superior to the scapula, and the index and middle fingers contact the second rib lateral to its chondro-

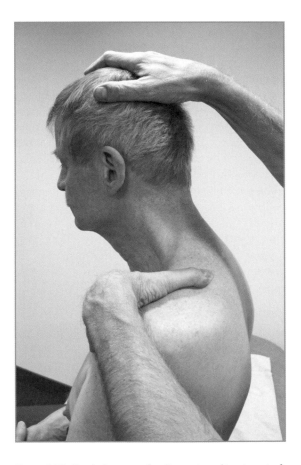

Figure 3.57: Hand placement for diagnosis and treatment of second rib dysfunction

sternal joint. Your right hand rests on the top of the patient's head. Listen to the motion of the rib, and adjust the position of the patient's head and neck using sidebending and rotation until a point of balanced ligamentous and myofascial tension is obtained. Because of the insertion of the posterior scalene muscle upon the second rib a decrease of tension can frequently be obtained by sidebending the head and neck to the left and rotating to the right. Monitor the patient's breathing and identify the phase (most often inspiratory) in which further ease of tension occurs. Instruct the patient to slowly breathe, prolonging the respiratory phase that provides the greatest decrease of tension. Await a complete release.

### Alternative procedure

Patient seated on the side of the table.

Practitioner standing behind the patient.

Place your left hand in such a way that the pad of your thumb contacts the angle of the second rib just superior to the scapula. Your right thumb and index finger, or index and middle fingers contact either side of the spinous process of T2. Listen to the motion between the second rib and T2, and follow these motions in the direction of ease until a point of balanced ligamentous and myofascial tension is obtained, and await a complete release.

## Thoracic inlet procedure

### Indications

Dysfunction of the osseous and myofascial components of the thoracic inlet; thoracic outlet syndrome; decreased thoracic cage compliance complicating cardiopulmonary diseases; venous and lymphatic congestion. Because the thoracic cage is suspended from the thoracic inlet, dysfunction of the thoracic inlet can globally affect thoracic cage compliance.

### Procedure (Fig. 3.58)

**Patient supine.**

Practitioner seated at the head of the table.

Place your hands on the patient's shoulders so that your thumbs bilaterally contact the transverse processes of T2 and the second ribs, your index fingers bilaterally contact the first ribs, and your

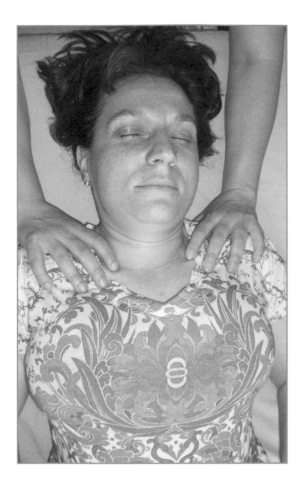

Figure 3.58: Hand placement for thoracic inlet release

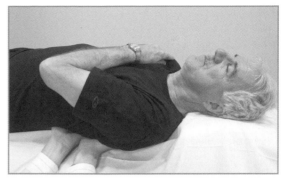

Figure 3.59: Hand placement for rib raising in the supine position

# Rib raising procedure

## Indications

Passive congestion of the lungs; pneumonia; bronchitis.

## Procedure (Fig. 3.59)

**Patient supine.**

Practitioner seated at the side of the table, at the level of the patient's chest.

Slide your hands, palms up, beneath the patient's chest with your fingers directed medially, so that they contact the posterior aspect of the ribs lateral to the costotransverse joints. Observe the patient's resting respiration. As they exhale, flex your fingers, lifting the patient's rib angles in an anterior direction, augmenting the expiratory motion of the thoracic cage. As the patient begins to inhale slowly relax your hands. This process may be repeated several times. Reposition your hands up, or down, along the rib cage and repeat the procedure. When one side of the chest has been treated, move to the patient's other side and apply the same procedure.

## Alternative seated procedure (Fig. 3.60)

Patient seated in a chair or on the side of the treatment table.

Practitioner standing facing the patient.

The patient folds their arms and leans forward, lifting their arms so that they may be placed upon your anterior chest at the pectoral level. With your hands, bilaterally reach around the patient's chest

other fingers rest upon the clavicles. Your thumbs follow rotation and sidebending of T2 and associated second rib motion. The remainder of each hand globally follows rotation left/right, anterior/posterior and lateral translation, and elevation/depression of the thoracic inlet.

When one side of the thoracic inlet is elevated, the opposite side is typically depressed. Listen to the motion of these structures, and follow them until a point of balanced ligamentous and myofascial tension is obtained. Observe the patient's breathing and identify the phase in which further ease of tension occurs. Ask the patient to breathe slowly, prolonging the respiratory phase that provides the greatest decrease of tension. Await a complete release.

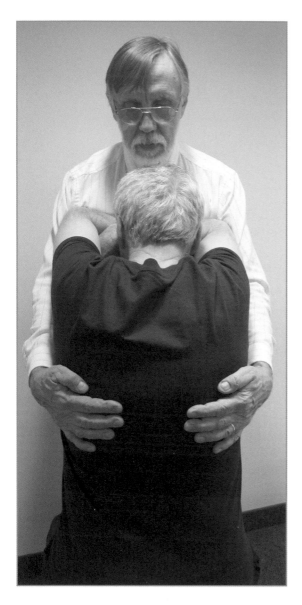

Figure 3.60: Hand placement for rib raising in the seated position

so that your finger tips are directed medially over the patient's paravertebral musculature. Instruct the patient to inhale and, as they do so, lean back, gently drawing your hands bilaterally in an anterolateral direction over the paravertebral muscles. This further flexes the patient's shoulders, decreases the thoracic kyphosis, and augments the patient's inspiratory effort. As the patient exhales,

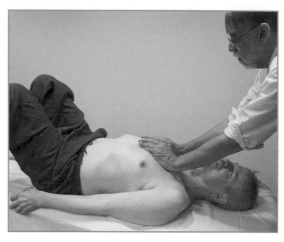

Figure 3.61: Hand placement for the thoracic pump

return to the starting position, move your hands up or down the spine, and repeat the procedure.

## Thoracic pump, oscillatory modification

### Indications

Pulmonary congestive disorders including bronchitis and pneumonia. Note: This procedure is contraindicated in the presence of pulmonary neoplasia; pneumothorax; pulmonary cancer; and thoracic cage injury.

### Procedure (Fig. 3.61)

**Patient supine.**
Practitioner standing at the head of the table.
    Place your hands palm down on the upper anterior chest wall just below the clavicles, with your fingers directed inferiorly and medially along and over the sternum. In female patients, the hand placement should be superior and medial to the breast tissue. Direct contact with the breast is not appropriate; it is often uncomfortable for the patient, and provides no therapeutic advantage. Instruct the patient to inhale and exhale deeply, and at the end of the exhalation, compress and relax the thoracic cage at a rate of 60–120 compressions per minute. This rate will be determined by the compliance and rebound of the

thorax to the pumping compressions. According to patient comfort, after three to five seconds, stop the compressions, and have the patient breathe deeply and repeat the process.

### Remarks

According to Facto, during the application of this procedure, the location of the sympathetic ganglia, in close relation to the heads of the ribs, will result in vasomotor, motor, and trophic reactions affect-ing the tissues supplied by them. This application may also have an influence upon the spinal cord, relieving congestion through increasing the venous and lymphatic drainage and thereby tending to normalize segmental function.[13]

The rate of application has ranged from 4–120 per minute. The consensus seems to be that the most comfortable, and probably the most useful rate is around the normal respiratory rate.[14]

# Thoracoabdominal diaphragm procedures

## Thoracoabdominal diaphragm procedure

### Indications

Thoracoabdominal diaphragm somatic dysfunction seen with decreased respiratory motion contributing to pulmonary dysfunction; cardiac dysfunction; venous and lymphatic congestion. Psychoemotional stress is frequently associated with thoracoabdominal diaphragm dysfunction.

Note: The practitioner is urged to recognize that this procedure, and any other procedure, when employed to address pulmonary, cardiac, and psychoemotional disorders must be used in an adjunctive or integrative fashion. Underlying pulmonary, cardiac, and psychiatric disorders and disease must first be diagnosed and treated with appropriate recognized medical management.

### Procedure (Fig. 3.62)

**Patient supine.**
Practitioner standing to either side of the table at the level of the patient's abdomen facing toward the patient's head.

Place your hands bilaterally upon the patient's lower thoracic cage in such a manner that the thumbs, pointed cephalically, contact the inferior medial edge of the costal cartilages of ribs seven to ten. Your fingers should extend posterolaterally along the bodies of the ribs bilaterally. As the patient breathes quietly, visualize the dome shaped diaphragm and listen to the motion of its

components (sternal, ribs, and lumbar). When a portion of the diaphragm is found to demonstrate restricted motion, follow that portion into expiration, thereby unloading the muscular fibers between their circumferential origin and their insertion upon the central tendon. When a position of myofascial balance is obtained, instruct the

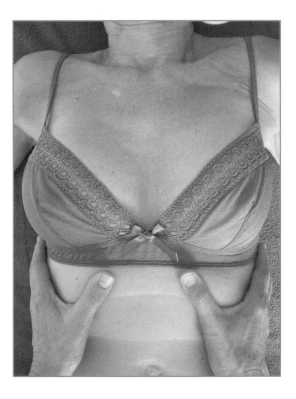

Figure 3.62: Hand placement for diagnosis and treatment of diaphragmatic dysfunction

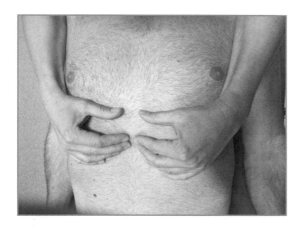

Figure 3.63: Alternative hand placement for diagnosis and treatment of diaphragmatic dysfunction

patient to slowly exhale and to hold their breath in exhalation as long as comfortably possible, and await a release.

### Alternative hand placement (Fig. 3.63)

Practitioner standing at the head the table facing toward the patient's chest.

Place your hands bilaterally upon the patient's lower thoracic cage in such a manner that the pads of the index, middle, ring, and small fingers bilaterally contact the inferior costal margins. The palms of the hands and the thumbs rest comfortably upon the anterior aspect of the lower rib cage. As the patient breathes quietly, listen to the motion of the diaphragm and rib cage. When one side of the diaphragm is found to demonstrate restricted motion, follow that portion into expiration. When a position of myofascial balance is obtained, instruct the patient to slowly exhale and to hold their breath in exhalation as long as comfortably possible. It may be necessary to repeat this process several times in order to obtain a complete release.

### Remarks

If the practitioner listens to the tissues and follows them effectively into the position of myofascial balance, spontaneous respiratory cooperation, on the part of the patient, frequently occurs with perfect timing and dosage, making it unnecessary to request respiratory cooperation. This process often occurs in synchrony with the PRM.

When diaphragmatic dysfunction involving the crura is identified, it is often the result of thoracolumbar spinal dysfunction that must be addressed before release of the diaphragm can be obtained. Conversely, primary diaphragmatic dysfunction can result in thoracolumbar spinal dysfunction that is resistant to treatment.

Because of the link between the three diaphragms (cranial, thoracolumbar, pelvic), any dysfunction affecting one of these diaphragms can affect the other two. As such, any of the bones upon which the cranial or pelvic diaphragms attach may be a source for dysfunction of the thoracoabdominal diaphragm. This is frequently encountered with temporal bone dysfunctions.

## Thoracoabdominal hemidiaphragm procedure

Although this procedure can effectively treat all portions of the diaphragm, it allows the practitioner to more readily address dysfunctions involving the crura and posterior portion of the diaphragm.

### Procedure (Fig. 3.64)

**Patient supine.**

Practitioner seated on the side of the dysfunctional hemidiaphragm at the level of the patient's abdomen facing toward the patient's head.

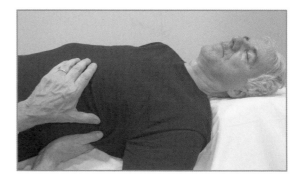

Figure 3.64: Hand placement for diagnosis and treatment of hemidiaphragmatic dysfunction

One hand is placed palm up, upon the table, beneath the patient's lower thoracic cage in such a manner that the index, middle, and ring fingers contact the spinous processes of T12–L2. The other hand is placed anteriorly over the ipsilateral lower thoracic cage, with the fingers pointing medially toward the sternum, and the thumb directed posteriorly along the inferior costal margin. As the patient breathes quietly, visualize the hemidiaphragm and listen to the motion of its components (sternal, costal, and lumbar). Follow the dysfunctional portion of the hemidiaphragm into expiration, unloading the muscular fibers between their circumferential origin and their insertion upon the central tendon. When a position of myofascial balance is obtained, instruct the patient to slowly exhale and to hold their breath in exhalation as long as comfortably possible and await a release. Once one side has been treated, repeat the procedure, as necessary, with the other hemidiaphragm.

# Cervical procedures

Because dysfunction in the cervical area can be the result of viscerosomatic reflexes, it should prompt the practitioner to seriously look for, and rule out, underlying visceral pathology. See further: 'Vertebral somatic dysfunction' in 'Section 4: Clinical considerations, Chapter 1: Musculoskeletal dysfunctions, Part 1: Axial system,' p. 183.

Additionally, because of the potential for vertebral artery compression and resultant cerebral ischemia, extreme caution should be exercised when employing combinations of extension, side-bending, and rotation when manipulating the cervical spine. Treatment procedures should never be applied to or through areas of spinal instability, hypermobility, or spinal levels with neurological compression.

## Occipitoatlantal procedures

### Indications

Occipitoatlantal dysfunction; suboccipital headaches; high cervical proprioceptive dysfunction; greater occipital nerve (nerve of Arnold) entrapment; pharyngeal and anterior myofascial dysfunction, as might be seen in sleep apnea, snoring, and swallowing dysfunction; vagal and trigeminal somatovisceral reflexes.

### Supine procedure (Fig. 3.65)

Patient supine with the top of their head in contact with the practitioner's sternum.

Practitioner seated at the head the table.

Place both hands beneath the occiput in such a way that the distal pads of the index, middle, and

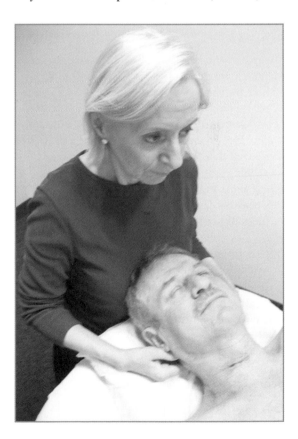

Figure 3.65: Hand placement for diagnosis and treatment of occipitoatlantal dysfunction in the supine position

ring fingers are in contact with, and extend as low as possible on, the squamous portion of the occiput, medial to the occipitomastoid suture. Compressive forces over the occipitomastoid suture are to be avoided. Contact the lateral masses of C1 with the tips of your thumbs. Visualize the occipital condyles and the articulation between C0 and C1. Listen to the motion to identify any dysfunctional pattern (restricted flexion, extension, rotation, and sidebending right/left; translatory motion right/left, or anterior/posterior, or both). Follow the identified motions in the direction of ease until a point of balanced ligamentous and myofascial tension is obtained. You may facilitate the introduction of occipital sidebending through the contact between the top of the patient's head and your sternum. The release of the dysfunction may be enhanced by the use of a pumping action that respects the inherent motility of the PRM. Await a complete release.

### Remarks

The occipital condyles are not accessible for direct palpation; therefore, their relationship with the atlas should be visualized during the entire procedure. When holding the skull one has to recognize that the condyles are not caudal to the tips of the examiner's fingers but rather are located anteriorly deep and somewhat superior to the tips of the fingers.

When examining the occiput and atlas, the movements induced are, too often, transmitted to the level of C3 or lower because of lack of precision in palpation and the use of force and amplitude that is too great. Because of the frequent restriction of mobility in the craniocervical junction, the movements induced must be very small.

Occipital rotation is most often associated with contralateral sidebending. During this procedure, a finding of heterolateral sidebending may be indicative of a dysfunction involving a lower cervical articulation.

### Seated procedure (Fig. 3.66)

**Patient seated on a chair.**
Practitioner standing to either side of the patient.
Place the pads of the thumb and index finger of your posterior, listening hand at the level of C1, between the occipital squama and the spinous

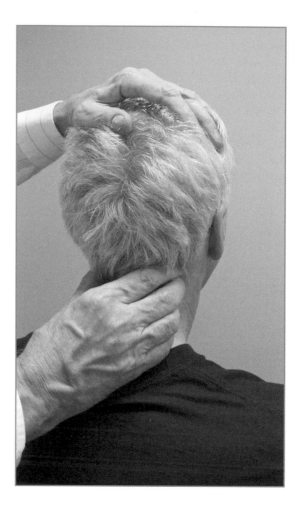

Figure 3.66: Hand placement for diagnosis and treatment of occipitoatlantal dysfunction in the seated position

process of C2. Place your anterior, active hand lightly on the top of the patient's head. Listen to the motion between C0 and C1, to identify any dysfunctional pattern (restricted flexion, extension, rotation, and sidebending right/left; translatory motion right/left, or anterior/posterior, or both). Follow the identified motions in the direction of ease until a point of balanced ligamentous and myofascial tension is obtained, and await a complete release.

### Remarks

Hand placement must be accomplished with the lightest possible touch that still allows for effective listening. Patients are often fragile and compression of the occipitoatlantal joint and the remainder of the cervical spine must be avoided. Because of the effort on the part of the patient holding their head up, the associated muscular tension can interfere with listening. Too heavy hand placement will cause the patient to increase muscular tone further limiting effective listening. Light touch not only facilitates listening, but it also helps to establish trust on the part of the patient between the patient and practitioner.

Following prolonged periods of somatic dysfunction with limitation of motion, patients often develop functional amnesia. They lose the ability to move the dysfunctional area through its full range of motion and consequently lose proprioception. Although this is true throughout the body, it is particularly significant in the high cervical region, and even though the dysfunction may have been effectively resolved, the patient will continue to move in the dysfunctional pattern and demonstrate continued proprioceptive impairment. For this reason it becomes imperative to rehabilitate the patient's capacity to move consciously through the full range of motion thereby regaining optimal proprioception.[15]

## Atlantoaxial procedure

### Indications

Atlantoaxial dysfunction; suboccipital headaches; high cervical proprioceptive dysfunction; greater occipital nerve (nerve of Arnold) entrapment; vagal and trigeminal somatovisceral reflexes.

### Procedure (Fig. 3.67)

Patient supine with the top of their head in contact with the practitioner's sternum.

Practitioner seated at the head the table.

Place both hands beneath the occiput in such a way that you contact the lateral masses of C1 with your thumbs and the lateral aspects of C2 with your index or middle fingers. Visualize the articulation between C1 and C2. Listen to the motion to identify any dysfunctional pattern (restricted flexion, extension, rotation, and sidebending right/left; translatory motion right/left, or anterior/posterior, or both). Follow the identi-

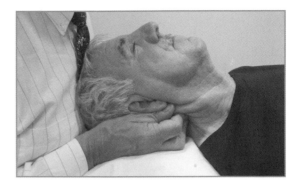

Figure 3.67: Hand placement for diagnosis and treatment of atlantoaxial dysfunction

fied motions in the direction of ease until a point of balanced ligamentous and myofascial tension is obtained. You may facilitate the introduction of atlantal sidebending through the contact between the top of the patient's head and your sternum. The release of the dysfunction may be enhanced by the use of a pumping action that respects the inherent motility of the PRM. Await a complete release.

### Remarks

Contact between the top of the patient's head and the practitioner's sternum allows one to establish a functional unit between C0 and C1. This permits you to relax your hands and to more effectively listen to C1–C2. It must be recognized that this should be done with the lightest possible contact between the patient and the practitioner's sternum.

Although the major motion of C1 upon C2 is rotation, it has long been recognized that sidebending and translations are present as minor motions in the articular relationship.[16] The incorporation of the minor motions into the procedure greatly enhances the efficacy of the treatment.

## Typical cervical vertebrae procedures

### Indications

Cervical somatic dysfunction; torticollis; headaches; anterior myofascial dysfunction, as might be seen in sleep apnea, snoring, and swallowing

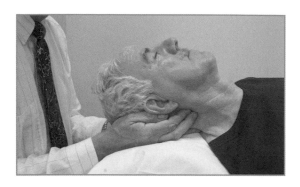

Figure 3.68: Hand placement for diagnosis and treatment of cervical dysfunction in the supine position

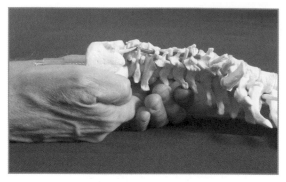

Figure 3.69: Alternative hand placement for diagnosis and treatment of cervical dysfunction in the supine position

dysfunction; cervico-ocular reflex dysfunction; C2, vagal, and trigeminal somatovisceral reflexes; C3–C5 phrenic nerve dysfunction.

### Supine procedure

(Example: C3–C4 dysfunction. (Fig. 3.68))

**Patient supine.**
Practitioner seated at the head the table.

Cradle the patient's head with both hands in such a way that the tips of the index fingers contact the transverse processes of C3 and the tips of the middle fingers monitor the intervertebral space between C3 and C4. Visualize the articular relationship between C3 and C4. Listen to the motion to identify any dysfunctional pattern (restricted flexion, extension, rotation, and sidebending right/left; translatory motion right/left, or anterior/posterior, or both). If necessary, to clarify the dysfunctional pattern, you may employ the palms of your hands through contact with the patient's head to gently introduce motion down to C3–C4. Follow the identified motions in the direction of ease until a point of balanced ligamentous and myofascial tension is obtained. If necessary, the use of a pumping action that respects the inherent motility of the PRM will enhance the acquisition of a release.

### Alternative supine procedure

(Example: C3–C4 dysfunction. (Fig. 3.69))

**Patient supine.**
Practitioner seated at the head the table.

Cradle the patient's head by placing one hand, palm up, transversely beneath the occiput, using caution not to compress the occipitomastoid sutures. This hand is your active hand. Place the other hand, your listening hand, palm up transversely upon the table, so that the pads of the index and middle fingers respectively contact the spinous processes of C4 and C3. Visualize the articular relationship between C3 and C4. Listen to the motion to identify any dysfunctional pattern (restricted flexion, extension, rotation, and sidebending right/left; translatory motion right/left, or anterior/posterior, or both). Employ indirect principles and take C3 upon C4 in the direction of ease, by introducing flexion or extension, sidebending, and rotation from above using your active hand. With your listening hand, monitor C3–C4 until a point of myofascial and ligamentous balance is established. If necessary, a pumping action maintaining synchronicity with the PRM will facilitate the release.

### Seated procedure

(Example: **C5–C6** dysfunction. (Fig. 3.70))
Patient seated on a chair.

Practitioner standing on either side of the patient.

Place the pads of the index and middle fingers of your posterior, listening hand, in such a manner that they are on each side of the spinous process of C5. Place your anterior, active hand lightly upon the top of the patient's head. Listen to the motion between C5 and C6, to identify any dysfunctional pattern (restricted flexion, exten-

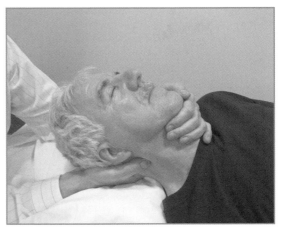

Figure 3.71: Hand placement for cervical fascia release

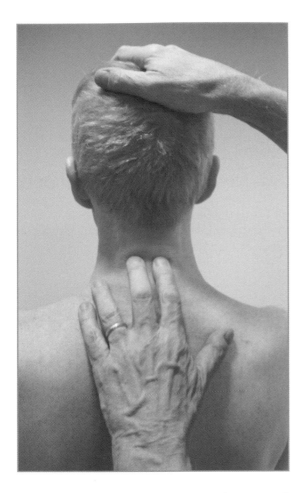

Figure 3.70: Hand placement for diagnosis and treatment of cervical dysfunction in the seated position

sion, rotation, and sidebending right/left; translatory motion right/left, or anterior/posterior, or both). If necessary, to clarify the dysfunctional pattern, you may introduce subtle motions from above with your anterior, active hand. Follow the identified motions in the direction of ease until a point of balanced ligamentous and myofascial tension is obtained. Wait for a complete release.

## Remarks

When introducing motion from above, it is extremely important that you focus upon the level of cervical dysfunction. Failure to do this can potentially provide confusing information involving structures above the area being diagnosed or treated.

## Anterior cervical fascial procedures

### Indications

Dysfunctional tensions in the cervical fasciae as might be seen in sleep apnea, snoring, swallowing, and vocal dysfunction; thoracic inlet syndrome; torticollis; headaches; lymphatic and venous congestion of the head and neck. Cervical fascial balancing may be appropriate when treating dysfunctions affecting any of its osseous attachments, including the clavicles, sternum, occiput, temporal bones, mandible, hyoid bone, and cervical vertebrae.

### Supine procedure (Fig. 3.71)

**Patient supine.**
Practitioner seated at the head the table.

Cradle the patient's occiput with one hand, and place your other hand palm down transversely in contact with the anterior aspect of the patient's neck. Listen to the tension within the cervical soft tissues and with both hands, using indirect principles, follow the tissues until myofascial balance is obtained. Await a release.

### Alternative supine procedure (Fig. 3.72)

**Patient supine.**
Practitioner seated at the head of the table.

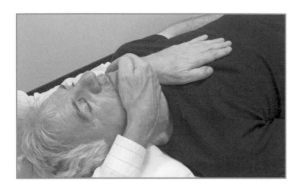

Figure 3.72: Alternative hand placement for cervical fascia release

Cradle the mandible with one hand and place the other hand palm down upon the sternum in such a manner that the fingers are directed caudally, and the thenar and hypothenar eminences contact the medial aspects of the clavicles. Listen to the tension within the cervical soft tissues and with both hands, using indirect principles, follow the tissues until myofascial balance is obtained. Await a release.

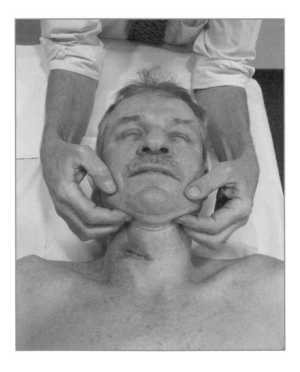

Figure 3.73: Hand placement for submandibular release

## Submandibular procedure (Fig. 3.73)

### Patient supine.

Practitioner seated at the head the table.

Curl your fingers bilaterally around the inferior border of the body of the mandible in such a manner that the pads of your fingers contact the mandibular attachment of the superficial cervical fascia. Yours thumbs should contact the lateral aspects of the mandible in the area of the mental foramina. With your fingers, palpate for areas of dysfunctional fascial tension. Listen to the mandibular and submandibular soft tissues and, using indirect principles, follow them until myofascial balance is obtained. Await a release.

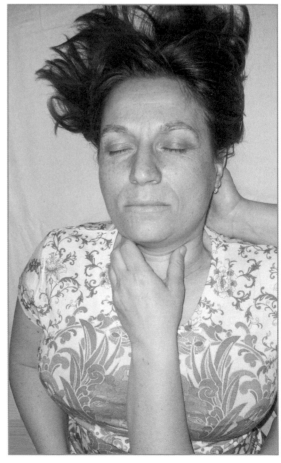

Figure 3.74: Hand placement for diagnosis and treatment of hyoid bone dysfunction

### Hyoid bone procedure (Fig. 3.74)

**Patient supine.**
Practitioner seated at the side of the table.

Cradle the patient's occiput with your cephalic hand, and with your caudal hand bilaterally contacting the greater cornua, hold the hyoid bone between your thumb and index finger. Listen to the tension within the soft tissues surrounding the hyoid bone. If necessary, subtly introduce superior/inferior, lateral right/left, and torsional motions to clarify the pattern. Using both hands, employ indirect principles to follow the tissues until myofascial balance is obtained. Await a release.

### Laryngeal procedure

Using the patient and practitioner positioning described above for the hyoid bone, the larynx may be treated by shifting the position of the caudal hand from contact with the hyoid to contact with the laryngeal cartilages and following the procedure as described.

### Remarks

The anterior structures of the neck, the larynx, trachea, and carotid arteries, are vulnerable to compression. The carotid sinus, in particular, can be stimulated by palpation, resulting in large decreases in heart rate, blood pressure, or both. Consequently, these procedures must be performed using the very lightest contact to avoid compression, or even the patient's perception of possible compression. If the patient is concerned, they will not relax.

## Upper extremity procedures

## Upper extremity global myofascial release

### Indications

Myofascial, or articular pain, or both and dysfunction anywhere within the upper extremity, including rotator cuff syndrome, lateral and medial epicondylitis, ulnar nerve entrapment, radioulnar dysfunction, and carpal tunnel syndrome.

### Procedure (Fig. 3.75)

**Patient seated.**
Practitioner seated beside the patient on the side of the dysfunction.

Hold the wrist with your caudal hand. Place your cephalic hand on the patient's shoulder, with your thumb contacting the acromion and your fingers directed anteriorly contacting the clavicle. Listen, and paying attention to the PRM, allow the entire extremity to move into a position of myofascial and ligamentous ease—most often a torsional pattern along the long axis of the limb that may require various positional combinations of the wrist, forearm (pronation or supination), elbow, and shoulder. Await a release.

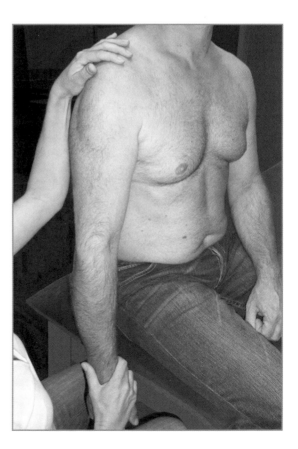

Figure 3.75: Hand placement for upper extremity global myofascial release

### Remarks

This hand position allows you also to monitor the acromioclavicular joint, and if necessary, you may position the upper extremity in such a way to act upon the acromion to normalize the acromioclavicular joint.

## Clavicular procedures

### Indications

Acromioclavicular, or sternoclavicular dysfunction, or both, often presenting as shoulder, neck or anterior chest complaints and potentially affecting upper extremity, head, and neck mechanics; thoracic outlet syndrome; rotator cuff syndrome; subclavius muscle spasm. The treatment of clavicular dysfunctions may be employed when addressing venous and lymphatic congestion in the upper extremity and upper respiratory tract condition.

### Sternoclavicular procedure

(Example: sternoclavicular dysfunction right.)

**Patient supine.**
Practitioner seated at the head of the treatment table.

With the thumb and index finger of your left hand, hold the clavicle at the sternoclavicular joint. With your right hand, hold the patient's right elbow in such a manner that you cradle the olecranon process. Introduce flexion/extension, abduction/adduction, external/internal rotation, and elevation/depression of the shoulder until optimal myofascial and ligamentous balance of the sternoclavicular joint is obtained, and await release.

### Remarks

The above procedure may be performed with the patient seated and the practitioner standing beside or behind the patient, on the side of the dysfunction.

The motions introduced through the arm should be very small, but sufficient enough to affect sternoclavicular myofascial and ligamentous tension.

By positioning the fingers in contact with the sternoclavicular joint, in such a way that they also contact the anterior chest as low as the second or third ribs, this procedure can be employed to address sternoclavicular, upper sternocostal, subclavius muscle, and clavipectoral fascia dysfunctions. (Fig. 3.76)

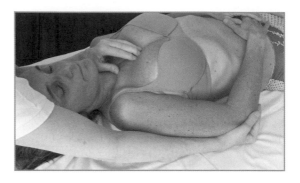

Figure 3.76: Hand placement for sternoclavicular joint and clavipectoral fascia release

### Bilateral sternoclavicular procedure (Fig. 3.77)

**Patient supine.**
Practitioner seated at the head of the treatment table.

With the thumb and index finger of both hands, hold the clavicles at the sternoclavicular joints bi-

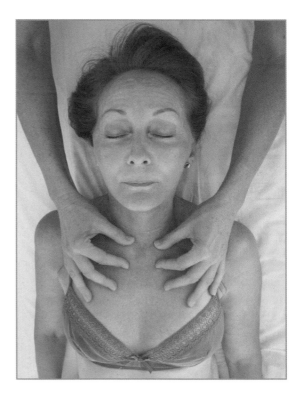

Figure 3.77: Hand placement for bilateral sternoclavicular procedure

laterally. Listen to the motion between the clavicles and sternum, and between the two clavicles. Follow it to the position of optimal myofascial and ligamentous balance of the sternoclavicular joints, and await release.

### Remarks

The above procedure may be performed with the patient seated and the practitioner standing directly behind the patient.

This procedure is particularly useful when addressing cervical fascial dysfunctions.

### Acromioclavicular procedure

(Example: left acromioclavicular dysfunction. (Fig. 3.78))

**Patient supine.**
Practitioner standing on the side of the dysfunction.

With the middle finger of your right hand upon the acromion, hold the lateral portion of the left clavicle with your thumb and index finger. With the patient's left elbow flexed, cradle the extensor surface of their arm with your left hand. Introduce flexion/extension, abduction/adduction, external/internal rotation, and elevation/depression of the shoulder until optimal myofascial and ligamentous balance of the acromioclavicular joint is obtained, and await release.

### Remarks

The above procedure may be performed with the patient seated and the practitioner standing beside or behind the patient, on the side of the dysfunction.

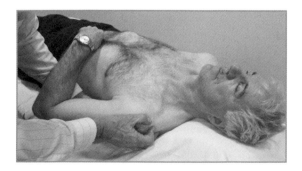

Figure 3.78: Hand placement for diagnosis and treatment of acromioclavicular dysfunction

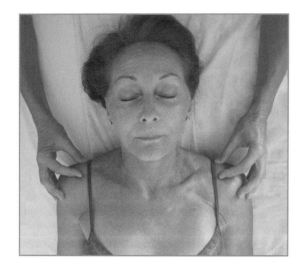

Figure 3.79: Hand placement for bilateral acromioclavicular procedure

The motions introduced through the arm should be very small, but sufficient enough to affect acromioclavicular myofascial and ligamentous tension.

### Bilateral acromioclavicular procedure (Fig. 3.79)

**Patient supine.**
Practitioner seated at the head of the treatment table.

With the thumb and index finger of both hands, bilaterally hold the lateral portions of the clavicles. Listen to the motion between the clavicles and acromion processes, and between the two clavicles. Follow it to the position of optimal myofascial and ligamentous balance of the acromioclavicular joints and await release.

### Remarks

The above procedure may be performed with the patient seated and the practitioner standing directly behind the patient.

This procedure is particularly useful when addressing cervical fascial dysfunctions.

### Combined sternoclavicular and acromioclavicular procedure

(Example: right clavicular dysfunction. (Fig. 3.80))

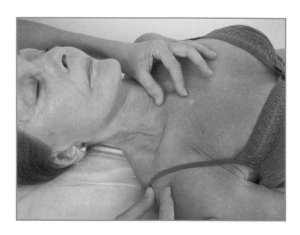

Figure 3.80: Hand placement for combined sternoclavicular and acromioclavicular procedure

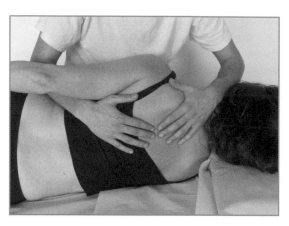

Figure 3.81: Hand placement for scapular release

**Patient supine.**
Practitioner seated at the head of the table.

With the thumb and index finger of your left hand, hold the clavicle at the sternoclavicular joint. With the thumb and index finger of your right hand, hold the clavicle at the acromioclavicular joint. Follow in the direction of unrestricted clavicular motion until a point of myofascial and ligamentous balance is obtained. Maintain synchronicity with the PRM and await a release.

### Remarks

The above procedure may be performed with the patient seated and the practitioner standing behind the patient on the side of the dysfunction.

## Scapular procedure

### Indications

Scapulothoracic dysfunction with resultant levator scapulae, glenohumeral, acromioclavicular, or thoracic or cervical spinal dysfunctions; myofascial or articular pain, or both and dysfunction of the shoulder including rotator cuff syndrome.

### Procedure

(Example: left scapular release. (Fig. 3.81))

Patient lying on their right side with their hips and knees flexed for comfort and positional stability, and with one or several pillows, as necessary, supporting their head and cervical spine.

Practitioner standing beside the treatment table in front of the patient, at the level of the shoulder.

Place your right forearm between the patient's left arm and thoracic cage, allowing your thumb to contact the lateral scapular border, and your index finger, the medial border, thereby giving you control of the inferior angle of the scapula. Your left hand should rest palm down, with your fingers directed caudally along the medial scapular border and your thumb resting upon the superior border of the scapular spine. This hand placement allows you to listen to the scapula and scapulothoracic myofascial structures. Listen and visualize these structures and follow the motion felt (superior/inferior, medial/lateral, and clockwise/counter clockwise glides) into the position of ligamentous and myofascial balance. Wait for a release. If necessary, the release may be enhanced by employing a pumping action between your two hands.

## Glenohumeral procedure

### Indications

Myofascial or articular pain, or both and dysfunction of the shoulder including rotator cuff syndrome.

### Procedure (Fig. 3.82)
**Patient seated.**
Practitioner seated or standing beside the patient on the side of the dysfunction.

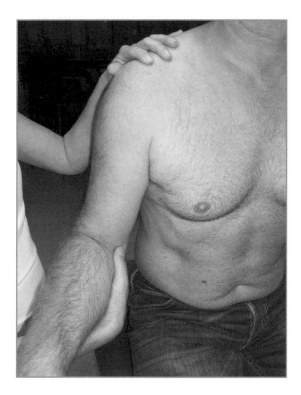

Figure 3.82: Hand placement for diagnosis and treatment of glenohumeral dysfunction

Place your posterior hand upon the patient's shoulder with your thumb contacting the acromion, and your fingers resting upon the clavicle. With your other hand, flex the patient's elbow and cradle their forearm in such a way that you hold the distal humerus between your thumb and fingers. From this position, listen to the motions at the glenohumeral joint (flexion/extension, abduction/adduction, external/internal rotation, and the minor motions of anterior/posterior glide, lateral/medial glide, cephalocaudal glide, and compression/distraction). Visualize the relationship between the humeral head and the glenoid fossa during this process. Follow each of the coupled motions in the direction of unrestricted motion, stacking them until the final position of ligamentous and myofascial balance is obtained. At this point, while maintaining the position of balance, listen to and follow the PRM, and wait for a release.

### Remarks

The hand placement with fingers contacting the acromion and lateral portion of the clavicle allows the practitioner to monitor the acromioclavicular as well as the glenohumeral joints. By approximating the spine of the scapula and the clavicle, you reduce tension in the coracoacromial arch, facilitating release of the rotator cuff.

This procedure may also be performed with the patient supine.

## Elbow procedures

### Indications

Lateral or medial epicondylalgia; epicondylitis; forearm tightness; wrist pain.

### Ulnohumeral procedure

(Example: left ulnohumeral dysfunction. (Fig. 3.83))

**Patient seated.**
Practitioner seated or standing in front of the patient toward the side of the dysfunction.

The patient's left elbow should be sufficiently flexed and their forearm neutrally positioned, in such a manner that you can hold their hand between your lateral chest and arm with their palm contacting the inner aspect of your left arm. With your left hand, hold their left olecranon process between your thumb and index, or middle finger. With your right hand placed just proximal to the el-

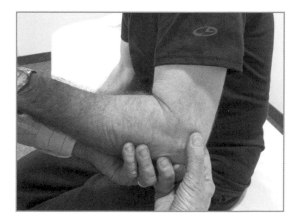

Figure 3.83: Hand placement for diagnosis and treatment of ulnohumeral dysfunction

bow and posteriorly upon the distal humerus, hold the medial and lateral epicondyles between your thumb and index, or middle finger. Listen to the ulnohumeral relationship from the perspective of the olecranon process. It may be assessed further by introducing very small amounts of ulnohumeral flexion/extension. Normally, flexion is combined with minor motions of adduction and external rotation of the ulna, while extension is combined with abduction and internal rotation. Follow each of the coupled motions in the direction of ease, stacking them until the final position of ligamentous and myofascial balance is obtained. Await a release.

### Remarks

Remember that when ulnar abduction is introduced, the tip of the olecranon process moves medially, and with adduction the olecranon process moves laterally.

### Radiohumeral procedure

(Example: left radiohumeral dysfunction. (Fig. 3.84))

**Patient seated.**
Practitioner seated or standing in front of the patient toward the side of the dysfunction.

The patient's left elbow should be sufficiently flexed and their forearm neutrally positioned, in such a manner that you can hold their hand between your lateral chest and arm with their palm

contacting the inner aspect of your left arm. With your left hand placed just proximal to the elbow, and posteriorly upon the distal humerus, hold the medial and lateral epicondyles between your thumb and index, or middle finger. With your right hand, hold the radial head between your thumb and index finger. Listen to the motion of the radial head in relation to the capitulum of the humerus, in the context of anterior/posterior glide, medial/lateral glide, external/internal rotation, and compression/decompression. Stacking the motions, follow them in the direction of ease, and await a release.

### Radioulnar procedure

(Example: left radioulnar dysfunction. (Fig. 3.85))

**Patient seated.**
Practitioner seated or standing in front of the patient toward the side of the dysfunction.

The patient's left elbow should be sufficiently flexed and their forearm neutrally positioned, in such a manner that you can hold their hand between your lateral chest and arm with their palm contacting the inner aspect of your left arm. With your left hand, hold their left olecranon process between your thumb and index, or middle finger. With your right hand, hold the radial head between your thumb and index finger. Listen to the motion of the radial head in relation to the radial notch of the ulna in the context of anterior/posterior glide and external/internal rotation. Follow

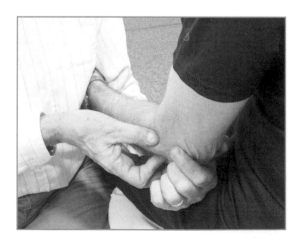

Figure 3.84: Hand placement for diagnosis and treatment of radiohumeral dysfunction

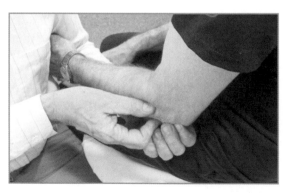

Figure 3.85: Hand placement for diagnosis and treatment of radioulnar dysfunction

the motions, stacking them in the direction of ease, and await a release.

### Remarks

The elbow constitutes a complex relationship between the humerus, ulna, and radius. The combination of motions between these bones results in flexion/extension of the elbow and pronation/supination of the forearm. Pronation is associated with flexion of the elbow and posterior glide of the radial head, while supination combines elbow extension and anterior glide of the radial head.

Although the major ulnohumeral motion is flexion/extension, the ulna often becomes dysfunctional in abduction/adduction. Ulnar abduction compresses the radial head against the humerus capitulum, forcing the radius distally, stressing the interosseous membrane and producing a tendency for adduction at the wrist. Ulnar adduction decompresses the radial head and capitulum, producing a tendency for abduction at the wrist.

Typically, ulnohumeral abduction or adduction will constitute the primary somatic dysfunction of the elbow. It should be treated or ruled out before addressing radiohumeral, radioulnar, interosseous membrane, and wrist dysfunctions. Similarly, radioulnar dysfunctions should be treated or ruled out before addressing interosseous membrane and wrist dysfunctions.

The visualization of tensions within the interosseous membrane greatly augments the diagnosis and treatment of the elbow (and wrist), often facilitating the release of otherwise resistant dysfunctions.

# Wrist and hand procedures

## Global wrist procedure

### Indications

Wrist dysfunction and pain; carpal tunnel syndrome; writer's cramp.

### Procedure

(Example: left wrist dysfunction. (Fig. 3.86))

Patient seated on a chair beside the treatment table in such a way that they can rest their forearm on the table with their wrist positioned beyond the edge of the table. This allows complete relaxation of the patient's forearm, wrist, and hand.
Practitioner seated in front of the patient.

Hold the radial aspect of the wrist with your left hand and the ulnar aspect with your right hand, in such a way that your thumbs contact the dorsal surface of the carpal bones and your fingers the palmar surface. Listen to the relationship between the ulna, radius, and carpal bones. If necessary, introduce the smallest amounts of flexion/extension and adduction/abduction. Follow these motions in the direction of ligamentous and myofascial balance and wait until a release is obtained.

## Myofascial palmar fascia procedure

### Indications

Wrist dysfunction and pain; carpal tunnel syndrome; writer's cramp; flexor retinaculum dysfunction.

### Procedure (Fig. 3.87)

Patient seated on a chair beside the treatment table in such a way that they can rest their forearm

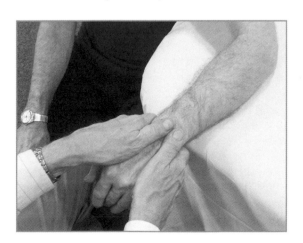

Figure 3.86: Hand placement for global wrist release

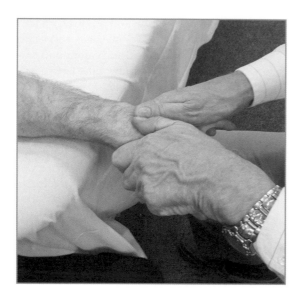

Figure 3.87: Hand placement for palmar fascia release

on the table with their wrist positioned beyond the edge of the table.

Practitioner seated in front of the patient.

Hold the radial aspect of the wrist with your left hand and the ulnar aspect with your right hand, so that your thumbs contact the dorsal surface of the carpal bones and your fingers, on the palmar surface, contact the medial and lateral ends of the flexor retinaculum. Listen to the myofascial tension within the flexor retinaculum and follow into the position of ligamentous and myofascial balance. Employ the pumping action of the PRM to facilitate a release.

### Remarks

The efficacy of this procedure may be augmented by combining it with the global wrist and upper extremity global myofascial procedures described above.

## First metacarpophalangeal joint procedure

### Indications

Treatment of the myofascial and ligamentous tensions that lead to the development and maintenance of thumb metacarpophalangeal pain.

### Procedure

(Example: left first metacarpophalangeal dysfunction. (Fig. 3.88))

Patient seated on a chair with their left forearm resting comfortably upon the treatment table, in such a manner that their wrist extends beyond the table's edge. The patient's arm should rest upon the ulna so that the forearm is in neutral position, neither pronated nor supinated.

Practitioner seated to the patient's left, facing the palmar aspect of the patient's left hand.

With the thumb and index finger of your left hand, hold the distal aspect of the patient's first metacarpal in such a manner that your thumb contacts the palmar surface and your index finger the dorsal surface. With the thumb and index finger of your right hand, hold the metacarpal phalangeal end of the patient's first proximal phalange. Follow metacarpal phalangeal motion in the direction of freedom, most often with the thumb in external rotation, flexion, and palmar glide, until a point of myofascial and ligamentous balance is obtained. From this position, while maintaining synchronicity with the PRM, await a release.

### Remarks

This procedure may also be applied to the other metacarpophalangeal and interphalangeal joints of all of the digits.

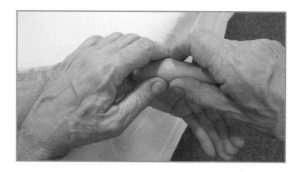

Figure 3.88: Hand placement for diagnosis and treatment of first metacarpophalangeal joint dysfunction

# Visceral procedures

"The first essential could well be voiced in Dr. Still's oft' repeated admonition, "No jabbing" the patient with the fingers. In other words, the approach should be one that would not cause the tissues of the patient to resist."[17]

Before applying any of the visceral manipulative procedures described below, a complete medical diagnosis must be obtained. Manipulative procedures should not be applied to areas of structural instability, acute inflammatory processes, or in any fashion that is inconsistent with, or disruptive to, the standard of medical care.

Inherent visceral motility is described below in the context of the Cartesian axes and cardinal planes of the body. These descriptions are reductionist simplifications of complex three-dimensional motions for the purpose of explaining the manipulative procedures.

## Gastric release procedures

### Indications

Ptosis; Glenard syndrome; delayed gastric emptying; gastroesophageal reflux.

### Supine procedure (Fig. 3.89)

**Patient supine.**
Practitioner standing beside the treatment table on the patient's left side, at the approximate level of the pelvis, facing toward the head of the table.

Place your left hand palm down with your fingers directed posterolaterally along the course of the patient's right lower ribs, and with your thumb directed cephalically contacting the lower sternum. This hand, although relatively passive throughout the procedure, is employed to monitor the right lower ribs and right hemidiaphragm. Place your right hand in a position that mirrors your left hand, but at a slightly less cephalic level, such that your thumb, directed cephalically, contacts the xiphoid process and your fingers are directed posterolaterally along the course of the left lower ribs, thus monitoring the left lower ribs and

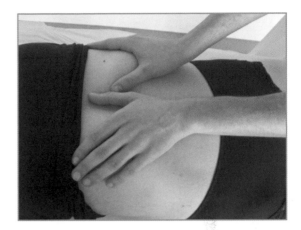

Figure 3.89: Hand placement for supine gastric release

left hemidiaphragm. The hypothenar aspect of the right palm, contacting the greater curvature of the stomach, monitors the inherent motion of the stomach.

Listen to this inherent motion, feeling for external and internal rotation, in the context of the major motion (rotation in the coronal plane, about a horizontal, anteroposterior axis, wherein the fundus is felt to move respectively in a caudal direction with an increase of the concavity of the lesser curvature of the stomach and in a cephalic direction, with a decrease of the concavity of the lesser curvature), and the minor motions (rotation in the sagittal plane, about a horizontal, transverse axis, wherein the fundus moves respectively in an anterior and posterior direction; rotation in the horizontal plane, about a vertical axis, wherein the lateral aspect of the greater curvature of the stomach alternately moves in an anterior and posterior direction).

While maintaining synchronicity with the inherent motility, follow the motion pattern of the stomach in the direction of ease, until fascial and ligamentous balance is obtained, and await a release.

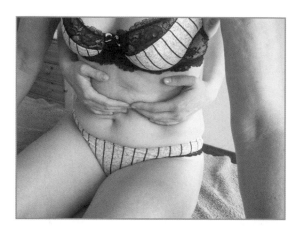

Figure 3.90: Hand placement for seated gastric release

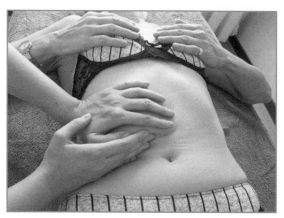

Figure 3.91: Hand placement for hepatic release and pump

### *Seated procedure* (Fig. 3.90)

**Patient seated.**

Practitioner standing behind the patient.

Place your hands bilaterally so that your hypothenar eminences cradle the inferior costal margins with your fingers directed medially. Listen to the position and inherent motion of the stomach, as described above. Maintain synchronicity with the inherent gastric motility and follow the motion pattern in the direction of ease, until fascial and ligamentous balance is obtained. Await a release.

### *Remarks*

During the process of establishing fascial and ligamentous balance, this procedure may be greatly improved by visualizing the relationship between the diaphragm and the stomach.

Gastric dysfunction may also be addressed by treating spinal somatic dysfunctions affecting the level of the spine responsible for somatovisceral influences: sympathetic, T5–T9 and parasympathetic, occiput–C2.

## Hepatic release and pump

### *Indications*

Conditions resulting in congestion of the liver; ligamentous and fascial dysfunction of the hepatic visceral peritoneum. This procedure is contraindicated in patients with hepatic malignancy, trauma, and acute hepatitis.

### *Procedure* (Fig. 3.91)

**Patient supine.**

Practitioner seated beside the treatment table on the patient's right side, at the level of the upper abdomen.

Place your left hand palm down with your fingers directed medially over the anteroinferior costal margin of the right hemithorax. Place your right hand such that the hypothenar portion of the palm and the little and ring fingers rest just below the costal margin or inferior edge of the liver. The inferior edge of the liver may be delineated by having the patient breathe deeply, while palpating with your right hand in the above position.

Listen to the inherent motion of the liver, feeling for external and internal rotation, in the context of the major motion (rotation in the coronal plane, about a horizontal, anteroposterior axis, wherein the right lobe is felt to move respectively in a caudal and cephalic direction), and the minor motions (rotation in the sagittal plane, about a horizontal, transverse axis, wherein the anterior edge of the liver moves respectively in a caudal and cephalic direction; rotation in the horizontal plane, about a vertical axis, wherein the lateral aspect of the liver alternately moves in an anterior and posterior direction).

Follow the motion pattern in the direction of ease until fascial and ligamentous balance is obtained and await a release. From this point of balance, a pumping action, which maintains synchronicity with the inherent motility of the liver, may be employed to induce further hepatic decongestion.

### Remarks

An alternative hand placement for the hepatic release and pump is to place one hand posteriorly, palm up beneath the lower ribs, and the other hand anteriorly with the hypothenar portion of the palm and the little and ring fingers just below the costal margin or inferior edge of the liver.

Hepatic dysfunction may also be addressed by treating spinal somatic dysfunctions affecting the level of the spine responsible for somatovisceral influences: sympathetic, T6–T9 and parasympathetic, occiput–C2.

## Splenic release and pump

### Indications

Conditions resulting in congestion of the spleen; ligamentous and fascial dysfunction of the splenic visceral peritoneum. This procedure is contraindicated in patients with trauma, splenic malignancy, and acute splenomegaly.

### Procedure (Fig. 3.92)

**Patient supine.**
Practitioner seated or standing beside the treatment table on the patient's left side, at the level of the upper abdomen.

Place your left hand palm down, with your fingers directed medially over the anteroinferior costal margin of the left hemithorax. Place your right hand palm up cradling the angles of the ninth, tenth, and eleventh ribs. Listen to the inherent motion of the spleen, feeling for external and internal rotation, in the context of the major motion (rotation in the coronal plane, about a horizontal, anteroposterior axis, wherein the superior border of the convex surface of the spleen is felt to move respectively in a medial and lateral direction), and

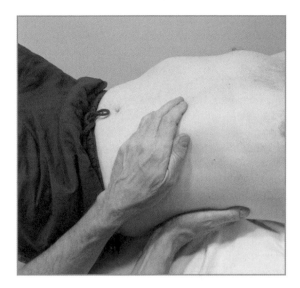

Figure 3.92: Hand placement for splenic release and pump

the minor motions (rotation in the sagittal plane, about a horizontal, transverse axis, wherein the superior border of the spleen moves respectively in an anterior and posterior direction; rotation in the horizontal plane, about a vertical axis, wherein the anterior border of the spleen alternately moves in a medial and lateral direction). Follow the motion pattern in the direction of ease until fascial and ligamentous balance is obtained and await a release.

### Remarks

An alternative hand placement for the splenic pump is to place the dorsum of the hand contacting the inferior costal margin of the left hemithorax at the midaxillary line. Similarly, place the other hand in the palm of the first hand, and using a rolling motion, introduce a medially-directed pumping compression against the left hemithorax at a rate of one to two compressions per second for 10–20 repetitions. This rate will be determined by the compliance and rebound of the left hemithorax to the pumping compressions.

Splenic dysfunction may also be addressed by treating spinal somatic dysfunctions affecting the level of the spine responsible for somatovisceral influences: sympathetic, T5–T12 and parasympathetic, occiput–C2.

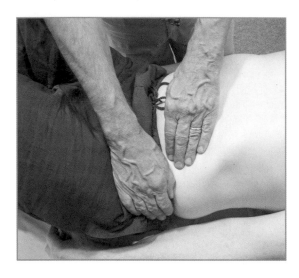

Figure 3.93: Hand placement for treatment of constipation

## Procedure for constipation

### Indications

Constipation.

### Procedure (Fig. 3.93)

**Patient supine.**
Practitioner seated or standing on the right side of the patient at the level of the abdomen.

Place your cephalic hand on the abdomen with your fingers contacting the left lower quadrant and listen and visualize the abdominal contents, using the pads of your fingers to identify the area of greatest tension within the descending and sigmoid colon. Your caudal hand lies on the left pelvic bone with the fingers directed posteriorly along the iliac crest. Listen and visualize the inherent motility of the pelvic bone. Using indirect principles, with both hands, follow the pelvic bone and colon to a position of balance and await a release.

## Cranial procedures

The following procedures respect the principles of tensegrity, wherein the membranes represent the prestressed tensioned components, and the bones,

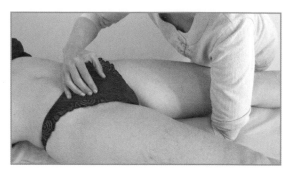

Figure 3.94: Hand placement for uterus release

### Remarks

Before using the above procedure you must first thoroughly identify and treat somatic dysfunction of the pelvic bone, sacrum, and lumbar spine as described above.

## Uterus release

### Indications

Uterine malposition; pelvic congestion.

### Procedure (Fig. 3.94)

**Patient supine.**
Practitioner standing on either side of the table, caudal to the level of the pelvis.

Place your caudal hand palm up beneath the patient's sacrum. With the thumb and index or middle finger of your cephalic hand, contact the uterine fundus. Listen to the position and inherent motion of the uterus and sacrum. Normally, the position of the uterus mirrors that of the sacrum. Follow the motion pattern in the direction of ease until a point of myofascial and ligamentous balance is obtained. Maintain synchronicity with the PRM and await a release.

the compressed components. For precise results, it is necessary to visualize these two elements individually and to differentiate between the restrictions affecting them. This involves identification of the location and depth of the primary dysfunction. Articular dysfunctions, although potentially resulting in far-reaching secondary dysfunction, are localized to the anatomic site of the compressed components. Membranous dysfunctions, because they affect the prestressed tensioned components, will affect all of the bones that they are attached to, resulting in a more global osseous dysfunctional pattern.

This having been said, although you must focus upon the precise location of the primary dysfunction, it must be recognized that, by its very nature, a tensegral system is a holistic system and working on any of its components ultimately affects everything within the system.

Before applying any of the cranial manipulative procedures described below, a complete medical diagnosis must be obtained. Manipulative procedures should not be applied to areas of trauma, acute inflammatory processes, circulatory compromise, or in any fashion that is inconsistent with, or disruptive to, the standard of medical care.

## Global equilibration of intracranial membranes

### Indications

Cranial dysfunction; intracranial venous sinus congestion; normalization of CSF fluctuation, facilitating function of the cerebrum, thalamus, hypothalamus, and pituitary gland.

### Vault hold procedure (Fig. 3.95)

**Patient supine.**
Practitioner seated at the head of the table.

Your hands bilaterally contact the lateral parts of the skull so that the pads of the index fingers are upon the lateral portions of the greater wings of the sphenoid. Your middle fingers contact the temporal squamae, anterior to the external auditory meatus and your ring fingers contact the mastoid portions of temporal bones behind the ear. Your little fingers rest upon the lateral angles of the squamous portion of the occiput. Interlock your thumbs over the sagittal suture without contacting the skull. Listen to the membranous

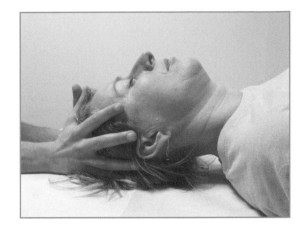

Figure 3.95: Hand placement for vault hold

pattern and inherent motility. Follow in the direction of ease, paying attention to the PRM and await a release, at which point a spontaneous respiratory cooperation often occurs in the form of a deep breath. If this does not happen, or if the release is incomplete, ask the patient to breathe deeply, inhaling and holding to augment the release of a flexion-external rotation dysfunctional pattern, or to exhale and hold for extension-internal rotation.

### Fronto-occipital hold procedure (Fig. 3.96)

**Patient supine.**
Practitioner seated at the side of the table.

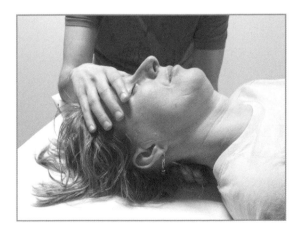

Figure 3.96: Hand placement for fronto-occipital hold

Place one hand transversely cradling the occiput while your other hand rests anteriorly upon the frontal bone in such a manner that the tip of your thumb is on the superior aspect of one sphenoidal greater wing and the tip of your index or middle finger is on the corresponding spot on the other side. Visualize, listen, and follow in the direction of ease as described above.

## Equilibration of the tentorium cerebelli

### Indications

Release of the tentorium cerebelli; release of the walls and contents of the laterosellar compartment; facilitation of cavernous sinus drainage.

### Procedure (Fig. 3.97)

**Patient supine.**
Practitioner seated at the head of the table.

Hold the temporal bones bilaterally, with your thumbs and index fingers respectively superior and inferior to the zygomatic processes. Your middle fingers should contact the external auditory meatus, your ring fingers the tips of the mastoid pro-

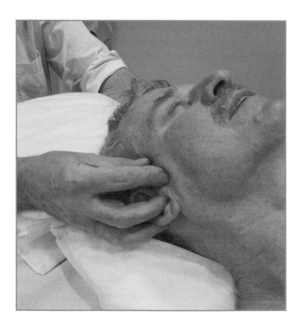

Figure 3.97: Hand placement for tentorium cerebelli equilibration

cesses and your little fingers the occiput, posterior to the asterion. Visualize and listen to the tentorium cerebelli, closely noting the motion of the temporal bones. Follow in the direction of ease, and paying attention to the PRM, wait until a release occurs.

### Remarks

By moving the thumbs to contact the lateral aspects of the greater wings of the sphenoid, you may add control of the sphenoid to this procedure. This allows you to focus attention on the anterior portions and attachments of the tentorium cerebelli, particularly the diaphragma sellae and the roof and lateral wall of the laterosellar compartment as they relate to the sphenoid and CNs III, IV, and V. The petrosphenoid ligament, sometimes considered to be a thickened portion of the anterior tentorium cerebelli, possibly affecting CN VI, may also be addressed with this procedure. See further below: 'Sphenotemporal procedure,' p. 149.

## Global cranial base release

### Indications

Cervical myofascial dysfunctions affecting the pharynx, deglutition, and respiration (including sleep apnea); temporomandibular joint (TMJ) dysfunctions.

### Procedure (Fig. 3.98)

**Patient supine.**
Practitioner seated at the head of the table.

Place one hand beneath the occiput. With your other hand cradle the mandible. Visualize and listen to the motion of the occiput in relation to the cervical spine. Visualize the TMJs and listen to the motion of the mandibular condyles in the mandibular fossae. Follow the occiput and mandible into a position of balanced myofascial and ligamentous tension. Following the intraosseous motion of the occiput and mandible will enhance the efficacy of the procedure. Await a release.

## Posterior cranial base release

### Indications

Dysfunction between the occiput and atlas, and occiput and temporal bones; postural compression at the level of the jugular foramen resulting in

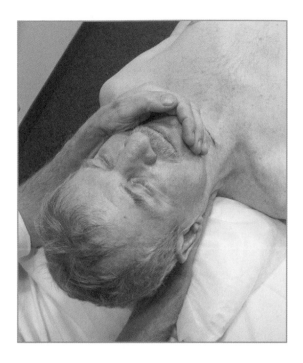

Figure 3.98: Hand placement for global cranial base release

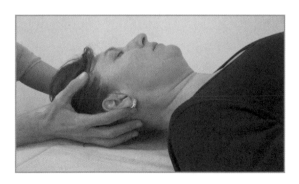

Figure 3.99: Hand placement for posterior cranial base release

cranial nerve entrapment syndromes (CNs IX, X, and XI) and intracranial congestion; stasis at the level of the hypoglossal foramen resulting in CN XII dysfunction; cervical myofascial dysfunctions affecting the pharynx, deglutition, and respiration (including sleep apnea).

## Procedure (Fig. 3.99)

**Patient supine.**
Practitioner seated at the head of the table.

Place your hands beneath the occiput in such a way that the ring and little fingers contact the occipital squama. The tips of your middle fingers are at the level of C1, your index fingers contact the mastoid processes, and your thumbs rest lightly on each side of the head. Listen and identify the pattern of occipitoatlantal flexion, extension, side-bending, and rotation, and follow it into the position of greatest ease. Next, listen to the relationship between the occiput and temporal bones and, using your index fingers, follow the temporal bones into their position of ease. Employ the inherent motility of the biphasic PRM to reinforce the previous two steps. In chronic cases, the release of the dysfunction may be facilitated by employing the pumping action of the PRM. Wait for a release.

### Remarks

It is necessary to use caution when performing this procedure in order to avoid adverse reactions such as nausea, vomiting, and headache due to the importance of the content of the jugular foramen.

## Sphenobasilar synchondrosis procedures

### Indications

Cranial base and membranous dysfunctional patterns secondary to sphenobasilar synchondrosis (SBS) dysfunction.

### Vault hold procedure (Fig. 3.100)

**Patient supine.**
Practitioner seated at the head of the table.

Your hands bilaterally contact the lateral parts of the skull so that the pads of the index fingers are upon the lateral portions of the greater wings of the sphenoid. Your middle fingers contact the temporal squamae anterior to the external auditory meatus and your ring fingers contact the mastoid portions of temporal bones behind the ear. Your little fingers rest upon the lateral angles of the squamous portion of the occiput. Interlock your thumbs over the sagittal suture without contacting the skull. Visualize and listen to the SBS. Use indirect principles to follow any identified pattern, while pumping the SBS in conjunction with the inherent forces of the PRM. Await a release.

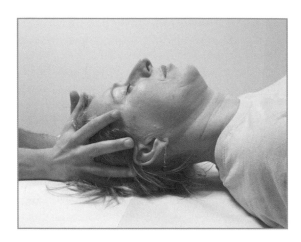

Figure 3.100: Hand placement for vault hold

### *Fronto-occipital hold procedure* (Fig. 3.101)

**Patient supine.**

Practitioner seated to one side at the head of the table.

Place one hand palm up, transversely beneath the occiput. Place your other hand palm down, transversely upon the frontal bone, in such a way that the pads of your thumb and middle finger bilaterally contact the lateral surfaces of the greater wings of the sphenoid. Visualize and listen to the SBS. Use indirect principles to follow any identified pattern, while pumping the SBS in conjunction with the inherent forces of the PRM. Await a release.

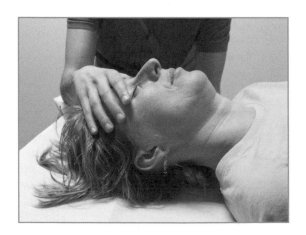

Figure 3.101: Hand placement for fronto-occipital hold

### *Cradling the skull* (Fig. 3.102)

**Patient supine.**

Practitioner seated at the head of the table.

Place your hands on each side of the head so that the distal pads of your index, middle, and ring fingers contact the lateral portions of the occipital squama. With the lateral aspects of the distal phalanges of your thumbs, bilaterally contact the greater wings of the sphenoid. Listen to the SBS and determine the pattern of ease. Using indirect principles in conjunction with the inherent forces of the PRM, follow the identified pattern to the point of balanced membranous tension. Await a release.

### *Remarks*

The three procedures described above are intended to address dysfunction of the SBS. It must be recognized, however, that the SBS is fused in the majority of individuals by the middle of the third decade of life. SBS dysfunction in elderly patients may be considered to be intraosseous dysfunction of the cranial base. Dysfunctional patterns of the SBS can go on to influence somatic dysfunctions throughout the body. Encouraging the cranial tissues to move toward, if not wholly into, their position of tensegrital ease will facilitate release of dysfunction in adjacent, as well as distant, areas of the body. The area may still be treated to enhance fluid motions within the skull and in the foramina of the cranial base.

The points of palpatory contact on the skull are distant from the SBS. It is a common mistake to

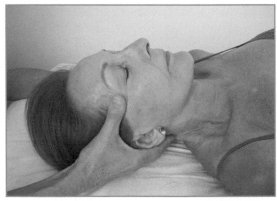

Figure 3.102: Hand placement for cradling the skull

palpate the superficial motion of the membranous skull and think that what is being perceived is SBS motion. A thorough knowledge of anatomy is necessary to visualize and focus one's attention to the SBS.

When treating cranial dysfunctions, it is always appropriate to have the patient in their most favorable position for myofascial and ligamentous balance. The patient will typically spontaneously assume this position. A common mistake is to begin a cranial treatment by straightening the patient's neck and placing their head in the midline of the table. This can create spurious palpatory findings if there is somatic dysfunction in the spine below.

One should pay particular attention to dysfunction in the cervicothoracic region. It is most appropriate to treat these dysfunctions before addressing cranial dysfunction. However, if this is not possible, leaving the patient in their position of ease (usually with their neck side bent and rotated away from the midline) will limit spurious palpatory finding. The acquisition of a cranial release and a total-body response will be facilitated by treating the patient in their position of optimal comfort. As such, the lower body should also accommodate the position of the sacrum, with flexion or extension of the legs, or both.

## Bilateral temporal bone release

### Indications

Temporal bone, vestibular, or pharyngotympanic (Eustachian or auditory) tube dysfunction with resultant headache, tinnitus, and hearing impairment; tentorium cerebelli dysfunction affecting the laterosellar compartment contents (cavernous sinus; internal carotid artery; CNs III, IV, V1, and VI).

### Procedure (Fig. 3.103)

**Patient supine.**
Practitioner seated at the head of the table.

Hold the temporal bones bilaterally, with your thumbs and index fingers respectively superior and inferior to the zygomatic processes. Your middle fingers, if possible, should contact the external auditory meati. Your ring fingers contact the tips

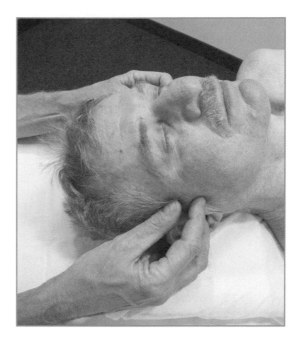

Figure 3.103: Hand placement for bilateral temporal release

of the mastoid processes and your little fingers the superior parts of the mastoid portions. Listen and follow the pattern to a point of balanced membranous tension. Await a release.

### Remarks

Magoun states: "With an external rotation lesion of the temporal, the (pharyngotympanic) tube may be held continuously open, and the patient complains of a low-pitched roar. With internal rotation, it may be held closed, accompanied by high-pitched humming or buzzing."[18]

When the temporal bones are externally rotated, the meati will be larger, whereas they are smaller with internal rotation. By listening to the tissues of the auditory meati with your middle fingers, as described above, you will feel motion that usually follows the external/internal rotation pattern of the temporal bones. Following the tissues of the auditory meati to a point of balanced tension may facilitate release of the tympanic membrane and, through its relationship with the ossicles, potentially enhance sound transmission by the middle ear.

By visualizing, following, and balancing the inherent motility of the inner ear within the petrous portions of the temporal bones, you may contribute to the circulation of perilymph and endolymph.

## Occipitomastoid suture procedure

### Indications

Occipitomastoid (OM) suture dysfunction affecting the jugular foramen and its contents, often the result of a fall upon the back of the head.

### Procedure (Fig. 3.104)

**Patient supine.**
Practitioner seated at the head of the table.

Place one hand palm up, transversely beneath the occiput, with the pads of the index, middle, and ring fingers contacting the occipital squama, medial to the OM suture on the side of the dysfunction. The other hand is placed on the temporal bone with the thumb and index finger superior and inferior to the zygomatic process. The middle finger contacts the external auditory meatus, the ring finger contacts the tip of the mastoid process, and the little finger the mastoid portion. Listen to the motion of the occiput and temporal bone. Using indirect principles, follow the dysfunctional pattern to the point of balanced membranous and associated myofascial tension. Await the release of the suture. In chronic cases, employ the inherent forces of

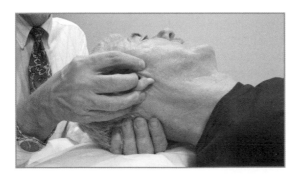

Figure 3.104: Hand placement for diagnosis and treatment of occipitomastoid suture dysfunction

the PRM to gently pump the area to facilitate a release.

## Petro-occipital procedure

### Indications

Petro-occipital suture dysfunction affecting the jugular and lacerum foramina and their contents; pharyngeal and soft palate dysfunctions including sleep apnea; hearing impairment.

### Procedure

**Patient supine.**
Practitioner seated at the head of the table.

Place your hands as described in the OM suture procedure above. Visualize the petro-occipital suture, the occiput, and the petrous portion of the temporal bone, its position and motion. Normally, the posterior border of the petrous portion goes up during cranial flexion-external rotation and down during extension-internal rotation. Use indirect principles and follow the dysfunctional pattern to the point of balanced membranous and associated myofascial tension. Await the release. If necessary, employ the inherent forces of the PRM to gently pump the area to induce a release.

### Remarks

The petro-occipital suture normally remains patent throughout life and as such should demonstrate motility in all individuals. Observations have been made however, associating ossification of this suture in older males with age-related conductive hearing loss.[19]

## Sphenoid procedure

### Indications

Cranial base and membranous dysfunctional patterns secondary to SBS dysfunction; ocular, hypothalamic-pituitary-adrenal axis, orofacial, and upper respiratory dysfunctions.

### Procedure (Fig. 3.105)

**Patient supine.**
Practitioner seated at the head of the table.

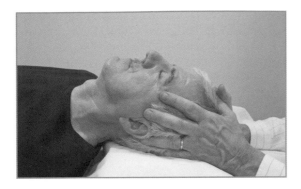

Figure 3.105: Hand placement for sphenoidal release

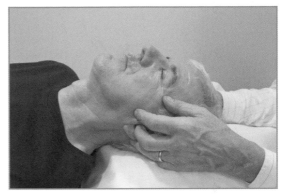

Figure 3.106: Hand placement for sphenotemporal release

Your hands bilaterally contact the lateral parts of the skull so that the pads of your index or middle fingers are upon the lateral portions of the greater wings of the sphenoid. The first sensation you will get reflects the motion of the greater wings and not necessarily what is happening at the level of the other parts of the sphenoid. When listening to the inherent motility of the sphenoid, visualization is helpful to define what portion of the sphenoid is dysfunctional. Follow the sphenoid in the direction of ease to the point of balanced membranous and associated myofascial tension, and paying attention to the PRM, await a release.

### Remarks

In the case of a dysfunction affecting one particular suture, a specific procedure as described below may be necessary.

## Sphenotemporal procedure

### Indications

Tentorium cerebelli dysfunction affecting the laterosellar compartment contents (cavernous sinus; internal carotid artery; CNs III, IV, V1, and VI); sphenopetrosal fissure dysfunction affecting the lacerum foramen and its contents; sphenosquamosal suture dysfunction; pharyngeal and soft palate dysfunctions including sleep apnea and upper respiratory dysfunctions; pharyngotympanic tube, ocular, and hypothalamic-pituitary-adrenal axis dysfunctions.

### Procedure (Fig. 3.106)

**Patient supine.**
Practitioner seated at the head of the table.

Place the lateral aspect of the pads of your thumbs upon the lateral portions of the greater wings of the sphenoid. Contact the temporal bones bilaterally, with your index finger inferior to the zygomatic processes and your middle fingers contacting the external auditory meati. Your ring fingers contact the tips of the mastoid processes and your little fingers the superior parts of the mastoid portions. Visualize the relationship between the temporal bones and the sphenoid, paying particular attention to the laterosellar compartments, and the diaphragma sellae. Listen and identify any articular or membranous dysfunction in the area. Follow the pattern of each temporal bone, and of the sphenoid, to the point of balance of articular and membranous tension. Await a release.

### Remarks

There is tensegrital relationship between the four areas of contact, the greater wings contacted with your thumbs, and the temporal bones contacted with your fingers. Under optimal functional circumstances the center of tensegrital balance between these points should be in the region of the laterosellar compartments, the sella turcica, and the diaphragma sellae.

Your index finger may be positioned inferior to the zygomatic processes to follow internal rotation

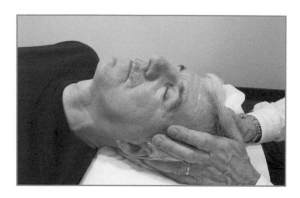

Figure 3.107: Hand placement for sphenosquamosal release

of the temporal bone, or superior to the zygomatic processes to follow external rotation.

In the laterosellar compartments there is a lot of fluid that is often responsible for stasis potentially affecting CNs III, IV, V1, and VI.

## Sphenosquamosal procedure

### Indications

Tension headaches; temporal muscles tension; intracranial venous sinus drainage.

### Procedure (Fig. 3.107)

**Patient supine.**
Practitioner seated at the head of the table.

Bilaterally palpate the sphenosquamosal suture in such a way that the pads of your index fingers contact the greater wings of the sphenoid and your middle fingers the temporal bones posterior to the suture. Listen and identify the pattern of motion demonstrated by the suture. Using indirect principles, follow the dysfunctional pattern to the point of balanced membranous and associated myofascial tension. Await the release of the suture.

### Remarks

Unilateral dysfunction may be treated by employing a 'V' spread. The fingers on the dysfunctional side are placed in contact with the sphenosquamosal suture as described above in order to receive the induced potentiation of the PRM. One or two fingers of the other inducing hand gently contact the skull

at a contralateral point, at the greatest possible distance from the dysfunction. While monitoring the PRM, gently employ a pumping action directed at the dysfunctional suture with the inducing hand to enhance potency of the PRM, and induce a release.

The sphenosquamosal suture is significantly affected by the temporalis muscle and as such by occlusal disorders, which when present should be addressed.

## Sphenofrontal procedure

### Indications

Ocular dysfunctions; frontal cephalalgia; sinusitis; maxillofacial and oral dysfunctions.

### Procedure (Fig. 3.108)

**Patient supine.**
Practitioner seated at the head of the table.

Place your hands bilaterally in such a way that the pads of your middle fingers contact the greater wings of the sphenoid and the pads of your index fingers contact the zygomatic processes of the frontal bones. Listen to the motion between the sphenoid and frontal bones. Using indirect principles, follow the motion in the direction of ease and await a release.

## Zygomatic procedure

### Indications

Dysfunction of the zygomata; upper respiratory tract, eye, and dental disorders.

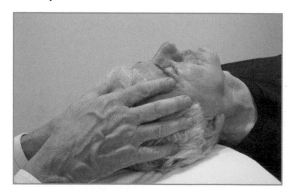

Figure 3.108: Hand placement for sphenofrontal release

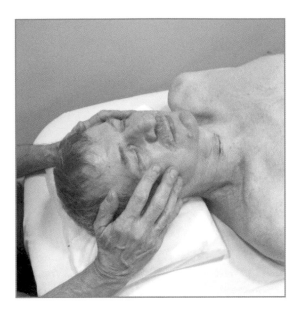

Figure 3.109: Hand placement for zygomatic release

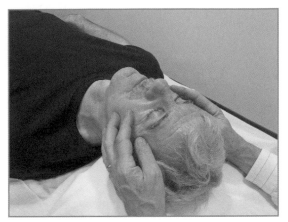

Figure 3.110: Hand placement for bilateral sphenozygomatic release

## *Procedure* (Fig. 3.109)

**Patient supine.**
Practitioner seated at the head of the table.

Place your hands bilaterally on the zygomata in such a way that your index fingers contact the orbital borders and your middle fingers, the inferior borders. Listen to their motion and follow it into the position of ease and await a release. In cases of chronic dysfunction the procedure may be augmented with pumping that follows the rhythm of the PRM.

### *Remarks*

Commonly, one zygoma will be found to be in external rotation and the other in internal rotation. This asymmetry is consistent with a torsion or sidebending rotation pattern of the SBS. It is important to pay attention to the quality of motion manifested by each zygoma. One will often be found to have significantly greater restriction. In this case, the location (spheno-, fronto-, temporo-, maxillozygomatic joint, or a combination of these joints) of zygomatic dysfunction should be identified and addressed.

## Sphenozygomatic procedure

### *Indications*

Dysfunction between the sphenoid and zygomatic bone; ocular dysfunctions; maxillary sinus dysfunctions.

### *Procedure* (Fig. 3.110)

**Patient supine.**
Practitioner seated at the head of the table.

Place your hands bilaterally in such a way that the lateral aspects of your thumbs contact the greater wings of the sphenoid and your index and middle fingers respectively contact the orbital and the inferior border of the zygomata. Listen to the movement of the sphenoid and zygomata, noting their inherent motility and the relationship between them. Follow the motion in the direction of ease and await a release

## Frontal procedure

### *Indications*

Dysfunction of the viscerocranium including eyes and nasal cavities; headaches; facial lymphatic congestion; dysfunction of the falx cerebri.

### *Procedure* (Fig. 3.111)

**Patient supine.**
Practitioner seated at the head of the table.

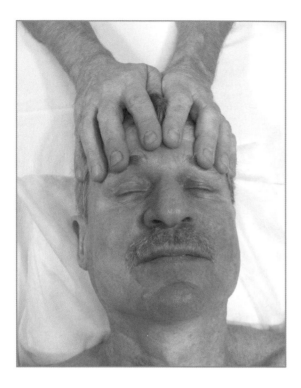

Figure 3.111: Hand placement for frontal release

Place the pads of your index fingers on the metopic suture, at the level of the ophryon (above the glabella). The pads of your middle and ring fingers should rest bilaterally upon the brow ridges and zygomatic processes of the frontal bone(s). Listen and note the inherent motility of the PRM, and any restriction therein. Follow the pattern using indirect principles and await a release. If necessary, employ the inherent forces of the PRM to gently pump the area to induce a release.

### Remarks

Anecdotally, it has been observed that frontal dysfunction may be associated with cognitive problems. This procedure is very relaxing and is often appreciated by the patient. Any frontal dysfunction should be effectively treated before addressing facial disorders.

## Frontozygomatic procedures

### Indications

Dysfunction of the viscerocranium including the eyes and nasal cavities; headaches; facial lymphatic congestion.

### Procedure (Fig. 3.112)

**Patient supine.**
Practitioner seated at the head of the table, at the side of the table opposite to the dysfunction, at the level of the patient's head.

Place the thumb and index finger of your cephalic hand on each side of the zygomatic process of the frontal bone, and the thumb and index finger of your caudal hand on each side of the frontal process of the zygomatic bone. Listen, and using indirect principles, follow the pattern of dysfunction. Await a release. If necessary employ the inherent forces of the PRM to gently pump the area to induce a release.

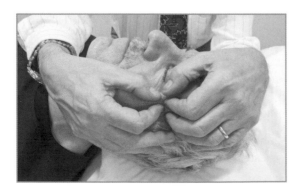

Figure 3.112: Hand placement for frontozygomatic release

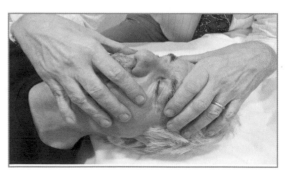

Figure 3.113: Hand placement for bilateral frontozygomatic release

### *Bilateral procedure* (Fig. 3.113)

To treat bilateral sphenozygomatic dysfunction, your cephalic hand should lie transversely upon the frontal bone, in such a way that the pads of your thumb and index finger bilaterally contact the lateral surfaces of the zygomatic process of the frontal bone. The thumb and index and middle fingers of your caudal hand contact the zygomatic bones bilaterally. Proceed to listen and treat as above.

# Vault procedures

## Coronal suture procedure

### *Indications*

Coronal suture dysfunction; intracranial congestion secondary to diminished CSF reabsorption and venous drainage.

### *Procedure* (Fig. 3.114)

**Patient supine.**
Practitioner seated at the head of the table.

Cross your thumbs and position them as far anterior as possible on either side of the sagittal suture. Place the pads of your index and middle fingers anteriorly to the coronal suture, in contact with the lateral portions of the frontal bone. Listen to the motion of the suture. During cranial inspiration (flexion-external rotation), the medial part of the parietal bones, upon which you have your thumbs, will descend and move slightly posterior, while the lateral parts of the frontal bone will move laterally and slightly anterior. The reverse occurs during cranial expiration (extension-internal rotation). Identify and follow the dysfunctional pattern in the direction of ease. Pay attention to the PRM and use its potency in a pumping fashion to induce a release.

## Lambdoid suture procedure

### *Indications*

Lambdoid suture dysfunction; intracranial congestion secondary to diminished CSF reabsorption and venous drainage.

### *Procedure* (Fig. 3.115)

**Patient supine.**
Practitioner seated at the head of the table.

Cross your thumbs and position them as far posterior as possible on either side of the sagittal suture. Place the pads of your middle, ring and little fingers posterior to the lambdoid suture, in contact with the lateral portions of the occipital squama.

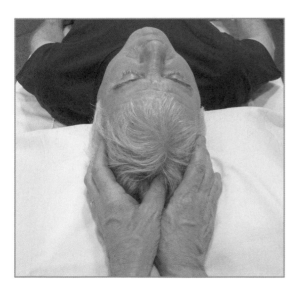

Figure 3.114: Hand placement for coronal suture release

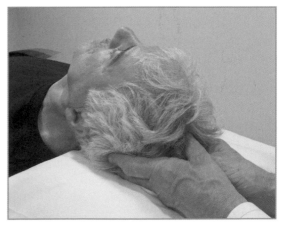

Figure 3.115: Hand placement for lambdoid suture release

Listen to the motion of the suture. During cranial inspiration (flexion-external rotation), the medial part of the parietal bones, upon which you have your thumbs, will descend and move laterally and posteriorly, while the lateral parts of the occiput will move laterally and posteriorly. The reverse occurs during cranial expiration (extension-internal rotation). Identify and follow the dysfunctional pattern in the direction of ease. Pay attention to the PRM and use its potency in a pumping fashion to induce a release.

### Remarks

In most cases, the anterior and posterior borders of the parietal bones have the same beveling, with an external bevel medially and an internal bevel laterally. The corresponding borders of the frontal and occipital bones demonstrate internal beveling medially and external beveling laterally. In order to disengage one bone from another, contact should be placed on the side of the suture that is externally beveled.

## Parietal procedure

### Indications

Parietal dysfunction; tension headaches; intracranial congestion secondary to diminished CSF reabsorption and intracranial venous sinus drainage.

*Procedure* (Fig. 3.116)

**Patient supine.**
Practitioner seated at the head of the table.

Your hands bilaterally contact the lateral parts of the skull so that the pads of all of your fingers are upon the lateral borders of the parietal bones. Interlock your thumbs over the sagittal suture without contacting the skull. Listen to the motion of the parietal bones and the PRM. Use indirect principles to follow any identified pattern, while pumping the parietals in conjunction with the inherent forces of the PRM. Await a release.

### Remarks

Because you are contacting only the parietal bones, this simple position allows you to concentrate upon the cranial rhythmic impulse (CRI) and PRM without being distracted by the complex motion pattern of multiple bones. This hand placement may be used to apply the same principles as those used in compression of the fourth ventricle (CV4) to enhance the power of the PRM.

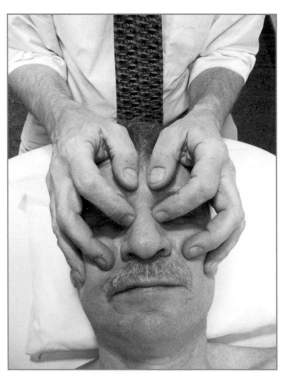

Figure 3.117: Hand placement for global facial release

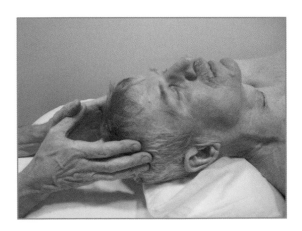

Figure 3.116: Hand placement for bilateral parietal release

# Facial procedure

### Indications

Orbital, ocular, upper respiratory, maxillofacial, and oral dysfunctions.

### Procedure (Fig. 3.117)

**Patient supine.**

Practitioner seated at the head of the table.

Place your hands on the patient's face with the pads of your thumbs upon the ophryon (above the glabella). Bilaterally, the pads of your index fingers should contact the frontal processes of the maxillae; your middle fingers, the bodies of the maxillae; and your ring and little fingers, the zygomata. Listen and visualize the global pattern of motion between the frontal bones, maxillae, and zygomata. Follow this pattern, noting the detailed relationship between these individual bones. Using indirect principles and the PRM, follow the motion of the bones into the position of balance and await a release. If necessary, employ the inherent forces of the PRM to gently pump the face to induce a release.

# Ocular procedures

## Orbital cavity pumping

### Indications

Congestion of the orbital veins; intraocular fluid stasis; compromise of the orbital fissure affecting its content; dysfunction of the extraocular muscles (EOM).

### Procedure (Fig. 3.118)

(Example: left orbital cavity.)

Patient supine, eyes closed.

Practitioner seated at the head of the table.

Place your right hand upon the frontal bone in such a manner that the pad of your middle finger contacts the left maxillary process of the frontal bone, and the pad of your index finger rests upon the brow ridge. The pads of your left index and middle fingers should respectively contact the orbital and inferior borders of the zygomatic bone. Listen to the inherent motility of the orbit. Follow it, and employ the PRM in a pumping fashion until a release occurs.

### Remarks

The diameter of the orbit is defined by a line connecting its superomedial and inferolateral angles. This pumping procedure facilitates increase and decrease of the orbital diameter.

## Ocular balance

### Indications

Release of the intra- and EOM. Intraocular fluid stasis might contribute to chronic glaucoma. (Note: Acute glaucoma is an emergency requiring immediate medical attention.)

### Procedure (Fig. 3.119)

Patient supine, eyes closed.

Practitioner seated at the head of the table.

Place the pads of your index fingers upon the patient's eyeball in such a manner that they rest gently upon the sclera on opposite sides of the cornea. Palpate the eyeball and listen, identifying any tension between the eyeball and any portion of the orbital cavity (frontal, sphenoid, zygomatic, and maxillary). Employing indirect principles, follow

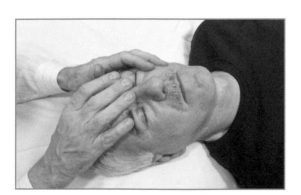

Figure 3.118: Hand placement for orbital cavity pumping

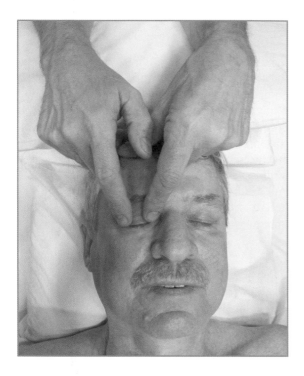

Figure 3.119: Hand placement for ocular release

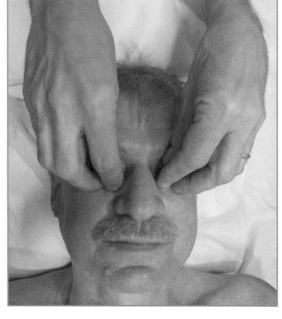

Figure 3.120: Hand placement for bilateral ocular release

the motion of the eyeball into a position of myofascial balance and await a release.

### Remarks

The test of listening and the balancing treatment procedure of the eyeballs can be performed by bilaterally placing the hands with the tips of the fingers and thumbs approximated in such a manner that you can palpate the sclera surrounding the cornea. (Fig. 3.120)

In the event that you feel a significant amount of tension between the eyeball and one of the bones of the orbit, one hand should remain upon the eyeball, and the other hand upon the identified orbital bone. In Figure 3.121, the orbital bone involved is the frontal bone.

## Intraocular fluid balancing

### Indications

Intraocular fluid stasis as might contribute to chronic glaucoma. (Note: Acute glaucoma is an emergency requiring immediate medical attention.)

### Procedure (Fig. 3.122)

Patient supine, eyes closed.

Practitioner seated at the head of the table.

Place the pads of your index fingers upon the patient's eyeball in such a manner that they rest gently upon the sclera on opposite sides of the cornea. Palpate the eyeball and listen, compar-

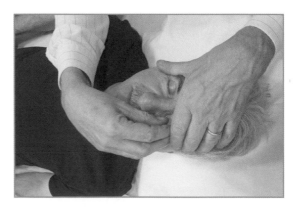

Figure 3.121: Hand placement for oculo-orbital release

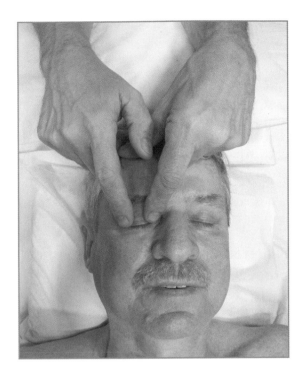

Figure 3.122: Hand placement for ocular release

ing the tension felt by each finger. Repeat this procedure, moving your fingers circumferentially around the sclera to identify areas of tension. Begin treatment in the area of least palpable tension, and follow the inherent motility of the eyeball. Enhancement of this motility may be accomplished with a light pumping procedure, alternating between your two fingers, until the motion is balanced and of increased amplitude. Continue the procedure, by moving your fingers to a new position and repeating the process until all points on the circumference of the eyeball are balanced and the motility has been optimized.

### Remarks

This procedure should be performed after the procedure for ocular balancing.

# Temporomandibular joint procedures

### Indications

Temporomandibular joint dysfunction often presenting as joint pain, malocclusion, headaches, ear pain, vertigo, cervical pain, and postural imbalance.

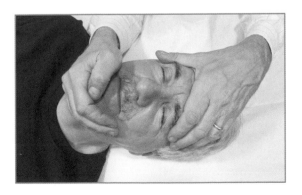

Figure 3.123: Hand placement for frontomandibular release

When treating TMJ dysfunctions it is always important that the patient have a full dental evaluation with particular attention to the diagnosis of malocclusion.

## Frontomandibular procedure (Fig. 3.123)

**Patient supine.**
Practitioner seated on either side of the treatment table.

Place one hand palm down upon the frontal bone in such a manner that your thumb and middle finger contact the greater wings of the sphenoid in the temporal fossae. With the palm of your other hand, cradle the patient's mandible. Listen to the global motion pattern between the mandible and the cranium. Follow the motion in the direction of ease, which most of the time involves a torsional pattern that is sensed between your two hands. Obtain optimal myofascial and ligamentous balance and await release.

## Remarks

The patient's facial area is very sensitive to tactile stimulus and as such the gentlest possible touch necessary to accomplish the treatment should be employed to ensure the patient's comfort and to avoid anxiety and the defensive responses of fight, flight, and freeze that can ensue. This is of particular importance when treating TMJ dysfunction because the fight, flight, and freeze response is commonly associated with clenching of the masticatory muscles.

The act of following the PRM through your hands often induces the patient's relaxation facilitating a release.

## Temporomandibular joint procedure

(Example: right TMJ dysfunction. (Fig. 3.124))

### Patient supine.

Practitioner seated on the left side of the treatment table.

With the index and middle fingers of your left hand, contact the right mandibular condyle. The index and middle fingers of your right hand contact the zygomatic process of the temporal bone over the mandibular fossa. Listen to the TMJ and follow the movements of the condyle until optimal myofascial and ligamentous balance of the TMJ is obtained and await release.

## Remarks

Temporomandibular joint dysfunctions are often extremely painful, and the articular innervation highly sophisticated, necessitating extreme precision when listening, identifying dysfunctional mechanics, and following the joint to the position of optimal myofascial and ligamentous balance.

When listening to the TMJ it is advantageous to visualize the articular disc. Dysfunctions can occur between the disc and the mandibular condyle or, more often, between the disc and the mandibular fossa. When treating these dysfunctions, it is appropriate to establish a functional unit between the fossa and disc in the instance of disc-condyle dysfunction or between the condyle and disc in the instance of disc-fossa dysfunction.

## Bilateral temporomandibular joint procedure (Fig. 3.125)

### Patient supine.

Practitioner seated at the head of the treatment table.

Place your hands bilaterally in such a manner that your thumbs contact the greater wings of the sphenoid in the temporal fossae, and your index and middle fingers contact the mandibular rami. Listen to the motion of the condyles. If necessary, introduce gentle motions (anterior/posterior glide, medial/lateral glide, compression/decompression) of the condyles. Follow these motions in the direction of ease until optimal myofascial and ligamentous balance of the TMJs are obtained and await release.

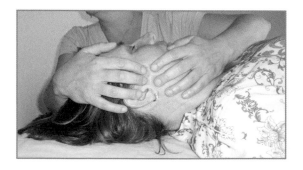

Figure 3.124: Hand placement for temporomandibular release

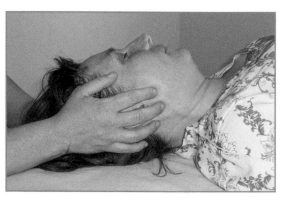

Figure 3.125: Hand placement for bilateral temporomandibular release

### Remarks

By positioning your index and middle fingers so that they contact the mandibular angles, this procedure may be employed to obtain relaxation of the muscles of mastication, particularly the medial and lateral pterygoid muscles. Properly applied, this is globally very relaxing for the patient.

In chronic TMJ dysfunctions an isometric modification may be added. After obtaining the position of optimal myofascial and ligamentous balance, ask the patient to translate their mandible in the direction of ease, very gently and briefly (about two seconds). The patient is then instructed to relax. At this point, listen carefully to the ease and degree of relaxation that occurs. This process may be repeated several times, as necessary, to obtain optimal muscular relaxation. For best results, each sequential contraction should employ slightly different amounts of anterior/posterior glide, medial/lateral glide, and compression/decompression, dependent upon the sensation of the ease and degree of relaxation, as observed by listening.

Note: This is not a traditional muscle energy procedure in that it is indirect and following the therapeutic contraction; the dysfunctional area is not stretched to directly take it to a new barrier.

Following prolonged periods of somatic dysfunction with limitation of motion, patients often develop functional amnesia and lose proprioception and the ability to move the dysfunctional area through its full range of motion. When this affects the TMJ, even though the dysfunction may have been effectively resolved, the patient will continue to move in the dysfunctional pattern and demonstrate continued proprioceptive impairment. For this reason it becomes imperative to rehabilitate the patient's capacity to consciously move through the full range of motion, thereby regaining optimal proprioception.[20][21]

# Procedures to modulate the primary respiratory mechanism

In all of the procedures described within this text in which the PRM is monitored, it may be modulated to varying extent by focusing upon it.

Primary respiratory mechanism procedures can be directed at globally balancing the PRM. Certain procedures may be specifically employed to increase or decrease its potency.

## Globally balancing the primary respiratory mechanism

### Procedure (Fig. 3.126)

**Patient supine.**
Practitioner seated at the head of the treatment table.

Place the palms of your hands bilaterally on the parietal bones. Evaluate the quality of the PRM, and its palpable sensation, the CRI. Assess the potency and the frequency of the PRM. Follow the CSF and the tissues of the skull to a point of balanced membranous tension, and let the potency of the PRM attain a still point.

In order to facilitate the acquisition of balance in the PRM, you must have the patience to allow it to go quietly through its complete cycle of inspiration and expiration, as many times as necessary, without trying to increase or decrease its potency.

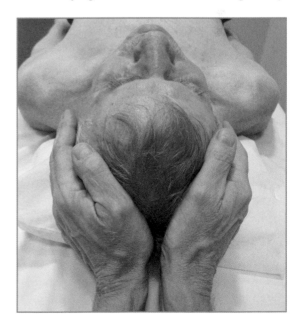

Figure 3.126: Hand placement for globally balancing the PRM

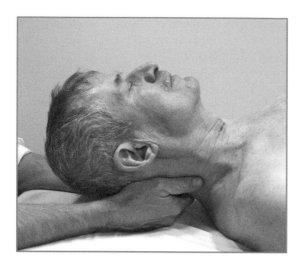

**Figure 3.127:** Hand placement for compression of the fourth ventricle

Your hands act as a fulcrum upon which the PRM is rebounding. The PRM will find its own balance if it is given a chance to do so.

# Compression of the fourth ventricle

## Indications

To increase the potency of the PRM using an occipital approach. This procedure tends to relax the patient. It is thought to stimulate the body's inherent recuperative ability by promoting fluid interchange, particularly lymphatic and CSF circulation.

## Procedure (Fig. 3.127)

**Patient supine.**

Practitioner seated at the head of the treatment table.

Place your hands palms up beneath the patient's head, with one hand resting in the palm of the other, in such a fashion that the thenar eminences are parallel, contacting the lateral angles of the patient's occiput, medial to the occipitomastoid suture. Allow the weight of the patient's head to rest upon your thenar eminences, resulting in medially-directed pressure upon the lateral angles of the occiput. Palpate and follow the occiput into extension and gently increase the medially-directed pressure of your thenar

eminences upon the lateral angles. When the occiput reaches full extension and is about to enter the flexion phase of the cycle, gently resist and maintain it in extension. This process is repeated with each cycle of the CRI. Track the amplitude of the CRI as it progressively decreases to reach a still point, when the CRI seems to palpably stop. After the still point, wait for the motion of the CRI to return and then follow it into the ensuing flexion and extension.

## Remarks

The CV4 procedure cannot be effectively performed in patients who have dysfunctional occipital flexion-external rotation.

The principles of the CV4 procedure may be applied through the parietals, the frontal(s), the temporals, or the sacrum. In fact it is appropriate to apply this procedure through the sacrum in cases of head trauma.

The average duration of CV4 of three to seven minutes,[22] has been demonstrated as 4.43 ± 2.22 minutes.[23]

# Bilateral rotation of the temporal bones

## Indications

To increase the potency of the PRM using a bitemporal approach. This procedure is stimulating and, according to Magoun, indicated to shift from parasympathetic dominance toward a more balanced sympathovagal tone.[24] However, one should be cautious not to overdo it. The aim is to reach a balance between sympathetic and parasympathetic tone, and not shift from one state to the opposite. This procedure should not be used in patients with vertigo.

## Procedure (Fig. 3.128)

**Patient supine.**

Practitioner seated at the head of the treatment table.

With your fingers interlaced, place your hands palms up beneath the patient's head in such a manner that your thenar eminences rest upon the most posterior aspects of the squamous portions of the temporal bones. Your thumbs should be directed inferiorly to bilaterally contact the mastoid processes. Listen to the PRM and follow it, very gently increasing temporal external rotation with your thumbs and temporal internal rotation with your thenar emi-

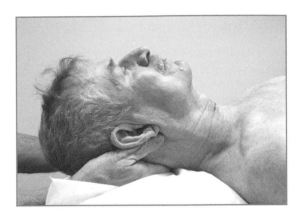

Figure 3.128: Hand placement for bilateral rotation of the temporal bones

nences. This process adds energy to the system increasing the amplitude of the palpable CRI.

## Remarks

Caution should be exercised not to overdo this intervention. As the amplitude of the CRI is felt to increase, it is appropriate to stop and observe the patient's response. It is better to progressively add to this process with subsequent treatments over time than to overdose the patient and have to deal with the sequelae.

This same procedure may be applied to any paired bones such as the parietal and pelvic bones.

## Alternating rotation of the temporal bones

### Indications

This is a repressant procedure, as compared to the incitant bilateral rotation of the temporal bones described above. It acts upon the lateral fluctuation of the CSF, and is indicated for intracranial venous congestion. This procedure should not be used in patients with vertigo.

### Procedure

**Patient supine.**
Practitioner seated at the head of the treatment table.

With your fingers interlaced, place your hands palms up beneath the patient's head in such a manner that your thenar eminences rest upon the most posterior aspects of the squamous portions of the temporal bones. Your thumbs should be directed inferiorly to bilaterally contact the mastoid processes. Listen to the PRM and the motion of the temporal bones. The majority of individuals will demonstrate some degree of asymmetrical temporal bone motion. Follow one temporal bone into external rotation while simultaneously taking the other one into internal rotation. Repeat this process alternating from side-to-side. This will start a lateral fluctuation pattern of the cranial mechanism. When this lateral fluctuation pattern is perceived, begin to gradually dampen its amplitude, allowing it to slow down in a fashion similar to CV4.[25]

### Remarks

This procedure cannot be effectively performed in patients who have temporal bone dysfunction.

This same alternating procedure may be applied to any paired bones such as the parietal and pelvic bones.

## References

1.  Still AT. Philosophy of Osteopathy. Kirskville, MO: A.T. Still; 1899. Reprinted, Indianapolis, IN: American Academy of Osteopathy; 1971:28.
2.  Fryette HH.Osteopathy. Year Book of the Academy of Applied Osteopathy. American Academy of Osteopathy. Indianapolis, IN. 1948;21-4.
3.  Seffinger MA, King HH, et. al. Osteopathic Philosophy. Chapt 1. In: Chila AG. ed. Foundations of Osteopathic Medicine. 3rd ed. Philadelphia: Wolters Kluwer/Lippincott Williams and Wilkins; 2011:7.
4.  Fuller DB. Osteopathy and Swedenborg. Swedenborg Scientific Association Press. Bryn Athyn PA, 2012.
5.  Glossary of Osteopathic Terminology. In: Chila AG. ed. Foundations of Osteopathic Medicine. 3rd ed. Philadelphia: Wolters Kluwer/Lippincott Williams and Wilkins; 2011:1098-9.
6.  Becker RE. Diagnostic touch: its principles and application. Part IV. Trauma and stress. Year Book of the Academy of Applied Osteopathy. American Academy of Osteopathy. Indianapolis, IN. 1965;2:165.
7.  Still AT. The Autobiography of A. T. Still. Chapter XXIV. Kirksville, MO: Published by the author, 1908:290.
8.  Jones LH. Spontaneous Release by Positioning. The DO, 1964; 4:109-16.
9.  Wales AL. Osteopathic dynamics. Year book of The Academy of Applied Osteopathy. American Academy of Osteopathy. Indianapolis, IN. 1946:42.
10. Lippincott HA. The osteopathic technique of WM. G. Sutherland, D.O. Year Book of the Academy of Applied Osteopathy. American

Academy of Osteopathy. Indianapolis, IN. 1949:1-24.

11. Sutherland WG. Contributions of thought. Fort Worth, TX : Sutherland Cranial Teaching Foundation, Inc.; 1998: 279.

12. Lippincott HA. The osteopathic technique of WM. G. Sutherland, D.O. Year Book of the Academy of Applied Osteopathy. American Academy of Osteopathy. Indianapolis, IN. 1949:1-24.

13. Facto LL. The osteopathic treatment for lobar pneumonia. J Am Osteopath Assoc. 1947 Mar;46(7):385-92.

14. Litton HE. Manipulative treatment of pneumonia. Year Book of the Academy of Applied Osteopathy. American Academy of Osteopathy. Indianapolis, IN. 1965:136-8.

15. Sergueef N. C0, C1, C2, Données physiologiques et normalisations. Paris: Spek; 1989.

16. Sergueef N. C0, C1, C2, Données physiologiques et normalisations. Paris: Spek; 1989.

17. Young MD. Head's law and its relation to treatment of the viscera. Year Book of the Academy of Applied Osteopathy. American Academy of Osteopathy. Indianapolis, IN. 1947:65-9.

18. Magoun HI. Osteopathy in the cranial field. 2nd ed. Kirksville, MO: The Journal Printing Company;1966:300.

19. Balboni AL, Estenson TL, Reidenberg JS, Bergemann AD, Laitman JT. Assessing age-related ossification of the petro-occipital fissure: laying the foundation for understanding the clinicopathologies of the cranial base. Anat Rec A Discov Mol Cell Evol Biol. 2005 Jan;282(1):38-48.

20. Sergueef N. C0, C1, C2, Données physiologiques et normalisations. Paris: Spek; 1989.

21. Sergueef N. Normaliser la colonne sans "manipulation vertébrale". Paris: Spek; 1994.

22. Becker RE. Life in motion. Portland, OR: Rudra Press; 1997:106.

23. Nelson KE, Sergueef N, Glonek T. The effect of an alternative medical procedure upon low-frequency oscillations in cutaneous blood flow velocity. J Manipulative Physiol Ther. 2006 Oct;29(8):626-36.

24. Magoun HI. Osteopathy in the cranial field. Kirksville, MO: The Journal Printing Company; 1951:86.

25. Magoun HI. Osteopathy in the cranial field. Kirksville, MO: The Journal Printing Company; 1951:88.

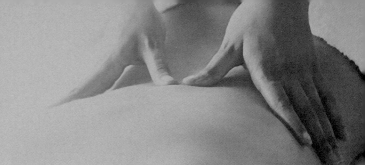

# SECTION 4

# Clinical considerations

# Musculoskeletal dysfunctions
# Part 1: Axial system

Back and neck pain are among the most frequently encountered complaints of older people. A thorough understanding of the anatomy and physiology of the vertebral column will facilitate comprehension of the mechanisms involved in the dysfunctional process of back and neck pain, and will help to treat the patients suffering with these symptoms.

## The vertebral column

The vertebral column supports the trunk and the upper extremities, protects the spinal cord, and offers strong attachment to the spinal muscles. At the same time, it allows movements between adjacent vertebrae, resulting in spinal mobility in all major planes.

In the sagittal plane, the vertebral column demonstrates four curvatures: cervical, thoracic, lumbar, and sacral.

Normally, in the cervical and lumbar regions the convexity of the curves is anterior and forms a lordosis. In the thoracic and sacral regions, the convexity of the curves is posterior and forms a kyphosis. As soon as 8 to 23 weeks gestation, radiographic examinations of human fetuses demonstrate the cervical curvature. Lumbar flattening has also been recognized as early as the eighth week.[1] In the coronal plane, any curvature of the vertebral column is pathological, with curvature greater than 10° constituting a scoliosis.

The vertebral column consists of a total of 33 vertebrae: seven cervical, twelve thoracic, five lumbar, five sacral, and four coccygeal. The five sacral vertebrae are fused to form the sacrum; sometimes, the coccygeal vertebrae are also fused.

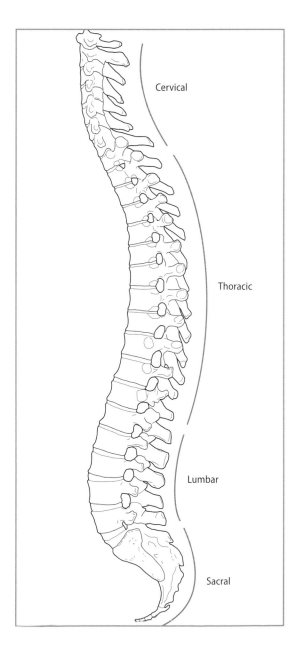

Figure 4.1.1: In the sagittal plane, the vertebral column demonstrates four curvatures

Cervical

Thoracic

Lumbar

Sacral

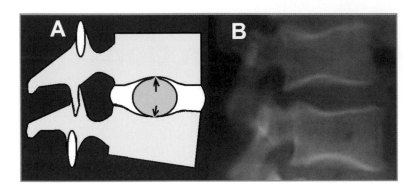

Figure 4.1.2: X-ray: (A) Schmorl's nodes—the herniation of the nucleus pulposus through the vertebral endplate, the result of excessive weight-bearing stress. (B) Lumbar X-ray demonstrating Schmorl's nodes.

With the exception of the first cervical vertebra (the atlas) each vertebra consists of a body, two pedicles, and two laminae that join posteriorly to form the spinous process. The atlas is a ring shaped bone, without a body. On each side of a vertebra, superior and inferior articular processes, also named zygapophyses, form synovial joints between adjacent vertebrae. Bilaterally, the transverse processes complete the vertebra. Numerous muscles insert on the spinous and transverse processes that act as lever arms.

Again, with the exception of the atlas upon the second cervical vertebra (the axis) in addition to the articulations present between the superior and inferior articular processes, there is also an intervertebral disc constituting another articulation between adjacent vertebrae.

A highly porous trabecular bone surrounded by a solid shell forms the architecture of a vertebral body. Between the cancellous core of the verte-bral body and the intervertebral disc, the vertebral endplate forms a structural boundary and prevents extrusion of the disc into the porous vertebral body. This arrangement evenly distributes load to the vertebral body and acts as a semipermeable interface, which permits the transfer of water and solutes but inhibits the loss of large proteoglycan molecules from the disc.[2] It seems to be the weakest part of the vertebral body and under excessive weight-bearing stress can deform allowing Schmorl's nodes, the vertical herniation of the nucleus pulposus through the vertebral endplate.

## Cervical vertebrae

There are seven cervical vertebrae. The third, fourth, fifth, and sixth are considered typical cervical vertebrae. The first, second, and seventh have special characteristics, and will be described independently.

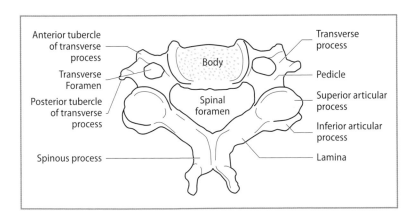

Figure 4.1.3: Typical cervical vertebra

Anterior tubercle of transverse process

Transverse Foramen

Posterior tubercle of transverse process

Spinous process

Body

Spinal foramen

Transverse process

Pedicle

Superior articular process

Inferior articular process

Lamina

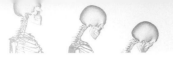

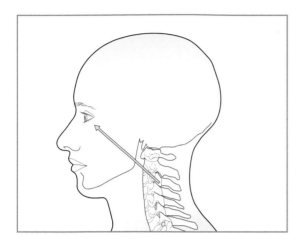

Figure 4.1.4: The plane of the cervical articular intervertebral facet joints points in the general direction of the patient's eye

## Typical cervical vertebrae

Typical cervical vertebrae have a small and broad vertebral body. The superior surface of the vertebral body is characterized by the uncinate processes expanding from the lateral circumference of the upper margin of the vertebral body. These processes restrict lateral gliding movements. Additionally, the superior, saddle-shaped surface of the body demonstrates several vascular foramina—the basivertebral foramina that convey basivertebral veins to the anterior internal vertebral veins. The inferior surface of the vertebral body is concave and the lowest part of the anterior margin projects inferiorly to partly cover the anterior surface of the intervertebral disc.

The anterior surface of the vertebral body is convex, whereas the posterior surface is slightly concave. On their superior and inferior borders, respectively, the anterior and posterior longitudinal ligaments are attached.

Because of the cervical enlargement of the spinal cord and the need for accommodation of a large vertebral canal, the cervical vertebral pedicles are directed posterolaterally and the longer laminae are directed posteromedially. On each side, an articular pillar, between the superior and inferior articular facets, also named the lateral mass, represents the junction between lamina and pedicle. Relatively flat, the superior articular facets are directed superoposteriorly; however, the inferior facets positioned closer to the coronal plane are directed anteriorly. As such, the plane of the cervical articular intervertebral facet joints points in the general direction of the patient's eye.

The spinous process is short and bifid, with two tubercles usually unequal in size. The transverse process is directed anterolaterally, presents a foramen transversarium for the vertebral artery, and ends with two tubercles: anterior and posterior. The anterior tubercle is developmentally homologous to the ribs in the thoracic spine, and as such the lower cervical segments have the potential for congenitally anomalous cervical ribs. The sixth anterior tubercle, the carotid tubercle of Chassaignac, is normally the longest. At this level, in the space between the vertebral body and the anterior tubercle, the carotid artery can be compressed.

## C1

The first cervical vertebra, the atlas, articulates with the occiput and supports the head. It consists of two lateral masses connected by an anterior and a posterior arch. Because the atlas does not have a vertebral body, it is often referred as the atlantal ring. Upper and lower borders of the anterior arch give insertion to the anterior atlanto-occipital membrane. The anterior surface of the anterior arch presents a tubercle where the anterior longitudinal ligament attaches. The posterior surface demonstrates an articular facet for the dens of the axis, maintained against the anterior arch by the transverse ligament.

On each side, the lateral mass is directed anteromedially and presents a superior articular facet, slightly concave, for the occipital condyle. The inferior articular facet of the lateral mass is flat and roughly circular. It is directed medially and very slightly backwards.

The posterior arch is longer than the anterior arch and represents three-fifths of the circumference of the atlantal ring. Just behind the lateral mass, a wide groove receives the vertebral artery and venous plexus. The posterior atlanto-axial

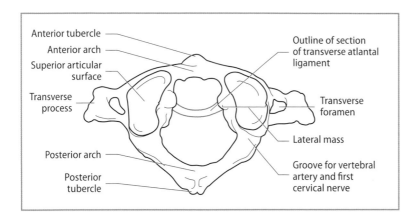

Figure 4.1.5: First cervical vertebra (atlas)

membrane attaches onto the superior border and the ligamenta flava to the inferior border. Posteriorly, a tubercle represents an undeveloped spinous process and gives insertion to the ligamentum nuchae.

Laterally, the transverse processes extend more than at the other cervical levels, with the exception of that of the seventh cervical vertebra. The apices of the transverse processes can be easily palpated bilaterally between the ramus of the mandible and the mastoid process, and are important landmarks in the normalization of the cervical spine.

## C2

The body of the second cervical vertebra (the axis) is fused with the ossification center of the body of the atlas above to form the dens, also named the

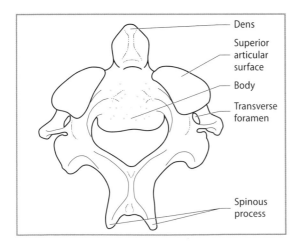

Figure 4.1.6: Second cervical vertebra

odontoid process. All through life, a synchondrosis persists between the body of the axis and the dens, and a rudimentary disc can often be seen. The posterior surface of the conically shaped dens displays a large groove for the transverse ligament, whereas its anterior surface demonstrates an ovoid articular facet for the anterior arch of the atlas.

Several ligaments attach to the dens that contribute to the maintenance of its position. From the apex arises the apical ligament that inserts onto the occiput. From the posterolateral surfaces above the transverse ligament the alar ligaments are attached. These are directed anteriorly and also insert onto the occiput.

On each side of the dens a sizeable ovoid, slightly convex, articular facet articulates with the atlas above. On the inferior border of the vertebral body anteriorly is the attachment of the anterior longitudinal ligament, whereas posteriorly, the inferior border gives attachment to the posterior longitudinal ligament and the membrana tectoria.

The transverse process is directed inferiorly and laterally. Its rounded tip can be palpated through the sternocleidomastoid muscle. The spinous process is big, bifid, and can be easily palpated. It is, in fact, the first spinous process palpable under the occipital bone and the ligamentum nuchae is inserted to its apical notch.

## C7

The seventh cervical vertebra, the vertebra prominens, has a long spinous process with a prominent tubercle usually well visible in the posterior

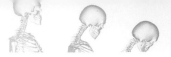 

midline at the lower part of the neck. It bears the attachment of the ligamentum nuchae and multiple muscles: trapezius, spinalis capitis, semispinalis thoracis, multifidus, and interspinales. Their traction explains the prominence of the tubercle. The transverse processes are wide and prominent and present at their anterior border the attachment of the suprapleural membrane.

## Thoracic vertebrae

There are twelve thoracic vertebrae. They provide attachment for the rib cage, which in turn reduces the thoracic spine mobility. At the upper and lower aspects of the thoracic region, thoracic vertebrae are somewhat atypical looking, like the cervical and lumbar vertebrae respectively.

The bodies of the vertebrae are more or less heart-shaped and their anteroposterior (AP) and transverse dimensions are almost identical. Their superior and inferior borders provide the attachment for the anterior and posterior longitudinal ligaments. On either side, the body of the typical thoracic vertebra exhibits two costal demifacets—the costocapitular facets that articulate with the head of the ribs: one above, near the root of the pedicle, the other below, in front of the inferior vertebral notch. The body of the ninth, tenth, eleventh, and twelfth thoracic vertebrae display only superior costal demifacets. Also, all but the lowest two or three transverse processes have articular facets, the costotubercular facets that articulate with the tubercle of the corresponding rib.

The superior articular processes are flat and face postero-supero-laterally, whereas the inferior articular processes face antero-infero-medially. At the level of the eleventh thoracic vertebra, or sometimes at the level of the twelfth, orientation of the articular processes typically changes so that while the superior articular processes are thoracic, more coronal, directed posterolaterally, the inferior articular processes become more lumbar, more sagittal, directed anteromedially. This transition in orientation of articular processes from thoracic to lumbar type marks the level of a sudden change of available intersegmental spinal motion from predominantly rotational to predominantly flexion/extension.

Thoracic transverse processes are long, thick, and strong, directed obliquely posteriorly and laterally. There is no foramen transversarium within the transverse process. At the front of each end of the upper five or six vertebrae, a tiny concave facet directed anterolaterally articulates with the rib. Below this level, the facets are more or less flat and directed superolaterally and somewhat anteriorly. If a line is drawn connecting the costovertebral and costotransverse articulations it forms an 'axis' for respiratory rib motion.

All ribs have 'pump handle' and 'bucket handle' motion.

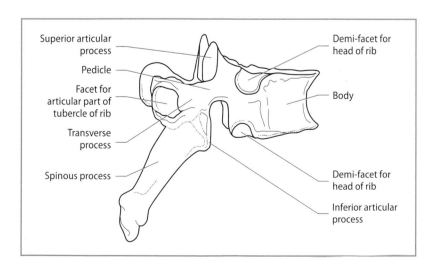

Figure 4.1.7: Thoracic vertebra

Superior articular process
Pedicle
Facet for articular part of tubercle of rib
Transverse process
Spinous process

Demi-facet for head of rib
Body
Demi-facet for head of rib
Inferior articular process

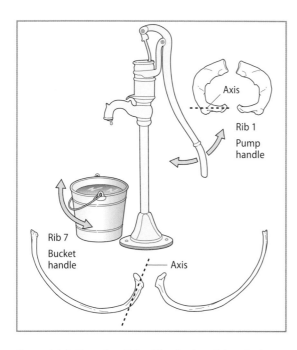

Figure 4.1.8: 'Pump handle' and 'bucket handle' motion'

The predominant respiratory motion is directly related to the positional relationship between the costovertebral and costotransverse articulations. For rib one the costovertebral costotransverse axis is nearly horizontal transverse, almost in the coronal plane. As such the upper ribs have pump handle motion as their major motion and demonstrate only a minor amount of bucket handle motion. For rib seven, the axis is about 45° below the horizontal transverse, and the costotransverse end of the axis is posterior relative to the costovertebral end. Consequently, the lower ribs have bucket handle motion as their major motion and demonstrate only a minor amount of pump handle motion. Respiratory rib dysfunctions tend to occur as restrictions of the minor motions between the thoracic vertebra and respective rib.

The spinous process is long and leans downward. At each level, supraspinous and interspinous ligaments are attached to the spinous process. The obliquity of the spinous process is at its maximum at the level of T7, where the tip of the spinous process reaches the level of the body of T9. Practically, the practitioner should always remember that the level of the tip of the spinous process does not al-

ways correspond with the level of the transverse process.

The approximate position of the transverse process of a given thoracic segment may be identified by using the location of the spinous process of the same vertebra. For T1–T3, the transverse processes are palpable at the same level as the tip of the respective spinous processes. For T4–T6, the transverse processes are palpable one half of a vertebral level above the tips of the spinous processes. For T7–T9, the transverse processes are found one full vertebral level above the tips of the spinous processes. The lowest three thoracic vertebrae reverse this positional sequence such that: the transverse process of T10 is one full vertebral level above the tip of its spinous process; the transverse process of T11 is one half of a vertebral level above the tip of its spinous process; and the transverse process of T12 is at the same level as the tip of its spinous process.

### T1

The first thoracic vertebra looks like a cervical vertebra, yet its body displays a round superior costal facet that articulates with the facet on the head of the first rib. Inferiorly, it presents a smaller facet that articulates with a demifacet on the head of the second rib. The spinous process is long, horizontal, and looks like the spinous process of the seventh cervical vertebra.

### T9

The body of the ninth thoracic vertebra displays only superior costal demifacets. Therefore, superiorly, it articulates above with the ninth ribs, but does not articulate inferiorly with the tenth ribs.

### T10

The tenth thoracic vertebra simply articulates with the tenth pair of ribs. Therefore it displays only superior demifacets. Also, the transverse process may not display a facet for the tenth rib tubercle.

### T11

The eleventh thoracic vertebral body approximates the size and form of a lumbar vertebra. It articulates only with the heads of the eleventh ribs, with large articular facets. The transverse processes

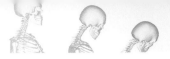

are very small and have no articular facets. The spinous process is short and almost horizontal.

### T12

The twelfth thoracic vertebra resembles the lumbar vertebrae. It articulates with the heads of the twelfth ribs. On either side, the transverse process displays three tubercles: superior, inferior, and lateral. The superior and inferior tubercles correspond to the mammillary and accessory processes of the lumbar vertebrae.

## Lumbar vertebrae

There are five lumbar vertebrae, recognized by their big size, absence of costal facets on the sides of the body, and lack of foramen transversarium within the transverse process. The body of each lumbar vertebra is large and wider transversely than it is antero-posteriorly. The short pedicles appear at the upper border of each body. They are directed posterolaterally and their inferior notches are well-marked whereas the superior notches are shallow.

The transverse processes are thin and long, apart from the fifth pair, which is thicker. They increase in length from the first to the third lumbar vertebra and then shorten. They are located in front of the articular processes instead of behind them as in the thoracic vertebrae, and the upper

three transverse processes are more horizontal than the lower two. They project posterolaterally. A tiny accessory process characterizes the posteroinferior aspect of the root of each transverse process.

The spinous process is thick, roughly horizontal, quadrangular, and its posterior and inferior borders are thickened.

The superior articular processes display articular facets that are vertical, concave, and directed posteromedially. On their posterior borders arise a rough tubercle (the mamillary process) where the multifidus and the medial intertransverse muscles are attached. The inferior articular processes exhibit articular facets that are vertical, convex, and directed anterolaterally.

The vertebral foramen is triangular, larger than at the thoracic levels, but smaller than in the cervical vertebrae. The conus medullaris of the spinal cord is enclosed within the spinal canal approximately at the level of the first lumbar vertebra. The spinal nerves below L1 form the cauda equina and exit through their respective intervertebral foramina, surrounded by the spinal meninges.

### L5

The fifth lumbar vertebra presents the largest body. It is also characterized by thick transverse processes and a small spinous process.

## Sacrum

The sacrum is a large, triangular bone at the base of the spine. It is the result of the fusion of five vertebrae inserted like a wedge between the two innominate bones and forms the posterosuperior wall of the pelvic cavity. Its upper wide base articulates with the fifth lumbar vertebra to form the prominent sacrovertebral angle, and its apex articulates with the coccyx. The five vertebrae are usually completely fused into a single bone by age 25.

It is curved upon itself with a convex dorsal surface and a concave pelvic surface that forms the roof of the pelvic cavity. Sexual dimorphism is typical. Usually, the sacrum of the female is smaller and wider, with a greater curve in its lower half than that of the male sacrum. The wide base of the sacrum is the upper surface of the first sacral vertebra. It is directed upward and forward, with an

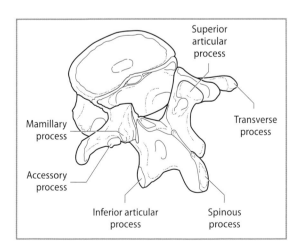

Figure 4.1.9: Lumbar vertebra

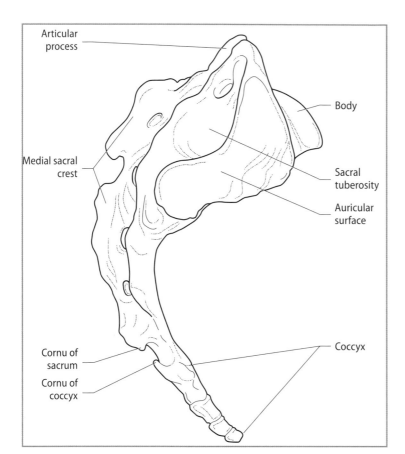

Figure 4.1.10: Sacrum

Labels on figure:
- Articular process
- Body
- Medial sacral crest
- Sacral tuberosity
- Auricular surface
- Cornu of sacrum
- Cornu of coccyx
- Coccyx

anterior border named the sacral promontory. The anterior and posterior longitudinal ligaments are inserted at the ventral and dorsal surfaces of the first sacral body.

On either side, the transverse processes are large, expanding laterally from the body of the sacral vertebra, and are referred to as the ala.

The superior articular processes directed superiorly display articular facets that are concave and face posteromedially. They articulate with the inferior articular processes of the fifth lumbar vertebra.

The laminae meet at a spinous tubercle. A median sacral crest on the posterosuperior portion of the dorsal surface, the result of fused sacral spines, consists of three or four spinous tubercles. In the posterior wall of the sacral canal, the failure of the laminae of the fifth sacral vertebra to fuse creates an arched sacral hiatus.

The fusion of the sacral vertebrae produces four pairs of anterior and posterior pelvic sacral

foramina. They lead into the sacral canal and the anterior pelvic sacral foramina convey ventral rami of the upper four sacral spinal nerves whereas the posterior pelvic sacral foramina transmit the dorsal ramus. On either side of the sacral hiatus, the inferior articular processes of the fifth sacral vertebra directed inferiorly form the sacral cornua. The sacral canal contains the cauda equina, the filum terminale, and the spinal meninges. The lower sacral spinal roots and filum terminale pierce the lowest part of the arachnoid and dura mater at the height of the middle of the sacrum. After that, the filum terminale becomes apparent under the sacral hiatus and reaches the coccyx.

The lateral surface of the sacrum is wide above, but narrowed into a thin edge in its lower part. Each of the lateral surfaces of the sacrum bears an auricular surface, a large L-shaped facet for articulation with the ilium of the pelvic bone. The area posterior to this facet is large and rough for the

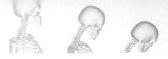

insertion of the strong interosseous sacroiliac (SI) ligaments. The auricular surface resembles an inverted letter L. The small cranial limb corresponds to the first sacral vertebra; the long caudal limb reaches the middle of the third sacral vertebra. Hyaline cartilage coats the auricular surface that turns out to be more grooved with age. Sacrotuberous and sacrospinous ligaments are fixed below the auricular surface at the level of the transverse processes of S4. The traction from these ligaments upon the lateral aspect of the sacrum results in a palpable bony prominence. This landmark is unique to osteopathic vocabulary and is referred to as the inferior lateral angle.

The inferior aspect of the fifth sacral vertebral body directed inferiorly is the apex of the sacrum, and presents an oval facet for articulation with the coccyx.

## Coccyx

The coccyx is the terminal part of the spinal column. It results from the fusion of three to five coccygeal vertebrae and has a triangular shape with its base projected superiorly. Occasionally, the first coccygeal vertebra is not fused with the second coccygeal segment.

The base or superior surface of the first coccygeal vertebral body supports an articular facet for articulation with the sacral apex. On either side, two horns or coccygeal cornua directed superiorly articulate with sacral cornua. Small, undeveloped transverse processes extend superolaterally

that sometimes articulate or fuse with the lower aspect of the inferolateral sacral angle. On the dorsum of the first coccygeal vertebra the filum terminale, located between the deep and superficial posterior sacrococcygeal ligaments, intermingle with these ligaments and the periosteum of the bone.

## Ligaments of the vertebral column

The ligaments of the vertebral column and the intrinsic muscles play an important role in the limit of vertebral motion. They also take part in the dysfunctions of the spine as well as in its degenerative processes.

### Anterior and posterior longitudinal ligaments

Two long ligaments link the occipital bone and the pelvis. They are the anterior and posterior longitudinal ligaments. The anterior longitudinal ligament attaches to the anterior surfaces of the vertebral bodies. Quite solid, it is slightly thicker and narrower over the vertebral bodies than at the levels of the intervertebral discs and generally in the thoracic region, when compared to the cervical and lumbar regions. Cranially, it inserts on the lower basilar part of the occipital bone, on the anterior tubercle of C1 and the anterior surface of the body of C2. Next it goes on to attach loosely to the anterior surfaces of the vertebral bodies, whereas it is more solidly adherent to the endplates and borders of vertebral bodies and the intervertebral

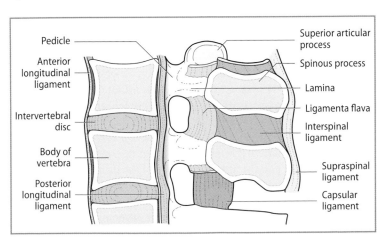

**Figure 4.1.11:** Sagittal section of two lumbar vertebrae and their ligaments

Pedicle

Anterior longitudinal ligament

Intervertebral disc

Body of vertebra

Posterior longitudinal ligament

Superior articular process

Spinous process

Lamina

Ligamenta flava

Interspinal ligament

Supraspinal ligament

Capsular ligament

discs. Caudally, the anterior longitudinal ligament inserts onto the front of the upper sacrum.

The posterior longitudinal ligament extends upon the posterior surfaces of the vertebral bodies from the axis to the sacrum and constitutes the anterior wall of the spinal canal. It is attached tightly to every intervertebral disc, and to the endplates and adjacent borders of vertebral bodies. Between the ligament and the posterior surface of the vertebral bodies, attachment is limited leaving space for the basivertebral veins. It is wide at the cervical and upper thoracic levels, and begins to narrow in the lower thoracic region. At the level of the lumbar spine it is denticulated, narrow over vertebral bodies and wide over the intervertebral discs. At the level of L5 it decreases to one half of its original, upper cervical width. Perivertebral ligaments can be described as deeper fibers extending between adjacent vertebrae.[3]

Above the axis, the posterior longitudinal ligament is continuous with the membrana tectoria that spreads out to the upper surface of the basilar occipital bone. It inserts on the anterior border of the foramen magnum, where its fibers intermingle with the cranial dura mater.

## Ligamenta flava

The ligamenta flava joins laminae of adjacent vertebrae in the vertebral canal. Above, it is attached to the anterior inferior surface of the laminae of the superior vertebral segment and below to the posterior superior border of the laminae of the vertebra below. Laterally, its fibers expand to the facet joint capsules. At the cervical level, the ligaments are thin, wide, and long; they thicken caudally to be the thickest at lumbar levels.

A high percentage of yellow elastin fibers give this structure its name and prevent separation of the laminae during vertebral flexion.[4] With age, this ligament can thicken, contributing along with other degenerative changes to spinal canal stenosis at the cervical and lumbar levels.[5]

## Ligamentum nuchae

Several descriptions have been reported for the ligamentum nuchae. In fact, several authors describe two structures: a dorsal raphe and a midline fascial septum. The posterior border of the dorsal raphe is superficial, expands over the cervical spine, and attaches to the external occipital protuberance and to the spine of C7. The fibroelastic fascial septum is fixed to the median part of the external occipital crest, the posterior tubercle of C1, and the medial aspects of the bifid spines of cervical vertebrae. It gives bilateral attachment to posterior cervical musculature and aponeurosis. There is also a midline continuity between the nuchal ligament and the posterior spinal dura at the atlanto-occipital and atlanto-axial intervals.

## Other vertebral ligaments

Other vertebral ligaments include interspinous and supraspinous ligaments that connect adjoining spinous processes. The former are slight, and more or less membranous. The latter is a stout fibrous cord expanding between the tips of spinous process from C7 to the sacrum. Above C7 the supraspinous ligament continues expanded as the ligamentum nuchae.

Above C2, the anterior and posterior atlanto-occipital membranes and fibrous capsules surround the occipital condyles and superior atlantal articular facets. The anterior atlanto-occipital membrane joins the anterior margin of the foramen magnum to the upper border of the anterior arch of the atlas. It is a solid fibrous structure that intermingles with the atlanto-occipital articular capsule and anteriorly with the median cord of the anterior longitudinal ligament. The posterior atlanto-occipital membrane joins the posterior margin of the foramen magnum to the upper border of the posterior atlantal arc. Wide and thin, it also blends with the atlanto-occipital articular capsule.

Behind the dens of the axis, the transverse atlantal ligament curves transversely in the atlantal ring, attached to each atlantal lateral mass on a small tubercle. Its mean length is 19.7 mm. A tough median longitudinal band bonds its upper border to the basilar part of the occipital bone, where it attaches between the membrana tectoria and the apical ligament of the dens. From its lower border, a delicate longitudinal band is connected to the posterior surface of the axis. This combined structure of the transverse ligament and its

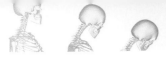
longitudinal parts is often referred to as the cruciform ligament. As such, the transverse atlantal ligament divides the ring of the atlas into an anterior and a posterior part. The anterior part holds the dens whereas the posterior part encloses the spinal cord and meninges.

Superiorly, the two alar ligaments stabilize the dens. Quite solid, they consist of a cord that connects the posterolateral aspect of the apex of the dens to the medial side of the occipital condyle on either side. From the apex of the dens, the apical ligament of the dens projects to the anterior border of the foramen magnum.

## Joints of the vertebral column

The anatomy of the vertebral column determines the motion patterns demonstrated by the vertebrae. Between C2 and S1, cartilaginous joints of the intervertebral discs provide articulation between the bodies of the vertebrae. Between the articular processes of the vertebrae (zygapophyses), the zygapophyseal joints are synovial joints, while the linkages between their laminae (the transverse and spinous processes) are fibrous joints. In the cervical area, additional unique articulations are present between the typical vertebrae. Between C3 and C7, uncovertebral joints, or joints of Luschka, exist between the uncinate processes of the upper margin of the superior surface of the vertebral bodies, and the inferior surface of the superior vertebral bodies. They display a synovial part, articular cartilage, and a partial capsule.[6]

Above C2, there is the junction between the vertebral column and the cranium. It consists of two articular units: the articulation of the occipital bone with the atlas, and the articulation between the atlas and the axis. This relationship allows precise movements that greatly enhance the mobility of the cervical spine. Between the occipital bone and the atlas there is a pair of synovial joints: the atlanto-occipital joints. The articular surfaces i.e., the occipital condyles and the lateral masses of the atlas are reciprocally curved: the occipital condyles are convex and the atlantal facets are concave.

Between the atlas and the axis there are three synovial joints: the atlanto-axial joints. Two of them are located between the lateral masses of the atlas and the axis and another one is located between the dens of the axis and the anterior arch of the atlas. On the anterior surface of the dens a vertically ovoid facet articulates with a facet on the posterior portion of the anterior atlantal arch.

## Intervertebral discs

Between the adjacent surfaces of vertebral bodies from C2 to the sacrum, the intervertebral discs are cartilaginous and articulating structures. They are the most important joints of the vertebral column that allow movement (flexion, extension, sidebending and rotation). At the cervical and lumbar levels the intervertebral disc represents approximately one-third of the height of the vertebral body, allowing for greater mobility than at the thoracic level where it corresponds to one-sixth of the vertebral body height. Although variable among individuals, the discs are about 0.7–1 cm thick. They consist of a dense outer ring of fibrous cartilage with concentric lamellae, the annulus fibrosus, which surrounds the nucleus pulposus, a more gelatinous center that consists of 88% of water in the healthy, young disc.[7] The collagen fibers of the annulus are arranged obliquely in layers, in alternating directions, and 15–25 distinct layers have been identified in the human lumbar spine.[8] With aging, the thickness of these layers differs circumferentially and radially, increasing noticeably.

Collagen fibers extend from the annulus fibrosus into the adjacent tissues, binding this fibrocartilaginous structure to the vertebral bodies at its rim, to the anterior and posterior longitudinal ligaments, and superiorly and inferiorly to the hyaline cartilage vertebral body endplates. At the same time, the cartilage endplates buttress into the osseous vertebral endplates via the calcified cartilage.[9]

At a molecular and cellular level, components of the lumbar intervertebral disc are similar to articular cartilage. The matrix of the nucleus pulposus and the cartilaginous vertebral endplate comes together from chondrocyte-like cells that synthesize type II collagen, proteoglycans, and non-collagenous proteins, whereas the annulus fibrosus develops from fibroblast-like cells.[10] Therefore, the properties of the matrix allow compression loads and support the annulus.

In the normal adult disc, nerves and blood vessels are present to a limited degree. The intervertebral disc is alymphatic,[11] avascular, and receives its nutrition by passive diffusion from vessels in the endplate regions and around the annulus.[12] Additionally, changes in the individual posture influences the fluid flow component of the nutrient supply.[13] [14] In sitting postures associated with flexion of the lumbar spine, more fluid is expressed from the lumbar discs than in erect postures. Additionally, changes in load between the day when the individual is weight-bearing and in motion and the night when they are resting also results in fluid exchange.

The nucleus pulposus has no nerve supply; only the outer lamellae of the annulus fibrosus contains nerve endings from the sinuvertebral nerves. A small number of mechanoreceptors are also found, having generally the morphology of Golgi tendon organs, a small number of Ruffini receptors, and fewer Pacinian corpuscles.[15]

## Vertebral canal

The vertebral canal extends from the foramen magnum to the sacral hiatus. Its size varies, adapting for changes in the diameter of the spinal cord. Typically, in the cervical region, the canal is large and triangular, its AP diameter being roughly 21 mm between C1–C3 and 18 mm between C4–C7. As a rule, the midsagittal diameter of the cervical spinal cord fills about 40% of the midsagittal diameter of the cervical canal.[16] However, a decrease of 2 to 3 mm occurs in the diameter of the cervical canal during extension of the neck.

As in the cervical region, the lumbar vertebral canal is large and triangular, its AP diameter being roughly 18 mm. Its size decreases progressively between L1–L5. In the thoracic region, the vertebral canal is small and circular.

## Intervertebral foramina

On either side of the vertebral column, the intervertebral foramina allow access into and out of the vertebral canal. Anteriorly, it is limited by

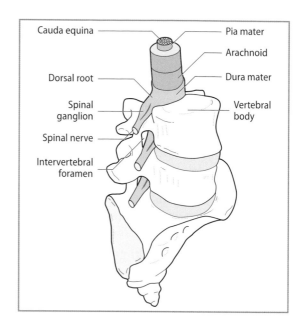

Figure 4.1.12: Intervertebral foramen

the posterolateral portion of the superior vertebral body above, the intervertebral disc, and the posterolateral portion of the body of the inferior vertebra below. Posteriorly, the limit is the zygapophyseal joint between the articular processes of the two vertebrae and part of the ventral aspect of the fibrous capsule of the facet synovial joint. Inferiorly, it is formed by the superior vertebral notch on the pedicle of the vertebra below, and superiorly by the inferior vertebral notch on the pedicle of the vertebra above.

Specific features exist depending upon the vertebral level that is considered. At the cervical level, the intervertebral foramina are directed anterolaterally, whereas at the thoracic and lumbar levels they are directed laterally. Furthermore, between the first to tenth thoracic vertebrae, the anteroinferior borders of the intervertebral foramina are shaped by the articulations of the heads of the ribs. Of clinical significance, at the lumbar level, vertebral insertions of the psoas major surround the foramina between T12–L1 and L4–L5. Consequently dysfunction of the psoas major might be responsible for compression of the structures, such as spinal nerves and blood vessels, as they enter and exit the vertebral canal.

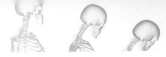

In fact, any structure enclosed in the intervertebral foramina may be affected by changes in the foraminal contour. Therefore the spinal nerve and its meningeal sheaths, the recurrent meningeal nerves, the spinal arteries, or the plexiform venous connections between the internal and external vertebral venous plexuses, may be impinged on by disc prolapse or degeneration, bony entrapment of facet joint osteoarthritis, and osteophyte formation. This can be further augmented by weight-bearing, pelvic unleveling, and muscle spasm.

With each movement of the spinal joints, the size of the intervertebral foramina varies. In the lumbar spine, flexion increases foraminal dimensions, whereas extension decreased foraminal dimensions. Sidebending considerably affects the intervertebral foramina, diminishing the foraminal width, height, and area on the side of the sidebending, while the opposite side displays an increase in its measurements. Rotation also produces a decrease of the foraminal measurements on the side of the rotation while the opposite side displays an increase of the same measurements.[17]

## Radicular canal

The space where the spinal nerve root runs from its point of emergence from the spinal cord to its exit through the intervertebral foramen is defined as the radicular canal. It has been extensively studied in the lumbar area. Shaped like a gutter directed vertically or somewhat obliquely downwards and backwards,[18] the lumbar radicular canal is typically divided into three portions: the retrodiscal portion, the parapedicular portion or lateral recess, and the intervertebral foramen.

- The retrodiscal portion is located between the intervertebral disc anteriorly, and the anterolateral surface of the superior articular process covered by the lateral part of the ligamentum flavum posteriorly.
- The parapedicular portion, or lateral recess, is medial to the entire height of the surface of the pedicle. Posteriorly, it is limited by the articular and isthmic part of the vertebra, where the nerve root is in direct contact with the ligamentum flavum. Anteriorly, it is limited by

the posterior surface of the body of the vertebra that is covered by the posterior longitudinal ligament.

- The intervertebral foramen differs in shape and dimensions according to the level of the lumbar spine. Above, it is limited by the concave, lower border of the pedicle, which is in close approximation to the nerve root. The inferior boundary of the radicular canal is defined by the superior border of the pedicle of the subjacent vertebra and the retrodiscal space. In its lower portion, the intervertebral foramen is limited anteriorly by the convexity of the disc and posteriorly by the ligamentum flavum covering the articular processes.

Within the lateral recess, the two roots of the spinal nerve, the anterior and posterior roots, run in the direction of the spinal ganglion, where they join. Typically, the spinal ganglion is located at the level of the intervertebral foramen. The spinal nerve roots are strongly ensheathed within the three layers of the meninges, which may be adherent to the lateral recess.[19] Beyond the intervertebral lumbar foramen, the meninges surrounding the spinal nerve roots extend for 6.7–8 mm.[20] Lymph vessels, arterioles, venous plexuses, and the sinuvertebral nerve travel along with the spinal nerve.

Bony compression of the spinal nerve may also occur in the lowest part of the parapedicular portion, or lateral recess. Anteriorly, it may be the bulging of the disc; posteriorly it may be osteoarthritis of the articular process or isthmic lysis. Furthermore, the size of the gutter in which the spinal nerve runs decreases at the level of the lower lumbar vertebrae, when the size of the lower spinal nerves increases, producing potentially more stress. This compression may also be aggravated by weight-bearing, pelvic unleveling, and muscle spasm.

## Innervation

The spinal nerves and the sinuvertebral nerves provide innervation to the spine. The ventral and dorsal rami of the spinal nerves appear in and just distal to the intervertebral foramina. Anteriorly, the sinuvertebral (recurrent meningeal) nerve is

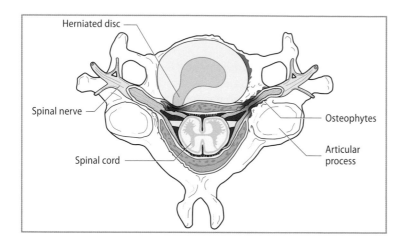

**Figure 4.1.13:** Spinal nerve compression

*Labels in figure:* Herniated disc, Spinal nerve, Spinal cord, Osteophytes, Articular process

formed by the merger of a somatic root from the ventral ramus of the spinal nerve and an autonomic root from the grey ramus communicans. The input from the sympathetic system comes directly from thoracic sympathetic ganglia.

The sinuvertebral nerve supplies structures within the vertebral canal. It goes into the vertebral canal through the intervertebral foramina, as a series of fine filaments. Branches ascend or descend one or more levels, interconnecting with the sinuvertebral nerves from other levels. The sinuvertebral nerve is distributed to the ventral aspect of the dural sac, the epidural soft tissues, the posterior longitudinal ligament, and the posterior portion of the annuli fibrosi. Its branches also encircle blood vessels and accompany the basivertebral veins into the vertebral bodies. Interestingly, from a clinical point of view, the lateral portions of the annuli fibrosi receive innervation from branches of the ventral rami and grey rami communicantes. The latter pass between and then deep to the attachments of the origin of the psoas major. As such, dysfunctions of the psoas may potentially be involved in mechanisms of low back pain through its relation with the annuli fibrosi. The anterior longitudinal ligament receives branches of the grey rami communicantes.

Posteriorly, medial branches of the dorsal rami provide innervation to the facet joints, periosteum of the posterior bony elements, overlying muscles, and skin. Each zygapophyseal or facet joint receives an innervation from at least two consecutive segments.

The outer third of the annulus of the intervertebral discs receives its innervation by the sinuvertebral nerves; the anterior and posterolateral aspects of the annulus receive direct branches from the sympathetic grey rami communicantes. In damaged and degenerated discs the nerves may infiltrate more centrally into the nucleus pulposus. In fact, nerve ingrowth is found in chronic back pain and because the sinuvertebral nerves consist of mixed polysegmental nerves and nerve plexuses, they facilitate a polysegmental signal and the spread of pain.

At the cervical level, innervation is provided by nerves, which have in part sympathetic and sensory nerve fibers. A projection from the spinal cord to the spinal trigeminal tract may play a role in neurogenic inflammation of the cranial dura. The overlap between trigeminal and upper cervical afferents throughout the trigeminocervical complex from the caudal trigeminal nucleus to the upper cervical segments provides understanding of referral mechanisms for cervical pain.[21]

## Vascularisation

### Blood supply

Blood supply of the cervical spine is derived from branches of the subclavian artery. The right subclavian artery starts from the brachiocephalic trunk, behind the upper border of the right

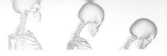

sternoclavicular joint, and passes superolaterally to the medial margin of the right scalenus anterior. The left subclavian artery arises from the aortic arch, at the level between the third and fourth thoracic vertebrae. It then ascends into the neck, curving laterally to contact the medial border of the left scalenus anterior.

The vertebral artery, one of the branches of the subclavian artery, originates from the superoposterior portion of the subclavian artery and ascends into the neck passing through the foramina of all the transverse processes of the cervical vertebrae with the exception of the seventh cervical vertebra. It arches back and medially behind the lateral masses of the first cervical vertebra to enter the skull via the foramen magnum. Several cervical spinal branches arise from the vertebral artery. These small spinal branches penetrate the vertebral canal through the intervertebral foramina to be distributed to the spinal cord, spinal dura, and vertebral bodies.

The blood supply to the thoracic spine is derived from branches of the thoracic aorta. As an extension of the aortic arch, the thoracic aorta starts at the level between the third and fourth thoracic vertebrae. It terminates at the level of the diaphragmatic aortic aperture, in front of the lower margin of the twelfth vertebra. It provides branches to the pericardium, lungs, bronchi, oesophagus, and to the thoracic wall. The dorsal branches of the posterior intercostal arteries have a spinal branch, which passes through the intervertebral foramen, enters the vertebral canal and supplies the vertebrae, spinal cord, and spinal dura.

The blood supply to the lumbar spine is derived from branches of the abdominal aorta. The abdominal aorta starts as a continuation of the thoracic aorta at the level of the aortic aperture of the thoracoabdominal diaphragm. From there it descends anterior to the vertebrae to the level of the fourth lumbar vertebra where it divides into the two common iliac arteries. The dorsal branches of the abdominal aorta are the lumbar and medial sacral arteries. Of these, the artery of Adamkiewicz provides significant blood supply to the lumbar and sacral spinal cord.[22] Damage to or obstruction of this arterial supply can result in anterior spinal artery syndrome.[23] This presents as urinary and fecal incontinence and lower extremities paraplegia, with sensory function often preserved to some extent.

Another dorsal branch arises from the lumbar artery to supply the dorsal muscles, joints, and skin and enters the vertebral canal supplying the spinal cord, meninges, fasciae, ligaments, vertebrae, and joints.

### Vascular drainage

Vascular drainage of the spine occurs via the vertebral veins.[24] These complex venous plexuses, external and internal to the vertebral canal, are present all along the entire spinal column. They have no valves, consist of many anastomoses, and connect to the intervertebral veins.

Anteriorly and posteriorly, the external vertebral venous plexuses are particularly well-developed in the cervical region. Anterior to the vertebral bodies, the anterior external plexuses are interconnected with basivertebral and intervertebral veins and receive branches from vertebral bodies. Posterior to the vertebral laminae, the posterior external plexuses surround the transverse and spinous processes. After joining the internal plexuses, the posterior external plexuses drain into the posterior intercostal and lumbar veins.

Between the dura mater and the vertebrae, the internal vertebral venous plexuses receive venous drainage from the vertebrae, red bone marrow, and spinal cord. They produce a compact network with two anterior and two posterior vertical connecting longitudinal vessels. Behind the vertebral bodies and intervertebral discs, the anterior internal plexuses form large plexiform veins running on the vertebral surfaces on either side of the posterior longitudinal ligament. Transverse branches receive the large basivertebral veins. On each side, anterior to the vertebral arches and ligamenta flava, the posterior internal plexuses connect with the posterior external plexuses through veins running among the ligaments.

The anterior external and internal vertebral venous plexuses receive the large and convoluted basivertebral veins that appear from the posterior foramina of the vertebral bodies. A large amount of haemopoietic tissue is found in the trabecular bone of the vertebral bodies.

External and internal vertebral venous plexuses connect to the intervertebral veins. The intervertebral veins go together with the spinal nerves through the intervertebral foramina. After they receive the spinal cord and internal and external vertebral plexuses, they drain into the vertebral, posterior intercostal, lumbar, and lateral sacral veins. The intercostal veins connect either with the caval or the azygos venous systems. After enveloping the vertebral bodies the lumbar veins may drain into the ascending lumbar veins or into the inferior vena cava.

Osteophyte formation and disc protrusion may impinge upon the vertebral nerve and venous system passing through the intervertebral foramina, with resultant stasis. Maintenance of the segmental mobility between vertebrae may consequently improve low pressure venous and lymphatic circulation. Disc protrusion may also compress the internal vertebral venous plexuses and be responsible for venous dilatation, and edema of the nerve root with resultant ischemia.

# Spinal motions

## Physiologic motion of the spine

Under normal circumstances, spinal motion is said to be physiological. Physiologic motion is motion demonstrated by the spine under normal weight-bearing circumstances. Motion restriction found in association with spinal somatic dysfunction commonly occurs within the normal range of motion manifested by the affected spinal articulation(s) in patterns consistent with the physiologic motion patterns. These patterns have been described in the osteopathic literature by authors like Harrison H. Fryette,[25][26] Fred L. Mitchell Sr.[27] and William L. Johnston.[28] When considering spinal somatic dysfunction, it is also important to differentiate between physiologic and non-physiologic motions. Non-physiologic motions result from exogenous forces, both macro- and micro-trauma, and are also found in association with alteration in normal anatomy, as seen in pathological conditions. As such, non-physiologic motion patterns are infinitely variable as determined by the direction of exogenous forces or the specific pathologic anatomic variations. Further, spinal dysfunction with ambiguous motion restriction is often the result of viscerosomatic reflexes. This is because it is a manifestation of a neurologically-mediated spinal cord reflex and not of mechanical origin. Consequently, when diagnosing somatic dysfunction, the identification of motion patterns that are inconsistent with the anticipated physiologic motion manifested in a given area should alert the examiner to the possibility of aberrant anatomic, traumatic, or viscerosomatic etiologies.

In both cases, complex physiologic and non-physiologic motion patterns are best understood by analyzing them in the context of simple motions occurring about, or along, the three dimensional (transverse, vertical, and AP) Cartesian axes.

- Motion (A) around the horizontal transverse (x) axis is flexion/extension.
- Motion (B) along the horizontal transverse axis is lateral translation to the left or right.

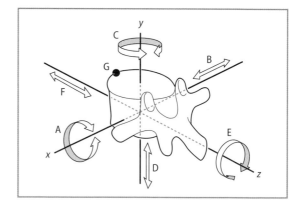

Figure 4.1.14: Motion upon the x axis: (A) flexion/extension, and along, (B) lateral translation to the left or right. Motion upon the y axis: (C) rotation to the left or right, and along, (D) superior or inferior translation. Motion upon the z axis: (E) sidebending to the left or right, and along, (F) anterior or posterior translation. (G) Point of reference for describing vertebral motion.

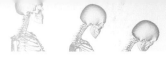
- Motion (C) around the vertical (y) axis is rotation to the left or right.
- Motion (D) along the vertical (y) axis is superior or inferior translation.
- Motion (E) around the horizontal AP (z) axis is sidebending to the left or right.
- Motion (F) along the horizontal AP (z) axis is anterior or posterior translation.
- Side bending left/right and lateral translation right/left are similar, but not identical motions.
- Flexion/extension and translation posterior/anterior are similar, but not identical motions.

In order to clearly communicate vertebral mechanics, a reference for the described motions must be defined. The motion of any spinal segment is described relative to the motion of a point on the most anterior superior aspect of the vertebral body of that segment.

When one is describing motion of a single vertebral segment, the reference is the vertebral segment immediately caudal. Thus, the motion being described and attributed to a given spinal segment is in fact a description of the motion between the segments of the vertebral unit, defined as two adjacent vertebrae, with their associated intervertebral disk, arthrodial, ligamentous, muscular, vascular, lymphatic, and neural elements.[29] When describing the motion of a group (three or more) of contiguous vertebrae the anatomic position is the reference. Since somatic dysfunction almost always is manifest as motion restriction, it may be described in the context of the direction in which the available motion is either unrestricted (free) or restricted. In this text, somatic dysfunction will be described in the context of the direction of motion freedom.

The physiologic motion encountered in all areas of the spine is a direct result of normal anatomy. Typical spinal vertebrae manifest segmental motion patterns as a result of their regionally unique intervertebral anatomy.[30] As such, cervical, thoracic, and lumbar (and lumbosacral) physiologic motion patterns are predictable. Segmental motion is determined in part by the relationship between adjacent vertebral bodies through the intervertebral disc. The unique anatomy of the vertebral bodies of typical segments within the cervical spine modifies this pattern somewhat when compared to the remainder of the spine and will be discussed below. The intervertebral range of motion is further modified by the anatomy of the intervertebral facets unique to each vertebral area. The facet orientation in the cervical spine that is between the coronal and transverse plane more readily permits rotation. The facet orientation in the thoracic spine in the coronal plane more readily permits sidebending and to a lesser degree rotation. The facet orientation in the lumbar spine, in the sagittal plane, more readily permits flexion and extension. The facet orientation at the lumbosacral junction being variable often results in individually variable motion predispositions within the neutral and non-neutral physiologic patterns. Potential facet asymmetry (facet tropism) is common at the lumbosacral junction, introducing the possibility of aberrant motion patterns.

It should be noted that the physiologic spinal motion patterns and all of the proposed axes of motion described herein are hypothetical. These motion patterns are observational and were first formally proposed over 90 years ago.[31] As such, they serve the purpose of providing a framework for clinical problem solving. The fact that they have been employed for almost a century attests to their usefulness. This chapter predominantly considers the motion patterns described by Fryette.[32] Where considered appropriate comparisons with other authors are made.

Fryette described neutral (type I) and non-neutral (type II) physiologic motion and consequently dysfunctional motion patterns for typical spinal segments. These principles of spinal physiologic motion apply only to motion patterns between typical spinal vertebrae. As defined by Fryette, this relationship occurs only between two or more spinal segments that possess articular facets and intervertebral discs. Under neutral circumstances, when the vertebrae behave as a group (three or more segments) and when sidebending forces are applied to the group, rotation occurs into the produced convexity. That is, sidebending and rotation occur in opposite directions relative to the anatomic position. Non-neutral mechanics occur when there is sufficient flexion or extension, for forces to become localized between two adjacent vertebrae. Then when sidebending forces are applied to the vertebral unit, rotation of the superior segment occurs into the produced concavity. That is, in the presence of significant flexion or extension, rotation and sidebending of the superior segment of the vertebral unit occur in the same direction relative to the inferior vertebral segment. See also 'Section 4: Clinical considerations, Chapter 2: Postural imbalance,' p. 242.

## Physiologic motion of the sacrum

Sacral mechanics can be considered relative to the ilia (anterior and posterior sacrum) or relative to the lumbar spine (forward and backward torsions). Under both circumstances, sacral rotation occurs about either the right or left oblique axis. Sacroiliac dysfunctions typically demonstrate the pattern of rotation and sidebending in opposite directions.[33] This coupled sacral sidebending and rotational relationship is described to be occurring as if the sacrum were rotating upon a hypothetical oblique axis. This oblique sacral axis, first described by H. I. Magoun Sr.[34] is currently said to pass from the superior pole of the SI articulation on one side to the inferior pole of the opposite SI articulation.

### The pelvis and the lumbar spine

*Lumbosacral mechanics:* Fryette stated that "anatomically the sacrum is part of the pelvis but physiologically it is part of the lumbar spine."[35] Sidebending of the lumbar spine upon the sacrum causes the sacrum to sidebend and rotate in such a way that the sacrum appears to be rotating upon the oblique axis on the side toward which the lumbar sidebending is occurring. That is, lumbar sidebending right engages the sacral right oblique axis and lumbar sidebending left engages the sacral left oblique axis. Under neutral weight-bearing circumstances (absence of significant forward or backward bending) the sacrum, relative to L5, will move forward on the side opposite the engaged oblique axis. This is referred to as a forward torsion

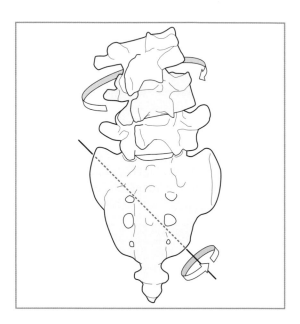

Figure 4.1.15: Fryette type I and forward torsion

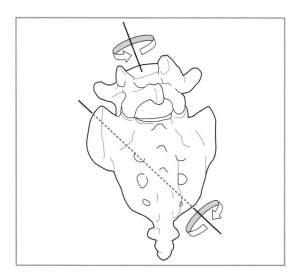

Figure 4.1.16: Fryette type II and backward torsion

and is further identified by the sacral mechanics on the involved oblique axis, that is: rotation right on the right oblique sacral axis or rotation left on the left oblique sacral axis. This is identical to the spinal motion seen in Fryette type I mechanics wherein the sacrum is acting as the lowest segment in a lumbar group curve.

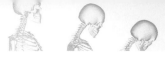

Under non-neutral circumstances (presence of significant forward or backward bending) the sacrum, relative to L5, will move backward on the side opposite to the engaged oblique axis. This is referred to as a backward torsion and is further identified by the sacral mechanics on the involved oblique axis, that is: rotation left on the right oblique sacral axis or rotation right on the left oblique sacral axis. This is identical to the spinal motion seen in Fryette type II mechanics wherein the sacrum is acting as the lower segment in a L5–S1 dysfunction.

### The sacrum and the ilium

*Anterior/posterior sacrum:* An anterior sacrum by definition is anterior to the ipsilateral ilium. Under these circumstances, if the ilium is described relative to the sacrum, it is posterior to the sacrum. This does not necessarily mean it is a 'posterior ilium.' The terms 'anterior ilium' and 'posterior ilium' may also refer to the position of one ilium relative to the contralateral ilium. This may result from asymmetrical soft tissue tensions, dysfunctional SI joint, pubic symphysis, or even lumbosacral mechanics. A similar relationship exists between the sacrum and ipsilateral ilium on the side of the posterior sacrum.

*As the sacrum moves so goes the ilium:* When rotational forces are applied to the sacrum from above and the sacrum rotates, the SI ligaments are tensed and the ilia move with the sacrum but to a lesser degree.[36]

*The symphysis pubis:* Superior and inferior shearing mechanics are most commonly seen in association with pubic dysfunction. This dysfunction, although relatively uncommon, is occasionally seen postpartum and following strenuous use of the adductor muscles of the thighs.

### The pelvis and the lower extremity

*Sacropelvic mechanics (the piriformis and gluteus medius):* As the sacrum rotates posteriorly, its ventral surface moves away from the greater trochanter on the side of posterior rotation, tensing the ipsilateral piriformis muscle. This initiates a stretch reflex, which results in the piriformis spasm found in association with a posterior sacrum.

The relationship between an anterior sacrum and gluteus medius tension is similar but not as immediately obvious. The anterior sacrum is anterior to the ipsilateral ilium. There is restriction of posterior movement of the sacrum relative to the ilium on the dysfunctional side. Under normal weight-bearing circumstances, forces acting upon the anterior sacrum from above, through the lumbar spine, tend to pull it posteriorly (toward a neutral position). Because of the SI restriction, the ilium is also pulled posterior relative to the femur. This places tension upon the gluteus medius (and minimus), which originates from the external surface of the ilium between the iliac crest and the posterior gluteal line above and anterior gluteal line below, and inserts upon the lateral aspect of the greater trochanter. The increased tension on the muscle results in spasm.

# Vertebral somatic dysfunction

Vertebral somatic dysfunction affects elder individuals involving any level of the spine. It will, however, be more commonly encountered in the lumbar, upper thoracic, and cervical regions. Although it can result from trauma, it commonly occurs from the accumulative effects of the stresses of day-to-day physical activities upon the individual's pattern of neutral weight-bearing mechanics. The initial complaint from vertebral dysfunction is usually localized or referred musculoskeletal pain.

The mechanics of vertebral somatic dysfunction that manifest in older adults typically demonstrate the coupled relationship between flexion-extension, sidebending, and rotation as described by Fryette.[37] Age-associated changes encountered in older patients, coupled with the possibility of concomitant illness, tends to lower their tolerance to osteopathic manipulative treatment. This does not necessarily mean that high velocity, low amplitude manipulation is contraindicated for these individuals. Rather, it requires that the practitioner thoroughly assess the patient and prescribe an effective dosage of manipulative treatment that the patient will tolerate without injury. The efficacy and comparative gentility of indirect procedures make these forms of manipulation ideal when treating frail or acutely ill individuals.

Because of the incidence of concomitant visceral pathology in older individuals, identified vertebral somatic dysfunction should be thoroughly evaluated to rule out a viscerosomatic origin. The effective treatment of viscerosomatic somatic dysfunction is predicated upon the appropriate treatment of the underlying visceral condition.

It is, consequently, imperative that the practitioner recognizes that somatic dysfunction can result as a reflex manifestation of visceral dysfunction and disease. Although the location of these reflexes may vary slightly from individual to individual, their locations are generally well recognized. While a reflex area may include multiple spinal segments, the clinical presentation of a viscerosomatic reflex may involve as few as two adjacent spinal segments within that larger area.[38] Reflex somatic dysfunction will demonstrate tenderness to palpation and associated palpable tissue texture abnormality, this latter finding being particularly identifiable in the subcutaneous tissues. It need not demonstrate associated altered anatomic position or motion restriction with clearly definitive barriers to normally available motion.

Viscerosomatic spinal somatic dysfunction is not mechanical in origin; it is the

# Viscerosomatic reflexes

The following locations are summarized from a review of the osteopathic literature.[1234567]

- Eyes, ears, nose, and throat: The sympathetic reflex is T1–T5. The trigeminal nerve is the final common pathway for both sympathetic and parasympathetic innervation of the upper respiratory tract. The muscles of mastication, commonly the temporalis muscles, receive motor innervation from the trigeminal nerve and serve as the somatic component for the upper respiratory tract sympathetic and parasympathetic reflexes. An additional reflex site is occiput–C2. This results from a reflex between the trigeminal nerve and upper cervical nerves.[8]
- Heart: The sympathetic reflex is T1–T5, left-sided greater than right. The parasympathetic reflex is vagal: occiput, C1, and C2.
- Lung: The sympathetic reflex is bilateral from T1–T4. Conditions involving both lungs result in bilateral reflex findings. Conditions involving one lung result in a reflex on the same side as the involved lung. The parasympathetic reflex is vagal: occiput, C1, and C2.

- Gastrointestinal tract:
  - The parasympathetic reflex from the gastrointestinal tract proximal to the mid-transverse colon is vagal: occiput, C1, and C2. The parasympathetic reflex from the distal half of the transverse colon to the rectum is sacropelvic, S2–S4.
  - The esophagus has a right-sided sympathetic reflex from T3–T6.
  - The stomach has a left-sided sympathetic reflex from T5–T10.
  - The duodenum has a right-sided sympathetic reflex from T6–T8.
  - The small intestine sympathetic reflex is from T8–T10, bilateral.
  - The appendix and cecum sympathetic reflex is from T9–T12 on the right.
  - The ascending colon sympathetic reflex is from T11–L1 on the right.
  - The descending colon to rectum sympathetic reflex is from L1–L3 on the left.
- Pancreas: The sympathetic reflex may be left-sided, or bilateral, and is T5–T9. The parasympathetic reflex is vagal: occiput, C1, and C2.

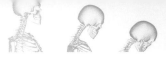

- Liver and gallbladder: The sympathetic reflex is right-sided from T5–T10. The parasympathetic reflex is vagal: occiput, C1, and C2.
- Spleen: The sympathetic reflex is left-sided from T7–T9.
- Kidney: The sympathetic reflex is on the same side as the involved kidney, from T9–L1. The parasympathetic reflex is vagal: occiput, C1, and C2.

- Urinary bladder: The sympathetic reflex is bilateral T11–L3. The parasympathetic reflex is sacropelvic, S2–S4.
- Ovaries (and testes): The sympathetic reflex is on the same side as the involved organ from T10–T11.
- Adrenal glands: The sympathetic reflex is on the same side as the involved gland from T8–T10.

## Endnotes

1. Pottenger FM. Symptoms of Visceral Disease. 5th ed. St. Louis, MO: C V Mosby; 1938.
2. Owens C. An Endocrine Interpretation of Chapman's Reflexes. 2nd ed. 1937. Reprinted by The Academy of Applied Osteopathy (American Academy of Osteopathy); Indianapolis, IN: 1963.
3. Beal MC. Viscerosomatic reflexes: a review. J Am Osteopath Assoc. 1985 Dec;85(12):786–801.
4. Kuchera ML, Kuchera WA. Osteopathic Considerations in Systemic Dysfunctions. 2nd ed. Columbus, OH: Greyden Press; 1994.
5. Dowling DJ. Neurophysiologic mechanisms related to osteopathic diagnosis and treatment. In: DiGiovanna EL, Schiowitz S, eds. An Osteopathic Approach to Diagnosis and Treatment. 2nd ed. Philadelphia, PA: J B Lippincott Co; 1997:29.
6. Van Buskirk RL, Nelson KE. Osteopathic family practice: An application of the primary care model. In: Ward RC, ed. Foundations for Osteopathic Medicine. 2nd ed. Philadelphia, PA: Lippincott Williams and Wilkins; 2002:289–97.
7. Sumino R, Nozaki S, Kato M. Central pathway of trigemino-neck reflex (abstract). In: Oral-facial sensory and motor functions. International Symposium. Rappongi, Tokyo. Oral Physiol. 1980:28.
8. Sumino R, Nozaki S, Kato M. Central pathway of trigemino-neck reflex (abstract). In: Oral-facial sensory and motor functions. International Symposium. Rappongi, Tokyo. Oral Physiol. 1980:28.

segmentally-related somatic response to increased general visceral afferent (GVA) neuronal activity, often associated with visceral inflammation. These GVA neurons return to the central nervous system (CNS) along the sympathetic and parasympathetic nerves that innervate the particular organ. As such, the respective viscerosomatic reflexes will be found in the spinal areas associated with the autonomic nervous system. The sympathetic reflexes are found between T1 and L2. The parasympathetic reflexes are sacral (pelvic splanchnic) and high cervical (occiput, C1, and C2, a reflection of vagal activity, possibly the result of direct vagal projections into the upper cervical spinal cord).[39] Thus, nociceptive afferent activity from a viscus results in sensitization of second-order neurons within the spinal cord. These sensitized neurons can also receive convergent nociception from somatic tissues, particularly deep somatic tissues, and other viscera. Consequently, within somatic tissues and visceral organs that demonstrate the same, or overlapping, segmental projections of their spinal afferent neurons into a given level of the spinal cord, a pattern of hyperalgesia and referred visceral pain is established.[40] Osteopathic practitioners can use referred pain complaints diagnostically. Their palpatory skills will allow the identification of the associated tissue texture changes, often well in advance of the clinical presentation of the visceral pathology.[41]

The facilitated state of the segmental spinal cord in the presence of visceral input can in turn result in a somatovisceral response. This can make it difficult, once the viscerosomatic/somatovisceral relationship is established, to determine which came first. It also provides complimentary treatment of the visceral condition, wherein the reduction of the associated somatic dysfunction is thought to have a salutary effect upon the visceral condition. The reader is cautioned that, in the presence of established visceral pathology, osteopathic manipulative treatment should not be considered as primary treatment of the underlying visceral pathology.

# Changes with aging

Typically, loss of flexibility with lower ranges of motion occurs with aging in most individuals. Previous somatic dysfunctions accumulated through the years added to the loss of elasticity of the connective tissue contribute to this decline.

Also, as a function of age, apparent bone density varies widely; some age-related osteoporosis may increase this process. Beginning as soon as the fourth decade of life this progressive demineralization is such that elderly men can gradually lose up to 30% of bone density, whereas elderly women can lose up to 50%.[42] As a result, between the ages of 30 and 80 years, individuals may experienced a loss of bone volume in the lumbar spine of 53%, in the thoracic spine a loss of 41%, and in the cervical spine 24%.[43]

Diminution of bone density associated with modifications in the architecture of the trabecular bone result in reduced structural strength. Normally, the trabeculae are oriented parallel to the lines of stress and vertical trabeculae predominate in the anterior two thirds of the vertebral body, while horizontal trabeculae are more apparent in the posterior part. The more porous cancellous bone aspect is the consequence of a greater loss of horizontal cross-linking components, which act as supporting cross-braces. With age, horizontal trabeculae significantly lose their thickness, become thinned, and perforated. On the contrary, the trabecular thickness of vertical trabeculae is independent of age, although the absolute loss of vertical trabeculae may be higher than that of horizontal trabeculae.[44]

The resultant architecture of the trabecular bone is more fragile and may collapse under normal compression loads. Morphological changes, with increased intratrabecular spacing and replacement of plate-like close trabecular arrangements with more open, rod-like structures, add to bone fragility.[45] As a result, vertebral bodies are less efficient in their capacity to bear weight and microfractures and micro-calluses become visible in the subchondral bone, with an augmentation of the concavity of the disc-vertebral junction.[46 47]

Changes with aging most often include osteoporosis, osteophytes or bony spurs, facet joint os-teoarthritis, degenerative disc disease, and spinal stenosis.

## Osteoporosis

In 1993, a consensus conference described osteoporosis as a systemic skeletal disease characterized by low bone mass and micro-architectural deterioration of bone tissue with a resultant increase in fragility and a consequent risk of fracture.[48] In its guidelines for diagnosis and management of osteoporosis the International Osteoporosis Foundation stated that more than 40% of middle-aged women in Europe will experience one or more osteoporotic fracture during their remaining lifetime.[49] These fractures have distressing health consequences because of their association with increased mortality and morbidity that in turn are a significant load to the healthcare system.

All living bone consists of a web of calcified connecting tissue of greater or lesser density depending upon the age and health of the individual. As a dynamic and living structure, the skeleton is under continuous adjustment. Among the cellular components of bone, osteoblasts are responsible for bone formation, and osteoclasts for bone resorption. A steady turnover takes place with bone formation and bone resorption. Normally, it is during the first two decades of life that most of the growth and mineralization of the skeleton occurs and that bone mass organizes. Later in life, during the fourth decade and after, loss of bone occurs. Environmental stimuli taking place throughout critical periods of early development, as early as intrauterine life, may be a factor for the risk of osteoporosis in later life.[50]

When there is an uncoupling between bone resorption and bone formation, with more bone resorption than bone formation, bone mass decreases, resulting in osteoporosis. Bony strength declines, which can lead to fracture from minimal trauma. In fact, only 25% of vertebral fractures follow a fall; others may result from daily activities involving bending, or the lifting of light objects, both of which involve a compressive component.[51] Most

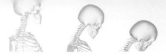

common fracture sites are the vertebra, wrist, and hip. At 50 years of age, a woman has a 17.5% risk of experiencing a hip fracture, and a 16% risk for a vertebral fracture, whereas a man has a 6% and 5% risk respectively.[52] Typically, primary vertebral fractures take place at the mid-thoracic or thoracolumbar spine and occur as wedge fractures. With progression of osteoporosis, fractures appear in the lumbar spine as biconcavity fractures.[53] Vertebral fractures are linked with significant intensification of back pain, loss of total height in the person, decreased physical function, disability, and social isolation. Furthermore, there is also an important increased mortality risk that persists up to five years after vertebral fracture in men and women.[54 55]

Vertebral pain may be associated with different conditions and because of that, vertebral fractures are sometimes overlooked and are not always diagnosed. Although height loss could be due to multiple fractures, it is considered an unreliable indicator of fracture status until it exceeds 4 cm.[56] In a multicenter study of osteoporotic fractures, a little more than two thirds of new radiographically detected vertebral fractures were not diagnosed clinically.[57] The practitioner must keep this fact in mind and always be very careful when treating back complaints in these patients.

Radiographic assessments for vertebral fractures should be performed by clinicians with precise expertise in the radiology of osteoporosis. Typically, osteoporotic vertebral fractures display a diminution of the height of the anterior wall of the vertebral body whereas the dimension of the posterior wall remains unchanged. Because of the resultant wedge-shaped deformity, a local kyphosis results. If there are several contiguous vertebral fractures, there will be an increase in the thoracic kyphosis and cervical lordosis. This is usually more severe in females, with the development of a 'dowager's hump' in the upper thoracic region.

Classically, vertebral deformities are described as wedge, crush, and biconcave deformities. Wedge deformities, the most frequent, and crush deformities, are found in the mid-thoracic and thoracolumbar portions of the spine in both men and women, whereas biconcave deformities are frequently located in the lumbar spine. These are the result of vertical herniation of the nucleus pulposus through the vertebral body endplates, often referred to radiographically as Schmorl's nodes. A vertebral deformity, however, does not always signify a vertebral fracture, although vertebral fractures consistently demonstrate vertebral deformity. Aging increases the prevalence of vertebral deformities, particularly in women.[58]

Most of the risk factors for osteoporosis cannot be avoided or modified. Nevertheless, it may be useful to identify patients at risk, to treat them, and propose preventive measures such as exercise and manipulative treatment to improve postural balance and function. Bone density, in order to be maintained, requires mechanical stress within its functional limits. Intelligent exercise programs can contribute to this goal.

Age, being female, genetics factors, cigarette smoking, and being thin are most often mentioned as risk factors in the epidemiology of osteoporosis.[59 60] Weight loss, particularly after age 50, is linked with lower bone mass and it has been observed than each 10 kg of weight loss may be associated with 3.9% lower bone mass.[61] Menopause occurring early in life in a natural fashion and delayed age at menarche appear to increase the risk of low bone density. However, breastfeeding does not seem to be a risk factor and sometimes may be protective.[62] Calcium or vitamin D supplementation has positive effects in some but not all studies.[63 64]

## Osteophytes

According to some authors, osteophytes, also named bony spurs, are outgrowths of healthy bone that develop as a defense mechanism against pressure.[65 66] In fact, osteophytes increase vertebral compressive strength by 17%.[67] Subsequently, they are more frequent with males who have often experienced higher compressive load-bearing by the spine. Although osteophytic spurs are asymptomatic most of the time, anterior vertebral osteophytes have been associated with lumbar intervertebral disc degeneration.[68 69] By progressively limiting motion, osteophyte formation may consequently improve spinal instability.[70] Besides arising in the periosteum covering the bone at the junction between cartilage and bone, osteophytes may also result from traction at the insertion of tendons and ligaments. They may be seen as inflammatory spurs (as with syndesmophytes) —bony growths originating inside a ligament and found at the attachment of ligaments and tendons to bone in conditions such as ankylosing spondylitis.

Even if individual disparities occur, osteophytes can appear on the anterior and lateral surfaces of the vertebral bodies, as soon as 20 years of age. By 60 years of age, 90% of individuals show osteophytes.[71] Anterior osteophytes are usually more frequent, particularly in the thoracic region, whereas posterior osteophytes are more frequent in the cervical and lumbar regions. Furthermore, it is noticeable that osteophytes appear in the concavities of the vertebral column where the pressure is the greatest and they are mostly found near the areas of greatest curvature of the spinal AP curves (C5, T8, and L3-L4), while they are infrequently present in areas of less pressure such as the intersections between the line of gravity and the spine (TI, T12, and L5–S1).[72]

Osteophytes may infiltrate every type of soft tissue surrounding the vertebrae. They can also develop in the vertebral ligaments, and anterior osteophytes are seen very often in the anterior longitudinal ligament, which covers a sizeable portion of the anterior surface of the vertebral bodies. Because there is less stress on the posterior longitudinal ligament, posterior osteophytes develop less commonly in this ligament. They are also found in the insertions of the prevertebral muscles, in the crura of the diaphragm, and in the attachments of the psoas muscle.[73]

As a defense mechanism against pressure, osteophytes may be asymptomatic. Nevertheless, sometimes they compress structures around the vertebrae, resulting in symptoms. Compression of the spinal cord and spinal nerves is frequent.[74] Osteophytes of L5–S1 vertebral bodies can produce lumbar radiculopathy caused by extraforaminal compression, with entrapment of the fifth lumbar nerve.[75 76] Because significant abnormal radiologic findings in the lumbar spinal canal are not always found, this may be misdiagnosed.[77] Osteophytic

compression in the cervical spine may produce compression of the esophagus and the trachea resulting in symptoms such as dysphagia, cough, shortness of breath, or throat tightness.[78 79] Symptomatic vertebral artery compression caused by anterior cervical osteophytes has also been reported.[80] Because the sympathetic trunk is located anterolaterally on the body of the vertebrae, it may be compressed by anterior osteophytes. Most often, it is the sympathetic trunk and the rami communicantes that are under pressure in the abdomen,[81] while the splanchnic nerves are frequently impinged upon in the thorax, with the greatest frequency at the T8-T10 level.[82]

## Facet joint osteoarthritis

Facet joints are among the spinal structures where degeneration may occur. With aging, as in other diarthrodial joints, osteoarthritis of facet joints may develop progressively. Osteoarthritis or degenerative arthritis is defined by the National Collaborating Centre for Chronic Conditions as "a metabolically active, dynamic process that involves all joint tissues: cartilage, bone, synovium/capsule, ligaments, and muscle." Usually, some pathological changes occur such as loss of hyaline cartilage and remodeling of contiguous bone with formation of osteophytes. Symptoms may include pain, tenderness, and stiffness. The numerous risk factors are usually divided into genetic factors (despite the fact that to date no responsible genes are known); constitutional factors such as aging, female sex, obesity; and biomechanical factors such as joint overuse or traumas.

Multiple studies have demonstrated an increase of the facet area, particularly in the lumbar spine, associated with age and most likely secondary to increased weight-bearing at the facet joint.[83] A significant correlation between sagittal orientation and osteoarthritis of the lumbar facet joints is also reported.[84] It suggests either that the facet joint with more sagittal orientation is likely to develop osteoarthritis, or that the remodeling course of osteoarthritis modifies the appearance of the facet joints, resulting in a sagittal orientation. Optimal postural balance should be addressed in all individuals as soon as possible to encourage efficient weight-bearing and decrease the risk of osteoarthritis.

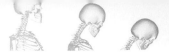

Osteoarthritis may be painful and may play a part in the development of radiculopathy. However, multiple reports suggest that mechanical compression of the nerve is not the only cause of radiculopathy and that chemical factors generated by facet joint inflammation may spread to nerve roots to induce radiculopathy. Interleukin-1 beta (IL-1β) and tumor necrosis factor-alpha (TNF-α) are the principal proinflammatory cytokines synthesized during the osteoarthritic process. An increase of the TNF-α protein expression in the dorsal root ganglion occurs during the acute inflammatory phase and is associated with the duration of mechanical allodynia.[85] The presence of increased levels of TNF-α can produce aberrant axonal electrophysiological activity independent of peripheral receptor involvement.[86][87]

## Degenerative disc disease

Although any portion of the musculoskeletal system—muscles, articular cartilage, intervertebral discs, tendons, ligaments, and joint capsules—may be impaired by the aging process, no musculoskeletal tissue undergoes more striking age-related transformations than the intervertebral disc.[88] Changes that occur in the disc include dehydration, remodeling of the nucleus pulposus, and stiffening of the annulus fibrosus. These degenerative alterations begin with fine biochemical changes that lead to micro-structural modifications to end with gross structural transformation of the intervertebral segment. However, considerable individual differences exist and differentiating modifications associated with aging from premature aging or degeneration occurring at any age is very difficult.

As soon as the end of the first decade of life, significant age-related alterations in the intervertebral disc can be seen. In the first half of the second decade, the three anatomic portions of the disc i.e., the nucleus pulposus, the annulus fibrosus, and the cartilaginous endplates are more or less affected.[89]

In a healthy disc, synthesis and degradation of the matrix elements are balanced. Therefore the first signs of aging are loss of aggrecan and water, a diminished collagen organization, and a reduction of disc height. Multiple factors can explain these changes in the metabolic equilibrium, including genetic predisposition.[90] The most important of these factors seems to be decreasing nutrition of the central disc. In fact, a diminution of the blood supply to the intervertebral disc appears to instigate disc tissue breakdown.[91] Normally, in healthy individuals the disc is avascular, except for minimal vascularization at the outer part of the annulus. It is by passage through the contiguous vertebral endplate that most of the nutrition of the disc occurs. In the aging disc, a diminished blood supply of the endplate results in tissue breakdown starting in the nucleus pulposus. Rim lesions of the body of the vertebrae, endplate fissure formation and tears at the annulus attachment are found associated with cracks and radiating ruptures of the annulus from the peripheral to the central regions. Blood vessels penetrate through the developing rim lesions and new blood vessels form from the pre-existing vessels. At this stage, vascular cells of the invading vessels produce cytokines and proteases thus enhancing the destructive pathway.[92] Actually, in degenerated disc and in herniated disc tissue, a vascular penetration is demonstrated.

At birth, multiple perivascular and free nerve endings are located on and among the peripheral layers of the annulus. During normal development, the innervation of the intervertebral discs decrease and the adult nucleus pulposus has no nerve supply. However, when degenerative processes begin, as innervation follows the distribution of vessels, an ingrowth of nerves accompanies the ingrowth of blood vessels.[93] Indeed, in unhealthy intervertebral discs the nerves are associated with blood vessels, and nociceptive nerve fibers are found in the annulus and nucleus.[94] This may be a source of associated back pain.

Intervertebral disc degeneration is not always symptomatic. It seems that several factors are necessary to produce the pain associated with disc degeneration. These include: weight-bearing damage to the annulus fibrosus, disc nutrition, inflammation, neoinnervation, nociceptive sensitization, and genetic predisposition.

The sinuvertebral nerves supply the outer third of the annulus of the intervertebral discs, whereas direct branches from the sympathetic grey rami communicantes supply the anterior and posterolateral aspects of the annulus. Immunocytochemical experiments in rats reveal two routes existing between the annulus and the dorsal root ganglia: one from the sinuvertebral nerve, and another along the paravertebral sympathetic trunk.[95] Consequently, two groups of symptoms may be present with a degenerated disc. One is a radicular pain that may result from stenosis and nerve root or cauda equina irritation and the other is a discogenic pain following internal disc disruption.[96] Additionally, compression of the nerve root produces local edema and ischemia that affect axoplasmic transport.[97]

Discogenic low back pain is now believed to have afferent pathways in the sinuvertebral nerves, mostly originating from the ventral rami of the spinal nerves. Current studies demonstrate that many of the nociceptive fibers emanating from the annulus fibrosus of the lower vertebral discs go through the sympathetic trunk in a non-segmental fashion and may be considered as sympathetic sensory afferents.[98] Consequently, similarities appear between sensory nerve supply of the disc and some enteric structures, and discogenic pain may be considered as a visceral pain.[99] Additionally, because the sympathetic trunk originates from the myelomeres of only T1–L2 as well as the sympathetic nerves, it is suggested that "discogenic low back pain is transmitted non-segmentally by visceral sympathetic afferents mainly through the L2 spinal nerve root, and that this may be perceived as referred pain in the L2 dermatome."[100] Clinically, normalization of L2 somatic dysfunction should be considered when treating discogenic low back pain, inguinal pain, and anterolateral thigh pain. This relationship between low lumbar disc pathology and an associated upper lumbar 'viscerosomatic reflex' (actually a somatosomatic reflex) may provide further insight into the physiological splinting of the psoas major in the presence of lumbar disc disease.[101]

## Spinal stenosis

Spinal stenosis is a narrowing of the vertebral canal that happens at one or several spinal levels. Most of the time, the lumbar and cervical regions are involved, and it is asymptomatic and goes undiagnosed until X-rays reveal its presence. Typically, symptoms begin progressively and worsen over time, being different according to the site of the stenosis.

Prevalence of lumbar stenosis is more important than cervical stenosis and in both cases, the prevalence of acquired stenosis increases with age. Cervical stenosis is estimated in 4.9% of the adult population, 6.8% of the population 50 years of age or older, and 9% of the population 70 years of age or older;[102] this disorder is remarkably more frequent in the Japanese population.[103] It should be noted that considerable variation in cervical canal dimensions exist. Anteroposterior dimension of the cervical canal is narrowest at the C4 level for African-Americans and at C6 for Caucasians, whereas transverse dimension is usually narrowest at the C2–C3 level in both populations.[104] By comparison, the prevalence of lumbar spinal stenosis is estimated in 20% of the population aged less than 40 years and 47.2% in those 60–69 years old.[105]

The degenerative lesions with massive joint hypertrophy are a major factor in the narrowing of the spinal canal. Hypertrophy and sometimes ossification of the ligamentum flavum can also contribute to this narrowing.

On each side of the vertebrae, the ligamentum flavum expands from the superior border of the lamina below to the inferior half of the anterior surfaces of the lamina above. The superior part of the anterior surface of each lamina is habitually in contact with the dura mater and cervical root sheaths to which they may become loosely attached.[106] Because this structure constitutes a major portion of the posterior wall of the spinal canal, its hypertrophy can contribute significantly to the development of spinal stenosis. It is of interest to note that such stenosis is often found in areas of spinal lordosis where the ligament, on the posterior, concave, side of the curve is under less tension, but where more stress is present associated with greater motion than at other spinal levels.

Ossification of spinal ligaments, when it occurs, is most frequently encountered in the lower thoracic spine, at the T9-T10 level or lower.[107]

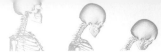

Repetitive mechanical stress is considered one of the significant factors that initiate the degenerative processes of the spinal ligaments and their ossification. In the spinal ligaments, elastic fibers are responsive to repetitive cyclical stretch stress and under such stress, mesenchymal fibroblastic cells change to chondrocytes and osteoblasts with an augmented expression of cytokines. Some investigators propose that hypertrophy happens also, due to scarring arising during the repair process in wound healing.[108] Other systemic factors for ossification of the ligamentum flavum include an irregular metabolism of growth hormone, calcitonin, and glucose, obesity, and genetic backgrounds.[109] Habitually, the ligamentum flavum displays a high content of elastic fibers with 60–70% of elastin and 30–40% of collagen in the extracellular matrix.[110] On the contrary, the hypertrophied ligamentum flavum demonstrates an increased number and size of collagen fibers, fibrocartilaginous cells between these collagen fibers, and ossification. In fact, the ligamentum flavum is also called the yellow ligament because it is usually yellow due to a larger content of elastic fibers than of collagen fibers.[111]

Ossification of the spinal ligaments, particularly the ligamentum flavum, is frequently present. It should be noted that associated ossification of the dura mater is not uncommon with ossification of the ligamentum flavum. At the level of spinal stenotic compression, the central canal that contains the spinal cord and the root canals that contain the spinal nerves are under pressure. Severe spinal stenosis may constrict the spinal cord and alter its arterial supply. Pain may be present, although cervical stenosis often causes no pain. Different symptoms are associated with spinal stenosis in the neck such as numbness, weakness, or tingling in a leg, foot, shoulder, arm or hand. Incoordination may be present with postural instability. Because the neurons contributing to the ascending dorsal spinal tracts enter the cord and run ventral to the neurons from lower segments, dorsal compression of the cervical cord will present, paradoxically, with lower extremity symptoms often before the development of upper extremity symptoms.

With spinal stenosis in the lower back, symptoms may be chronic low back pain with secondary radiating pain in the buttock or cramping in the legs, or both, after long periods of walking. Most of the time these symptoms improve when the patient bends forward, squats, or sits down. Patients may also report bowel or urinary dysfunction with dysaesthesia in the perineum area, and problems with the bladder ranging from extreme urgency to urinary delay. These last symptoms constitute a medical emergency and indicate that the patient should be immediately seen by a neurosurgeon.

Once the underlying pathology has been identified and appropriately addressed, the treatment goals are to maintain flexibility and stability of the spine, with exercise and manual procedures to optimize postural balance. Manipulative procedures are typically employed to reduce motion restriction and consequently are not appropriate for areas of structural instability. Under these circumstances, stabilizing exercises should be employed, along with manual interventions using the gentlest of indirect procedures and specifically limited to areas of motion restriction adjacent to the instability. By judiciously addressing these areas, the compensatory stresses placed upon the unstable area may be decreased. Surgery to relieve the pressure on the spinal cord or nerve roots should be performed emergently under the circumstances described above and should be further considered when conservative treatments do not improve the condition.

## The osteopathic contribution to the physical examination and treatment

The physical examination begins at the very first moment you observe the patient. This could be the moment you first walk into the examination room, or, better yet, as the patient comes from the waiting area to the examination room. At this time, and at all times afterward, observe them for areas of restricted mobility as they walk and perform transitional movements (sitting to standing, standing to sitting, getting onto the treatment table) and generally move. When they are static, standing, seated, or lying down, look for spontaneous positioning, particularly noting positional asymmetries of the torso, head and neck, shoulders, arms, and legs.

During examination of the neuromusculoskeletal system begin, if at all possible, with the patient standing and observe them from the front, side, and back. From the front observe the position of the head and symmetry of the anterior thorax, abdomen, and pelvis. Note whether or not the patient appears to bear weight equally on the lower extremities. From the side, look at postural balance. The ear, shoulder, hip, knee, and lateral malleolus should be in alignment. Observe the cervical and lumbar lordoses and the thoracic kyphosis for gross and discrete areas of increase or flattening.

From behind the standing patient, again observe postural landmarks: mastoid processes, acromion processes, iliac crests, greater trochanters, popliteal creases, and medial malleoli. Look for, either active or passive, pelvic sideshift, the deviation of the pelvis to either side of the midline. This can be the result of muscle pull mechanics with sideshift away from the tight muscles, a lumbar type I group curve with sideshift toward the side of the concavity of the curve, or anatomic short leg with sideshift toward the long leg side.

Now, look for the asymmetry of the torso. Observe the position of the shoulders, scapula, and any asymmetric paravertebral prominence. This latter observation is augmented by having the patient forward bend from the hips. Asymmetric prominence of the paravertebral area is most often a manifestation of spinal rotation on the convex side of neutral type I spinal mechanics.

Next, examine the pelvis and sacral base to assess weight-bearing imbalance that could affect the vertebral column. If necessary, in the presence of pelvic unleveling or lower extremity asymmetry, place a pad under the foot of the leg that appears to be short. Then re-evaluate the spine in the standing position after the influence of leg or pelvic imbalances has been reduced or eliminated. Similarly, when you observe the patient in the seated position you can put a pad, in the same manner, under one ischiatic tuberosity to level the pelvis.

Progress to the seated, prone, and supine portions of the examination. Do a complete examination for somatic dysfunction of the spine, sacrum, pelvis, lower extremity pectoral girdle, and upper extremity as necessary. The seated position facilitates the examination of the upper thoracic spine. With the patient in the prone position, sacropelvic mechanics, particularly SI articular motion, can be further evaluated. Finally, with the patient supine assess the pelvis (ilio-iliac and pubic symphysis mechanics), thoracoabdominal diaphragm, thoracic cage and inlet, anterior neck muscles, cervical spine, and cranial region.

In each area palpate for membranous, myofascial, and interosseous somatic dysfunction contributing to the functional restrictions that were initially visually observed. For the treatment of somatic dysfunction in these individuals it is appropriate to begin by using indirect principles to release any restriction of motion identified. Areas of dysfunction commonly encountered and of particular importance include the pelvis, upper thoracic spine, ribs, sternum, thoracoabdominal diaphragm, pectoral girdle, cervico-occipital area, and cranium. Also keep in mind that the goal of the treatment is to restore the best function possible according to the state of the patient, and not to correct any asymmetry connected to structural modification. Dosage is extremely important. When inflammation is present, special attention should be given to the use of the very gentlest treatment procedures. Extreme caution should be exercised when treating conditions associated with structural instability. The goal of essentially all manual treatment procedures is to eliminate dysfunctional limitations of motion. This is arguably dangerous in areas with underlying instability. It should also be stressed that with this age group, as with any other group of patients, any underlying organic pathology should be identified and appropriately addressed as part of the complete treatment of the individual. This often necessitates diagnostic laboratory and radiographic evaluation as appropriate.

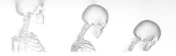

# Advice to the patient

Everyone can benefit from programs to improve gait, balance, strength, and confidence. Movement, like walking and swimming, if at all possible, should be encouraged. Dosage is of paramount importance and exercise programs must be individualized.

It has been demonstrated that bone strength may be increased with weight-bearing aerobic exercise if the program lasts at least a year.[112] In particular, strengthening the back extensors may load the transverse trabeculae of the vertebrae and help to prevent vertebral fracture. Balance exercises should also be encouraged to reduce falls and fall-related fractures.[113]

Nutrition is very important as well. Adequate hydration is of primary importance. Refined foods should be avoided as much as possible, while a diet rich in fresh fruits and vegetables, and antioxidants, such as vitamins C and E, is recommended. A diet high in probiotics that promote the growth of beneficial bacteria (*Bifidobacterium, Lactobacillus,* and *Bacteroides*) is advised. Lactose and gluten intolerances should be considered.

Sleeping positions should be discussed. Patients should avoid the use of multiple pillows that tend to project the head forward and affect the neck, cranial base, and mandibular balance. They should pay attention to chronic resting positions when watching the television, or reading with the head always rotated to the same side. They should be encouraged to employ symmetry of position as much as possible.

# References

1. Standring S. Ed. Gray's Anatomy: The anatomical basis of clinical practice. 39th ed. Edinburgh: Churchill Livingstone; 2004.
2. Ferguson SJ, Steffen T. Biomechanics of the aging spine. Eur Spine J. 2003 Oct;12 Suppl 2:S97-S103.
3. Standring S. Ed. Gray's Anatomy: The anatomical basis of clinical practice. 39th ed. Edinburgh: Churchill Livingstone; 2004.
4. Benoist M. Natural history of the aging spine. Eur Spine J. 2003 Oct;12 Suppl 2:S86-9.
5. Crock HV. Normal and pathological anatomy of the lumbar spinal nerve root canals. J Bone Joint Surg Br. 1981;63B(4):487-90.
6. Standring S. Ed. Gray's Anatomy: The anatomical basis of clinical practice. 39th ed. Edinburgh: Churchill Livingstone; 2004.
7. Devereaux MW. Anatomy and examination of the spine. Neurol Clin. 2007 May;25(2):331-51.
8. Marchand F, Ahmed AM. Investigation of the laminate structure of lumbar disc anulus fibrosus. Spine (Phila Pa 1976). 1990 May;15(5):402-10.
9. Roberts S, Evans H, Trivedi J, Menage J. Histology and pathology of the human intervertebral disc. J Bone Joint Surg Am. 2006 Apr;88 Suppl 2:10-4.
10. Hadjipavlou AG, Tzermiadianos MN, Bogduk N, Zindrick MR. The pathophysiology of disc degeneration: a critical review. J Bone Joint Surg Br. 2008 Oct;90(10):1261-70.
11. Malko JA, Hutton WC, Fajman WA. An in vivo magnetic resonance imaging study of changes in the volume (and fluid content) of the lumbar intervertebral discs during a simulated diurnal load cycle. Spine (Phila Pa 1976). 1999 May 15;24(10):1015-22.
12. Brown MF, Hukkanen MV, McCarthy ID, Redfern DR, Batten JJ, Crock HV, Hughes SP, Polak JM. Sensory and sympathetic innervation of the vertebral endplate in patients with degenerative disc disease. J Bone Joint Surg Br. 1997 Jan;79(1):147-53.
13. Adams MA, Hutton WC. The effect of posture on diffusion into lumbar intervertebral discs. J Anat. 1986 Aug;147:121-34.
14. Bibby S, Jones DA, Lee RB, Jing YU, Urban J. Biochimie. Biologie et physiologie du disque intervertébral. Rev Rhum. 2001; 68:903-08.
15. Roberts S, Evans H, Trivedi J, Menage J. Histology and pathology of the human intervertebral disc. J Bone Joint Surg Am. 2006 Apr;88 Suppl 2:10-4.
16. Devereaux MW. Anatomy and examination of the spine. Neurol Clin. 2007 May;25(2):331-51.
17. Fujiwara A, An HS, Lim TH, Haughton VM. Morphologic changes in the lumbar intervertebral foramen due to flexion-extension, lateral bending, and axial rotation: an in vitro anatomic and biomechanical study. Spine (Phila Pa 1976). 2001 Apr 15;26(8):876-82.
18. Vital JM, Lavignolle B, Grenier N, Rouais F, Malgat R, Senegas J. Anatomy of the lumbar radicular canal. Anat Clin. 1983;5(3):141-51.
19. Latarjet A, Magnin F. Etude anatomique des rapports des racines rachidiennes lombaires avec l'étui dural et le système ostéoarticulaire vertébral. J Med Lyon. 1941: 347-57.
20. Senegas J, Guerin J, Carles CL. Rapports du foureau dural et des racines lombaires et sacrées avec les vertèbres et les disques intervertébraux. Congrès International d'Anatomie. Manchester. 1974. In Vital JM, Lavignolle B, Grenier N, Rouais F, Malgat R, Senegas J.
   Anatomy of the lumbar radicular canal. Anat Clin. 1983;5(3).141-51.
21. Phelan KD, Falls WM. The spinotrigeminal pathway and its spatial relationship to the origin of trigeminospinal projections in the rat. Neuroscience. 1991;40(2):477-96.
22. Hyodoh H, Shirase R, Kawaharada N, Hyodoh K, Sato T, Onodera M, Aratani K, Hareyama M. MR angiography for detecting the artery of Adamkiewicz and its branching level from the aorta. Magn Reson Med Sci. 2009;8(4):159-64.
23. Glaser SE, Shah RV. Pain Physician. Root cause analysis of paraplegia following transforaminal epidural steroid injections: the 'unsafe' triangle. 2010 May-Jun;13(3):237-44.
24. Standring S. Ed. Gray's Anatomy: The anatomical basis of clinical practice. 39th ed. Edinburgh: Churchill Livingstone; 2004.
25. Fryette HH. Physiologic movements of the spine. Osteopath Man Ther and Clin Res Assn. Reprinted in Year Book of the Academy of Applied Osteopathy. American Academy of Osteopathy. Indianapolis, IN. 1942:54-7.
26. Fryette HH. Principles of Osteopathic Technic. Academy of Applied Osteopathy, Carmel CA (American Academy of Osteopathy, Indianapolis IN); 1954.
27. Magoun H.I. A Method of Sacroiliac Correction. J. Amer Osteopath. Assc. June 1940. Reprinted in Year Book of the Academy of Applied Osteopathy. American Academy of Osteopathy. Indianapolis, IN. 1965(2):200-3.
28. Johnston WL. Segmental definition: Part I. A focal point for diagnosis of somatic dysfunction. J Am Osteopath Assoc. 1988 Jan;88(1):99-105.
29. Glossary of Osteopathic Terminology. In: Ward RC, ed. Foundations for Osteopathic

Medicine. 2nd ed. Baltimore: Williams et Wilkins; 2003.

30. Fryette HH. Principles of Osteopathic Technic. Academy of Applied Osteopathy, Carmel CA. (American Academy of Osteopathy, Indianapolis IN.); 1954.

31. Fryette HH. Physiologic movements of the spine. J Amer Osteopath Assoc. 1918;18(1).

32. Fryette HH. Principles of Osteopathic Technic. Academy of Applied Osteopathy, Carmel CA (American Academy of Osteopathy, Indianapolis IN); 1954.

33. Strachan WF, Beckwith CG, Larson NJ, Grant JH. A study of the mechanics of the sacroiliac joint. J Am Osteopath Assoc. 1938;37(2):575-8.

34. Magoun H.I. A Method of Sacroiliac Correction. Year Book of the Academy of Applied Osteopathy. American Academy of Osteopathy. Indianapolis, IN. 1965(2):200-3.

35. Fryette H.H.: Principles of Osteopathic Technic, Academy of Applied Osteopathy, Carmel CA (American Academy of Osteopathy, Indianapolis IN); 1954.

36. Strachan, J Amer Osteopath Assoc. August 1938:576-8.

37. Fryette HH. Principles of Osteopathic Technic. Academy of Applied Osteopathy, Carmel CA. (American Academy of Osteopathy, Indianapolis IN); 1954.

38. Beal MC. Viscerosomatic reflexes: a review. J Am Osteopath Assoc. Dec Dec;1985(12):786-801.

39. McNeill DL, Chandler MJ, Fu QG, Foreman RD. Projection of nodose ganglion cells to the upper cervical spinal cord in the rat. Brain Res Bull. 1991 Aug;27(2):151-5.

40. Jänig W. Visceral pain-still an enigma? Pain. 2010 Nov;151(2):239-40.

41. Korr IM. Skin resistance patterns associated with visceral disease. Fed Proc. 1949 Mar;8:87.

42. Mazess RB. On aging bone loss. Clin Orthop Relat Res. 1982 May;(165):239-52.

43. Grote HJ, Amling M, Vogel M, Hahn M, Pösl M, Delling G. Intervertebral variation in trabecular microarchitecture throughout the normal spine in relation to age. Bone. 1995 Mar;16(3):301-8.

44. Thomsen JS, Ebbesen EN, Mosekilde LI. Age-related differences between thinning of horizontal and vertical trabeculae in human lumbar bone as assessed by a new computerized method. Bone. 2002 Jul;31(1):136-42.

45. Ferguson SJ, Steffen T. Biomechanics of the aging spine. Eur Spine J. 2003 Oct;12 Suppl 2:S97-S103.

46. Barnett E, Nordin BE. The radiological diagnosis of osteoporosis: a new approach. Clin Radiol. 1960 Jul;11:166-74.

47. Twomey L, Taylor J, Furniss B. Age changes in the bone density and structure of the lumbar vertebral column. J Anat. 1983 Jan;136(Pt 1):15-25.

48. Consensus development conference: diagnosis, prophylaxis, and treatment of osteoporosis. Am J Med. 1993 Jun;94(6):646-50.

49. Kanis JA, Delmas P, Burckhardt P,Cooper C, Torgerson D. Guidelines for diagnosis and management of osteoporosis. The European Foundation for Osteoporosis and Bone Disease. Osteoporos Int. 1997; 7(4):390-406.

50. Walker-Bone K, Walter G, Cooper C. Recent developments in the epidemiology of osteoporosis. Curr Opin Rheumatol. 2002 Jul;14(4):411-5.

51. Dennison E, Cole Z, Cooper C. Diagnosis and epidemiology of osteoporosis. Curr Opin Rheumatol. 2005 Jul;17(4):456-61.

52. Lips P. Epidemiology and predictors of fractures associated with osteoporosis. Am J Med. 1997 Aug 18;103(2A):3S-8S; discussion 8S-11S.

53. Sinaki M, Pfeifer M, Preisinger E, Itoi E, Rizzoli R, Boonen S, Geusens P, Minne HW. The role of exercise in the treatment of osteoporosis. Curr Osteoporos Rep. 2010 Sep;8(3):138-44.

54. Nevitt MC, Ettinger B, Black DM, Stone K, Jamal SA, Ensrud K, Segal M, Genant HK, Cummings SR. The association of radiographically detected vertebral fractures with back pain and function: a prospective study. Ann Intern Med. 1998 May 15;128(10):793-800.

55. Bliuc D, Nguyen ND, Milch VE, Nguyen TV, Eisman JA, Center JR. Mortality risk associated with low-trauma osteoporotic fracture and subsequent fracture in men and women. JAMA. 2009 Feb 4;301(5):513-21.

56. Ettinger B, Black DM, Nevitt MC, Rundle AC, Cauley JA, Cummings SR, Genant HK. Contribution of vertebral deformities to chronic back pain and disability. The Study of Osteoporotic Fractures Research Group. J Bone Miner Res. 1992 Apr;7(4):449-56.

57. Nevitt MC, Ettinger B, Black DM, Stone K, Jamal SA, Ensrud K, Segal M, Genant HK, Cummings SR. The association of radiographically detected vertebral fractures with back pain and function: a prospective study. Ann Intern Med. 1998 May 15;128(10):793-800.

58. Ismail AA, Cooper C, Felsenberg D, Varlow J, Kanis JA, Silman AJ, O'Neill TW. Number and type of vertebral deformities: epidemiological characteristics and relation to back pain and height loss. European Vertebral Osteoporosis Study Group. Osteoporos Int. 1999;9(3):206-13.

59. Bauer DC, Browner WS, Cauley JA, Orwoll ES, Scott JC, Black DM, Tao JL, Cummings SR. Factors associated with appendicular bone mass in older women. The Study of Osteoporotic Fractures Research Group. Ann Intern Med. 1993 May 1;118(9):657-65.

60. Scott JC. Epidemiology of osteoporosis. J Clin Rheumatol. 1997 Apr;3(2 Suppl):9-13.

61. Bauer DC, Browner WS, Cauley JA, Orwoll ES, Scott JC, Black DM, Tao JL, Cummings SR. Factors associated with appendicular bone mass in older women. The Study of Osteoporotic Fractures Research Group. Ann Intern Med. 1993 May 1;118(9):657-65.

62. Fox KM, Magaziner J, Sherwin R, Scott JC, Plato CC, Nevitt M, Cummings S. Reproductive correlates of bone mass in elderly women. Study of Osteoporotic Fractures Research Group. J Bone Miner Res. 1993 Aug;8(8):901-8.

63. Riggs BL, Wahner HW, Melton LJ 3rd, Richelson LS, Judd HL, O'Fallon WM. Dietary calcium intake and rates of bone loss in women. J Clin Invest. 1987 Oct;80(4):979-82.

64. Riggs BL, Wahner HW, Melton LJ 3rd, Richelson LS, Judd HL, O'Fallon WM. Dietary calcium intake and rates of bone loss in women. J Clin Invest. 1987 Oct;80(4):979-82.

65. Nathan H. Osteophytes of the vertebral column. An anatomical study of their development according to age, race and sex with considerations as to their etiology and significance. J Bone Joint Surg Am 1962;44:243–68.

66. O'Neill TW, McCloskey EV, Kanis JA, Bhalla AK, Reeve J, Reid DM, Todd C, Woolf AD, Silman AJ. The distribution, determinants, and clinical correlates of vertebral osteophytosis: a population based survey. J Rheumatol. 1999 Apr;26(4):842-8.

67. Al-Rawahi M, Luo J, Pollintine P, Dolan P, Adams MA. Mechanical Function of Vertebral Body Osteophytes, as Revealed by Experiments on Cadaveric Spines.Spine (Phila Pa 1976). 2010 Jul 30.

68. Vernon-Roberts B, Pirie CJ. Degenerative changes in the intervertebral discs of the lumbar spine and their sequelae. Rheumatol Rehabil. 1977 Feb;16(1):13-21.

69. Hassett G, Hart DJ, Manek NJ, Doyle DV, Spector TD. Risk factors for progression of lumbar spine disc degeneration: the Chingford Study. Arthritis Rheum. 2003 Nov;48(11):3112-7.

70. Kirkaldy-Willis WH, Farfan HF. Instability of the lumbar spine. Clin Orthop Relat Res. 1982 May;(165):110-23.

71. Nathan H. Osteophytes of the vertebral column. An anatomical study of their development according to age, race and sex with considerations as to their etiology and significance. J Bone Joint Surg Am 1962;44:243-68.

72. Nathan H. Osteophytes of the vertebral column. An anatomical study of their development according to age, race and sex with considerations as to their etiology and significance. J Bone Joint Surg Am 1962;44:243-68.

73. Nathan H. Osteophytes of the vertebral column. An anatomical study of their development according to age, race and sex with considerations as to their etiology and significance. J Bone Joint Surg Am 1962;44:243-68.

74. Morton SA. Localized hypertrophic changes in the cervical spine with compression of the spinal cord or of its roots. J Bone joint Surg Am 1936;18:893-98.

75. Nathan H, Weizenbluth M, Halperin N. The lumbosacral ligament (LSL), with special emphasis on the 'lumbosacral tunnel' and the entrapment of the 5th lumbar nerve. Int Orthop. 1982;6(3):197-202.

76. Matsumoto M, Chiba K, Nojiri K, Ishikawa M, Toyama Y, Nishikawa Y. Extraforaminal entrapment of the fifth lumbar spinal nerve by osteophytes of the lumbosacral spine: anatomic study and a report of four cases. Spine (Phila Pa 1976). 2002 Mar 15;27(6):E169-73.

77. Matsumoto M, Chiba K, Nojiri K, Ishikawa M, Toyama Y, Nishikawa Y. Extraforaminal entrapment of the fifth lumbar spinal nerve by osteophytes of the lumbosacral spine: anatomic study and a report of four cases. Spine (Phila Pa 1976). 2002 Mar 15;27(6):E169-73.

78. Meeks LW, Renshaw TS. Vertebral osteophytosis and dysphagia. Two case reports of the syndrome recently termed ankylosing hyperostosis. J Bone Joint Surg Am. 1973 Jan;55(1):197-201.

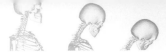

79. Aronowitz P, Cobarrubias F. Images in clinical medicine. Anterior cervical osteophytes causing airway compromise. N Engl J Med. 2003 Dec 25;349(26):2540.

80. Citow JS, Macdonald RL. Posterior decompression of the vertebral artery narrowed by cervical osteophyte: case report. Surg Neurol. 1999 May;51(5):495-8; discussion 498-9.

81. Rawat SS, Jain GK, Gupta HK. Intra-abdominal symptoms arising from spinal osteophytes. Br J Surg. 1975 Apr;62(4):320-2.

82. Nathan H. Osteophytes of the spine compressing the sympathetic trunk and splanchnic nerves in the thorax. Spine (Phila Pa 1976). 1987 Jul-Aug;12(6):527-32.

83. Otsuka Y, An HS, Ochia RS, Andersson GB, Espinoza Orías AA, Inoue N. In vivo measurement of lumbar facet joint area in asymptomatic and chronic low back pain subjects. Spine (Phila Pa 1976). 2010 Apr 15;35(8):924-8.

84. Fujiwara A, Tamai K, An HS, Lim TH, Yoshida H, Kurihashi A, Saotome. Orientation and osteoarthritis of the lumbar facet joint. Clin Orthop Relat Res. 2001 Apr;(385):88-94.

85. Tachihara H, Kikuchi S, Konno S, Sekiguchi M. Does facet joint inflammation induce radiculopathy?: an investigation using a rat model of lumbar facet joint inflammation. Spine (Phila Pa 1976). 2007 Feb 15;32(4):406-12.

86. Sorkin LS, Xiao WH, Wagner R, Myers RR. Tumour necrosis factor-alpha induces ectopic activity in nociceptive primary afferent fibers. Neuroscience. 1997 Nov;81(1):255-62.

87. Igarashi T, Kikuchi S. Shubayev V, Myers RR. 2000 Volvo Award winner in basic science studies: Exogenous tumor necrosis factor-alpha mimics nucleus pulposus-induced neuropathology. Molecular, histologic, and behavioral comparisons in rats. Spine (Phila Pa 1976). 2000 Dec 1;25(23):2975-80.

88. Buckwalter JA, Woo SL, Goldberg VM, Hadley EC, Booth F, Oegema TR, Eyre DR. Soft-tissue aging and musculoskeletal function. J Bone Joint Surg Am. 1993 Oct;75(10):1533-48.

89. Boos N, Weissbach S, Rohrbach H, Weiler C, Spratt KF, Nerlich AG. Classification of age-related changes in lumbar intervertebral discs: 2002 Volvo Award in basic science. Spine (Phila Pa 1976). 2002 Dec 1;27(23):2631-44.

90. Benoist M. Natural history of the aging spine. Eur Spine J. 2003 Oct;12 Suppl 2:S86-9. Epub 2003 Sep 5.

91. Boos N, Weissbach S, Rohrbach H, Weiler C, Spratt KF, Nerlich AG. Classification of age-related changes in lumbar intervertebral discs: 2002 Volvo Award in basic science. Spine (Phila Pa 1976). 2002 Dec 1;27(23):2631-44.

92. Benoist M. Natural history of the aging spine. Eur Spine J. 2003 Oct;12 Suppl 2:S86-9. Epub 2003 Sep 5.

93. Palmgren T, Grönblad M, Virri J, Kääpä E, Karaharju E. An immunohistochemical study of nerve structures in the anulus fibrosus of human normal lumbar intervertebral discs. Spine (Phila Pa 1976). 1999 Oct 15;24(20):2075-9.

94. Freemont AJ, Peacock TE, Goupille P, Hoyland JA, O'Brien J, Jayson MIV. Nerve ingrowth into diseased intervertebral disc in chronic back pain. Lancet. 1997;350:178-81.

95. Nakamura SI, Takahashi K, Takahashi Y, Yamagata M, Moriya H. The afferent pathways of discogenic low-back pain. Evaluation of L2 spinal nerve infiltration. J Bone Joint Surg Br. 1996 Jul;78(4):606-12.

96. Lotz JC, Ulrich JA. Innervation, inflammation, and hypermobility may characterize pathologic disc degeneration: review of animal model data. J Bone Joint Surg Am. 2006 Apr;88 Suppl 2:76-82.

97. Devereaux MW. Anatomy and examination of the spine. Neurol Clin. 2007 May;25(2):331-51.

98. Edgar MA. The nerve supply of the lumbar intervertebral disc. J Bone Joint Surg Br. 2007 Sep;89(9):1135-9.

99. Ohtori S, Takahashi Y, Takahashi K, Yamagata M, Chiba T, Tanaka K, Hirayama J, Moriya H. Sensory innervation of the dorsal portion of the lumbar intervertebral disc in rats. Spine (Phila Pa 1976). 1999 Nov 15;24(22):2295-9.

100. Nakamura SI, Takahashi K, Takahashi Y, Yamagata M, Moriya H. The afferent pathways of discogenic low-back pain. Evaluation of L2 spinal nerve infiltration. J Bone Joint Surg Br. 1996 Jul;78(4):606-12.

101. Nelson KE, Rottmen J. The female patient, Chapt. 9. In: Somatic Dysfunction in Osteopathic Family Medicine. Nelson, Glonek, eds. Baltimore, MD: Lippincott, Williams & Wilkins; 2007;111-2.

102. Lee MJ, Cassinelli EH, Riew KD. Prevalence of cervical spine stenosis. Anatomic study in cadavers. J Bone Joint Surg Am. 2007 Feb;89(2):376-80.

103. Muthukumar N. Dural ossification in ossification of the ligamentum flavum: a preliminary report. Spine (Phila Pa 1976). 2009 Nov 15;34(24):2654-61.

104. Tatarek NE. Variation in the human cervical neural canal. Spine J. 2005 Nov-Dec;5(6):623-31.

105. Kalichman L, Cole R, Kim DH, Li L, Suri P, Guermazi A, Hunter DJ. Spinal stenosis prevalence and association with symptoms: the Framingham Study. Spine J. 2009 Jul;9(7):545-50. Epub 2009 Apr 23.

106. Standring S. Ed. Gray's Anatomy: The anatomical basis of clinical practice. 39th ed. Edinburgh: Churchill Livingstone; 2004.

107. Aizawa T, Sato T, Sasaki H, Kusakabe T, Morozumi N, Kokubun S. Thoracic myelopathy caused by ossification of the ligamentum flavum: clinical features and surgical results in the Japanese population. J Neurosurg Spine. 2006 Dec;5(6):514-9.

108. Sairyo K, Biyani A, Goel VK, Leaman DW, Booth R Jr, Thomas J, Ebraheim NA, Cowgill IA, Mohan SE. Lumbar ligamentum flavum hypertrophy is due to accumulation of inflammation-related scar tissue. Spine (Phila Pa 1976). 2007 May 15;32(11):E340-7.

109. Muthukumar N. Dural ossification in ossification of the ligamentum flavum: a preliminary report. Spine (Phila Pa 1976). 2009 Nov 15;34(24):2654-61.

110. Evans JH, Nachemson AL. Biomechanical study of human lumbar ligamentum flavum. J Anat. 1969 Jul;105(Pt 1):188-9.

111. Kosaka H, Sairyo K, Biyani A, Leaman D, Yeasting R, Higashino K, Sakai T, Katoh S, Sano T, Goel VK, Yasui N. Pathomechanism of loss of elasticity and hypertrophy of lumbar ligamentum flavum in elderly patients with lumbar spinal canal stenosis. Spine (Phila Pa 1976). 2007 Dec 1;32(25):2805-11.

112. de Kam D, Smulders E, Weerdesteyn V, Smits-Engelsman BC. Exercise interventions to reduce fall-related fractures and their risk factors in individuals with low bone density: a systematic review of randomized controlled trials. Osteoporos Int. 2009 Dec;20(12):2111-25.

113. Sinaki M, Itoi E, Wahner HW, Wollan P, Gelzcer R, Mullan BP, Collins DA, Hodgson SF. Stronger back muscles reduce the incidence of vertebral fractures: a prospective 10 year follow-up of postmenopausal women. Bone. 2002 Jun;30(6):836-41.

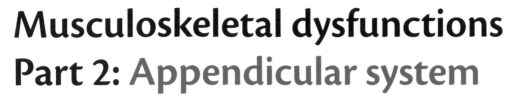

# Musculoskeletal dysfunctions
# Part 2: Appendicular system

The normal aging process is accompanied by anatomic changes that are currently inevitable. This does not mean, however, that there is nothing that can be done when caring for the aged patient. When considering the appendicular disease and dysfunction affecting these individuals, it must be recognized that somatic dysfunction results in frequently subtle functional compromise that can add to physical limitations in the presence of chronic diseases. Additionally the cumulative effect of a lifetime of such functional compromise most likely establishes areas of greater degenerative vulnerability. Thus the earliest possible diagnosis of somatic dysfunction should enhance the patient's current functional capacity and at the same time reduce physical stress, decreasing the progression of degenerative processes. Since it is a fundamental osteopathic principle that the body, when unencumbered by somatic dysfunction, can optimally exert its self-healing processes, it is reasonable to conclude that, when somatic dysfunction is effectively treated, some degree of reversal of chronic degenerative musculoskeletal disease processes should be possible.

Degenerative musculoskeletal disease processes can affect all areas of the upper and lower extremities. To describe them all is beyond the scope of this section. However, certain categories repeatedly manifest and we shall consider them in the context of specific examples. These categories include:

- Degenerative arthritis, e.g., osteoarthritis (OA) of the hip and knee.
- Overuse syndromes, e.g., rotator cuff syndrome.
- Entrapment syndromes, e.g., carpal tunnel syndrome (CTS).

## Degenerative arthritis: osteoarthritis of the hip and knee

In humans, the lower limbs provide mobility, allowing the individual to move from one place to another. Somatic dysfunction affecting any of the structures of the lower limbs, or the functionally related torso, will cause, or contribute to, lower extremity musculoskeletal impairment with pain, limited joint range of motion, muscle weakness, and ultimately reduced function. When these dysfunctions go untreated they can result in chronic joint conditions. As the individual gets older, functional limitations appear, such as inability to walk satisfactory distances or climb stairs frequently, leading to disability with impaired quality of life. Osteoarthritis, frequently the result of a lifetime of wear and tear (macro and micro trauma), often contributes to disability in the elderly and this disability can be further amplified by reversible somatic dysfunction. The degenerative changes of OA can affect any joint in the body. The knees and hips are commonly affected.

### Osteoarthritis of the knee

The knees are particularly subject to the development of OA. When people are asked what area of their body is the most affected with pain, swelling, or stiffness, most often they answer the knee and the back. The prevalence of knee disorders is over 16% in adults over 55 years of age.[1] For a discussion of the dysfunction of the knee, as well as foot imbalance and leg length inequality see further: 'Section 4: Clinical considerations, Chapter 2: Postural imbalance,' p. 237.

Osteoarthritis of the knee is a disease process that demonstrates progressive destruction of the articular cartilage, thickening of the subchondral bone, and new bone formation, resulting in articular deformation. Radiography has typically been used for diagnosis, because the results of the pathological processes of OA—joint space narrowing, subchondral sclerosis, and osteophyte formation—are readily seen on X-ray.[2] Population surveys, however, illustrate that a distinction must be made between the X-ray findings and the clinical condition. It has been shown that 50% of patients with X-ray evidence of knee OA do not have pain. Further, 50% of patients, who are 55 years or older, who complain of knee pain do not have X-ray findings consistent with OA.[3] These observations should lead one to seriously look for functional impairment that can be responsible for patients' pain complaints.

Risk factors for OA of the knee, and other weight-bearing joints, are obesity and injury. Athletic activities and heavy labor requiring repetitive bending of the knees, probably increases the risk of knee OA.

Three key physical attributes that contribute to OA of the knees are: obesity, knee alignment, and foot type. A person who is overweight increases their knee joint load, wearing out articular cartilage faster than a person of ideal body weight. Patients with genu varus, or valgus, have uneven compression of the articular surfaces of the knee. Either the outer or inner aspect of the knee will, respectively, absorb most of the weight-bearing load causing more wear and tear to that area. Patients with pes planus, or whose feet overpronate, induce genu valgus stresses, while those with pes cavus induce genu varus. Additionally, patients with pes cavus, or whose feet underpronate, will absorb less impact with each step, sending greater force up through the leg and necessitating that their knees cushion that increased impact.

Weakness and functional imbalance of the muscles surrounding the knee will compromise the patient's capacity to buffer the impact of walking or running, thereby causing the knee joint to absorb the remaining forces of the impact. Increased muscle tension, particularly affecting the quadriceps, hamstrings, and calf muscles, draws the tibia and femur closer together. In a patient with OA of the knee, whose joint space is reduced, muscle tension increases compression of the already compromised joint space. Increased muscle tension further reduces articular flexibility, decreases, coordination, and slows reaction time.

The quadriceps muscles function to significantly support the weight of the body and help to absorb the load placed upon the knee joints. When pain deters the patient from loading the knee, it is common for the quadriceps to develop atrophy of disuse. This will gradually lead to the inability to cushion the impact of weight-bearing, and establishes a vicious cycle of pain, disuse, and weakness that will progress unless it is effectively addressed.

Weakness of the gluteus medius will destabilize gait, causing the patient to waddle, demonstrating increased side-to-side hip sway. This loss of gluteus medius function that normally maintains hip joint stability, especially when walking, can further contribute to OA of the knee. The thigh muscles will have to work harder to stabilize the hip, causing imbalance of weight-bearing stress through the knee joints.

## Osteoarthritis of the hip: coxarthrosis

After 55 years of age, the prevalence of coxarthrosis is between 3% and 12% in the Western world, an occurrence that is half that of OA of the knee.[4] A genetic influence is suspected through multiple studies showing that a European gene component is required for the expression of the phenotype.[5] Indeed, primary OA leads to total hip replacements in 65% to 70% of individuals with European genes, while it is almost non-existent in Asia, South Asia, and Africa.

In addition to the genetic influence, epigenetic factors are found. This is the case of developmental or acquired hip deformities happening in infancy or childhood that contribute to the development of hip OA. Unrecognized childhood hip disorders such as Legg-Calvé-Perthes disease, slipped capital femoral epiphysis, or hip dysplasia are biomechanical factors disrupting the congruency of the joint.[6] Abnormal joints are associated with increased intra-articular stress with microdamage and remodeling that is detrimental to articular function.[7]

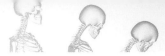
Any load increase on the weight-bearing joints, such as that which occurs with obesity, is a risk factor as well.[8] Consistent with this, a BMI among older individuals less than 24.8 is associated with the absence of hip OA.[9] Accumulation of micro-trauma following increase in intra-articular stress is considered to be a common mechanical factor underlying OA.[10] Several studies have highlighted such mechanical factors in the etiopathogenesis of this disease. For instance, the influence of a life-time exposure to physical activity, either recreational or professional, with related joint-loading has been well-studied showing moderate to strong evidence that it is a risk factor for OA.[11] Athletic activities with strenuous loading may be associated with hip OA.[12] Occupational activities with heavy lifting or climbing stairs or ladders and exposure to heavy lifting combined with kneeling or squatting may contribute to the development of hip OA.[13] [14] A force equal to one third of the body's weight is applied to the hip in the standing position. When climbing stairs, however, the burden totals five to seven times the body's weight.[15]

## The evolution of the hip and pelvis

To fully understand hip mechanics, one should recall the phylogenesis of the hip and pelvis. Besides encephalization, the other characteristic of humanity's evolution is bipedal gait that transformed the structure and function of the pelvis. When compared with australopithecines or modern apes, the modern human pelvis is wider, with hip joints that are relatively further apart. Pelvic evolution has also been greatly influenced by childbirth, since a larger pelvic outlet allows birth of infants with bigger brains. With a larger pelvis, the hip joints are under more mechanical stress from the weight of the torso. This has led to the development of: strong abductor muscles, to stabilize the pelvis during bipedal gait; changes in the femoral head that became larger making it capable of absorbing more stress; and a longer femoral neck that increases the power of the abductor muscles.

Another big difference between human and chimpanzee during bipedal gait is that the chimpanzee walks with flexion of both hips and knees to compensate for a forward bent position of the torso. Humans differ clearly from the chimpanzee in having flexible lumbar spines that allows lordosis. Thus

they are able to maintain a vertical position during upright locomotion with the head, arms, and trunk vertically above the joints of the lower limb. The lumbar lordosis became a significant advantage, allowing the individual the possibility to sustain their hips and knees in more extended positions.[16] [17] Indeed, because extension in the hip takes place in both the hip joint and in the pelvis through the backward tilting associated with bipedalism, it has been described as a 'double extension.'[18] As a result, the femoral head displays an 'anterior uncovering' in its relationship with the acetabulum.

According to the theory of recapitulation, ontogeny recapitulates phylogeny. This process extends into infancy and childhood. As such, the child is first creeping, and then crawling, before walking at about 15 months. At 18 months the acetabulum is fairly flat. Cupping of the acetabulum is visible at three years, and continues to deepen over the following years, with the posterior wall always showing greater ossification than the anterior wall. After the closure of the triradiate cartilage, between the ages of 11 and 13, no further conformational change occurs.[19] At this point, more than half of the femoral head displays an 'anterior uncovering.' Normally, the mouth of the human acetabulum faces anteriorly, laterally, and inferiorly, with the hip joint displaying the best congruency when the femur is in flexion, abduction, and external rotation. However, when humans are in an upright position, the 'double extension' and 'anterior uncovering' do not permit such congruency.

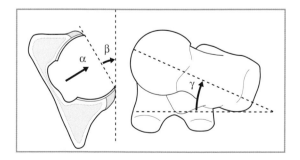

Figure 4.1.17: Orientation of the right acetabulum and femoral head
α Normally, the mouth of the acetabulum faces anteriorly, laterally, and inferiorly
β Acetabular anteversion angle
γ Femoral neck anteversion angle

As a result, the transmission of forces from weight-bearing is concentrated only upon a small portion of the cartilage surface of the femoral head. While a force spread over a large articular surface would produce no injury, a minimal force transmitted to a small contact area may cause stresses and lead to cartilage damage.[20]

## Coarthrosis anatomopathology

Although coxarthrosis results from an interaction between multiple factors, mechanical and structural changes play an important part. During early childhood, before ossification of the three parts of the pelvic bone occurs, any stress applied to the acetabulum can lead to intraosseous dysfunction of the pelvic bone and developmental displacement of the hip.[21] Uterine constraint and the sleeping position of the infant, with a preference to lie on one side, are examples of contributing factors.[22] Some studies associate hip OA with developmental displacement of the hip.[23] Indeed, patients with developmental dysplasia of the hip display deficiency of the acetabular coverage of the femoral head in its anterior and anterosuperior portions.[24] Additionally, hip dysplasia may be associated with an acetabular retroversion,[25] where the mouth of the acetabulum faces laterally, inferiorly, and more posteriorly than normal. Acetabular retroversion can increase femoroacetabular impingement between the femoral neck and anterior acetabular edge, a cause for hip OA, which is found in 20% of patients with idiopathic hip OA, while it is seen in only 5% of the general population.[26][27]

Indeed, two main types of femoroacetabular impingement are frequently described as part of the etiopathogenesis for OA of the hip.[28] In the first, the aspherical portion of the femoral head gets jammed against the acetabular rim during hip flexion, which ultimately leads to chondral abrasion. In the second, there is contact between the acetabular rim and the junction between the femoral head and neck. Besides a history of groin pain and radiographic evidence, decreased range of motion can be observed during clinical examination. Additionally, in most cases, the 'impingement test' (passive movement of the thigh into full flexion, adduction, and internal rotation) will elicit pain.[29] During this motion the proximal and anterior part of the femoral neck contacts the rim of the acetabulum, usually where the labrum is damaged.

## Coxarthrosis and somatic dysfunction

From an osteopathic point of view, postural dysfunctions contribute largely to weight-bearing imbalance. In fact, any dysfunction in the body may affect posture and weight-bearing. It may be a somatic dysfunction in the limbs, a vertebral dysfunction, a visceral dysfunction, or a cranial dysfunction. Small anatomic inequities of leg length, that are present in over half of the adult population, can be responsible for the development and maintenance of postural dysfunction.[30] (See further: 'Section 4: Clinical considerations, Chapter 2: Postural Imbalance,' p. 237.)

The hips are of paramount importance in the support of the body's weight, and in its distribution to the lower limbs. Both the pelvic bone and the femur must be considered in the study of the hip joint. From above, the pelvic bones on each side constantly adjust the acetabula upon the femoral heads to allow for different postures. From below, during standing, walking, or running, the femur heads fine-tune their position to fit into the acetabula.

As a paired structure, the femurs demonstrate craniosacral external and internal rotation motions. Dysfunctions of the femur may include restriction of flexion/extension, abduction/adduction, external/internal rotation, and the minor motions of medial/lateral glide and cephalocaudal glide. In the presence of dysfunction, the congruence between the femoral head and acetabulum is compromised, with resultant abnormal stress upon the articular cartilage.

Normally, when the sacrum demonstrates craniosacral flexion and extension, the pelvic bones respectively demonstrate craniosacral external and internal rotation, a combination of three components that can be described in the context of the three cardinal planes.[31] During craniosacral external rotation, the inspiratory phase of the primary respiratory mechanism (PRM), the motion of the pelvic bones is as follows:

- In the sagittal plane, there is a major component of motion (anterior rotation) wherein the

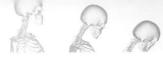
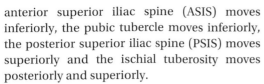

anterior superior iliac spine (ASIS) moves inferiorly, the pubic tubercle moves inferiorly, the posterior superior iliac spine (PSIS) moves superiorly and the ischial tuberosity moves posteriorly and superiorly.

- In the coronal plane, there is a minor component of motion—abduction of the iliac crest and adduction of the ischial tuberosity.
- In the transverse plane, there is a minor component of motion, where the entire iliac crest moves laterally but to a greater degree at the PSIS than at the ASIS.

During craniosacral internal rotation, the expiratory phase of the PRM, the reverse occurs.

Somatic dysfunctions of the sacrum, as occur in sacral torsions, will have an effect upon the position of the pelvic bones, modifying the orientation of the acetabula. Similarly, acetabular positional change will occur with leg length inequality or from any myofascial imbalance affecting structures inserting upon the pelvic bone or the femur.

(See further discussion of 'Physiologic motion of the sacrum' in 'Section 4: Clinical considerations, Chapter 1: Musculoskeletal dysfunctions, Part 1: Axial system,' p. 182, and of 'Leg length inequality' in 'Section 4: Clinical considerations, Chapter 2: Postural Imbalance,' p. 237.)

With aging, loss of lumbar lordosis occurs, particularly in the lower portion of the lumbar spine.[32] At the same time, there is a loss of hip extension.[33]

Because of the tensegrital relationship between the different parts of the body, myofascial imbalance can affect the pelvis from above, or from below. From above, the pelvis may be affected by asymmetric spasm of the psoas major, producing a pelvic sideshift toward the side opposite to the spasm. From below it may be dysfunction of the knee or foot causing myofascial imbalance in the iliotibial tract. Once again, in each case, congruence in the hip joint is affected, and for this reason a complete postural and functional assessment of the patient must be performed.

## The osteopathic contribution to the physical examination and treatment

When treating the patient with OA of the weight-bearing joints of the lower extremities, functional imbalance of the pelvis, hip, and knee should be sought out and appropriately treated with osteopathic manipulative treatment (OMT). A complete postural examination should be performed. See 'Section 2: Osteopathic assessment,' p. 37. Start with the patient standing. Observe the posture and the weight-bearing distribution that should be distributed equally upon both feet. Observe the alignment of the patient's feet, which should normally form an angle of 30°, open anteriorly. Somatic dys-

function of the femur or of the pelvic bone in external or internal rotation may result respectively in an increase or decrease of this angle. Observe the alignment of the patient's lower extremities. Then observe structures above as they may interfere with pelvic balance.

Next proceed to tests of listening of the pelvis in the standing position and in the supine position, as described in 'Section 2: Osteopathic assessment,' p. 50. Evaluate hip joint motion, and assess myofascial structures in relation with the pelvis. Address any identified dysfunctions.

## Advice to the patient

Since obesity significantly increases the possibility of developing OA in the weight-bearing joints, encourage your patient to maintain a healthy weight. Encourage them to follow a regular exercise routine to improve flexibility and range of motion of the hips. Exercises should release myofascial tension in the

tight muscles, most often the hip flexors, hip adductors, hamstrings, rectus femoris, tensor fascia lata, and piriformis. Improvement of muscle strength in the gluteus maximus and medius is recommended.

Explain to your patient that remaining in a seated position for prolonged periods is not recommended, and that getting up from time to time to stretch, particularly the hips and iliopsoas muscle group, is a good habit. Teach your patient to walk using as much hip extension as possible while avoiding forward tilting of the pelvis.

Since there is a risk of hip fracture with hip OA,[34] a program of exercises to improve balance performance is indicated. Give advice for preventing falls such as elimination of home hazards, having sufficient light in the rooms, and wearing properly fitting, secure non-slippery shoes.

Concern should be employed to exercise weakened muscles without causing excessive stress to the arthritic joints. Studies of patients, however, who were self-selected for exercise and followed for substantial periods of time, have demonstrated no evidence of accelerated development of OA, provided injury was avoided. Further, there is good evidence that appropriately dosed exercise reduced pain and disability as compared to controls. Patients with established OA, who performed muscle-strengthening, aquatic, or physiotherapy-based exercise modalities, derived functional benefit, with reduction of pain and disability.[35]

# Overuse syndromes: rotator cuff syndrome

With the acquisition of the upright posture the upper limbs were no longer involved in weight-bearing. Thereby, humans developed new functions, requiring additional performance from pre-existing structures, and in the process gaining greater mobility but losing stability. Newly acquired motions including abduction, supination, and pronation allow humans to achieve manual dexterity. These motions are frequently, however, the first to be lost and the most difficult to regain in upper limb disorders.

Among the general population, between 16% and 26% of individuals complain of shoulder pain.[36] This number increases with age, and in people over 65, 34% have shoulder complaints, with 30% having motion restriction and disability.[37] In fact the shoulder has the largest range of motion of all of the articulations in the body. Consequently, any shoulder pain, or restriction of mobility, considerably affects quality of life, and activities of daily living such as feeding and dressing become difficult. With age, degenerative disorders increase. Osteoarthritis of the shoulder and rotator cuff syndromes are the most common causes of pain and disability in the older population.

## Rotator cuff syndrome

As with any other shoulder problem, the incidence of rotator cuff disease increases with age. The precise incidence of this disease is, however, difficult to establish because many subjects are asymptomatic. During an evaluation of asymptomatic individuals with magnetic resonance images of the shoulders, 54% of individuals over 60 years of age had a tear of the rotator cuff.[38]

### Rotator cuff anatomopathology

In order to diagnose and treat any shoulder dysfunction, one must have a real appreciation for the anatomical considerations pertinent to the area, and how somatic dysfunction may affect function.

On each side, the pectoral, or shoulder girdle, anatomically consists of three bones (scapula, clavicle, and humerus). These three bones are united with one another and to the axial skeleton by five joints:

- The glenohumeral joint between the head of the humerus and the glenoid cavity of the scapula is the main articulation; it permits adduction, abduction, medial and lateral rotation, flexion, and extension of the arm.
- The acromioclavicular joint is the articulation between the acromion process of the scapula and the lateral end of the clavicle. It allows translatory and rotation motions between the acromion of the scapula and the acromial surface of the clavicle.
- The sternoclavicular joint is the articulation between the manubrium of the sternum and the first costal cartilage with the medial end of the clavicle. It is the joint joining the pectoral girdle to the thorax.
- The scapulocostal joint or scapulothoracic joint is not a true anatomical joint, but rather a

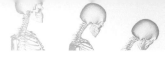

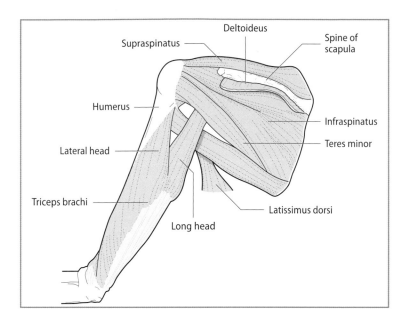

**Figure 4.1.18:** Left shoulder muscles (posterior view)

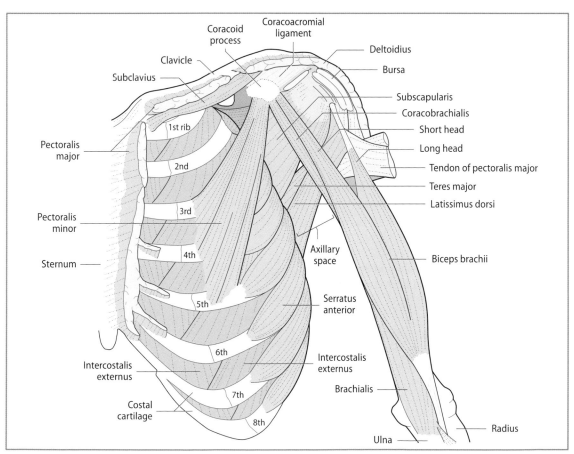

Figure 4.1.19: Left shoulder muscles (anterior view)

physiological joint, sometimes referred to as a 'false' joint. It consists of the relation between the anterior scapula and the posterior thoracic rib cage, allowing gliding movements of the scapula.

- The suprahumeral joint or subacromial joint is also a physiological or 'false' joint between the head of the humerus and the coracoacromial ligament, containing the subacromial bursa and the tendon of supraspinatus.

**The rotator cuff muscles**

While the shoulder joints are designed for mobility, their muscles and ligaments provide stability. Among the numerous muscles of the shoulder, the rotator cuff is of paramount importance. It consists of muscles: the supraspinatus, infraspinatus, teres minor, and subscapularis, and tendons that stabilize the head of the humerus in the glenoid fossa. All of these muscles originate on the scapula and insert on the humerus. The supraspinatus arises from the fossa above the spine of the scapula and inserts on the upper part of the greater tubercle of the humerus. The infraspinatus arises from the fossa below the spine of the scapula and inserts on the middle part of the greater tubercle. The teres minor arises from the lateral border of the scapula, in its upper two thirds and inserts on the lower part of the greater tubercle. The subscapularis arises from the ventral aspect of the scapula and inserts on the lesser tubercle of the humerus.

On the head of the humerus, the tendons of the rotator cuff muscles splay out and interdigitate to form a continuous cuff.[39] Overlapping exists between the infraspinatus and supraspinatus and between the infraspinatus and teres minor that makes them difficult to separate from one another. This arrangement distributes load from the contraction of one muscle to the attachment of neighboring tendons, in both normal function, and dysfunction. Additionally, fibers from the subscapularis and supraspinatus tendons surround the biceps tendon leading some authors to consider the long head of the biceps tendon as a part of the rotator cuff.[40] It is also suggested that subscapularis tendon integrity is necessary for biceps tendon stability.[41]

One of the major functions of the rotator cuff muscles is their contribution to 'concavity

compression,' i.e., the compression of the humeral head against the glenoid cavity. Normally, antagonistic forces between the subscapularis anteriorly and the infraspinatus and teres minor posteriorly, stabilize the glenohumeral joint. The rotator cuff muscles maintain the humeral head in its centered position and control humeral translatory motions. Conversely, any dysfunction of these muscles leads to shoulder instability.

The rotator cuff muscles perform multiple additional movements. These include humeral abduction by the supraspinatus, lateral rotation by the infraspinatus and teres minor, and medial rotation by the subscapularis.

**The coracoacromial arch**

Above the rotator cuff is the coracoacromial arch that consists of the bony acromion, the coracoacromial ligament (CAL), and the coracoid process. It forms the roof of a space, the supraspinatus outlet, through which the supraspinatus tendon traverses, and contains a bursa that lies between the supraspinatus tendon and the acromial arch. Any change in the relationships between the coracoacromial arch components can compress the supraspinatus tendon between the coracoacromial arch above and the humeral head below. Of all the components of the coracoacromial arch, the

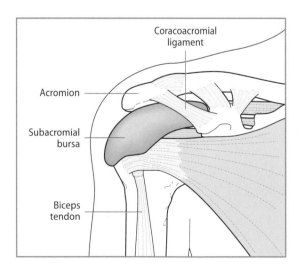

Figure 4.1.20: The coracoacromial arch

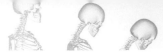

coracoid process is thought to contribute the most to changes in the space under the arch.[42]

The CAL is at the center of the coracoacromial arch. V-shaped, it originates from the anterior margin of the acromion, and runs anteriorly and inferiorly to insert onto the posterior aspect of the coracoid process. Medially, the CAL is continuous with the clavipectoral fascia (costocoracoid membrane) that encloses the subclavius muscle, connects to the clavicle, and blends with the deep cervical fascia. Laterally, the CAL is continuous with the fascia covering the undersurface of the deltoid. Multiple myofascial connections influence the coracoacromial arch and their dysfunction can contribute to rotator cuff impingement.

## Changes with age

Although the etiology of rotator cuff damage is still debated, whether it is caused by extrinsic or intrinsic factors, degeneration with age is one of the multiple etiopathogenetic factors. Extrinsic factors are thought to most commonly occur from hooking of the acromion process with bony impingement, causing mechanical compression of tendons and the surrounding soft tissue of the coracoacromial arch. Intrinsic factors consist of degenerative changes in the cuff tendons.

Aging is associated with the development of small acromial spurs.[43] Acromion enthesopathy, i.e., spur formation within the coracoacromial ligament (CAL) where it attaches to the acromion, is commonly encountered. This may result from increased traction upon the CAL associated with pectoral girdle imbalance.[44] Aging is usually associated with degenerative changes of the coracoacromial arch, even when the rotator cuff is normal.[45] Additionally, the supraspinatus tendon becomes thickened with age, and is more likely to tear.[46] This loss of elasticity, with repeated friction from contact with the acromion, results in damage to the tendon.

Normally, collagen type I is the most abundant in the rotator cuff, providing tensile strength. Collagen type III is weaker and increases with aging and tendon degeneration.[47] As with the changes occurring in other tendons in the body associated with aging, these variations can lead to rotator cuff tendinous impairment. As elsewhere in the body, reduction of collagen synthesis is also associated with oxidative stress.[48]

A 'critical area' in the distal 10 mm of the supraspinatus tendon is recognized as the commonest site for rotator cuff tears.[49] This area demonstrates hypovascularity that may be a predisposing factor for tears, although some hypervascularity appears to develop in this 'critical area' secondary to mechanical impingement.[50] Indeed, inflammation is significant in the genesis of rotator cuff rupture, as demonstrated by inflammatory swellings of the subacromial bursa.[51]

## Rotator cuff syndrome and somatic dysfunction

Among individuals, multiple anatomical and morphological variations exist in the scapular components. Multiple studies have examined the differences in size and shape of the acromion and coracoid process among patients with rotator cuff syndrome, in an attempt to define the predisposing characteristics. Simple observation of postural differences in shoulder girdles among the general population, however, shows that the scapula rests differently upon the thorax. Scapular position is the result of multiple influences through myofascial relationships. Such fascial influences emanate from the cervical, thoracic, and lumbosacral spine and the ribs as well as some viscera. The osteopathic principle of the relationship between function and structure is well-illustrated in this case. Any resultant dysfunction of the scapula will affect the position of its components and the mechanical stress applied to them, leading to acromial spurs, or modifications of their size and shape. In addition, in order for the rotator cuff to function at an optimal level, the scapula must be well-positioned, and as such scapular dysfunction may contribute to rotator cuff syndrome.

The acromioclavicular articulation is a site of articular somatic dysfunction that can significantly affect the shoulder. Acromioclavicular dysfunction slightly changes the neutral resting position of the scapula thereby not only producing symptoms referable to the acromioclavicular joint but also potentially to any of the scapulothoracic muscles.

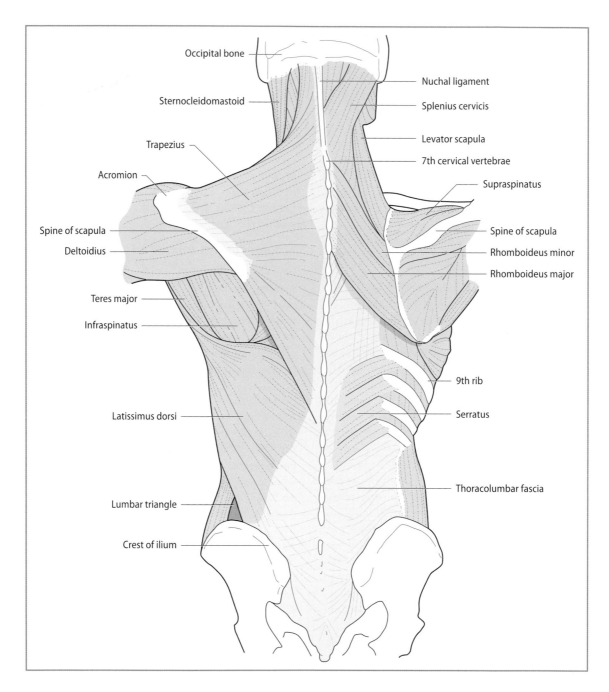

Figure 4.1.21: Posterior view of the myofascial influences upon scapular position

Shoulder complaints may also result from dysfunction affecting the cervical spine, as the innervation of the muscles and other tissues of the shoulder, arm, and hand come from the cervical spine. Complaints may also follow thoracic somatic dysfunction because of associated segmental facilitation. The sympathetic supply for the upper extremities emanates from the mid- to upper thoracic

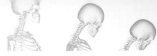

region. Segmental facilitation affects the sympathetic cell bodies in the lateral cell column. This results in increased vasomotor tone, producing decreased peripheral tissue perfusion. Slight alteration of the blood supply to peripheral nerves can be enough to produce dysesthesias and paresthesias.[52,53]

# The osteopathic contribution to the physical examination and treatment

Osteopathic manipulative treatment, integrated with appropriate treatment according to accepted standards of medical practice, should be used for its contribution to the treatment of the various presentations of rotator cuff syndrome to facilitate the body's inherent capacity for self-healing, to enhance the patient's functional capacity, and to provide comfort. A holistic assessment should include the psychosocial and occupational issues of the patient as well as a physical examination. Inquire if the patient has pain, instability, weakness, or loss of range of motion. Complaints of paresthesias may be associated with neurovascular disorders, requiring appropriate neurological assessment for radiculopathy, neuropathy, and structural anomalies, as might result in thoracic outlet compromise. The demonstration of any neurological deficit necessitates a complete evaluation for organic pathology.

Observe the patient, during and after the acquisition of their history. Look at the pectoral girdle to assess its relationship with other parts of the body. Shoulder dysfunctions may follow dysfunctions of the cervical, thoracic, and lumbosacral spine, ribs, pelvis, and visceral dysfunctions.

Next, proceed to a test of listening of the scapula. This can be done with the patient seated. Place the palm of your hand upon the scapula, with your fingers directed cephalically. This hand placement allows you to listen to the scapula and assess its motility. As a paired bone, in the absence of any dysfunction, the scapula should present craniosacral external and internal rotation components of motion in each of the three cardinal planes. During craniosacral external rotation—the inspiratory phase of the PRM—the motion is as follows:

- In the sagittal plane, there is posterior rotation where the superior angle moves posteriorly and the inferior angle moves anteriorly.

- In the coronal plane, the superior angle moves laterally and the inferior angle medially.
- In the transverse plane, the axillary border moves posteriorly to a greater degree than the vertebral border.

During craniosacral internal rotation—the expiratory phase of the PRM—the motion is reversed.

Listen and identify the degree of craniosacral external or internal rotation dysfunction of the scapula globally and in each of the cardinal planes. Determine also if distant somatic dysfunction is affecting the motion of the scapula through the influence of myofascial structures. In such a case the scapula will be drawn toward the location of the dysfunction. If this is present the distant dysfunction must be addressed before the scapula can be effectively treated. Myofascial dysfunction should be treated, following its tensegrital sensations of ease and bind to a point of fascial balance. The scapula must be free of any dysfunctional influences in order to provide correct support for all the myofascial structures that attach upon it and to allow correct function of all its aspects.

Assess the clavicle, and the acromioclavicular and sternoclavicular joints. The acromioclavicular joint is an arthrodial joint, where the lateral clavicular articular surface faces inferolaterally to cover a corresponding facet on the medial acromial border. Clavicular motion is an anteroposterior glide. The sternoclavicular joint is a double-plane synovial joint with two portions, separated by an articular disc that allows the clavicle to move predominantly anteroposteriorly with a small degree of rotation on the long axis of the clavicle.

Identify and treat the dysfunctions that may be present. The clavicle is a key bone affecting several myofascial structures that attach to it. It binds the shoulder to the thorax, the craniocervical area, and the lower half of the body. As such, the clavicle is part of a tensegral relationship, acting as a compression-bearing rigid 'girder' stretching flexible, tension-bearing myofascial 'cables.'

With the patient seated or in the supine position, test the humerus relative to the scapula at the glenohumeral joint. Begin with a test of listening. During the inspiratory phase of the PRM, the humerus demonstrates craniosacral external rotation (the same as its anatomic motion), while there is internal rotation during the expiratory phase. Most of the time, with a dysfunctional shoulder, there is a somatic dysfunction at the level of the glenohumeral joint. The head of the humerus is found in external or internal rotation with limitation also affecting the balance between the minor motions of anterior/posterior, lateral/medial, cephalocaudal glide, or any combination of the minor motions. If necessary, proceed next to range of motion testing. Be respectful of the capacities of the patient and remember that stiffness may indicate adhesive capsulitis, arthritis, or both and that crepitus may be associated with OA, bursa, or rotator cuff pathology. Address any somatic dysfunction found.

Several orthopaedic tests are described. However, not all of them demonstrate the same level of reliability.[54 55] Usually, the 'empty can,' or Jobe, test is used to evaluate the strength and integrity of the supraspinatus muscle and tendon. The patient is seated or standing. The practitioner is standing in front of the patient, on the side of the complaint. Abduct the patient's arm to 90° in the coronal plane, with adduction of 30° in the transverse plane, in order to place the arm in the scapular plane. Instruct the patient to keep their elbow extended, and to internally rotate their arm with the thumb directed towards the floor, as if they were emptying a can or glass. Stabilize the scapula with your posterior hand, place your anterior hand upon the patient's forearm, and ask the patient to perform shoulder abduction against the resistance of your anterior hand. The test is positive when pain or weakness prevents the patient from performing as requested. This test performed with shoulder abduction in the coronal plane of 30° instead of 90°, allows one to test the supraspinatus.

Most of the time, non-surgical treatments are used first in rotator cuff syndrome, before considering surgery. Osteopathic manipulative treatment has a place of choice among these treatments, and studies suggest that manual therapy in conjunction with a program of strengthening and stretching is more beneficial than strengthening and stretching alone.[56] Treatment should address associated spinal, scapulothoracic, and clavicular dysfunctions as well as consideration of glenohumeral mechanics. For optimal results it is often beneficial to assess and address the patient's global functional pattern as well.

It should be remembered that after prolonged periods of somatic dysfunction with limitation of motion and pain, patients quite often develop functional amnesia. They lose proprioception and the ability to move the dysfunctional area through its full range of motion. This may be addressed with conscious rehabilitation of the patient's capacity to move the dysfunctional structures. Begin by explaining to the patient how to visualize the motion that needs to be addressed, and then instruct them to gently perform that motion, progressively reaching the full range of motion, thereby regaining optimal proprioception.[57] Rehabilitation can be completed with exercises to improve global posture, flexibility, and strength of the shoulder.

# Advice to the patient

Explain to your patient that many times, rotator cuff syndromes result from overuse, and that some adjustments will be necessary in their daily routine and activities to reduce stress to the shoulder. Identify with them injurious movements or sustained positions that they are repeatedly exposed to during the day, and in particular look for positioning where the elbow is raised above the shoulder level.

Stress the importance of a good posture and how it affects the pectoral girdle. Teach them how to retract their shoulders and avoid positions

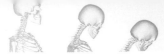

combining flexion, adduction, and internal rotation of the shoulder, the position most frequently causing subcoracoid impingement.[58] Because this can occur at times of inactivity, when they are relaxing, it is not readily recognized as deleterious. Such a slouched position is often taken when seated on a sofa to watch TV for instance. Frequently, this is also the position of the shoulder when sleeping in a lateral decubitus position. Indeed, a correlation has been demonstrated between the side of the shoulder pain and the side that the individual selectively sleeps upon.[59] For this reason, encourage them to sleep supine or to avoid the lateral decubitus position on the side of the dysfunctional shoulder.

Encourage your patient to follow a program of supervised exercises with an experienced physical therapist, and then to continue exercises alone to further increase strength, decrease pain, and improve function. Classical exercises include pendulum exercises where the patient is forward bent, with the dysfunctional arm hanging directed toward the floor, in a very relaxed manner, and their other arm supports their torso upon a table. Rotations of the arm are performed in a clockwise pattern ten times, and then repeated counterclockwise ten times. Additional forward, backward, and side-to-side movements are included. Gradual increase of the range of motion is recommended, and these exercises must be done at least three times per day.

After successfully using these exercises, the patient may then progress to active assisted motion, where they can use their unaffected arm to assist the dysfunctional side. Next, they may move on to more active range of motion exercises. To do so in front of a mirror is recommended to avoid ineffective positional compensations.

# Entrapment syndromes: carpal tunnel syndrome

Carpal tunnel syndrome is an entrapment neuropathy of the median nerve that represents about 90% of all entrapment neuropathies.[60] The prevalence of electrophysiologically confirmed, symptomatic CTS is approximately 3% among women and 2% among men.[61] It occurs more often in women with peaks between 50 and 59 years of age. For men, there is an additional peak between 70 and 79 years.[62]

Carpal tunnel syndrome is associated with activities of the hand and wrist, where repetition, force, external pressure, and vibration are involved as in, for example, keypunching, typing, scrubbing, or using air-powered hand tools. Indeed since 2003, CTS has been listed in the European Union's list of occupational diseases. Particular anthropometric characteristics such as short and wide hand with square wrist increase the liability for CTS.[63] Obesity is another risk factor,[64] as well as tobacco, caffeine, and alcohol consumption.[65] In addition, several medical conditions are linked to CTS, including inflammatory arthritis, wrist fracture, hypothyroidism, diabetes mellitus, and use of corticosteroids and estrogens.[66]

## Carpal tunnel anatomopathology

The carpal tunnel is a space located between the concave arch of the carpus and the flexor retinaculum, through which the flexor tendons of the digits

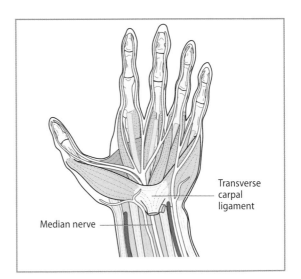

Figure 4.1.22: Left hand with median nerve passing through carpal tunnel

and the median nerve pass. Its volume, depending on the size of the hand, is approximately 5 ml.[67]

Median nerve entrapment is the hallmark of CTS. The median nerve arises from the brachial plexus (spinal nerves C5–T1). The brachial plexus courses through the neck, between the anterior and middle scalene muscles, and then passes between the first rib and clavicle to reach the axilla and the arm. In the arm, it runs on the medial side of the humerus between the biceps brachii and brachialis. It traverses the elbow in the antecubital fossa deep to the bicipital aponeurosis where it usually enters the forearm between the two heads of the pronator teres, to descend between the heads of the flexor digitorum superficialis and pass under the flexor retinaculum, entering the hand through the carpal tunnel. As it passes through the carpal tunnel, the median nerve conveys sensory impulses from the skin of the palmar aspects of the thumb, index, middle, and radial half of the ring finger, and the terminal parts of their dorsal aspects. The nerve also supplies the abductor pollicis brevis, the opponens pollicis, part of the flexor pollicis brevis, and the two lateral lumbrical muscles.

The flexor retinaculum is a strong band of connective tissue, 2.5-3 cm long, firmly fused with four bones of the wrist: medially to the pisiform and the hook of the hamate; and laterally to the tubercle of the navicular, the crest of the trapezium, and sometimes the radial styloid process. The transverse carpal ligament represents the central portion of the flexor retinaculum.

One of the theories of CTS—the mechanical compression theory—proposes that the symptoms of CTS are due to compression of the median nerve in the carpal tunnel. Indeed, any decrease in the space of the carpal tunnel may contribute to compression of the nerve, including repetitive flexion extension of the wrist, finger flexion, or forearm supination, trauma, and inflammatory or metabolic processes. It is also possible that edema of the contents of the carpal tunnel can compromise the median nerve in the absence of any decrease in carpal tunnel volume.

Neural compression has pathophysiological effects upon neuronal microanatomy as well as upon surrounding tissues. All peripheral nerves include sensory, motor, general visceral afferent, and sympathetic nerve fibers. Myelinated and unmyelinated fibers are present within both motor and sensory nerves. They are surrounded by a layer of connective tissue (CT) that forms the perineurium, while all the fascicles of a nerve are encased by the external epineurium and the mesoneurium. Neural compression may result in thickening of these connective tissues. In fact, the mesoneurium plays a critical role in the gliding of the nerve, a function that can be limited in the presence of fibrosis. With chronic nerve compression, intraneural microcirculation, via the vasa nervosa, and nerve fiber structure are modified, with an increase in vascular permeability that results in edema formation, deterioration of anterograde and retrograde axonal transport, and alteration in nerve function.[68] Scarring, with the development of fibrous tissue eventually occurs within the nerve. The symptoms of CTS, described as tingling, numbness, severe pain, and reversible loss of nerve conduction are associated with a possible vascular dysfunction and ischemia of the affected nerve segment.

In addition, serial impingements can occur involving a peripheral nerve. In 1973, Upton and McComas described the 'double crush' theory, which stated that serial impingements can act in a cumulative manner to cause a symptomatic distal entrapment neuropathy.[69] Proximal impingement, e.g., at the level of the cervical spine, is thought to alter axoplasmic flow and increase the susceptibility of nervous fibers at a distal site to be damaged by a distal compression. For this reason, when treating CTS, any somatic dysfunction along the course of the brachial plexus must also be addressed.

## Carpal tunnel and somatic dysfunction

The flexor retinaculum is part of a tensegrital model. Proximally, the flexor retinaculum is a direct continuation of the deep antebrachial fascia, which is continuous above with the brachial fascia, while the brachial fascia is continuous with the fascia covering the deltoid and the pectoralis major muscle, which attaches above to the clavicle, acromion, and spine of the scapula. Distally, the

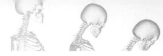

flexor retinaculum is continuous with the palmar aponeurosis. As such, any dysfunction of the segmentally-related spine and shoulder can tensegritally affect the flexor retinaculum.

As one of the neurological syndromes affecting the brachial plexus, CTS may, in the context of the 'double crush' theory, have associated dysfunction affecting the spinal nerve roots, the brachial plexus as it traverses the neck, and the peripheral median nerve.[70] The motor neurons of peripheral nerves are located in the ventral horn in the spinal cord, and the sensory cell bodies in the dorsal root ganglion. As such, any spinal somatic dysfunction of the vertebral units from C4–C5 through T1–T2, involving the brachial plexus, may facilitate the development of CTS.

As the brachial plexus traverses the neck and passes between the anterior and middle scalene muscles, the first rib, and clavicle, the median nerve is vulnerable to somatic dysfunction affecting any of these structures, while peripherally it is vulnerable to myofascial compression anywhere along its course, particularly at the elbow and in the forearm. Dysfunction of the radius or the ulna may also be involved in carpal tunnel compromise.

At the level of the wrist, somatic dysfunction of any of the carpal bones, particularly the lunate bone, can decrease the volume of the carpal tunnel, and contribute to CTS.[71] This dysfunction is often an extension dysfunction of the lunate and may follow a fall on the hyperextended wrist. Extension of the wrist is associated with more pressure on the median nerve.[72]

The preganglionic fibers of the sympathetic division concerning the upper extremities have their cell bodies in the intermediolateral horn of the spinal cord in the mid- to upper thoracic spinal segment. Somatic dysfunctions of these areas may contribute to sympathetic dysfunction and result in vasospasm, with decreased arterial perfusion through the vasa nervosa, and impaired venous and lymphatic drainage, increasing the pathophysiological effects seen in CTS.[73][74] Decrease of the power of the baroreflex component of the PRM may further contribute to impairment of peripheral circulation.[75]

## The osteopathic contribution to the physical examination and treatment

Most of the time, non-operative treatment options are proposed in patients diagnosed with CTS. The reduction of inflammation, and consequently edema of the carpal tunnel contents with non-steroidal anti-inflammatory drugs is the first line of medical treatment. Then local steroid injections and, or, splinting are suggested, and after that surgery.[76] Therefore OMT can be proposed integratively as a non-operative option.

Because of all the potential sites where somatic dysfunction may contribute to CTS, the osteopathic structural examination and subsequent treatment with OMT should start at the level of the thoracic spine and ribs, and then continue to the cervical spine. The soft tissues of the neck, with attention to the scalene muscles should follow. Next, the pectoral girdle and shoulder should be examined for their relationship with the brachial plexus. The mechanics of the elbow and forearm should be evaluated. After that, the carpal and metacarpal bones should be examined, with particular attention to the lunate, and any identified somatic dysfunction should be appropriately treated.

Myofascial release of the neck, shoulder, arm, wrist, and finger structures may complete the treatment. In particular, the release of the flexor retinaculum, which extends from the distal aspect of the radius, which is the proximal wrist flexion crease, to the proximal aspect of the third metacarpal, should be considered to alleviate pressure from the median nerve. Apply indirect procedure, listening to the connective tissue with great attention to the tissue response, especially in the presence of inflammation.

The 'Opponens roll maneuver' may also be applied to stretch the flexor retinaculum. This procedure can be taught to the patient as an exercise to repeat at home. Hold the patient's thenar with one hand, and the hypothenar with your other hand, so that bilaterally your thumbs are upon the palmar surface of the patient's hand, contacting the medial and lateral ends of the flexor retinaculum, and your fingers are on the dorsal surface of the carpal bones. Progressively pull the patient's thenar area laterally, bringing the thumb into a retroposition with lateral rotation in order to lift the transverse carpal ligament up and off the nerve.[77] Dosage of application of this particular procedure is an issue. Because this is a direct procedure and when done properly can be forceful, extreme respect must be exercised for the level of tolerance of aged tissues. The principles of dosage, discussed earlier in this text, must be rigorously adhered to. (See further: 'Section 3: Treatment of the patient,' p. 77.) The precaution when employing direct procedures is to obtain the optimal therapeutic response without exceeding tolerance and injuring the patient. Caution coupled with intelligent palpation is the watchword.

Neural release can be applied to median nerve adhesions with its surrounding connective tissue to restore neural gliding.[78] Myofascial procedures should be applied to thenar muscles and flexor tendons, as well, because tension in these structures can contribute to the compression of the median nerve.

## Advice to the patient

First, explain to your patient the importance of rest for the affected hand and the need to avoid any activity that contributes to CTS. When using their hands, encourage them to take breaks and to avoid continuous repetitive activities.

Vitamin B-6 may be used as a conservative and adjunct therapy, at 200 mg daily, unless symptoms progress.[79] When employing one of the B complex vitamins therapeutically it is always a good idea to provide some supplementation of the entire vitamin complex as well. This will tend to reduce the possibility of producing a secondary deficiency of unsupplemented B vitamins due to renal clearance of the entire group of water soluble vitamins. The homeopathic remedy, arnica gel, may also be used to contribute to the relief of pain and inflammation. A balanced diet stressing unrefined foods is always recommended to improve the health of connective tissues.

Wrist splints may be employed at night. If tolerated without discomfort they can be useful to relieve nighttime symptoms of tingling and numbness.

Encourage your patient to stretch their myofascial structures, in particular neck, shoulders, arms, wrists, and fingers, without triggering any pain or symptoms of CTS. This can be done simply by sidebending the neck on one side, maintaining the position during three or four slow respirations, and repeating the same movement on the other side. This cycle should be repeated about five times at least three times a day. Encourage your patient also to gently rotate the wrists in both directions, and to stretch the palms and fingers. Yoga has shown to bring some improvement and can be recommended.[80] When employing any exercise it should be stressed that the patient should not experience pain while exercising. If pain occurs, the exercise should be stopped and alternative exercises considered. Post-exercise soreness of tolerable levels may be acceptable but this should not last more than 24 hours, or 48 hours in the very elderly. Prolonged post-exercise soreness indicates that, although the activity may be appropriate, the dosage of exercise is too great and should be reduced. As the patient progresses, increase of the exercise dosage may be cautiously attempted.

## Conclusion

The recognition of the contribution of somatic dysfunction to appendicular conditions of the elderly is of paramount value in the care of these individuals. Even though the impact of a lifetime of activity may have resulted in irreversible structural change with loss of function, somatic dysfunction

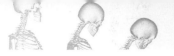

is reversible and its effective treatment will inevitably lead to functional gains that are not only physically beneficial but emotionally powerful.

The principles of treatment of the myriad of conditions that result in upper and lower extremity complaints in the context of osteopathic principles are strikingly similar and exemplified by the conditions discussed above. When treating these problems it is all too easy to become focused upon the site of the patient's complaint and lose the holistic perspective that is distinctly osteopathic. One should always remember W.F. Strachan's observation that "Diagnosis of any complaint in a peripheral part is not complete without analysis of the region of the spine segmentally related."[81] This should then be expanded to include the relationship of the complaint to the PRM.

# References

1. Badley EM, Tennant A. Changing profile of joint disorders with age: findings from a postal survey of the population of Calderdale, West Yorkshire, United Kingdom. Ann Rheum Dis. 1992 Mar;51(3):366-71.

2. Peat G, McCarney R, Croft P. Knee pain and osteoarthritis in older adults: a review of community burden and current use of primary health care. Ann Rheum Dis. 2001 Feb;60(2):91-7.

3. McAlindon TE, Snow S, Cooper C, Dieppe PA. Radiographic patterns of osteoarthritis of the knee joint in the community: the importance of the patellofemoral joint. Ann Rheum Dis. 1992 Jul;51(7):844-9.

4. Lequesne M. Coxarthrose et coxopathies de l'adulte. Diagnostic et traitement. Encycl Méd Chir (Elsevier, Paris): Appareil locomoteur, 14-308-A-10, 2009.

5. Hoaglund FT. Primary osteoarthritis of the hip: a genetic disease caused by European genetic variants. J Bone Joint Surg Am. 2013 Mar 6;95(5):463-8.

6. Goodman DA, Feighan JE, Smith AD, Latimer B, Buly RL, Cooperman DR. Subclinical slipped capital femoral epiphysis. Relationship to osteoarthrosis of the hip. J Bone Joint Surg Am. 1997 Oct;79(10):1489-97.

7. Radin EL. Osteoarthrosis--the orthopedic surgeon's perspective. Acta Orthop Scand Suppl. 1995 Oct;266:6-9.

8. Sellam J, Berenbaum F. Arthrose et obésité. Rev Prat. 2012 May;62(5):621-4.

9. Goekoop RJ, Kloppenburg M, Kroon HM, Dirkse LE, Huizinga TW, Westendorp RG, Gussekloo J. Determinants of absence of osteoarthritis in old age. Scand J Rheumatol. 2011 Jan;40(1):68-73.

10. Brandt KD, Dieppe P, Radin EL. Etiopathogenesis of osteoarthritis. Rheum Dis Clin North Am. 2008 Aug;34(3):531-59.

11. Bierma-Zeinstra SM, Koes BW. Risk factors and prognostic factors of hip and knee osteoarthritis. Nat Clin Pract Rheumatol. 2007 Feb;3(2):78-85.

12. Papavasiliou KA, Kenanidis EI, Potoupnis ME, Kapetanou A, Sayegh FE. Participation in athletic activities may be associated with later development of hip and knee osteoarthritis. Phys Sportsmed. 2011 Nov;39(4):51-9.

13. Kaila-Kangas L, Arokoski J, Impivaara O, Viikari-Juntura E, Leino-Arjas P, Luukkonen R, Heliövaara M. Associations of hip osteoarthritis with history of recurrent exposure to manual handling of loads over 20 kg and work participation: a population-based study of men and women. Occup Environ Med. 2011 Oct;68(10):734-8.

14. Andersen S, Thygesen LC, Davidsen M, Helweg-Larsen K. Cumulative years in occupation and the risk of hip or knee osteoarthritis in men and women: a register-based follow-up study. Occup Environ Med. 2012 May;69(5):325-30.

15. Jensen LK. Hip osteoarthritis: influence of work with heavy lifting, climbing stairs or ladders, or combining kneeling/squatting with heavy lifting. Occup Environ Med. 2008 Jan;65(1):6-19.

16. Lovejoy CO. The natural history of human gait and posture. Part 1. Spine and pelvis. Gait Posture. 2005 Jan;21(1):95-112.

17. Hogervorst T, Bouma HW, de Vos J. Evolution of the hip and pelvis. Acta Orthop Suppl. 2009 Aug;80(336):1-39.

18. Hogervorst T, Bouma HW, de Vos J. Evolution of the hip and pelvis. Acta Orthop Suppl. 2009 Aug;80(336):1-39.

19. Weiner LS, Kelley MA, Ulin RI, Wallach D. Development of the acetabulum and hip: computed tomography analysis of the axial plane. J Pediatr Orthop. 1993 Jul-Aug;13(4):421-5.

20. Hunter DJ, Wilson DR. Role of alignment and biomechanics in osteoarthritis and implications for imaging. Radiol Clin North Am. 2009 Jul;47(4):553-66.

21. Sergueef N. Cranial Osteopathy for Infants, Children and Adolescents. Churchill Livingstone Elsevier, Edinburg, UK: 2007.

22. Wynne-Davies R. Acetabular dysplasia and familial joint laxity: two etiological factors in congenital dislocation of the hip. A review of 589 patients and their families. J Bone Joint Surg 1970;52(4):704-16.

23. Murray RO. The aetiology of primary osteoarthritis of the hip. Br J Radiol. 1965 Nov;38(455):810-24.

24. Fujii M, Nakashima Y, Yamamoto T, Mawatari T, Motomura G, Matsushita A, et al. Acetabular retroversion in developmental dysplasia of the hip. J Bone Joint Surg Am. 2010 Apr;92(4):895-903.

25. Reynolds D, Lucas J, Klaue K. Retroversion of the acetabulum. A cause of hip pain. J Bone Joint Surg Br. 1999 Mar;81(2):281-8.

26. Giori NJ, Trousdale RT. Acetabular retroversion is associated with osteoarthritis of the hip. Clin Orthop Relat Res. 2003 Dec;(417):263-9.

27. Ezoe M, Naito M, Inoue T. The prevalence of acetabular retroversion among various disorders of the hip. J Bone Joint Surg Am. 2006 Feb;88(2):372-9.

28. Ganz R, Parvizi J, Beck M, Leunig M, Nötzli H, Siebenrock KA. Femoroacetabular impingement: a cause for osteoarthritis of the hip. Clin Orthop Relat Res. 2003 Dec;(417):112-20.

29. Klaue K, Durnin CW, Ganz R. The acetabular rim syndrome. A clinical presentation of dysplasia of the hip. J Bone Joint Surg Br. 1991 May;73(3):423-9.

30. Nelson KE, Schilling Mnabhi AK. The patient with back pain: Short leg syndrome and postural balance. Chapt. 26. In: Nelson, Glonek, eds. Somatic Dysfunction in Osteopathic Family Medicine. Lippincott, Williams & Wilkins, Baltimore, MD; 2007:408-33.

31. Sergueef N. L'odyssée de l'iliaque. Paris: Spek; 1985.

32. Gelb DE, Lenke LG, Bridwell KH, Blanke K, McEnery KW. An analysis of sagittal spinal alignment in 100 asymptomatic middle and older aged volunteers. Spine (Phila Pa 1976). 1995 Jun 15;20(12):1351-8.

33. Kerrigan DC, Lee LW, Collins JJ, Riley PO, Lipsitz LA. Reduced hip extension during walking: healthy elderly and fallers versus young adults. Arch Phys Med Rehabil. 2001 Jan;82(1):26-30.

34. Cumming RG, Klineberg RJ. Epidemiological study of the relation between arthritis of the hip and hip fractures. Ann Rheum Dis. 1993 Oct;52(10):707-10.

35. Bosomworth NJ. Exercise and knee osteoarthritis: benefit or hazard? Can Fam Physician. September 2009 55:871-878.

36. Urwin M, Symmons D, Allison T, Brammah T, Busby H, Roxby M, Simmons A, Williams G. Estimating the burden of musculoskeletal disorders in the community: the comparative prevalence of symptoms at different anatomical sites, and the relation to social deprivation. Ann Rheum Dis. 1998 Nov;57(11):649-55.

37. Chakravarty K, Webley M. Shoulder joint movement and its relationship to disability in the elderly. J Rheumatol. 1993 Aug;20(8):1359-61.

38. Sher JS, Uribe JW, Posada A, Murphy BJ, Zlatkin MB. Abnormal findings on magnetic

resonance images of asymptomatic shoulders. J Bone Joint Surg Am. 1995 Jan;77(1):10-5.

39. Clark JM, Harryman DT 2nd. Tendons, ligaments, and capsule of the rotator cuff. Gross and microscopic anatomy. J Bone Joint Surg Am. 1992 Jun;74(5):713-25.

40. Barr KP. Rotator cuff disease. Phys Med Rehabil Clin N Am. 2004 May;15(2):475-91.

41. Arai R, Mochizuki T, Yamaguchi K, Sugaya H, Kobayashi M, Nakamura T, Akita K. Functional anatomy of the superior glenohumeral and coracohumeral ligaments and the subscapularis tendon in view of stabilization of the long head of the biceps tendon. J Shoulder Elbow Surg. 2010 Jan;19(1):58-64.

42. Renoux S, Monet J, Pupin P, Collin M, Apoil A, Gasc JP, Jouffroy FK, Doursounian L. Preliminary note on biometric data relating to the human coraco-acromial arch. Surg Radiol Anat. 1986;8(3):189-95.

43. Ogawa K, Yoshida A, Inokuchi W, Naniwa T. Acromial spur: relationship to aging and morphologic changes in the rotator cuff. J Shoulder Elbow Surg. 2005 Nov-Dec;14(6):591-8.

44. Barr KP. Rotator cuff disease. Phys Med Rehabil Clin N Am. 2004 May;15(2):475-91.

45. Panni AS, Milano G, Lucania L, Fabbriciani C, Logroscino CA. Histological analysis of the coracoacromial arch: correlation between age-related changes and rotator cuff tears. Arthroscopy. 1996 Oct;12(5):531-40.

46. Yu TY, Tsai WC, Cheng JW, Yang YM, Liang FC, Chen CH. The effects of aging on quantitative sonographic features of rotator cuff tendons. J Clin Ultrasound. 2012 Oct;40(8):471-8.

47. Kumagai J, Sarkar K, Uhthoff HK. The collagen types in the attachment zone of rotator cuff tendons in the elderly: an immunohistochemical study. J Rheumatol. 1994 Nov;21(11):2096-100.

48. Longo UG, Berton A, Papapietro N, Maffulli N, Denaro V. Epidemiology, genetics and biological factors of rotator cuff tears. Med Sport Sci. 2012;57:1-9.

49. Brooks CH, Revell WJ, Heatley FW. A quantitative histological study of the vascularity of the rotator cuff tendon. J Bone Joint Surg Br. 1992 Jan;74(1):151-3.

50. Chansky HA, Iannotti JP. The vascularity of the rotator cuff. Clin Sports Med. 1991 Oct;10(4):807-22.

51. Ko JY, Wang FS. Rotator cuff lesions with shoulder stiffness: updated pathomechanisms and management. Chang Gung Med J. 2011 Jul-Aug;34(4):331-40.

52. Larson NJ. Functional vasomotor hemiparasthesia syndrome. Year Book of the Academy of Applied Osteopathy. American Academy of Osteopathy. Indianapolis, IN. 1970:39–44.

53. Larson NJ. Osteopathic manipulation for syndromes of the brachial plexus. J Am Osteopath Assoc. 1972 Dec;72(4):378-84.

54. Hegedus EJ, Goode A, Campbell S, Morin A, Tamaddoni M, Moorman CT 3rd, Cook C. Physical examination tests of the shoulder: a systematic review with meta-analysis of individual tests. Br J Sports Med. 2008 Feb;42(2):80-92; discussion 92.

55. Cadogan A, Laslett M, Hing W, McNair P, Williams M. Interexaminer reliability of orthopaedic special tests used in the assessment of shoulder pain. Man Ther. 2011 Apr;16(2):131-5.

56. Bang MD, Deyle GD. Comparison of supervised exercise with and without manual physical therapy for patients with shoulder impingement syndrome. J Orthop Sports Phys Ther. 2000 Mar;30(3):126-37.

57. Sergueef N. C0, C1, C2, Données physiologiques et normalisations. Paris: Spek; 1989.

58. Gerber C, Terrier F, Zehnder R, Ganz R. The subcoracoid space. An anatomic study. Clin Orthop Relat Res. 1987 Feb;(215):132-8.

59. Zenian J. Sleep position and shoulder pain. Med Hypotheses. 2010 Apr;74(4):639-43.

60. Aroori S, Spence RA. Carpal tunnel syndrome. Ulster Med J. 2008 Jan;77(1):6-17.

61. Atroshi I, Gummesson C, Johnsson R, Ornstein E, Ranstam J, Rosén I. Prevalence of carpal tunnel syndrome in a general population. JAMA. 1999 Jul 14;282(2):153-8.

62. Mondelli M, Giannini F, Giacchi M. Carpal tunnel syndrome incidence in a general population. Neurology. 2002 Jan 22;58(2):289-94.

63. Chiotis K, Dimisianos N, Rigopoulou A, Chrysanthopoulou A, Chroni E. Role of anthropometric characteristics in idiopathic carpal tunnel syndrome. Arch Phys Med Rehabil. 2013 Apr;94(4):737-44.

64. Becker J, Nora DB, Gomes I, Stringari FF, Seitensus R, Panosso JS, Ehlers JC. An evaluation of gender, obesity, age and diabetes mellitus as risk factors for carpal tunnel syndrome. Clin Neurophysiol. 2002 Sep;113(9):1429-34.

65. Nathan PA, Keniston RC, Lockwood RS, Meadows KD. Tobacco, caffeine, alcohol, and carpal tunnel syndrome in American industry. A cross-sectional study of 1464 workers. J Occup Environ Med. 1996 Mar;38(3):290-8.

66. Solomon DH, Katz JN, Bohn R, Mogun H, Avorn J. Nonoccupational risk factors for carpal tunnel syndrome. J Gen Intern Med. 1999 May;14(5):310-4.

67. Richman JA, Gelberman RH, Rydevik BL, Gylys-Morin VM, Hajek PC, Sartoris DJ. Carpal tunnel volume determination by magnetic resonance imaging three-dimensional reconstruction. J Hand Surg Am. 1987 Sep;12(5 Pt 1):712-7.

68. Mackinnon SE. Pathophysiology of nerve compression. Hand Clin. 2002 May;18(2):231-41.

69. Upton AR, McComas AJ. The double crush in nerve entrapment syndromes. Lancet. 1973 Aug 18;2(7825):359-62.

70. Larson NJ. Osteopathic manipulation for syndromes of the brachial plexus. J Am Osteopath Assoc. 1972 Dec;72(4):378-84.

71. Ott F, Mattiassich G, Kaulfersch C, Ortmaier R. Initially unrecognised lunate dislocation as a cause of carpal tunnel syndrome. BMJ Case Rep. 2013 Mar 18;2013. pii: bcr2013009062. doi: 10.1136/bcr-2013-009062.

72. Robbins H. Anatomical study of the median nerve in the carpal tunnel and etiologies of the carpal tunnel syndrome. J Bone Joint Surg Am. 1963 Jul;45:953-66.

73. Functional vasomotor hemiparasthesia syndrome. Year Book of the Academy of Applied Osteopathy. American Academy of Osteopathy. Indianapolis, IN. 1970:39–44.

74. Ramey KA. Carpal tunnel syndrome: more than just a problem at the wrist. AAO Journal. Fall 2000;10 (3):25-7.

75. Nelson KE. The primary respiratory mechanism. AAO Journal. Winter 2002;12(4):25-34.

76. American Academy of Orthopaedic Surgeons. Clinical practice guideline on the treatment of carpal tunnel syndrome. Available at http://www.aaos.org/research/guidelines/ctstreatmentguideline.pdf. Accessed May17, 2013.

77. Sucher BM. Palpatory diagnosis and manipulative management of carpal tunnel syndrome. J Am Osteopath Assoc. 1994 Aug;94(8):647-63.

78. Mackinnon SE. Pathophysiology of nerve compression. Hand Clin. 2002 May;18(2):231-41.

79. Holm G, Moody LE Carpal tunnel syndrome: current theory, treatment, and the use of B6. J Am Acad Nurse Pract. 2003 Jan;15(1):18-22.

80. O'Connor D, Marshall S, Massy-Westropp N. Non-surgical treatment (other than steroid injection) for carpal tunnel syndrome. Cochrane Database Syst Rev. 2003;(1):CD003219.

81. Strachan W.F. J Am Osteopath Assoc. October 1940; 2(2):59-60.

# Chapter 2
# Postural imbalance

Posture may be defined as the spatial relationship between the different parts of the body in order to maintain a stable position. Although several postures may be described, most of the time the term posture refers to the body in a standing position. As a state of balance, posture may, at first, seem to be a static positional interrelationship between the different body areas. But particularly from the osteopathic perspective, it is actually dynamic, requiring continuous accommodation to gravitational influences as the individual moves through their activities of daily living. As such, posture is a constantly changing functional—and consequently potentially dysfunctional—state of the body. Many factors influence the postural aspect of the individual, and they reflect their psychology as well as their motor skills. The observation of an individual's static posture in different positions provides the examiner with insight into the etiology of many dysfunctional conditions.

As a rule, an individual demonstrates a good posture when their body is erect, chin in, shoulders straight with a full chest, a flat abdomen and the weight of the body equally balanced on the heads of the femora. Observed in the sagittal plane the cervical, thoracic, and lumbar curves are not exaggerated and a vertical line dropped from the level of the external auditory meatus falls through the humeral head, femoral head, mid-knee, and lateral malleolus. The line of gravity extends from the external auditory meatus, through the dens of the axis just anterior to the body of the second thoracic vertebra, through the centre of the body of the twelfth thoracic vertebra, and through the rear of the body of the fifth lumbar vertebra to lie anterior to the sacrum.[1]

In a well-adjusted posture, in the coronal plane, the gravity line divides the body into two parts; it passes through the glabella, the middle of the suprasternal notch, the pubic symphysis, and on the ground is equidistant between both feet.

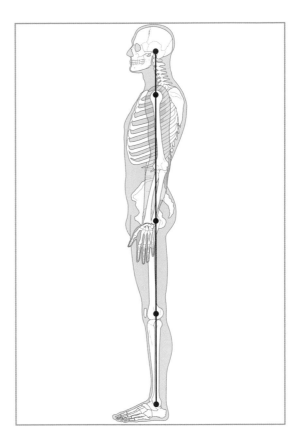

Figure 4.2.1: Sagittal postural balance

A balanced posture is a requisite to be able to stand, to walk, and to perform daily activities in a safe manner. With aging, the individual's posture quite often declines. In fact an estimation of the age of the individual can be made through their posture. Bad posture can make the person look older while good posture makes them look younger. An imbalanced posture is a potentially severe functional compromise, with the resultant incapacity to walk safely, to climb stairs, or to dress autonomously. The risk of falls with the possibility of injuries is increased.

Maintenance of the posture is a non-volitional activity and depends on a complex interaction of physiological mechanisms. On the basis of selective and fast integration of sensory information from multiple sources, the central nervous system (CNS) produces appropriate and complex motor responses. Because of the age-related decline of the musculoskeletal and sensory systems, neural processing, and conduction of information, good posture becomes more difficult to maintain as the individual gets older. Conversely, reduction of dysfunction of the musculoskeletal and sensory systems can enhance posture allowing greater stability of the body's mass against gravity.

The CNS controls and coordinates posture and balance with several processes that produce reactive musculoskeletal changes in response to variations in the external environment. Three sensory systems—vestibular, visual, and somatosensory/proprioceptive—provide indispensable information for the regulation of an individual's postural balance. The vestibular apparatus provides information about gravitational, linear, and angular accelerations of the head. Visual information establishes the orientation of the eyes and head in relation to the surrounding elements. Somatosensory/proprioceptive input supplies information about the position of the body in relation to external surfaces of contact and the orientation of the different parts of the body in relation to one another.

Understanding the anatomy and physiology of the vestibular, visual, and somatosensory/proprioceptive sensory systems, helps the practitioner to better understand the posture- and balance-impaired patient and how therapeutic procedures may address their dysfunctions.

# The vestibular sensory system

The vestibular apparatus is the sensory organ that perceives sensations of equilibrium. On each side of the skull, it is located within the petrous portion of the temporal bone, enclosed in bony cavities named the bony labyrinth. Within these cavities, membranous ducts and sacs form the *membranous labyrinth*—the functional part of the vestibular apparatus. The membranous labyrinth is filled with endolymph and is separated from the periosteum that covers the walls of the bony labyrinth by perilymph.

The membranous labyrinth consists of three semicircular ducts and two large sacs—the *utricle* and *saccule*—all components of the equilibrium system. It consists also of the *cochlear duct*, the sensory organ of hearing. Anteriorly, is the cochlear duct within the cochlea of the bony labyrinth; posteriorly are the three semicircular ducts within the three semicircular canals of the bony labyrinth; and in between are the saccule and utricle within the vestibule of the bony labyrinth.

The three semicircular ducts empty into the utricle. The *utriculosaccular duct* unites the utricle and saccule and creates a link between all the parts of the membranous labyrinth. The *endolymphatic* duct comes out of the utriculosaccular duct and passes into the *vestibular aqueduct* through the temporal bone to appear on the posterior surface of the petrous part of the temporal bone in the posterior cranial fossa. At this point, the endolymphatic duct enlarges to form the endolymphatic sac, an extradural pouch that is an intracranial expansion

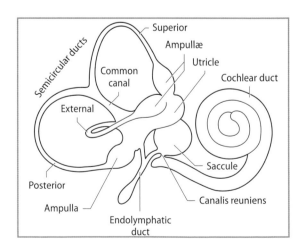

Figure 4.2.2: The membranous labyrinth

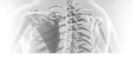
of the membranous labyrinth. It helps to maintain the constant volume and steady electrochemical composition of the endolymph, indispensable phenomena for hearing and vestibular function.[2]

## Sensory receptors for equilibrium

Sensory receptors for equilibrium are found in each of the components of the vestibular apparatus i.e., in the utricle and saccule and in the three semicircular ducts. Each of the components of the equilibrium system is intended to detect specific types of motion. The utricle and saccule detect gravitational forces and linear accelerations of the head in space, while the semicircular canals transmit afferent input about angular acceleration, such as head rotation.

### Utricle and saccule

On the inner surface of the utricle and saccule are the *macula of utricle* and *macula of saccule*, respectively. These are tiny sensory areas, about 2 mm in diameter. Each has a different orientation and therefore a different function. The macula of

the utricle is positioned mostly in the transverse plane on the inferior surface of the utricle, and as a result contributes in detecting orientation of the head when the head is upright. The macula of the saccule is situated mostly in the vertical plane and detects head orientation when the person is lying down.

Each macula is covered with a neurosensory epithelium consisting of thousands of hair cells that synapse with sensory endings of the vestibular nerve. Covering this epithelial surface, a gelatinous layer forms the *otolithic membrane* in which many small calcium carbonate crystals—the *statoconia*—are embedded. Because of their weight, the statoconia bend the cilia—the projections of the hair cells up into the gelatinous layer—in the direction of gravitational pull (Fig. 4.2.4).

Each hair cell has multiple rows of small cilia called *stereocilia* and one large cilium, the *kinocilium*. The kinocilium is constantly positioned on one side of the hair cell, and the stereocilia are gradually shorter in the direction of the opposite side. Each stereocilium's tip is connected to the next longer stereocilium and, ultimately, to the

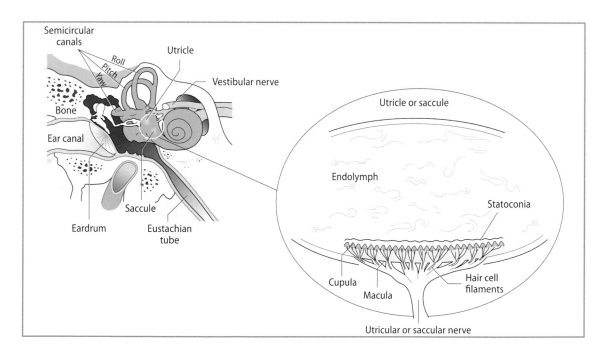

Figure 4.2.3: The inner surface of the utricle and saccule

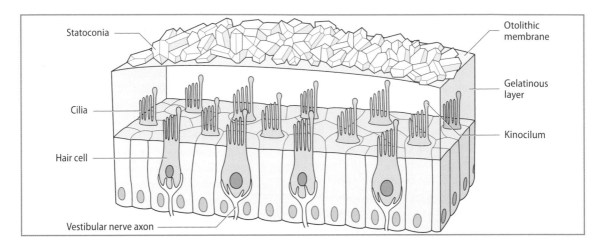

Figure 4.2.4: The epithelium of the macula

kinocilium, with tiny filamentous attachments. Therefore, movement or shearing of the stereociliary bundle in the direction of the kinocilium drags the stereocilia away from the cell body. As a result, several hundred fluid channels in the neuronal cell membrane around the bases of the stereocilia are opened, producing a depolarization of the hair cells, the release of neurotransmitters from the base of the hair cell, and an increased neural discharge in the primary afferent neurons. With the contrary movement of the stereociliary bundle away from the kinocilium, a hyperpolarization of hair cells, reduced neurotransmitter release, and decreased neural firing results.

Movement of the stereociliary bundle is critical for sensory transduction, and the orientation of the head in space determines the signals conveyed to the brain to regulate equilibrium. Additionally, because hair cells have different orientations, a number of them are stimulated with the bending of the head forward, while others are stimulated with bending backward or laterally.

### Semicircular ducts

In each temporal bone, the three semicircular ducts are located within the three semicircular canals of the bony labyrinth to which they are, to a large extent, firmly attached. They are named the anterior, posterior, and lateral (horizontal) semicircular ducts, and are organized at right angles to one another so that they represent all three planes in space. When forward bending the head approximately 30°, the lateral semicircular ducts are almost horizontal; the anterior ducts are in the vertical plane directed forward and 45° outward; and the posterior ducts are in the vertical plane directed backward and 45° outward.

Before entering the utricle, the medial ends of the superior and posterior ducts combine to form a common canal—the *crus commune*. Each semicircular duct is dilated at one of its ends to form the *ampulla*. Both the ducts and ampulla are filled with endolymph.

The membranous wall of each ampulla displays a transverse septum with a sensory area—the *ampullary crest* in the middle. A loose gelatinous tissue collection, the *cupula*, is attached along the free edge of the crest. Because it projects far into the ampulla, flow of endolymph within the duct promptly bends the cupula and the stereocilia of the sensory cells inserted into its base. Rotation of the head in one direction deflects the cupula to one side while rotation of the head in the opposite direction provokes bending of the cupula to the opposite side. Hair cells located on the ampullary crest project into the cupula. When bending of the cupula occurs in the direction of the kinocilia of these hair cells, it causes their depolarization;

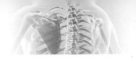

conversely, bending it in the reverse direction produces hyperpolarization of the cells. Therefore, the three semicircular canals sense angular accelerations during tilting or turning movements of the head that may occur in any direction. From these hair cells signals are sent by way of the vestibular nerve to the CNS.

It should be emphasized that both ears function in a complementary fashion. The semicircular canals work as pairs: the two horizontal canals are positioned in the same plane, while the anterior canal on one side is coupled in the same plane as the posterior canal on the contralateral side. There is also a coupled relationship between the utricles and saccules. This mode of action is of paramount importance for oculomotor control and overall muscular and somatosensory/proprioceptive postural control. In cases of dysfunction of one of the components of the vestibular system, inappropriate or inaccurate signals are sent out to the brain that contribute to balance disorders. Dysfunction of the temporal bones with asymmetry of the two petrous portions and their contents may produce ambiguous signals. For this reason procedures to address somatic dysfunctions of the temporal bones are recommended in the treatment of balance disorders. According to Magoun: "Lesions may interfere with free fluctuation, or they may disturb the parallelism of the semicircular canals and so the equilibrium."[3]

## Vestibular nerve

Most of the *vestibular nerve* (CN VIII) fibers enter the brainstem at the junction of the medulla and the pons, where they synapse in the vestibular nuclear complex of the brainstem. The vestibular primary afferent neurons synapse in the vestibular nuclei with second-order neurons that convey fibers into the cerebellum, the vestibulospinal tracts, the medial longitudinal fasciculus, and other areas of the brain stem, especially the reticular nuclei. Other vestibular nerve fibers have collaterals that synapse directly in the cerebellum. Signals to the spinal cord from the cerebellum control the relationship between facilitation and inhibition of the

multiple antigravity muscles, consequently automatically monitoring equilibrium.

The *vestibular nuclear complex* (VNC) consists of the *vestibular nuclei* and nearby neuronal groups. It is a location for neural integration of information from multiple sensory, motor, and higher level cognitive systems.[4] From the VNC information is sent for control of eye, head, and body movements. In addition, there is a vestibular influence on oculomotor and motor coordination abilities engaged in daily cognitive tasks that demonstrates cognitive-vestibular interactions.[5] There is also evidence that the vestibular system influences the development of spatial memory through areas of the brain like the hippocampus,[6] and that vestibular-autonomic responses regulate blood pressure and respiratory function during movement and postural variations. This regulation of blood pressure in response to postural change has been shown to be impaired in patients at the outset of vestibular dysfunction.[7] This latter observation is of particular interest to the osteopathic practitioner in that the cranial rhythmic impulse (CRI), the palpable component of the primary respiratory mechanism (PRM), has been demonstrated to be associated with baroreflex physiology.[8] Further, cranial manipulation affects low frequency oscillations in blood flow velocity that are manifestations of baroreflex physiology.[9 10]

Vestibular mechanisms for stabilizing the eyes, to preserve a constant image on the retinas, are necessary when the head is moved rapidly or bent forward, backward, or laterally. Reflexes are transmitted through the vestibular nuclei and the medial longitudinal fasciculus to the oculomotor nuclei. Thus, when the head is rapidly rotated, signals from the semicircular ducts produce an equivalent motion of the eyes in the direction opposite to the rotation of the head so that the eyes stay fixed on a particular visual object. (See below for further discussion of the vestibulo-ocular reflex – VOR.) Ascendant signals to the cerebral cortex that terminate in a primary cortical center for equilibrium situated in the parietal lobe deep in the Sylvian fissure, also contribute to consciousness of the equilibrium status of the body.

# The visual sensory system

Vision is a critical source of information on spatial orientation that maintains posture and balance. Subjects who have had destruction of the vestibular apparatus or lost much of their proprioceptive awareness can still retain equilibrium through the visual mechanisms.

## Sensory receptors

The sense of vision is extremely complex, allowing us to perceive the world around us. Several processes occur concurrently. Light and images of external objects pass through various refracting media in the eye, the aqueous humor, the lens, and the vitreous body before reaching the retina. They are received upon the retinal receptors, stimulating a chemical reaction and action potentials transmitted through the *optic nerve* (CN II) to the visual cortex within the occipital lobe where information can be processed. On each side of the skull, CN II passes through the optic canal where the two roots of the lesser wing of the sphenoid join the sphenoidal body. Both optic nerves unite to form the *optic chiasma*. Typically, the optic chiasma is situated directly above the sella turcica of the sphenoid bone, anterior to the pituitary stalk, and inferior to the hypothalamus and third ventricle. Within the chiasma, the optic nerve fibers from the nasal halves of the retinas cross to the opposite side, where they join the fibers from the contralateral temporal retinas to form the optic tracts. Therefore, posterior to the chiasma, each optic tract contains fibers originating in the ipsilateral temporal retina and contralateral nasal retina. Next, fibers of each of the optic tracts synapse in the dorsal lateral *geniculate nuclei* of the thalamus. Finally, the *geniculocalcarine* fibers follow the optic radiation to the primary *visual cortex* in the calcarine fissure area of the medial side of the occipital lobe.

The chemical reactions and resultant action potentials generated in the different photoreceptors by light passing through the eye construct a two-dimensional representation of a visualized object that is transmitted to the brain. Subsequently, the brain restructures a three-dimensional representation with information from both eyes. As a result of the activity of the visual system, we experience sensations that represent the object and its surroundings.

## Extraocular muscle proprioceptors

Because the eyes and the visual world move, extraretinal information is involved to establish gaze direction. It seems this information is necessary in monitoring eye movements and to allow the brain to define the direction of gaze and the relationship of the organism to its environment.[11] Evidence of a non-visual afferent feedback signal appears to come from proprioceptors within the *extraocular muscles* (EOM).[12] This works in such a manner that both eyes are directed to the same point.

Muscular control of eye movements is under the influence of three pairs of muscles: the *medial* and *lateral recti*, the *superior and inferior recti*, and the *superior and inferior obliques*. These muscles interact with one another, and do not function as isolated units. Each of the three arrangements of muscles for both eyes is reciprocally innervated in order that one muscle of the pair relaxes while the other contracts. The superior and inferior recti adduct the eyeball, in association with elevation and medial rotation (intorsion) from the superior rectus, whereas the inferior rectus depresses and laterally rotates (extorsion) the eyeball. The medial rectus adducts the eyeball while abduction is the result of contraction of the lateral rectus. Both the superior and inferior oblique muscles abduct the eye, with a component of depression from the superior oblique and elevation from the inferior oblique.[13]

With ageing, the horizontal rectus muscles are displaced inferiorly, with a larger displacement for the medial rectus than the lateral rectus, while the superior rectus and inferior rectus do not change their position. This may be the consequence of an inferior location of the corresponding muscle pulleys and may contribute to the impaired ability to elevate the eyes frequently observed in older

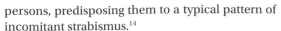

persons, predisposing them to a typical pattern of incomitant strabismus.[14]

Innervation of the EOM comes from the *oculomotor* nerve (CN III), the *trochlear nerve* (CN IV), and the *abducens nerve* (CN VI). Cranial nerve III supplies the superior, medial, and inferior rectus muscles, while CN IV carries somatic efferent fibers to the superior oblique muscle and CN VI to the lateral rectus muscle. These nerves all traverse the lateral sellar compartment and pass through the superior orbital fissure, between the greater and lesser wings of the sphenoid bone. Thus, osseous dysfunction of the sphenoid and membranous dysfunctions affecting the components of the lateral sellar compartment can functionally compromise these nerves.[15]

## Vestibulo-ocular reflex

The role of the VOR, also called the *oculovestibular reflex*, is to stabilize images on the retina during head movement by producing an eye movement in the direction opposite to head movement. Thus, when the head turns to the right, the eyes move to the left and vice versa.

Eye movement is under the control of the EOM. In the transverse plane, the lateral rectus moves the eye laterally, and the medial rectus moves the eye medially. Normally, they work in pairs to move the eyes in the same direction. For instance, in order to move the eyes horizontally together to the right, the lateral rectus muscle of the right eye and the medial rectus of the left eye both contract to pull both eyes to the right.

Head displacement triggers signals from the vestibular apparatus in the inner ear that produce the VOR. Head rotation is perceived by the semicircular canals, while head translation is perceived by the utricle and saccule. During head rotation to the right, the ampullary crest of the lateral (horizontal) semicircular duct is excited on the right side, while the ampullary crest on the left is inhibited. Impulses are sent from the right side via CN VIII to the vestibular nuclei in the brainstem where the right vestibular nuclear complex collects increased peripheral input as compared to the left. Second order neurons are, consequently, activated

on the right. They stimulate CN III neurons at the oculomotor nuclei on the right side, and crossing the midline, CN VI neurons are stimulated at the left abducens nucleus. In the left vestibular nuclear complex the opposite actions occur.

Therefore, during head rotation to the right, motor neurons from the right oculomotor nuclei produce a contraction of the medial rectus muscle on the right side of the head that moves the right eye to the left. At the same time, motor neurons from the left abducens nucleus stimulate the lateral rectus muscle on the left side of the head, resulting in a movement of the left eye to the left. Conversely, the medial rectus of the left eye and the lateral rectus of the right eye rest because of decreased stimulatory input.

## Vision and balance

Multiple studies demonstrate the influence of vision on posture and balance. Decreased visual acuity, restrictions of the visual field, increased susceptibility to glare, and poorer depth perception cause an increased postural instability.[16] [17] Aging is frequently associated with visual impairments such as different vision in the two eyes, which decreases stereo acuity and consequently depth perception. Commonly, aging individuals develop cataracts with resultant decreased visual acuity and contrast sensitivity.[18] Age-related macular degeneration is quite frequent as well, with changes in central vision and visual acuity.[19] Retinopathy, sometimes associated with diabetes, diminishes central vision and glaucoma impairs field vision.

Typically, after the age of 50 years, in the absence of ocular pathology, visual acuity and dark adaptation worsen. Transparency of the lens decreases and the nucleus becomes stiffer, diminishing its ability to change shape, which is necessary for accommodation. As a result, there is an inability to focus at near distances. This condition is known as presbyopia, a prevalent form of visual impairment in people over 40.[20] Presbyopia can be corrected by either separate single lens glasses for distant and near vision or, for convenience, a single pair of multifocal glasses that can be, most commonly, bifocal, trifocal, or progressive lenses. Nevertheless, with multifocal glasses, distant objects in the lower visual field are indistinctly perceived, a factor particularly important for older people. In fact, studies show that multifocal glasses reduce depth perception and edge-contrast sensitivity at critical distances for detecting obstacles in the environment.[21] Walking up or down stairs becomes more challenging, increasing the risk of falls, in particular when the person is aging.[22] Therefore, older people may benefit from wearing non-multifocal glasses when walking up or down stairs or when in unfamiliar settings outside the home as an effective fall prevention strategy.[23][24] If possible, improvement of depth perception and distant edge-contrast sensitivity should be considered as significant factors necessary to preserve balance and stay away from surrounding hazards.[25]

In any case, vision impairment affects postural control, particularly if acquired and not congenital.[26] Healthy individuals are able to adjust the sway of their center of mass in response to external forces applied to their body, floor surface circumstances, and modifications in the surrounding environment. On the other hand, diminished visual acuity affects the magnitude of anteroposterior (AP) sway and the sway spectrum.[27]

Because poor visual acuity roughly doubles the risk of falls,[28] visual influence on balance should be considered and improved as much as possible.[29] Compensatory mechanisms exist through the vestibular and somatosensory systems. They participate in the maintenance of balance and compensate for frail or absent visual input. However, when standing on a compliant surface, in the presence of inadequate visual acuity and contrast sensitivity that are associated with inadequate proprioceptive information, postural sway intensifies, therefore increasing the risk of falls.[30] Programs designed to improve postural deficit should include visual improvement as much as vestibular and somatosensory rehabilitation, in order to gain a better posture and balance and reduce the risk of falls, which in the end can increase morbidity.[31]

## The somatosensory/proprioceptive sensory system

Somatic sensations may be classified according to their territory as exteroceptive sensations, proprioceptive sensations, and interoceptive sensations. *Exteroceptive sensations* are related to the surface of the body. *Proprioceptive sensations* are connected with position sensations and tendon and muscle sensations. *Interoceptive sensations* or visceral sensations originate from the viscera of the body. Somatic sensations may also be classified according to the characteristics of the stimulus such as thermal, mechanical, or chemical. Somatic sensations may also be categorized according to the nature of their perception, such as pain, temperature, or deep sensations consisting, for instance, of pressure or vibration from deep tissues including fascia, muscle, and bone.

Postural control corresponds to a continuous interaction between the sensory and motor systems. Subjects must sense environmental stimuli, adjust to variations in the body's orientation, and maintain the body's center of gravity within its base of support.

Somatosensory/proprioceptive input provides information about orientation of the different parts of the body in relation to one another and about the status of the body within the environment. Peripheral afferent mechanisms related to postural control come primarily from exteroceptive and proprioceptive input. These two systems allow the individual to preserve normal unperturbed stance and to safely achieve most daily activities. When postural stability is challenged, multiple sensory systems such as the visual and vestibular systems are also involved.

The exteroceptive sensations of touch, pressure, vibration, and tickle are detected through the cutaneous mechanoreceptors of the somatosensory system. These senses are usually classified as *tactile senses*. The proprioceptive senses, or the *senses of position*, include senses that perceive static position and movement rates of the different parts of the body. Input comes from receptors, in large quantities, located in joint, muscle, connective, and ligamentous tissue, usually referred to as proprioceptors.

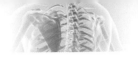

## Tactile sense

Cutaneous mechanoreceptors contribute to tactile sense and are found in the skin. They consist of fast adapting Meissner's corpuscles, rapidly adapting Pacinian corpuscles, slow adapting Merkel's discs, and the slowly adapting Ruffini endings. Also, in areas of hairy skin, there are hair end-organs, while glabrous or hairless skin contains free nerve endings.

*Hair end-organs* perceive either the movement of objects on the surface of the body or any first contact with the body. *Free nerve endings* are located everywhere in the skin as well as other tissues; they perceive touch, pressure, and pain. *Meissner's corpuscles* adapt in a fraction of a second following stimulation. Thus, they are especially sensitive to objects moving over the surface of the skin and to low frequency vibration. *Pacinian corpuscles* are located directly beneath the skin and in the depth of fascial tissues. They react in a few hundredths of a second to brisk local compression of the tissues. Their role is predominantly to perceive tissue vibration or any fast changes in the tissues. *Merkel's discs*, found under the epithelium of the skin participate in locating tactile sensations, in particular surface areas of the body, and in identifying the consistency of what is felt. *Ruffini endings* adapt very slowly. They are found in the subcutaneous tissues and indicate conditions where tissues are under constant deformation. They are also located in joint capsules.

Studies demonstrate that cutaneous mechanoreceptors present in the feet might play a significant role in the control of upright stance.[32] [33] During static stance, awareness of the footpads' receptors indicates the distribution of the body weight between the two feet, as well as its distribution between the anterior and posterior parts of the foot. Furthermore, stimulation of foot cutaneous mechanoreceptors prompts extensive reflex actions on multiple muscles through the lower extremities, mainly the ipsilateral limb, with some modulation dependent on the task that the subject is assuming. Thus, plasticity in the expression of cutaneous reflex activity is present.[34]

## Sense of position

Senses of position are frequently named proprioceptive senses. Proprioception includes two categories: the sense of static position and the sense of the rate of movement also named *kinaesthesia* or *dynamic proprioception*. The sense of static position represents the conscious perception of the orientation of the different parts of the body in relation to one another. 'Kinaesthesia,' a term coined by Henry C. Bastian in 1888, represents the aptitude to sense the position and movement of our limbs and trunk.[35]

Different types of receptors are involved in the awareness of position of the different parts of the body, either from a static or a dynamic perspective. They include mostly the participation of the *muscle spindles*, but also participation of the *Golgi tendon organs*, *skin tactile receptors*, and *deep receptors* near the joints.

### Muscle spindles

Muscle spindles are part of complex functional systems.[36] As stretch-sensitive mechanoreceptors, they supply information to the CNS regarding a muscle's length and velocity of contraction. Therefore, they contribute to the unconscious, automatic reflex regulation of posture as well as to the sense of kinaesthesia. However, debates exist about the complete function of muscle spindles as position sensors because they produce impulses in response to muscle length variations and also from fusimotor activity during muscle contraction. Therefore, the CNS has to differentiate both activities.[37] [38]

Muscle spindles are embedded in parallel within the contractile muscular elements. They measure 3–10 mm in length and are enclosed in a capsule of connective tissue consisting of two sheaths. Each spindle consists of particular primary and secondary afferent nerve endings surrounding 3–12 very small intrafusal muscle fibers. The muscle spindle intrafusal fibers are organized into two types to form either the *nuclear bag* or the *nuclear chain* fibers. They convey afferent information on dynamic and static muscular conditions to the CNS. *Intrafusal fibers* are side by side and parallel to the large *extrafusal fibers*, or regular skeletal muscle, to which they are attached.

Muscle spindles are distinctive organs, having both afferent and efferent innervation. The sensory innervation is of two types, primary and secondary, and consists of the unmyelinated terminations of large myelinated axons. The primary sensory afferent innervation consists of the endings of large sensory fibers, the group Ia afferents. Also named annulospiral endings, they are located on the equator of the muscle spindles, organized in spirals around the nucleated parts of intrafusal fibers. The secondary sensory afferent neurons are the endings of thinner myelinated afferents, the group II afferents. Spray-shaped as flower spray or annular, they are mainly limited to nuclear chain fibers. While the primary endings respond rapidly, the secondary endings adapt more slowly to static stretch.

The motor innervation of muscle spindles is of three types. Two come from gamma myelinated fusimotor efferent neurons, and the third comes from beta myelinated efferent neurons. When the gamma and beta efferent neurons are stimulated, they produce a contraction of the intrafusal fibers and excitation of their sensory endings.

Because the central region of the intrafusal muscle fibers has little or no actin and myosin filaments, the muscle spindles are only contractile on the end and non-contractile centrally. Small gamma efferent fibers originate from small type A gamma motor neurons in the anterior horns of the spinal cord. In contrast, large alpha efferent fibers innervate the extrafusal skeletal muscle. Gamma efferent motor neurons synapse on the contractile region of the intrafusal fibers. Any muscular contraction pulls on the central regions of the intrafusal fibers. Thus, when the muscle is actively shortened, the gamma efferent motor neurons adjust the sensitivity of the muscle spindles by controlling the level of contraction in the intrafusal fibers.

Non-contractile, the central region functions as the sensory organ of the apparatus. Stretching of the central region portion as a result of lengthening of the whole muscle excites the sensory fibers. Furthermore, even if the length of the whole muscle does not change, contraction of the end portions of the spindle's intrafusal fibers stretches the mid-portion of the spindle. This allows an adjustment of the muscle spindles' sensitivity by controlling the level of contraction in the intrafusal fibers,

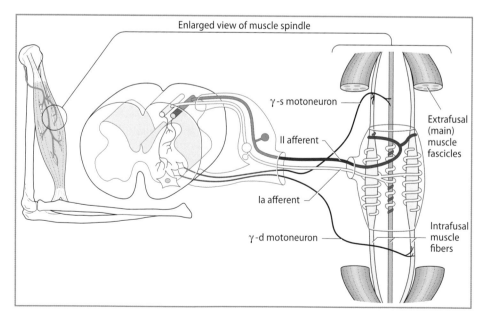

Enlarged view of muscle spindle

γ-s motoneuron

II afferent

Ia afferent

γ-d motoneuron

Extrafusal (main) muscle fascicles

Intrafusal muscle fibers

Figure 4.2.5: The muscle spindle

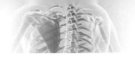

thus increasing their sensitivity to variations in muscle length.

When gamma neuron stimulation is associated with alpha motor neuron activation by the CNS, the process is called 'alpha-gamma coactivation.' Additionally, alpha and gamma motor neurons get information from articular and cutaneous receptors, spinal interneurons (the site of segmental facilitation associated with spinal somatic dysfunction)[39][40], and higher centers. This provides an accurate feedback about the muscle length and velocity of contraction.

Stabilization of body position is one of the significant functions of the muscle spindle. It is the result of excitatory signals from the bulboreticular facilitatory area located in the pons, and associated segments of the brainstem sent out through the gamma nerve fibers to the intrafusal muscle fibers of the muscle spindles. As a consequence, the ends of the spindles are shortened and the central region is stretched, exciting its sensory fibers and intensifying their signal output. When spindles on both sides of a joint are activated simultaneously, muscles on both sides are stimulated becoming taut and tense. Thus, the position of the joint becomes effectively stabilized.

## Golgi tendon organs

Constant feedback of sensory information to the spinal cord reveals each muscle's functional status, i.e., the muscular length or the muscular state of tension. Besides the muscle spindles, another particular type of sensory receptor, the Golgi tendon organ, provides this information. These are located in the muscle tendons and relay afferent information about tendon tension or rate of change of tension.

The Golgi tendon organ is an encapsulated sensory receptor located at the muscle-tendon interface. Every Golgi tendon organ is typically associated with 10–15 muscle fibers. Golgi tendon organs are sensitive to very small changes. Thus, they are responsive to every muscular contraction or stretch, sending to the nervous system immediate information about the amount of tension present in the muscle. Where the muscle spindle senses muscle length and modifications in muscle length, the Golgi tendon organ identifies muscle tension as indicated by the tension in the Golgi tendon organ itself. It provides a dynamic intensive response when the muscular tension abruptly increases, and a static response within a fraction of a second, reaching a lower level of steady-state firing, when the muscular tension decreases.

Activation of the Golgi tendon organ results in activation of large, rapidly conducting type Ib afferent neurons. This afferent information synapses in the dorsal horn of the spinal cord. The local cord signal excites a single inhibitory interneuron that inhibits the alpha motor neuron of the associated muscle. As a result, tension decreases within the particular muscle and tendon without affecting adjacent muscles. This inhibitory reflex establishes a negative feedback system, inducing relaxation in a muscle that is being overstretched. This prevents the development of too much tension with resultant tearing of muscular or tendinous fibers or avulsion of the tendon.

## Joint proprioceptors

Located in the joint capsule and ligaments the joint proprioceptors sense mechanical deformation.[41] They consist of the rapidly adapting Pacin-

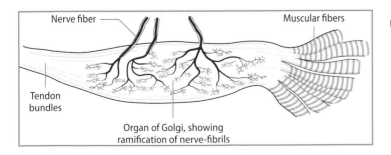

Nerve fiber — Muscular fibers

Tendon bundles

Organ of Golgi, showing ramification of nerve-fibrils

Figure 4.2.6: The Golgi tendon organ

ian corpuscles, slower-adapting Ruffini endings, ligament receptors, and free nerve endings. *Pacinian corpuscles* react to mechanical stimulation during movement; they do not react when the joint is maintained in a constant position. Conversely, Ruffini endings respond at the extremes of joint movement and even more to passive motion. Comparable to the Golgi tendon organs the Ruffini endings react to ligamentous tension. Free nerve endings respond to great mechanical deformation and inflammation.

The mechanoreceptors present in and around the joints are in charge of preserving postural control and joint position sense. Associated with visual and auditory input, which expand our spatial perception even further, the mechanoreceptors contribute to the maintenance of postural stability. Foot, knee, and neck proprioceptors are of particular importance. Foot proprioceptors contribute to information about the distribution of weight between the two feet, and pressure between the feet and the ground. However, every part of the body provides proprioceptive information for the maintenance of equilibrium. For instance, a person who is running is aware of the air pressure against the front of the body that indicates a force being applied to the body. As a result the person may bend forward to resist.

One of the most important sources of proprioceptive information, essential to the preservation of equilibrium, is the signals sent out from the *neck proprioceptors*. While the vestibular apparatus detects orientation and movement of the head, neck proprioceptors inform the CNS about the position of the head compared to the position of the body. Information is conveyed directly to the vestibular and reticular nuclei in the brainstem and indirectly by way of the cerebellum. Every time a subject bends their head signals from the neck proprioceptors counterbalance the signals from the vestibular apparatus, diffusing signals accurately contrary to the signals from the vestibular apparatus. This avoids perception of disequilibrium. Osteopathic procedures that balance the joints and associated tissues contribute to more accurate proprioceptive information and tuning of sensorimotor control.

# Central integration

Human balance and posture relies on a synchronized integration of sensory input from the vestibular and visual systems, and the somatosensory/proprioceptive sensory system, which provide information as to the position and movement of specific joints and the body as a whole. Information about muscle contraction and other sensory information from the peripheral portions of the body is constantly sent to the cerebellum from other brain motor control areas. In this manner, variations in position, rate of movement, or stressful conditions involving any part of the musculoskeletal system are identified and sent to the cerebellum. Subsequently, the cerebellum compares movement sensed from peripheral sensory feedback information with the movements expected by the motor system. When they do not match, corrective signals are sent back into the motor system resulting in the activation of appropriate muscles.

Three levels of the cerebellum are in charge of these synchronized motor control functions. These are the vestibulocerebellum, the spinocerebellum, and the cerebrocerebellum. The *vestibulocerebellum* consists principally of small flocculonodular cerebellar lobes located under the posterior cerebellum and contiguous portions of the vermis. Neural paths for most of the body's equilibrium movement are found there, and failure of the vestibulocerebellum triggers severe equilibrium and postural problems. The vestibulocerebellum, in particular, plays a significant role in the management of balance between agonist and antagonist muscular contractions involving the spine, hips, and shoulders. This allows for rapid accommodation for fast variations in body position as mediated by the vestibular apparatus.

The *spinocerebellum* consists of most of the vermis, of the posterior and anterior cerebellum, and the contiguous transitional zones on each side of the vermis. The coordination of the distal portions of the limbs comes from the spinocerebellum.

The *cerebrocerebellum* consists of the bulky lateral regions of the cerebellar hemispheres, lateral to the transitional zones. Nearly all of its input comes from the cerebral motor cortex and

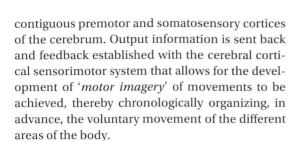

contiguous premotor and somatosensory cortices of the cerebrum. Output information is sent back and feedback established with the cerebral cortical sensorimotor system that allows for the development of '*motor imagery*' of movements to be achieved, thereby chronologically organizing, in advance, the voluntary movement of the different areas of the body.

Neuroimaging techniques provide an understanding of which sites in the brain are processing kinaesthetic information. A central integration of sensory information from multiple origins, such as vision, touch, and kinaesthesia seems to be occurring, and it is the cerebellum that demonstrates this critical function.[42]

# Age-related changes

## Muscle strength and somatosensory/proprioceptive perception

Diminution of all somatosensory and physiological functions takes place as part of the normal aging process. Proprioception is no exception, and, as such, a decline in cutaneous sensation in the lower extremities has a negative impact on balance and mobility in the aging adult.[43] Several studies have shown differences between young and older persons in somatosensory/proprioceptive perception such as a decrease in somatosensory sensitivity,[44] higher thresholds for vibratory stimuli,[45] and increased joint position error.[46 47 48]

Diminished muscle strength is also associated with aging and contributes to diminished proprioception. Thus it may cause impairment in physical performance and loss of independence in the aging patient. Globally, age-related modifications in muscle function and structure are rather minor until the age of 60–70 years, whereas after 70 years, alterations increase significantly.[49] Concentric peak torque strength levels begin to decline, however, in the fourth decade.[50] It should be emphasized that variations exist between individuals and several muscles in healthy subjects do not demonstrate an age-related weakening in function. Loss of strength differs from muscle to muscle, and some, such as non-weight-bearing muscles, are less affected by age than weight-bearing muscles.[51] Decline in muscle function may also be due to the influence of factors extrinsic to aged skeletal muscle fibers such as restrictions in diet, exercise and immobility, and comorbidities.[52] Factors resulting in the aging of skeletal muscle are, in fact,

multifaceted, also involving intrinsic biochemical transformations in muscle metabolism, variations in the distribution and size of muscle fibers, and an overall loss of muscle mass. Other factors like the control of muscle contraction by the motor neural system and denervation atrophy of skeletal muscles may also be major mechanisms for muscle degeneration in the aging individual.[53]

According to Vladimir Janda, muscles can be classified into two groups based upon their functional roles: the *postural* and *phasic muscles*.[54] The postural group consists of muscles involved in patterns where anatomic flexion, adduction, and internal rotation are combined. Conversely, the phasic group supports patterns with an association of anatomic extension, abduction, and external rotation. In their function as anti-gravitational muscles, the two groups should balance each other in order to maintain an erect posture. When there is a disorder of the CNS, such as cerebral palsy and stroke, Janda observed that postural muscles are more predisposed to tightness and phasic muscles to weakness. Interestingly, most of the time, the same patterns of imbalance are present in chronic musculoskeletal pain.

Among the phasic muscles inclined to weakness are the following: peroneus longus, brevis, and tertius; tibialis anterior; vastus medialis and lateralis; gluteus maximus and medius; transversus and rectus abdominis; and multifidus. Among the postural muscles more predisposed to tightness are the following: hip adductors, hamstrings, rectus femoris, tensor fascia lata, and piriformis.

Multiple studies support the observation of imbalance in the muscular strength of aging patients.

Quadriceps strength, for instance, diminishes with advanced age,[55] and is frequently employed as a marker of lower limb strength.[56] Hip abductors and adductors display reduction in both the magnitude and rate of torque production with aging.[57] These losses may impair rapid lateral stepping movement that plays a significant role in the maintenance of balance. In fact, mediolateral stability is considerably reduced in women between their forties and sixties.[58] This represents a risk factor for lateral falls that are frequent in aging adults and related to the increased possibility of hip fracture.[59] Also among the muscles stabilizing the pelvis in the coronal plane is the gluteus medius. Together with step movement time, gluteus medius onset times appear to be the variable best able to predict a patient's increased potential to suffer a lateral fall.[60] As such, programs consisting of weight-bearing exercises, including balance exercises in the sagittal plane as well as in the coronal plane, should be combined with osteopathic manipulative treatment (OMT) procedures for a complete therapeutic protocol.

From an osteopathic perspective, a correlation may be observed between the anatomic flexion, adduction, and internal rotation demonstrated by the *postural* muscles and the anatomic extension, abduction, and external rotation of the *phasic* muscles, as described by Janda and the PRM of Sutherland. The cyclic phenomenon of the PRM consists of two phases: cranial inspiration and cranial expiration. During the inspiratory phase, the midline unpaired structures of the skull and pelvis move in the direction of the fetal curve, termed craniosacral flexion, while associated paired anatomic structures externally rotate. In the reciprocal expiratory phase of the PRM, the midline structures move in the direction of craniosacral extension, and the paired structures internally rotate. It should be emphasized that the craniosacral flexion and extension movements described, in some instances, are different from, and should not be mistaken with, anatomic flexion and extension.

The different vertebral segments exhibit craniosacral flexion and craniosacral extension. The overall motion of the spine, in synchrony with the PRM, demonstrates a decrease of the normal AP curves in connection with the inspiratory phase and an increase of the AP curves in connection with the expiratory phase. The structures of the upper and lower limbs also exhibit a biphasic motion in association with the inspiratory and expiratory phases of the PRM, with external rotation in association with the inspiratory phase and internal rotation with the expiratory phase. From that perspective, a somatic dysfunction of craniosacral flexion anywhere in the midline unpaired structures of the skull, vertebral spine, or pelvis would be associated with a tendency toward a pattern of external rotation in the paired structures. Conversely, a somatic dysfunction of craniosacral extension would be associated with an increase pattern of internal rotation. These patterns in the aging patient may be chronic and in the whole-body approach, associated with muscular imbalances. Craniosacral flexion somatic dysfunction would be associated with a predominance of the phasic muscles prevailing during association of anatomic extension, abduction, and external rotation. On the other hand, craniosacral extension somatic dysfunction would be found with a dominance of the postural muscles leading during association of anatomic flexion, adduction, and internal rotation.

## Osteoarthritis

Changes in the muscular function and therefore in proprioception may be associated with arthritic conditions, sequelae of previous injuries, or neuropathies. Injuries and inflammation may produce direct or indirect modifications in transmission of information sensed by mechanoreceptors. Damage may affect the ligaments, joint capsule, and nerve fibers with a decline in control of balance, associated with an increased risk of falling.

Osteoarthritis (OA) quite often develops in the knees. Radiographic evidence of OA of the knee occurs in approximately 27% of individuals before the age of 70 and increases to 44% in subjects age 80 or older.[61] Besides the presence of significant pain, the quality of life for patients suffering from knee OA is impaired. There is reduction of articular mobility, with resultant disability and the increased risk of falls. Indeed, decreased proprioception is clearly

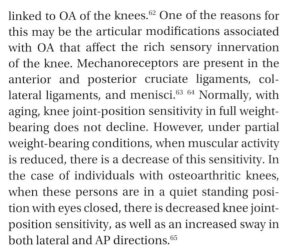

linked to OA of the knees.[62] One of the reasons for this may be the articular modifications associated with OA that affect the rich sensory innervation of the knee. Mechanoreceptors are present in the anterior and posterior cruciate ligaments, collateral ligaments, and menisci.[63] [64] Normally, with aging, knee joint-position sensitivity in full weight-bearing does not decline. However, under partial weight-bearing conditions, when muscular activity is reduced, there is a decrease of this sensitivity. In the case of individuals with osteoarthritic knees, when these persons are in a quiet standing position with eyes closed, there is decreased knee joint-position sensitivity, as well as an increased sway in both lateral and AP directions.[65]

Osteoarthritis of the knees may be more or less painful. When comparing individuals suffering from this condition with and without pain, the individuals with pain, as compared to those who are pain-free, demonstrate reduced proprioceptive acuity, reduced quadriceps strength, and increased postural sway. The pain-free individuals do, however, reveal poorer proprioceptive acuity than healthy subjects.[66] The perceived reduction of knee pain, using either a peripheral local anesthetic, or central placebo mechanism results in intensified maximum voluntary contraction of the quadriceps, but does not result in increased proprioception.[67]

Any decline in proprioceptive acuity in the knee alters the distribution of forces at the articular level and may promote further degenerative changes in the joint. Furthermore, with inflammation, such as occurs in OA, there are increases in the spontaneous activity and the responsiveness of nociceptors. Typically, high-threshold nociceptive afferents, located in the synovium and periosteum, are silent. They normally become active when joint movements are induced that take the articulation beyond its physiological limits. With joint inflammation, the mechanical sensitivity of articular nociceptors is changed and many afferent neurons that were totally non-excitable in a healthy joint become responsive, demonstrating a decrease of their mechanical threshold. Additionally, sensitization of articular nociceptors is increased by inflammatory mediators released into the joint that combine with the receptors on the nerve endings.[68]

Because OA is considered to be the result of joint loading, in the context of systemic and local susceptibility, the effect of muscle activity upon knee joint load is significant. The role of muscle function in structural disease development has been widely studied. Muscle vulnerability, as an augmentation to joint loading, is recognized as a potential risk factor for the development of OA.[69] For this reason, osteopathic procedures that address somatic dysfunction of the lower limb joints, particularly the knee, should be associated with exercise, with attention to the quadriceps, to improve the muscular strength.

## Vestibular disorders

### Benign paroxysmal positional vertigo

Dizziness is the third most frequent complaint among outpatients.[70] Dizziness and poor balance can be caused by multiple pathologies affecting the pathways of the vestibular apparatus. These pathologies may be central or peripheral, affecting respectively the pathways in the brain or the organs in the inner ear or CN VIII, or both. Peripheral pathologies are quite frequent and they most commonly manifest as benign paroxysmal positional vertigo (BPPV).[71]

Vertigo is a reaction following head rotation where there is a disruption of equilibrium, a sensation of spinning, and of dizziness. Benign paroxysmal positional vertigo is one of the most common causes of vertigo with a prevalence of 2.4% in the general population.[72] Although this mechanism is not fully understood, some conditions are associated with secondary BPPV such as head trauma, vestibular neuritis, Menière's disease, and post-operative sequelae.[73] Normally, BPPV is an episodic vertigo without hearing loss, whereas Menière's disease presents as an episodic vertigo with hearing loss. Vertigo, coupled with blurred vision during head rotation, may be caused by a vertebral artery compression that is usually diagnosed by angiography.[74] Vertebral artery compression must be considered and excluded before performing the following BPPV tests or any other manipulation of the cervical spine.

Benign paroxysmal positional vertigo occurs when dislodged statoconia (otoconia) (calcium carbonate particles) from the macula of the utricle enter one of the semicircular canals of the inner ear. Any of the semicircular canals can be involved, but most usually it is the posterior canal, with a prevalence of more than 91%, as compared to 8% for the horizontal canal and less than 1% for the anterior canal.[75] When dislodged statoconia break free, they either float freely in one of the semicircular canals to produce a condition called *canalithiasis*, or they stick to and move with the hair cells of the cupula of the canal, leading to *cupulolithiasis*. During head movements, the statoconia shift and abnormally stimulate the ampullary crest of the affected canal. In response to the resultant amplified neural activity on one side relative to the other, the VOR reflex circuit sets off compensatory eye movements. This explains the association of brief nystagmus and vertigo in patients suffering from BPPV.

The various types of *nystagmus* are described according to their fast phase. Thus a horizontal nystagmus with a fast phase pulsing in the direction of the patient's right ear is referred to as a rightward horizontal nystagmus. For the practitioner looking at their patient, a torsional nystagmus, pulsing in the direction of the patient's left ear is a clockwise nystagmus and a torsional nystagmus, pulsing towards the patient's right ear, is a counterclockwise nystagmus.

A nystagmus differs according to the affected semicircular canal. Nystagmuses associated with disorders of the horizontal semicircular canal are horizontal, with a fast phase toward the involved side, and a slow phase in the opposite direction. Nystagmuses associated with disorders of the posterior canal are upward and torsional in the direction of the affected ear. Finally, nystagmuses associated with disorders of the anterior canal are downward and torsional toward the affected ear.

Dix and Hallpike, in 1952, described a maneuver to diagnose this disorder referred to as the *Dix-Hallpike maneuver:* "The patient is laid supine upon a couch with his head just over its end. The head is then lowered some 30° below the level of the couch and turned some 30–45° to one side. In taking up this position, the patient is first seated upon the couch with the head turned to one side and the gaze fixed upon the examiner's forehead. The examiner then holds the patient's head firmly between his hands and briskly pushes the patient back into the critical position."[76]

Most of the time, this maneuver is practiced with some variants.[77] Generally, at the beginning of the maneuver, the patient is in an upright seated position, without any eye glasses, with the practitioner standing at their side. The patient is told to keep the eyes open. In order to test for involvement of the posterior canal on the right, the practitioner rotates the patient's head 45° to the right. This head position is maintained and, rather rapidly, the patient is moved into the supine position, with their right ear down, their neck extended about 20° below the transverse plane, and their head, maintained by the practitioner's hands, hanging off the edge of the treatment table. A diagnosis of BPPV is made if the patient develops vertigo and nystagmus. Afterwards, the patient is gradually positioned back in the seated position. The same process is repeated for the left ear.[78]

Once a diagnosis of BPPV has been established, treatment is usually rapid, simple, and effective in more than 90% of cases.[79] Most of the time, a 'modified' version of the maneuver developed by Epley is used. In the *Epley maneuver*, the patient is initially positioned in an upright seated position, with the legs extended and their head turned 45° toward the affected ear, i.e., the ear that was positive on the Dix-Hallpike maneuver. The patient is then quickly laid back into a supine position with their affected ear down, and with about a 30° neck extension. This position is maintained for 20–30 seconds. The head is then turned 90° toward the opposite side and kept in this position for another approximately 20–30 seconds. The patient next rolls from the supine position to the lateral decubitus position, toward the non-affected ear, and maintains this position for 20–30 seconds. Lastly, the patient is gradually brought into the upright sitting position, while maintaining the 45° rotation of the head. This maneuver must be repeated two more times, and during this process, the patient may be subjected to some dizziness. As a precaution, the patient should be instructed to refrain, if possible, from flexing, extending, sidebending, or rotating their head after the procedure, although the need for postural restrictions after the treatment is debated.[80]

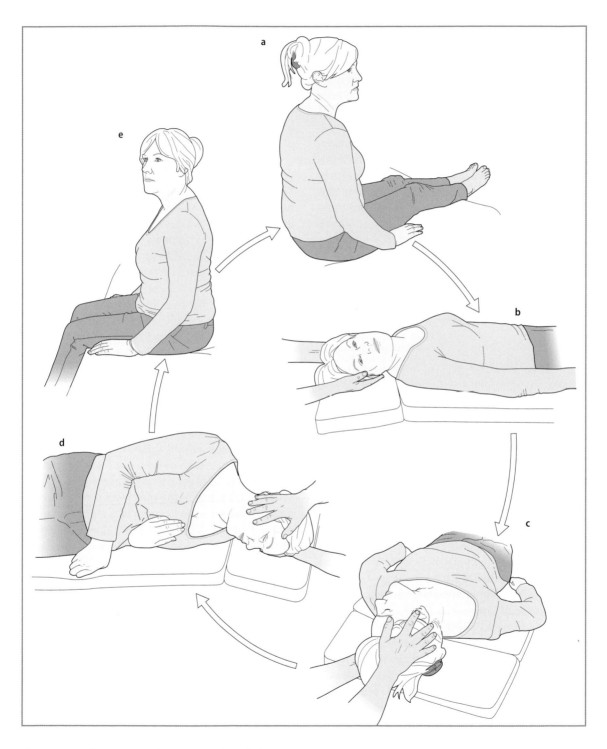

Figure 4.2.7: Epley maneuver for a right sided ear dysfunction

In 1988 Semont described another procedure to treat posterior canal cupulolithiasis, the *Semont maneuver*, or *freeing maneuver*.[81] The patient is initially seated in the upright position, with their head turned 45° toward the side opposite the affected ear. They then rapidly lie down towards the affected side while keeping the cervical rotation. This position is maintained for about 30 seconds. Next, the patient is rapidly moved to the opposite lateral decubitus position, without pausing in the seated position, and always keeping the same cervical rotation. This position is maintained for about 30 seconds, and always keeping the head fixed, the patient returns slowly to the upright seated position.

Osteopathic manipulative treatment to address any somatic dysfunction identified in the thoracic and cervical spine, the temporal bones, and other components of the cranial base and meninges discussed elsewhere contributes to the treatment of BPPV.

## Menière's disease

In 1861, Prosper Menière described a disease with episodic vertigo, ringing in the ears, and hearing loss.[82] At this time, it was accepted that the disease resulted from a disorder of the brain, and its name was apoplectic cerebral congestion. Menière disputed this theory and proposed that it was, rather, a disorder associated with the peripheral organ of the inner ear like 'glaucoma of the inner ear.'

The etiology of Menière's disease is multifactorial with a genetic predisposition.[83] Most of the time, its onset occurs around the age of 40, with the incidence increasing with age thereafter.[84] In 1995, the American Academy of Otolaryngology–Head and Neck Surgery defined a precise set of criteria for the diagnosis of this disease.[85] A triad of symptoms describes Menière's disease: vestibular symptoms, auditory symptoms, and aural pressure. The vestibular symptoms consist of vertigo that is recurrent, spontaneous, and episodic. It lasts at least 20 minutes to several hours, is frequently prostrating, and is associated with disequilibrium that can persist for several days, and also with nausea or vomiting, or both, but with no loss of consciousness. In every instance horizontal rotatory nystagmus is observed. The auditory symptoms include hearing loss and tinnitus. Aural pressure may or may be not associated with the tinnitus.

Typical Menière's disease usually refers to the presence of both cochlear symptoms, i.e., hearing loss, tinnitus, aural pressure, and vestibular symptoms i.e., vertigo. Atypical Menière's disease displays either cochlear or vestibular symptoms.

Multiple hypotheses to explain the etiopathogenesis of Menière's disease have been set forth. For some authors, allergies, autoimmune reactions,[86] and viral infections,[87][88] could cause the disease. Others propose that the same pathophysiological mechanisms resulting in vascular constriction responsible for migraine headaches cause Menière's disease.[89] Generally, it is accepted that the pathophysiology of Menière's disease is an endolymphatic hydrops i.e., an abnormal accumulation of endolymph, although there is a lack of consistency of finding endolymphatic hydrops in the temporal bones of affected patients.[90]

All the parts of the membranous labyrinth are filled with endolymph and separated by perilymph from the periosteum that covers the walls of the bony labyrinth. The endolymph drains into the endolymphatic duct and the endolymphatic sac, and, through the specialized epithelium of the sac, into the adjacent vascular plexus. The role of the endolymphatic sac is of great importance; it controls the immune response of the inner ear, the removal of endolymphatic waste products by phagocytosis, and the volume and pressure of the endolymph. Any decline in the resorptive capacity of the endolymphatic sac that results in a rise of the amount of fluid in the endolymphatic compartment, creating an endolymphatic hydrops, can be part of the pathophysiology of Menière's disease.[91]

Normally, homeostatic mechanisms prevail between the different fluid compartments containing perilymph and endolymph in the inner ear, the perilymphatic tissue, and the cerebrospinal fluid. This affects the production and resorption of perilymph and endolymph. Disruption of these mechanisms causes an endolymphatic hydrops and an impediment in the normal functioning of the inner ear.[92] As such, impairment of the venous

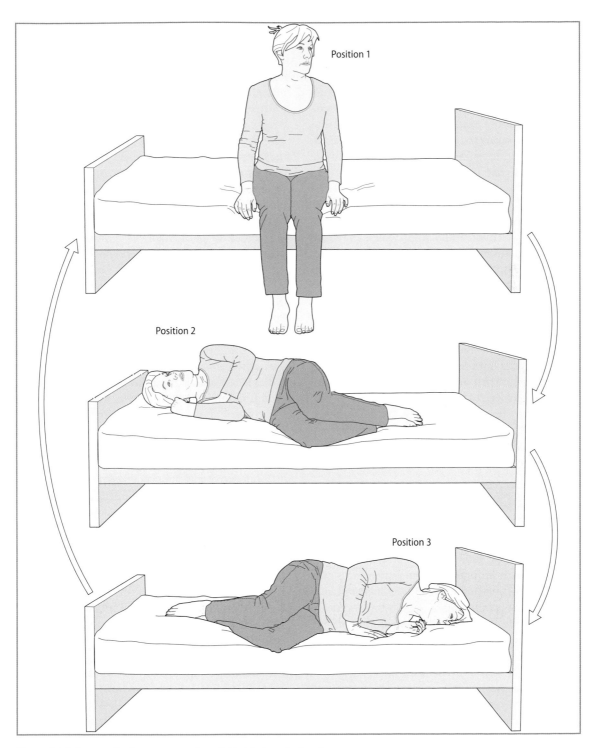

Position 1

Position 2

Position 3

**Figure 4.2.8:** Semont freeing maneuver for a right sided ear dysfunction

drainage may cause accumulation of fluid in the inner ear. A deficiency in the endolymphatic sac's resorptive capacity will contribute to impaired endolymphatic homeostasis. Indeed, the size of the vestibular aqueduct and endolymphatic sac is reduced in Menière's disease, and less tubular epithelial structures are found in their intraosseous portion.[93] In some individuals, endolymphatic hydrops may demonstrate a peripheral extension of alterations in the hemodynamics within the central CNS.[94]

According to Magoun, Sutherland stated: "With every fluctuation of the cerebrospinal fluid there is created a wave in the endolymph which augments fluid movement in the internal ear. The connection of the duct with both the saccule and the utricle is of significance in vertigo, deafness and the like."[95]

Medical treatment of Menière's disease is mostly empiric.[96] Osteopathic procedures addressing the cerebrospinal fluid fluctuation, membranous tension, and inter- and intraosseous dysfunctions of the temporal bones should be considered. If the disease progresses, in spite of conservative management, surgery can be an option. Surgical procedures may be conservative, like endolymphatic sac enhancement, and if this fails, destructive procedures such as labyrinthectomy and vestibular neurectomy may be attempted.[97 98]

## Neck proprioception

Proprioceptors associated with the cervical spine are linked, significantly, to the vestibular and the visual apparatus. They are all integrated at the level of the CNS for an internal representation of postural and spatial orientation. This interrelationship facilitates the production of appropriate motor responses to the challenges of the environment.

Neck proprioceptors contribute to the coordination of eye, head, and body, particularly the sensorimotor control of the head-on-trunk stabilization. As such, they influence spatial orientation and postural control. The proprioceptive system of the cervical spine is particularly rich in mechanoreceptors that are located in the cervical joint capsules, ligaments, and muscles. Predominantly located in the upper part of the cervical spine, most

of them are the muscle spindle afferents in the short muscles, such as the suboccipital muscles.[99] These short muscles demonstrate very high spindle content and spindle density, when compared with other human muscles. Among these upper cervical muscles, the obliquus capitis inferior and obliquus capitis superior muscles have significantly higher spindle density than the rectus capitis posterior major and rectus capitis posterior minor.[100] Because they are close to the joints of the upper cervical spine, and because of their very high spindle content and density, these muscles perceive joint position and movements of craniovertebral joints. They therefore participate in the fine control of the positional sense of the head and neck.

Sensory information from the proprioceptive system of the cervical spine enters the CNS through the dorsal root ganglia of the spinal cord. From there it passes through interneurons that synapse with the dorsal root ganglia to ascending and descending tracts, or to α motor neurons in the ventral horn, forming polysynaptic or monosynaptic reflex arcs. Input from the proprioceptive system connects with the VNC and the superior colliculus, where coordination between vision and neck movement occurs.[101] Additionally, it joins the central cervical nucleus, a pathway to the cerebellum where integration of vestibular, ocular, and proprioceptive information takes place.[102]

Musculoskeletal functional capacity typically decreases with age. In males, musculoskeletal function, balance, and mobility are often reduced significantly by the seventh decade of life.[103] The stresses encountered throughout life will have accumulated by this time and the cervical region is particularly vulnerable. Trauma can be the result of repetitive microstresses, as might occur from the chronic postural stress of working with a computer for years. Or, it can be the result of a single episode of macrostress as can occur in whiplash injuries that are the result of relative acceleration between the head and thorax during motor vehicle collisions. Following a whiplash injury, a patient may experience greater balance disturbances than normal.[104] Deficits in the motor system, such as decreased cervical range of movement, may also be present.[105] In fact, dysfunction affecting cervical proprioceptors, particularly joint proprioceptors and muscle spindles, in musculoskeletal disorders of the neck can alter afferent input into the CNS, disrupting the integration, timing, and tuning of sensorimotor control.[106] Studies also suggest that the initial peripheral nociceptive input subsequent to a cervical trauma, such as whiplash injury, can produce disturbances in motor function in the acute phase of the injury that can persist over time.[107] Disorders in pain processing may also be associated with affiliated sensory changes following cervical trauma.[108]

In neck disorders, sensorimotor disturbances, such as poor balance, are found more frequently in patients with chronic cervical pain than in controls. Interestingly, it appears that sensorimotor impairment is greater in patients enduring pain from the upper, rather than the lower cervical spine. One explanation for this observation may be the anatomical and neurophysiological link between the sensorimotor control system and the upper cervical region.[109] Patients with chronic pain also have more somatic dysfunction in the cervical region than asymptomatic subjects, again with greatest occurrence at the level of the upper cervical region, specifically the cervico-occipital joint, rather than the lower level.[110] Somatic dysfunction of the upper cervical spine, an "impaired or altered function of related components of the somatic (body framework) system: skeletal, arthrodial, and myofascial structures and their related vascular, lymphatic, and neural elements,"[111] contributes to decreased proprioception.

The link between sensorimotor disturbances in neck disorders and postural instability, dysfunction of head and eye movement control, dizziness, and unsteadiness has been demonstrated.[112] Generally, in aging individuals, the deterioration of vestibular function may be counterbalanced with neck proprioception.[113] Normally, following rotation of the neck, input from the muscles and the facet joints of the cervical spine produce a cervico-ocular reflex that operates with the vestibulo-ocular reflex to control the EOM with an ocular response that maintains visual stability. In older individuals who have stiffer necks or somatic dysfunction with reduced range of motion, however,

neck proprioceptor input during neck rotation and, consequently, this compensatory response, may be decreased.[114] The concept of facilitation as associated with spinal somatic dysfunction was originally identified by Denslow et al.[115] Somatosensory input as a source of spinal somatic dysfunction has been described.[116] Spinal somatic dysfunction is, as such, associated with an exaggerated central response to sensory input. The spinal cord level facilitation of somatic dysfunction can consequently disrupt proprioceptive input through the ascending spinal pathways. As such, spinal somatic dysfunction should be identified and treated. Osteopathic manipulative procedures directed at the treatment of the somatic dysfunction, along with sensorimotor retraining, should be considered in order to improve cervico-ocular reflex dysfunction. Under these circumstances, the efficient function of the upper cervical spine, in particular the occipital bone, where many of the muscles from the neck attach, is of paramount importance.

## Stomatognathic system

Among the different factors that affect body posture the stomatognathic system (SS) can play a significant part. The SS is a functional arrangement that includes several components: the maxilla and mandible, with their dental arches, soft tissues, and vasculoneural structures; the temporomandibular joint (TMJ); and the masticatory muscles.[117] Additional muscular relationships exist between the mandible, the hyoid bone, the skull, and the sternum.[118] They constitute a 'kinetic chain' wherein every structure is interdependent with the others as part of a system that influences postural balance. The structural and functional interrelationships between the cervical region, the skull, and the TMJ form a complex system, referred to as the 'craniocervical-mandibular system.'

Occlusion is the relationship between the occlusal surfaces of the maxillary and mandibular teeth when they are in contact. Occlusion is identified according to the respective positions of the teeth. A centric occlusion is present when the relation of opposing occlusal surfaces of mandibular and maxillary teeth provides the maximum contact or intercuspation. In such a case, the mandible is in centric relation to the maxillae. Normally, this allows a better positional and functional symmetry of the associated myofascial structures. With age, alterations in dental structure often happen. Teeth may be replaced with crowns, bridges, or implants, with the potential for occlusal changes and TMJ disorders.

Natural teeth have extremely sensitive tactile sensors: the periodontal mechanoreceptors. Located in the middle of the collagen fibers in the ligaments that fix the root of the tooth to the alveolar bone, the periodontal mechanoreceptors supply information about tooth load.[119] They demonstrate sensory discriminative capabilities of the magnitude, direction, and rate of occlusal load application. With associated feedback mechanisms, the periodontal mechanoreceptors contribute to oral stereognosis and modulation of the neuromotor control of jaw function.[120] Loss of periodontal mechanoreceptors contributes to changes in proprioceptive sensations and jaw function. Oral kinesthetic and proprioceptive sensations are described as the "perceptions of static jaw position and velocity of jaw movement and forces generated during contractions of the jaw muscles."[121]

Tooth loss is generally associated with loss of some periodontal mechanoreceptors and, quite often, with modification of occlusion. In the aging individual, this loss is considered to be a risk factor for postural instability.[122] Studies demonstrate that modification of the occlusal relationship is associated with decreased lower extremity dynamic strength and diminution in the amount of time that the individual is able to stand on one leg with opened eyes.[123]

When occlusal dysfunction is present, TMJ disorder may follow. TMJ disorder may also be the consequence of a direct trauma to the joint, or an indirect trauma, such as during a whiplash injury or an intubation during surgery when the mouth is opened and the cervical spine positioned in hyperextension. TMJ disorder, one of the significant disorders affecting the craniocervical-mandibular system, is associated with balance disorders.[124]

TMJ disorder contributes to musculoskeletal modifications of the craniocervical-mandibular system, often associated with musculoskeletal disorders. Subjects with TMJ disorders, as compared to asymptomatic subjects, demonstrate a significant difference in the measurement of the C0–C1 joint space.[125] They present with an increased cervical lordosis and a head position that is displaced excessively forward.[126] [127]

In fact, the TMJs influence posture and vice versa. For instance, modification of the plantar arches results in changes in the occlusal plane.[128] Also, postural changes, particularly at the level of the craniocervical junction, impact occlusion.[129] [130]

For some authors, the association between TMJ disorders and balance and gait disorders may be explained through the anatomical and physiological pathways of the trigeminal nerve and its connections with the dorsal horn of the cervical spinal cord bilaterally from C1–C5, the reticular formation, the vestibular nuclei, and the cerebellum.[131] [132] These connections may be part of the reciprocal influence between the SS and posture. This is illustrated by the fact that, after receiving unilateral conduction anesthesia of the mandibular nerve, postural control in human subjects significantly deteriorated.[133]

## Pelvic imbalance

One of the prerequisites for good posture is a well balanced body. Throughout life, however, everybody accumulates somatic dysfunction that may affect their ability to stand effectively in the fight against gravity. Each part of the body: the lower limbs, pelvis, spine, upper limb, and skull, may be affected by any other part.

Four bones constitute the pelvis: the sacrum, the two pelvic bones, and the coccyx. Perfect pelvic symmetry is exceptional. Beginning in intrauterine life, the fetus adopts asymmetrical positions. Most of the time, in the last months of pregnancy, the fetus is in a position where their pelvis demonstrates a pattern of torsion to the left. This is because, at this time, the fetus is most often in a cephalic presentation, with their left pelvic bone against the maternal spine, and the right pelvic bone against the maternal abdominal wall. In a pattern of pelvic torsion to the left, the fetal sacrum demonstrates a combination of sacral sidebending and rotation in opposite directions. Thus, a left sacral torsion occurs when the sacrum is positioned into coupled left rotation and right sidebending. In this instance, the right pelvic bone accompanies the left sacral torsion, with external rotation, wherein the major component of the movement is anterior rotation, and the left pelvic bone demonstrates internal rotation with a major component of posterior rotation. At birth, the same pattern is often present, incorporated into a whole-body pattern, where the child seems to be positioned in a complete spiral between the head and pelvis. Therefore, with a *left pelvic torsion*, the infant's head is quite often rotated to the right. In a study of 649 children, a pattern of left sacral torsion was present in 60.2% of the cases and right sacral torsion in 32.4%. The occipital bone was side bent to the left and rotated to the right in 56.0% of the cases, while the opposite pattern was found in 43.7%.[134]

Because of the resiliency and flexibility of their tissues, children adapt considerably. And even though there is pelvic asymmetry, the motion of the pelvis may still be possible in both directions, despite the fact that there is a better quality in the direction of the left torsion. Later during childhood, somatic dysfunctions may occur as the result of various traumas, like sports injuries. These acquired somatic dysfunctions stack upon the initial pattern of pelvic torsion present at birth, making their diagnosis sometimes troublesome for the inexperienced practitioner. In adults, nevertheless, an asymmetrical pelvic pattern that reflects the childhood pattern of pelvic torsion to the left is quite frequent. Out of 100 cases Mitchell found 72 with a posterior pelvic bone on the left and only six with a posterior pelvic bone on the right.[135]

Pelvic asymmetry from pelvic torsion, with associated sacral torsion, must be differentiated from other pelvic asymmetries. Pelvic asymmetry may also be the result of somatic dysfunction at the level of the sacroiliac (SI) joint or any joint in the lower extremity. It can also result from structural changes such as fracture or intraosseous dysfunction resulting in asymmetrical development. Here it should be recognized that, whereas structural changes may be appreciated through a palpation of the anatomy, somatic dysfunction is diagnosed through palpation for function.

The difference between the pelvic motion patterns associated with pelvic torsions and those associated with pelvic asymmetry from SI somatic dysfunction can be readily appreciable through palpation for function, in particular through tests of listening. Some experience is, however, necessary. In the presence of a pelvic torsion pattern, one pelvic bone moves without difficulty into external rotation and returns to demonstrate a less prominent internal rotation phase. At the same time, the other pelvic bone moves easily into internal rotation, with less prominence in the external rotation phase. A sense of unity of pelvic girdle motion is well established, with the sensation that when one pelvic bone moves, the other side moves as well in synchrony, although, in the opposite direction.[136] Most commonly, this pattern is the result of a dysfunction between the sacrum and L5. In this case, the sacrum demonstrates coupled rotation and sidebending in opposite directions, the rotation demonstrated by the sacrum being opposite to the rotation of L5. Pelvic torsion may also follow any dysfunction in the axial skeleton above, including possibly the cranial base. In this instance, the pelvis is not primarily dysfunctional; the pattern is an accommodation to dysfunction above. (See further discussion of 'Physiologic motion of the sacrum' in 'Section 4: Clinical considerations, Chapter 1: Musculoskeletal dysfunctions, Part 1: Axial system,' p. 182.)

Conversely, if during palpation the sense of pelvic girdle unity is not present, with the sensation that both pelvic bones are moving out of synchrony, the somatic dysfunction is in the lower limbs, including the pelvic bones or the SI joints.[137]

# Leg length inequality

Leg length inequality (LLI) is quite often associated with pelvic torsion and may be its cause or its consequence. Leg length inequality is very common with a prevalence of 90% in the population and an average inequality of 5.2mm.[138] Generally, the right leg is the shorter leg.[139] [140] It is generally accepted that for most individuals, anatomical LLI of less than 20 mm is most of the time not clinically significant, with no need for heel lifts to compensate for the LLI.[141]

That having been said, musculoskeletal symptoms, particularly, but not limited to, low back pain, as the result of pelvic unleveling from LLI as small as 3–6 mm tend to become more prevalent as individuals age. This is because the unlevel pelvis necessitates that asymmetrical spinal mechanics in the coronal plane be established in order to maintain postural balance. This places an asymmetrical workload upon the core musculature, particularly the paravertebral muscles. As the patient ages, they progressively lose the muscular strength necessary to compensate for the postural response to the LLI. As such, they become vulnerable to muscular fatigue with resultant pain and functional compromise. This process tends to begin to manifest after the fourth decade of life and often presents at the same time every day, as the patient decompensates to weight-bearing stress.[142] As such, although LLI may be of little consequence in the majority of patients, it should be seriously considered as a contributory factor, particularly in aged patients where offending somatic dysfunction is recurrent in spite of other conservative management attempts.

Leg length inequality is described as either anatomical or functional. *Anatomical LLI* corresponds to measured differences in the bony anatomy of the lower extremity, and may be the consequence of structural changes such as unequal development, unilateral coxa vara, fracture with shortening or lengthening, and hip replacement. *Functional LLI*, on the contrary may be found with somatic dysfunction of the pelvis, such as pelvic torsion or iliosacral somatic dysfunction, lumbar asymmetries, imbalances in muscular, fascial, or ligamentous tensions such as psoitis, or somatic dysfunction in the lower limb joints.[143] [144]

Interestingly, studies of simulated LLI result in pelvic torsion. Usually, the pelvic bone contralateral to the side of the elevation rotates more likely in a movement of anterior rotation and the pelvic bone ipsilateral to the side of the elevation rotates in a movement of posterior rotation.[145] [146] Additionally, lumbar sidebending becomes greater toward the side of the elevation.[147]

Pelvic torsion is associated with sidebending of the sacrum. This pattern creates a postural imbalance. This baseline unleveling potentially results in compensatory lumbar, thoracic, and cervical lateral curves, with concomitant increase in the pre-existent spinal AP curves. There will be stress at the apexes of resultant lateral curves, where spinal rotation changes direction. Flattening of the spinal AP curvature is found at the crossover points between adjacent lateral curves where spinal sidebending changes direction. At these crossover points Fryette type II spinal dysfunctions, opposite the normal AP curve, are often encountered.

Most frequently, pelvic torsion is found with rotation toward the side of the long leg.[148] This pattern is, however, not present all the time and pelvic torsion and lumbar curvatures are identified in patients with equal leg length suggesting that other mechanisms can be involved.[149] Understanding the patterns present at birth and postural evolution throughout life may help to differentiate between a) total-body asymmetry resulting in a functional LLI and pelvic torsion, where unencumbered motion is present at the level of the SI joints and L5–S1, and b) localized somatic dysfunction affecting the pelvis, lower limb joints, or both that need to be addressed.

The pelvic accommodation to LLI has been described in the osteopathic literature. In the description of the cycle of walking, Mitchell explained that asymmetrical weight-bearing, as is encountered with LLI, causes the sacrum to rotate posteriorly on the side that the weight is borne.[150] In the patient with LLI, this will be chronically on the side of the long leg. Similar sacral accommodation is found on the side of the concavity produced by lumbar sidebending that, when the result of LLI, is found on the long leg side. As the sacrum rotates posteriorly on the side of the anatomic long leg and anteriorly on the side of the short leg, it pulls the pelvic bones with it, posteriorly and anteriorly respectively.[151] This sacral rotation occurs such that the sacrum pulls the ilia with it, but not as far. Under these

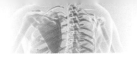

circumstances, sacroiliac articular dysfunction should be anticipated, with the sacrum posterior relative to the ilium on the long leg side, or anterior relative to the ilium on the short leg side.[152] Thus it is important to differentiate between the global dysfunctional pattern of the pelvis and articular dysfunctions that may manifest within the greater pelvic pattern.

## Examination for leg length inequality

The examination for LLI is a common screening and diagnostic procedure. Several methods are used for this assessment, either through physical examination or radiographic imaging. Physical examination is frequently performed using a tape measure to assess the length of each lower extremity by measuring the distance between the anterior superior iliac spine and the medial malleolus. Valuation of reliability covers considerable variations and the accuracy of this method for determining differences in leg length has always been questioned,[153] although it may be considered with large asymmetries.[154] Some authors propose a variation of this procedure, by measuring the true length of the leg, from the pelvis to the bottom of the heel, taking into account therefore, a possible shortening distal to the ankle.[155]

The attempt to measure leg length using a tape measure may suffice for determining orthopedic (20 mm or greater) anatomic inequities of leg length. The inequities dealt with when treating the somatic dysfunction secondary to LLI are most often significantly smaller. The act of placing a tape measure, upon whichever anatomic structures in question, has an inherent potential error of at least plus or minus several millimeters, thus invalidating this measurement for assessing minor LLI.

If the majority of LLIs are to be identified by physical examination, it is best to examine the patient from behind in the standing position with their knees fully extended and bearing weight equally on both legs. The floor, thus, becomes a fixed point of reference. After the symmetry of the hips, knees, ankles, and feet has been evaluated, a constellation of bilateral anatomic landmarks is observed and compared for symmetry. These landmarks include the following:

- Tops of the greater trochanters, the most direct indicator of LLI.
- Posterior superior iliac spines.
- Sacral dimples (dimples of Venus).
- Most lateral aspect of the iliac crests.

The examination continues by having the patient forward bend at the hips and observing for asymmetric lumbar paravertebral prominence, indicative of spinal rotation found in association with spinal lateral curves. Finally, the patient may be observed for pelvic sideshift.

Using this examination sequence, the presence of LLI can be identified by recognizing a constellation of physical findings. Typically, the greater trochanters and all of the pelvic landmarks will be high on the side of the long leg. The paravertebral prominence will be present on the side of the short leg and the pelvis will sideshift more freely toward the long leg. It must be recognized that these findings can vary greatly from patient to patient depending upon individual anatomic variations (congenital asymmetries, traumatic structural changes, and independent scoliosis) and dysfunctional muscle pull mechanics (particularly psoas spasm). The identification of inconsistencies in the identified pattern should lead the examiner to look further for muscle pull mechanics or anatomic variations. Further, although this examination sequence can identify the possibility of LLI, it does not provide a measurement of the extent of LLI. Precise measurements are best obtained radiographically.

Of the different evaluation methods, radiographic measures such as scanograms are acknowledged as reliable for the evaluation of anatomical LLI.[156] Like supine radiographs, however, where the patient must stay immobile between the different radiographic exposures, risk of error is possible with scanograms, if the patient repositions between the exposures. As such, a more effective method of measuring LLI, and at the same time obtaining an assessment of the patient's postural accommodation, is the standing postural X-ray series.[157] [158] [159] [160] [161]

It has been stated that with LLI of less than 20 mm difference, there is no need for compensation with heel lifts.[162] This may be so in the general population. However, with the functional decompensation that normally occurs with aging, LLI as small as 3–6 mm can prove to be of clinical significance.[163][164]

To find out if and how much heel lift would be appropriate, it is useful to place a series of small shims (with 1 mm thickness increments) under the short leg, until the pelvis is functionally level and the test of listening of the pelvis gives the sensation of a balanced motion. The implementation of a heel lift may be helpful when the use of the shims under the short leg results in qualitatively and quantitatively more balanced motions of the sacrum and the two pelvic bones. If postural X-rays have been employed, it is appropriate to begin the assessment using a shim of approximately one half the radiographically measured LLI, and progress from there. The thickness of the shim that results in functional balance determines the thickness of the heel pad to be employed. A complete sole adapted to the patient's shoe may be better than a heel lift, when the correction is one centimeter or greater, in order to avoid unnecessary compensatory stresses being placed upon the joints of the foot. In any case, before using a lift, the practitioner should make any corrections to dysfunctional mechanics that are achievable, and after that clinically re-evaluate the patient, and, if suitable, apply a lift.[165] Then, osteopathic procedures must be provided until the patient is able to maintain clinical improvement. As the patient accommodates to their lift therapy it may be appropriate to reassess them, and increase (or rarely decrease) the height of the heel pad in 1 mm increments to maintain functional balance. The accommodation to lift therapy progresses slowly as the pelvis adjusts to its new balance. The area of dysfunctional stress often progressively ascends the axial skeleton.

# Foot imbalance

Functionally, the foot serves to support the body and to propel the individual forward when walking. In addition to the simple hinge action of the ankle joint, the multiple joints of the foot form a sophisticated complex able to adapt to the different surfaces of the ground, and through proprioception, to allow for proper bipedal posture. In order to fulfill this role, the foot must be compliant, and, with great sensitivity, constantly responsive to minute ground surface deformations.[166] Any somatic dysfunction in the foot disrupts this complex function. Postural balance is compromised. Conversely, postural dysfunction can affect the static and dynamic properties of the foot.

Aging is associated with an increased incidence of foot disorders. Over the age of 70 years, more than one third of the population has disabling foot pain.[167] Most of the time, this continues to increase with age.[168][169] As a demonstration of applied holistic principles, subjects who suffer from disabling foot pain also complain of pain in other parts of their bodies, including the back, hips, knees, and hands or wrists.[170]

In individuals over 50 years of age, the feet are more pronated, flatter, and have a decreased range of motion in the ankle and in the first metatarsophalangeal joints. Hallux valgus and other toe deformities, toe plantar flexor weakness, and lessened plantar tactile sensitivity are more frequent than in younger subjects.[171] As a result, plantar loading patterns during gait are modified and the risks of losing postural balance and falling are increased.[172]

The cause of foot symptoms in aging individuals is multifactorial. Some factors are intrinsic to the feet, such as pes planus, hallux valgus deformities, hammer toes, calluses, or corns, while others are extrinsic, such as ill-fitting footwear, or systemic conditions such as obesity and generalized OA.[173]

## Hallux valgus

Hallux valgus, or hallux abducto valgus, is a deviation (abduction) of the first toe (hallux) toward the midline of the foot. An abductus angle of the hallux greater than 15° with respect to the first metatarsal bone is considered abnormal.

Several etiologies exist to explain this deformation. Footwear, in particular high heels, is frequently mentioned, but different studies challenge this view.[174] A genetic predisposition may exist, as well as a sexual dimorphism, as a more rounded and smaller first metatarsal head articular surface contributes to a less stable joint

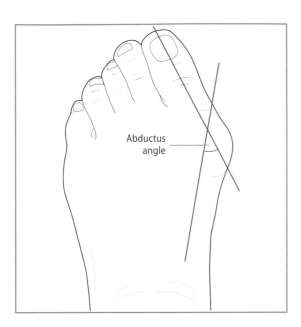

Figure 4.2.9: Abductus angle

in female individuals.[175] Indeed, hallux valgus is twice as frequent in women as in men.[176]

The foot normally demonstrates three arches: two longitudinal (medial and lateral) and one transverse. These arches transform the foot from a rigid lever into a dynamic spring mechanism. Ligaments and muscles maintain this arrangement, holding the bones together, although allowing the dynamic deformations and spring actions necessary during locomotion. The medial arch depends upon the integrity of the first ray, i.e., the distal phalanx, first metatarsal, first cuneiform, and navicular bones. Although the cause of hallux valgus is multifactorial, failure anywhere along the first ray, including the talonavicular joint, can result in hallux valgus.[177] Any restriction of mobility in the subtalar and talocrural joints, as well, may predispose to hallux valgus. This may be the result of reversible somatic dysfunction or the consequence of a lifelong series of traumas upon the ankle with ensuing structural change. The loading under the first metatarsal head is increased, when the calcaneus is everted.[178] Since the talus is greatly influenced by the fibula, any dysfunction at the level of the superior or inferior tibiofibular joints must be

considered in individuals with first ray disruption. Hallux valgus may also occur with a tight Achilles tendon and decreased dorsiflexion of the ankle.

When the foot is in pronation, the first ray rotates on its longitudinal axis and loading is increased on the medial margin of the hallux, in particular during heel rise. This may be a contributing factor for hallux valgus. Typically, pronation of the foot is combined with dorsiflexion and abduction motions. The association of these three motions is referred to as eversion. In the craniosacral concept, during the motion of extension-internal rotation associated with cranial expiration, the internal rotation of the lower limb produces an eversion pattern in the foot. Therefore, any total-body somatic dysfunction pattern that exaggerates the eversion pattern of the foot may facilitate the development of hallux valgus. For instance, a pattern of sacral extension that is associated with internal rotation in the lower limbs may predispose to bilateral hallux valgus.

An increase of the eversion pattern of the foot may also result from postural imbalance, with resultant displacement of the gravity line anterior to the spine as is frequently encountered in individuals over 40 years of age. [179] Normally, 60% of the body's weight is transmitted to the posterior part of the foot, and 40% to the anterior part. By shifting the gravity line anteriorly, individuals increase the amount of pressure applied on the anterior part of the foot. During weight-bearing, the first toe tends to be pulled into valgus; normally the ligaments, the muscles, and the two sesamoid bones located beneath the head of the first metatarsal prevent this deformation. However, as soon as the metatarsal head is no longer maintained in correct position, tightening of the muscles contributes to the increase of the deformity.

Hallux valgus can be a progressive condition that becomes increasingly painful. Pressure on the metatarsophalangeal joint from shoes can produce swelling and a bunion with the formation of a fluid filled sac at the base of the big toe. Initial treatment is conservative directed at decreasing the abductus angle and preventing additional deformity. Osteopathic manipulative treatment procedures directed at the elimination or reduction of somatic dysfunction should be employed. Although the dysfunctional pattern will be individual, it is appropriate to address local dysfunctional mechanics in the foot, leg, pelvis, and spine remembering that: "Diagnosis of any complaint in a peripheral part is not complete without analysis of the region of the spine segmentally related."[180] The patient's global functional pattern including: pelvic unleveling, postural accommodation, and whole-body cranial pattern must also be taken into consideration. Ultimately, with severe deformity, pain, and functional compromise, surgical correction may become necessary. Surgery is not, however, a panacea. Post-operatively the osteopathic practitioner must still address the functional compromise that follows surgery.

### Toe deformities

Each ray of the foot consists of a metatarsal bone and a proximal, middle, and distal phalanx. Because the metatarsophalangeal, proximal interphalangeal, and distal interphalangeal articular surfaces are so very small, the role of ligaments and muscles is of paramount importance in the stabilization of these joints.

Toe deformities include mallet toe, hammer toe, and claw toe. As with hallux valgus, they result from disruption of the balance between the structures of the foot that may be aggravated with poor footwear.

Mallet toe is a flexion deformity at the distal interphalangeal joint, giving the toe a mallet-like appearance. The proximal interphalangeal and metatarsophalangeal joints remain in neutral position, although the distal phalanx may deviate medially or laterally.

Hammer toe is characterized by a flexion deformity of the proximal interphalangeal joint, most of the time with the distal interphalangeal joint held in extension.

Claw toe deformity consists of flexion deformities of the proximal and distal interphalangeal joints associated with a hyperextension at the metatarsophalangeal joint. Claw toe deformity may be indicative of an underlying neurological condition.

# Vertebral imbalance

As we grow older, our posture changes, having a tendency to decompensate. The vertebral column is one location where these changes occur. Ideally, no spinal curvature should be present in the coronal plane. Any lateral curvature of the vertebral column greater than 10° is classified as a scoliosis and is considered to be pathological. However, any asymmetry can be stressful, and because of the propensity of minor pelvic unleveling from LLI, and other environmental influences, like chronically maintained postures associated with different types of work, spinal lateral curvatures of less than 10° are ubiquitous in the general population.

In the sagittal plane, the four AP curvatures of the vertebral column are cervical, thoracic, lumbar, and sacral. Typically, the sagittal profile of the spine is described as being lordotic between C1–C7 and L1–L5, and kyphotic between T1–T12, and at the level of the sacrococcygeal region.

Although variations between normal and pathologic curvatures are well defined in the coronal plane, less attention is paid to the sagittal plane. However, spinal curvatures in the coronal plane are accompanied by increased sagittal plane curves and minor functional spinal imbalance is as common in the sagittal plane as it is in the coronal plane. Mainstream medical literature notes that most spinal degenerative disease takes place in spines that are well aligned in the coronal plane but are compromised in the sagittal plane.[181] From the osteopathic perspective, however, it is appropriate to address spinal imbalance in both the coronal and the sagittal planes before these stressors induce pathology or, if degenerative disease has begun, reduce its progression.

### Spinal lateral curves

In order to effectively diagnose and treat spinal dysfunction it is of value to understand spinal anatomy and functional physiology. Whether pathological (scoliosis) or the result of minor postural accommodation, spinal curvatures in the coronal plane (lateral curves) demonstrate a predictable coupled relationship between spinal sidebending and the resultant vertebral rotation that occurs under weight-bearing circumstances, as the result of the normal physiologic motion of the spine. These spinal mechanics are commonly encountered in association with spinal somatic dysfunction, and should be differentiated from dysfunction resulting from trauma. The latter demonstrates highly variable dysfunctional motion patterns dependant, to a great extent, upon the exogenous forces of the trauma. The physiologic motions of the spine associated with somatic dysfunction were originally described by Fryette—who was a student of Littlejohn—as neutral and non-neutral, and are limited in their incidence to typical vertebrae.[182][183] Typical vertebrae are those spinal segments that possess superior and inferior articular facets and rest upon an intervertebral disc. As such, these physiologic motions, with some variation in the cervical spine (see discussion of cervical spinal neutral mechanics below), apply from C2 upon C3 to L5 upon S1.

Fryette neutral mechanics (also referred to as 'type I' or 'physiologic principle I') are a description of the motion of a group of three or more contiguous typical vertebrae and define the mechanics of functional spinal lateral curves. To be clearly understood, these mechanics must be considered both in terms of the motion pattern demonstrated by the entire group, and that of each of the individual segments that comprise the group.

As a description of the mechanics of spinal lateral curves, Fryette's first principle of physiologic motion states that when the spine is neutral (absence of significant flexion or extension), and sidebending is introduced, rotation will occur in the direction of the produced convexity. Simply stated, Fryette neutral (type I), or group mechanics demonstrate sidebending and rotation in opposite directions, with maximum rotation within the group occurring at the apex (most central segment) of the curve. As with most simplifications, the actual vertebral mechanics are more complex than the statement implies. When the group of vertebrae is considered relative to the anatomic position, sidebending and rotation of the entire group does, in fact, occur in opposite directions. It is when the mechanics of the individual segments within the group are analyzed that the complexity is discovered.

It is important that one has a thorough understanding of these individual vertebral mechanics, because it is only with such an appreciation that manipulative procedures may be employed intelligently and effectively, and dysfunctional patterns associated with the physiological response of the spine to weight-bearing can be differentiated from traumatic dysfunctional patterns, functional patterns resulting from structural abnormalities and viscerosomatic reflexes.

To illustrate this, it is appropriate to consider the pattern of physiologic motion of a five segment spinal lateral curve (see 'Figure 4.2.10: Fryette type I, group lateral curve,' p. 244).

Relative to the anatomic position, the entire group is side bent left and rotated right. Each of the individual segments in the curve contribute to this pattern, although each somewhat differently. Segments one and five are located at the junctions of the curve with adjacent lateral curves above and below. These segments are said to be at the crossover points between two curves, where sidebending mechanics change. At the crossover points there is no rotation (0° rotation) relative to the anatomic position.

Segment three is located at the apex of the curve. The apex of a curve is, by definition, the segment that has rotated the most, relative to the anatomic position. For the purpose of this example, arbitrarily assume that segment three is rotated 10° to the right from the anatomic position of 0° rotation. Segments two and four are also rotated to the right more than segments one and five, but not as much as segment three. Assume that segments two and four are rotated 5° to the right from the anatomic position.

Consider now, the individual mechanics between each of the five segments within the group. Here, individual segmental mechanics are described relative to the vertebral segment immediately below. For the sake of this analysis, begin at the base of the curve considering the mechanics of segment four relative to segment five, and work segmentally in a cephalad direction up through segment one relative to segment two. Relative to the anatomic position, the entire curve is side bent to the left, and as such each segment within the curve relative to the segment below is also side bent to the left. The base of the curve, segment five, is located at a crossover point with 0° rotation, and because the mechanics inferior to segment five are not under consideration this is all that needs to be said.

Relative to the anatomic position and relative to segment five with 0° rotation, segment four is rotated 5° to the right. Segment four, relative to segment five, is side bent left and rotated to the right.

Similarly, relative to the anatomic position, segment three (the apex of the curve) has rotated 10° to the right. This is 5° more right rotation than segment four. Relative to segment four, segment three is side bent left and rotated 5° to the right.

This next step is the one that can be confusing, but, when carefully considered, it is really quite simple. What must be remembered is that the rotational mechanics change at the apex of the curve. Segment two (the segment immediately above the apex) has only rotated 5° to the right (relative to the anatomic position), while segment three (the apex) has rotated 10° to the right. Consequently, segment two has rotated 5° less than segment three. Because segment two has rotated 5° less to the right than segment three, relative to segment three, segment two is rotated 5° to the left. Therefore segment two, relative to segment three, is side bent left and rotated 5° to the left.

Following the above logic it is readily apparent that segment one, the upper crossover point of the curve, with 0° rotation, is actually rotated 5° to the left relative to segment two, and as such, relative to segment two, segment one is side bent left and rotated left.

This exercise may seem pointless until it is realized that most OMT procedures introduce rotation in only one direction at a time. Consequently, when treating a group curve that is side bent left and rotated right with indirect principles, introducing sidebending left and rotation right will effectively treat the curve only at the apical segment and below. This can result in treatment failure, or rapid re-establishment of the dysfunctional mechanics of the entire curve.

Here, in the context of spinal lateral curves, it is appropriate to briefly discuss Fryette type II dys-

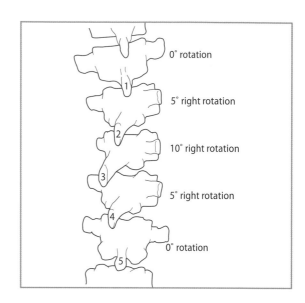

**Figure 4.2.10:** Fryette type I, group lateral curve

functional mechanics. Type II dysfunctions demonstrate non-neutral spinal physiologic motion and occur when the presence of inter-segmentally local flexion or extension engages the vertebral articular facet joints. Under these circumstances, when sidebending is introduced, the upper segment must first rotate before the sidebending can occur and the sidebending and rotation will occur coupled in the same direction. Type II dysfunctions are often found at transitional points within a type I pattern. At the crossover point between two type I curves, because the AP curve flattens, there is increased vulnerability for type II extension dysfunctions in the thoracic region and type II flexion dysfunctions in the lumbar region. Because type I curves are associated with an increase in the pre-existent AP (lordotic, kyphotic) curves, and intersegmental rotational mechanics change at the apex of a type I curve, intersegmental mechanics resembling type II (flexion mechanics) are found above the apex of a type I thoracic curve, and type II (extension mechanics) above the apex of a type I lumbar curve.

**Cervical spinal neutral mechanics**

There is some consensus that the typical vertebrae of the cervical spine do not manifest neutral mechanics.[184] This is debatable. Fryette did, in fact, describe neutral mechanics in the cervical region, noting: "As has been implied, in all movements that involve sidebending there is an accompanying twisting movement of the vertebral body toward the concavity and a tendency to sideshift toward the convexity. In sidebending-twisting-sideshift-ing, the facets interlock on the side of the concav-ity."[185] That is, relative to the anatomic position, the coupled relationship between sidebending and the resultant rotation of a group of typical cervical vertebrae (C2–C7) occurs in the same direction. In this case, the individual segmental mechanics within the group, as discussed above, demonstrate the same change above the apex of the curve. However, because of the rotational difference, in-tersegmental sidebending-rotation in the same di-rection is present in segments below the apex, and in opposite directions above the apex.

## Spinal anterior/posterior curves

### Lumbar lordosis

In the sagittal plane, alignment of the vertebral column and pelvis in a standing position exhibits a great variability among individuals. In subjects over the age of 40 without pathological spinal abnormality, the lumbar lordosis is around 64° +/- 10°.[186] To a great extent, the distinctiveness of the lumbar lordosis relies on the orientation of the sacral inclination and the pelvis. Generally, the upper portion of the lumbar lordosis stays rather constant. On the other hand, the lower portion of the lumbar lordosis, essential in the definition of the global lumbar lordosis, may vary.[187] With ag-ing, loss of lumbar lordosis occurs in particular in the lower portion of the lumbar spine.[188] This loss has been associated with chronic low back pain and orientation of the sacrum more vertically.[189] From an osteopathic perspective, when the base of the sacrum moves posteriorly, the long axis of the sacrum becomes more vertical and the superior surface of the sacral base becomes more horizon-tal. This motion, in cranial osteopathic terminol-ogy is sacral flexion (anatomic sacral extension). It occurs during the inhalation phase of the PRM (cranial flexion) and is associated with a lessen-ing of the lumbar lordosis. As such, when a patient presents a sacral (cranial model) flexion somatic dysfunction, the lumbar AP curvature is flattened.

Typically, compensation for sagittal imbalance in the vertebral column is knee flexion that is cor-related with a decrease of the lumbar lordosis.[190] Such a pattern alters the proper function of the weight-bearing joints, particularly the knee and its surrounding soft tissues, and is a risk factor for falls.[191] Quite frequently, knee flexion is also asso-ciated with increased tension in the posterior thigh muscles and hip flexors, with consequent decrease in hip mobility. Somatic dysfunction of the knee, on the other hand, may also cause postural im-balance. However, postural imbalances resulting from a somatic dysfunction of the pelvis or from the vertebral column will produce bilateral knee compensation, whereas a somatic dysfunction of the knee tends to be unilateral.

Psoas somatic dysfunction is also a major cause for lumbar lordosis decrease. Normally, the ilio-psoas group, particularly the psoas major, plays a role as both a flexor of the hip and as a dynamic stabilizer of the lumbar spine.[192] When the psoas is dysfunctionally contracted, lumbar spine exten-sion is decreased. Nevertheless, the L5–S1 level, free of psoas attachment, compensates for this decreased lordosis with increased extension, a potential source of lower back pain. As such, the appropriate treatment for these patients is the treatment of the psoas spasm, and not manipula-tion of the painful lumbosacral junction.

Psoas spasm may be classified as primary or sec-ondary. Primary spasm of the psoas major is most often bilateral, but one side commonly predomi-nates, producing a pelvic sideshift away from the predominantly tight psoas. Somatic dysfunction in the upper half of the lumbar spine will produce psoas spasm. Type II mechanics of L1 on L2 or L2 on L3, typically in flexion, with rotation and side-bending toward the side of the spastic psoas, are the most commonly encountered dysfunctional etiology. Treatment of the upper lumbar somatic dysfunction will alleviate the spasm. Secondary psoas spasm is encountered in the presence of lum-bosacral instability (herniated nucleus pulposus, spondylolisthesis) or inflammation (discitis). As a response, physiological splinting of the surrounding musculature results in psoas spasm. In this case, the definitive treatment is the effective stabilization of the unstable lumbosacral junction.[193]

Loss of muscle mass tends to occur with the aging process. While quadriceps strength diminishes with advanced age,[194] the muscle's size, as measured through cross-sections, is maintained until about 60 years of age. Psoas size, on the other hand, declines steadily from 20–60 years and significantly between 60 and 70 years.[195] As people age, they have a tendency to spend more time sitting, and less time practicing movements that would stretch the psoas. When different age groups of adults are observed standing, there are no statistically significant differences in hip extension. On the contrary, significant differences are found when subjects are walking. Older subjects demonstrate a decreased hip extension and an increased anterior pelvic tilt.[196] Therefore, in addition to OMT to balance the vertebral column and the psoas, advice should be given on proper walking, in a manner that provides control of pelvic tilt and sufficient hip extension.

**Thoracic kyphosis**

In older subjects, loss of lumbar lordosis is associated, on average, with increase of the thoracic kyphosis. Normally, the thoracic spine forms an anterior curvature, a kyphosis, associated with the shape of the vertebral bodies and intervertebral discs. In the aging individual, hyperkyphosis may result from multifactorial causes, such as vertebral fractures, inflammatory conditions, degenerative disc disease, or osteoporosis. Weakness of the thoracic paravertebral extensor muscles also contribute significantly to increased kyphosis. In healthy, post-menopausal women, back extensor strength shows a relationship with posture, such that the larger an individual's kyphosis, the greater their loss of back strength.[197] Hyperkyphosis may also be the result of compensation for somatic dysfunction elsewhere in the body, frequently in the upper thoracic and cervical spine. Dysfunction where the occipital condyles are anterior in relation to the superior atlantal facets, for instance, will oblige the patient to compensate with increased cervical lordosis and thoracic kyphosis.

Radiographically, the thoracic kyphosis is measured by the kyphosis angle. (See: 'Figure 4.2.11:

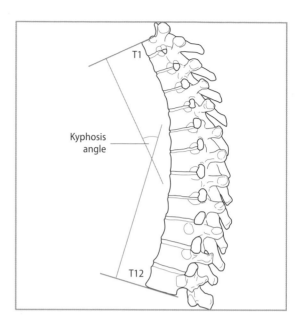

Figure 4.2.11: Kyphosis angle

Kyphosis angle.') Lines are drawn from the superior border of the uppermost vertebra of the kyphotic curve and from the inferior border of the lowermost vertebra. From these two lines, perpendicular lines are drawn. They intersect to form the kyphosis angle. Typically, kyphosis begins to increase after 40 years of age, more quickly in women than men.[198] [199] Between 55–60 years of age, the kyphosis angle measures an average of 43°, reaching 52° in women from 76–80 years of age.[200] In addition to increased upper and middle back pain, increased kyphosis is associated with impaired balance and decreased gait velocity—both risk factors for falls.[201] It is also associated with an increased risk of vertebral fracture, cardiopulmonary failure, and increased mortality.[202][203][204] As such, the quality of life decreases as the kyphosis angle increases.

Thoracic somatic dysfunction is commonly found in all patients. These dysfunctions may have their initial origin as early as the end of fetal life, or as a consequence of labor and delivery, when the head and cervical spine are excessively side bent, and the fetal head is compressed against the maternal pelvis, as a result of uterine contractions putting pressure upon the breech. Somatic dysfunction in

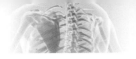

the cervical and upper thoracic regions may also occur during the delivery of the shoulders in a difficult birth. During childhood and adolescence, athletic injuries may also contribute to somatic dysfunction in the upper thoracic area. In adult life, poor posture is another potential etiology, or aggravating factor for thoracic dysfunction. As an individual ages, their head becomes more protracted forward, their shoulders more rounded, and their thoracic spine tends to develop increased kyphosis. This is particularly true in the upper thoracic region where these changes are sometimes referred to as dowager's hump.

These postural mechanics may be evaluated through a gravity line analysis. With the subject standing on a platform containing pressure sensors, the center of the distribution of force, in association with the position of the individual's feet, defines their projected center of gravity, or gravity line. In subjects over 40 years of age, this gravity line is anterior to the whole spine, whereas it passes through L4–L5 in younger individuals.[205] In the coronal plane, the gravity line shifts to the right of the spine. In several studies, the spine, pelvis, midpoint between the femoral heads, and midpoint between the heels are always located on the left of the gravity line, as a result of an unequal distribution of the body mass on either side of the sagittal plane.[206][207]

# The osteopathic contribution to the physical examination and treatment

The postural examination is a total-body examination as described in detail in 'Section 2: Osteopathic assessment,' p. 37. If possible, it should begin with the patient standing to assess their ability to deal with the forces of gravity. Further evaluation and treatment are done in the supine position. The general postural examination is intended to provide an overview of total-body functional mechanics and dysfunctional limitations. This is the context in which the patient's localized dysfunctional limitations responsible for, or contributing to, their chief complaint must be considered.

## Observation and palpation in the standing position

Observation and palpation in the standing position are achieved from the front, the side, and the back of the patient.

### From the front

Observe the global posture of the subject. Normally, the gravity line that joins the glabella, the middle of the suprasternal notch, and the pubic symphysis separates the body symmetrically into left and right halves. It should, when extended to the ground, fall halfway between the two feet.

Next, examine the symmetry of the pelvis, thorax, and anterior abdomen, and the symmetry and alignment of the lower limbs. Notice whether or not the patient appears to bear weight equally on both lower extremities. If weight-bearing is asymmetrical, try to define the cause of this asymmetry. It may be a dysfunction in the lower limb joint, or it may be related to a vertebral spinal dysfunction. Note any pelvic sideshift that may reveal a psoas dysfunction on the side opposite to the sideshift, or may be associated with an inequity of leg length toward the long leg side, or a complex combination of both.[208]

Look for inequity of the heights of the greater trochanters and iliac crests that may indicate LLI, or somatic dysfunction in the foot, knee, hip, and pelvic bone. Look for protraction or an associated asymmetrical pattern of the pectoral girdle. Compare the shoulder height.

Note any sidebending or rotation of the head that shifts the gravity line to one side. Become aware of the balance between the occipital bone and the atlas. Normally, the facial midline should be aligned with the thoracoabdominal midline. If the facial midline at the chin is deviated toward one side of the body, it may indicate a sidebending of the occipital bone toward the side opposite the direction that the facial midline deviates from. This sidebending is associated with an occipital rotation toward the side opposite the sidebending. Additionally, if the chin is displaced forward, the occipital condyle that is anterior (the condyle on the side opposite to the direction of occipital rotation) is dysfunctional. Similarly, if the chin is retracted, the dysfunction is on the side of the posterior condyle.

Observe the temporal bones. Look at the ears; they mirror the position of the temporal bones. When the ear is flared out, the ipsilateral temporal bone is habitually in external rotation. Conversely, when the ear is pinned against the side of the head, the temporal bone is in internal rotation. Next observe the position of the mandible and occlusion. Normally, the chin should be centered along the facial midline. In cases of deviation of the chin from the facial midline, as a rule, the chin is deviated toward the side of the temporal bone that is in external rotation. When this is not the case, a somatic dysfunction of the TMJ may be suspected.

### From the side

Look at lateral postural balance. Normally, the external auditory meatus, the humeral head, femoral head, mid-knee, and lateral malleolus should be in alignment. Evaluate the cervical and lumbar lordoses, and thoracic kyphosis for exaggeration of curves or gross and discrete areas of increase or flattening. Appreciate the posture of the neck; in particular, look at the upper cervical area. If there is an anteriorly displaced head position that increases the cervical lordosis and alters the facial profile, the occipital condyles are quite often positioned anteriorly. Consider also the relationship of an anteriorly displaced head posture with the cervical lordosis and the thoracic kyphosis. A forward displacement of the head could be indicative of a dysfunction of the upper cervical spine or compensation from increase of the thoracic kyphosis. Quite often, the aging patient, particularly female patients, demonstrates increased cervical and upper thoracic AP curves associated with somatic dysfunction involving the craniocervical junction or upper thoracic vertebrae. A dowager's hump—marked upper thoracic flexion with associated low

cervical extension—signals such a potential underlying dysfunction.

### From behind

Examine the symmetry of the anatomic landmarks: the ears, mastoid processes, scapular angles, shoulder heights, iliac crests, and popliteal folds. Consider the inferior hairline posteriorly that potentially reflects the position of the occiput and basicranium. Often, a pattern of occipital sidebending and rotation will be apparent. Note the alignment of midline structures: occipital protuberance, spinous processes of the vertebrae, and intergluteal fold. Ask the patient to forward bend at the hips. Asymmetric paravertebral prominences may be observed, indicative of spinal lateral curves—Fryette type I mechanics.

With the patient's arms in a relaxed position at their sides, observe the level of contact of their finger tips against the side of their legs., Unlevel finger tip position may indicate spinal sidebending, or dysfunction involving the upper limb, including the shoulder.

Palpate the shape and alignment of the spinous processes of the vertebrae. Palpate the iliac crests, sacral base, and greater trochanters. Proceed to the tests of listening (see 'Figure 2.1: Observation from behind,' in 'Section 2: Osteopathic assessment,' p. 50) to further identify previously recognized dysfunction and if necessary, also evaluate the grosser range of motion. Active and passive motion testing procedures, including the test for pelvic sideshift, may be employed. (See further: 'Section 2: Osteopathic assessment,' p. 52.)

### The Fukuda stepping test

This test may be used to identify labyrinthine dysfunction. Tadashi Fukuda described this test in 1959 to identify the weaker of the labyrinths. To do so, the subject, with their eyes closed and both arms extended, is invited to march in place for 50–100 steps. As they proceed, their rotational change in position is noted. Normally, the resultant deviation in position about the vertical axis is between 20° and 30°. A greater deviation indicates asymmetrical labyrinthine function with the impaired labyrinth on the side of the direction of rotation.[209]

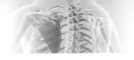

The Fukuda stepping test has been modified to assess the influence of dental occlusion upon posture. Here, the patient is asked to perform the stepping process sequentially with their teeth in contact and apart. When done before and after an osteopathic treatment, this test may also demonstrate the efficiency of the treatment. However, the reliability of this test to establish the side of vestibular dysfunction is disputed.[210]

## Observation and palpation in the supine position

Additional observation and palpation for structure and function may be accomplished with the patient in the supine position. Differences may be observed in the findings because in this position the patient does not have to respond to the forces of gravity. Somatic dysfunction will be detected, however, during the examination in both the standing and supine positions. If a restriction of motion observed in the standing position in a given area is not present during the non-weight bearing examination, it is indicative of an accommodation in this area to somatic dysfunction elsewhere.

Ask the patient to lie comfortably on the examination table. Assess their global attitude—the alignment of the different parts of their body. Consider any difficulty staying in a relaxed supine position that may reveal dysfunction. Then, observe the lower limbs to further evaluate leg length. Take hold of both feet with your hands so that your palms support the patient's heels. Compare the levels of the distal medial malleoli. Because this procedure is performed in a non-weight-bearing position it allows the examiner to assess the contribution of somatic dysfunction, which results in functional LLI, to inequity from anatomic LLI. Asymmetrical muscle spasm, particularly involving the quadrates lumborum or iliopsoas group, will result in the ipsilateral medial malleolus being pulled superiorly. The presence of a lumbar group curve will pull the lower extremity superiorly on the side of the concavity of the curve. Torsion of the pelvis will draw the acetabulum, and consequently the lower extremity, superiorly on the side

of posterior displacement of the pelvic bone, and inferiorly on the side of anterior pelvic bone displacement. These findings may then be compared to those of the standing structural examination. From the above it must be recognized that the clinical appreciation of LLI, and the differentiation between functional and anatomic LLI, is complex and, particularly when assessing for the small amount of LLI that is relevant in an osteopathic examination, if anatomic LLI is suspected, further radiological evaluation may be necessary.

Examine the feet. Look for asymmetries in the longitudinal and transversal arches. Quite often, in the aging patient the feet are flatter and more pronated. Compare the position of the ankles. Search for deformities such as hallux valgus, toe deformities, and hammer toes.

With tests of listening, evaluate the inherent motility of the PRM in the different bones of the feet. Assess the distal and proximal tibiofibular joints. Check the calcaneum, talus, cuboid, and navicular bones, as well as the subtalar, calcaneocuboid, cuneocuboid, and talonavicular articulations. Proceed to gross motion testing, if needed, and treat any identified somatic dysfunction with appropriately dosed OMT procedures. Remember that the feet affect posture, and conversely any postural dysfunction contributes to poor distribution of pressure on the feet, which promotes dysfunctions of the foot, and toe deformities.

Next, compare the knees. Look for malposition between the tibia, femur, and patella. Observe the alignment of the tibia and femur. Detect any genu varum or genu valgum, tibiofemoral rotation, and lateral or medial translation. Observe the position of the thighs, noting any asymmetry in hip flexion and external or internal rotation. When one thigh is slightly more flexed at the hip joint, with more external rotation, suspect a tight psoas muscle on that side.

Confirm observational information with tests of listening, and if necessary, further employ gross motion tests. Treat any somatic dysfunction identified. Treatment of the knees and feet are particularly important for postural balance. Most of the time, any dysfunction affecting the fibula should be considered before treatment of the knee or foot because of its influence upon knee and foot mechanics. Of the two tibiofibular articulations, the distal joint is most apt to be the site of primary articular dysfunction because it is the stronger of the two.[211] It is important here to remember the potential for the interosseous membrane to contribute to tibiofibular dysfunction.

Notice the position of the pelvis in relation to the examination table, the lower extremities below, and torso above. Lateral deviation of the pelvis from the midline may be associated with lumbosacral dysfunction. Note any asymmetry of the anatomic landmarks: anterosuperior iliac spines, iliac crests, and greater trochanters. Apply tests of listening to the pelvic bones, sacrum, and lumbar spine and treat any somatic dysfunction identified.

Observe the thoracic cage. Assess the resting pulmonary respiratory motion and diaphragmatic excursion. The pulmonary respiratory motion should be symmetrical, and diaphragmatic excursion unencumbered. Dysfunction of the pulmonary diaphragm may be present with postural imbalance, in particular when associated with lumbar and psoas somatic dysfunction. Next, assess the abdomen, and identify excessive obesity that may affect postural weight-bearing. With tests of listening, palpate the thoracic cage for dysfunction of the ribs, sternum, and diaphragm; palpate the abdominal wall and abdominal contents, and treat any identified somatic dysfunction.

Observe next the general contour and symmetry of the shoulders and clavicles. Notice any asymmetry of myofascial tension in the extremities. Observe the resting position of the head, looking for increased flexion or extension, sidebending, and rotation relative to the torso. Try to identify the origin of these positional malalignments: cervicothoracic, mid-cervical, or upper cervical. Sidebending and rotation in the same direction occurs in the upper thoracic or cervical spine; almost pure rotational dysfunctions occur between the atlas and axis; sidebending and rotation in opposite directions takes place at the occipitocervical junction. Assess the cervical, upper, mid-, and lower thoracic vertebrae,

ribs, and associated myofascial structures. Upper thoracic somatic dysfunction is frequent, often affecting the head and neck above and postural balance. Treat any somatic dysfunction that has been identified.

Observation and palpation of the neurocranium is also done in the supine position. With tests of listening, proceed to a complete examination of the skull with a vault hold approach. Appreciate the global quality of the tissues of the head, the state of tension in the intracranial and intraspinal membranes. Evaluate the different areas of reciprocal membranous tension and the quality of the PRM transmitted through the membranes. Define any areas of intracranial and intraspinal dysfunction with the membranes being tugged in that direction. Assess the frequency and potency of the CRI.

Pay particular attention to the cranial base, where the nerve supply to and from the cerebellum may be affected. Check the temporal bones, where entrapment of CN VIII can occur at the internal acoustic meatus, or as a result of dural membrane tension, increased endolymphatic pressure, or both.[212] Assess the position of the mastoid portion of the temporal bone, noting particularly the tip of the mastoid process. The mastoid process tip is posterior, medial, and high in external rotation of the temporal bone, and anterior, lateral, and low in internal rotation. Proceed to palpation for function with tests of listening. At a deeper level, evaluate the motility of intracranial fluid. Treat any identified dysfunction with indirect principles.

Observation and palpation of the orbits and eyeballs may follow. Observe the face for symmetry of the forehead, eyebrows, eyeballs, cheekbones, and temporal fossae. Palpate the frontal, sphenoid, zygomatic bones, and maxillae and employ tests of listening to confirm observational findings. Because of their muscular attachments, any dysfunction of these bones will affect the balance of the EOM. Further, the treatment of dysfunction affecting the facial bones and eyeballs promotes lymphatic drainage of the eyeballs. Follow indirect principles to treat any dysfunction.

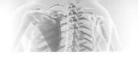
# Advice to the patient

Balance control is a complex interaction between sensory input (visual, vestibular, and proprioceptive), central processing, and neuromuscular responses. However, balance performance can be enhanced through the use of different exercises and physical activities that boost balance control while contributing to healthy aging.[213]

Proprioceptive exercises should be considered. They strengthen the proprioceptive capacity of musculoskeletal structures and provide ongoing stimulation to sensorimotor integration. For these reasons, they have the best impact upon balance regulation and fine tuning. They consist of the practice of balance exercises with and without the contribution of vision to enhance position sense in weight-bearing. They include yoga, tai chi and gymnastique douce, such as Autogenic Functional Balancing.[214]

Proprioceptive exercises focus on postural awareness and will allow the practitioner to help the patient to become self conscious of bad habits and to learn good posture. Proprioceptive exercises should start with the development of the awareness of good contact of the soles with the ground. More pressure must be distributed on the heels and less on the front of the feet. These exercises should be done on different types of surfaces to challenge proprioception. They should also include changes in the base of support such as standing with the feet more or less apart, or standing only on one foot. Strategies involving stepping or grasping movements of the limbs are recommended as well.[215] The patient's walking habits may need to be reconsidered—in particular, the tendency to walk with a forward leaning posture that maintains too much hip flexion and contributes to tightening of the hip flexors, particularly the iliopsoas muscles.

Encourage the patient to follow a regular exercise routine to improve flexibility and range of motion, in particular in the feet, toes, ankles, and hips, but also in the lumbar, thoracic, and cervical portions of the spine. Exercises should also be directed at the release of myofascial tension in the tight muscles, most often hip adductors, hamstrings, rectus femoris, tensor fascia lata, and piriformis. Encourage the patient to do gentle stretching, always within easy amplitudes, in order to avoid reflex mechanisms that increase muscle tension.

Improvements in the strength of the following muscles must be part of the program: vastus medialis and lateralis of the quadriceps femoris; the gluteus maximus and medius; the transversus and rectus abdominis; and the multifidi. The strengthening of the back extensor muscles in particular improves postural balance by reducing the tendency for increased kyphosis.

Persuade the patient of the need to wear shoes with low heels and large contact areas to reduce the risk of falls. This also helps prevent foot deformation. Encourage conservative treatments as much as possible for hallux valgus and other foot deformities. These include night splints to balance the pull of the surrounding ligaments, foot exercises to improve muscle flexibility and strength, and orthoses to correct foot function. An elastic bandage may be employed to facilitate knee proprioception. Surgical procedures may be necessary when function is affected.

Patients should be checked for visual acuity and wear appropriate eyeglasses. They should control their weight to avoid stress upon weight-bearing joints, the knees in particular.

# References

1. Standring S . Ed. Gray's Anatomy : The anatomical basis of clinical practice . 39th ed . Edinburgh : Churchill Livingstone ; 2004.

2. Couloigner V, Teixeira M, Sterkers O, Rask-Andersen H, Ferrary E. Le sac endolymphatique: ses fonctions au sein de l'oreille interne. Med Sci (Paris). 2004 Mar;20(3):304-10.

3. Magoun HI. Osteopathy in the cranial field. Kirksville, MO: The Journal Printing Company; 1951. p. 120.

4. Jones SM, Jones TA, Mills KN, Gaines GC. Anatomical and Physiological Considerations in Vestibular Dysfunction and Compensation. Semin Hear. 2009;30(4): 231-241.

5. Hanes DA, McCollum G. Cognitive-vestibular interactions: a review of patient difficulties and possible mechanisms. J Vestib Res. 2006;16(3):75-91.

6. Smith PF, Darlington CL, Zheng Y. Move it or lose it--is stimulation of the vestibular system necessary for normal spatial memory? Hippocampus. 2010 Jan;20(1):36-43.

7. Yates BJ, Bronstein AM. The effects of vestibular system lesions on autonomic regulation: observations, mechanisms, and clinical implications. J Vestib Res. 2005;15(3):119-29.

8. Nelson KE, Sergueef N, Lipinski C, Chapman A, Glonek T. Cranial rhythmic impulse related to the Traube-Hering-Mayer oscillation: comparing laser-Doppler flowmetry and palpation. J Am Osteopath Assoc. 2001 Mar;101(3):163-73.

9. Nelson KE, Sergueef N, Glonek T. The Effect of an Alternative Medical Procedure (CV-4) upon Low-Frequency Oscillations in Cutaneous Blood flow Velocity. J Manip Phys Ther. 2006; 29(8):626-36.

10. Glonek T, Sergueef N, Nelson KE. Physiological Rhythms/Oscillations. Chapt 11. In: Chila AG. ed. Foundations of Osteopathic Medicine. 3rd ed. Philadelphia: Wolters Kluwer/Lippincott Williams and Wilkins. 2011:162-90.

11. Donaldson IM.The functions of the proprioceptors of the eye muscles. Philos Trans R Soc Lond B Biol Sci. 2000 Dec 29;355(1404):1685-754.

12. Weir CR. Proprioception in extraocular muscles. J Neuroophthalmol. 2006 Jun;26(2):123-7.

13. Williams PL, editor. Gray's anatomy. 38th ed. Edinburgh: Churchill Livingstone; 1995.

14. Clark RA, Demer JL. Effect of aging on human rectus extraocular muscle paths demonstrated by magnetic resonance imaging. Am J Ophthalmol. 2002 Dec;134(6):872-8.

15. Magoun HI. Entrapment neuropathy of the central nervous system. II. Cranial nerves I-IV, VI-VIII, XII. J Am Osteopath Assoc. 1968 Mar;67(7):779-87.

16. Paulus WM, Straube A, Brandt T.Visual stabilization of posture. Physiological stimulus characteristics and clinical aspects. Brain. 1984 Dec;107 ( Pt 4):1143-63.

17. Mohapatra S, Krishnan V, Aruin AS. The effect of decreased visual acuity on control of posture. Clin Neurophysiol. 2012 Jan;123(1):173-82.

18. Ivers RQ, Cumming RG, Mitchell P, Attebo K. Visual impairment and falls in older adults: the Blue Mountains Eye Study. J Am Geriatr Soc. 1998 Jan;46(1):58-64.

19. Foran S, Wang JJ, Mitchell P. Causes of visual impairment in two older population cross-sections: the Blue Mountains Eye Study. Ophthalmic Epidemiol. 2003 Oct;10(4):215-25.

20. Patel I, West SK. Presbyopia: prevalence, impact, and interventions. Community Eye Health. 2007 Sep;20(63):40-1.

21. Lord SR, Dayhew J, Howland A.Multifocal glasses impair edge-contrast sensitivity and depth perception and increase the risk of falls in older people. J Am Geriatr Soc. 2002 Nov;50(11):1760-6.

22. Johnson L, Buckley JG, Scally AJ, Elliott DB. Multifocal spectacles increase variability in toe clearance and risk of tripping in the elderly. Invest Ophthalmol Vis Sci. 2007 Apr;48(4):1466-71.

23. Johnson L, Buckley JG, Harley C, Elliott DB. Use of single-vision eyeglasses improves stepping precision and safety when elderly habitual multifocal wearers negotiate a raised surface. J Am Geriatr Soc. 2008 Jan;56(1):178-80.

24. Haran MJ, Cameron ID, Ivers RQ, Simpson JM, Lee BB, Tanzer M. et al. Effect on falls of providing single lens distance vision glasses to multifocal glasses wearers: VISIBLE randomised controlled trial. BMJ. 2010 May 25;340:c2265.

25. Lord SR, Dayhew J. Visual risk factors for falls in older people. J Am Geriatr Soc. 2001 May;49(5):508-15.

26. Schwesig R, Goldich Y, Hahn A, Müller A, Kohen-Raz R, Kluttig A, Morad Y. Postural control in subjects with visual impairment. Eur J Ophthalmol. 2011 May-Jun;21(3):303-9.

27. Uchiyama M, Demura S. Low visual acuity is associated with the decrease in postural sway. Tohoku J Exp Med. 2008 Nov;216(3):277-85.

28. Harwood RH. Visual problems and falls. Age Ageing. 2001 Nov;30 Suppl 4:13-8.

29. Harwood RH. Visual problems and falls. Age Ageing. 2001 Nov;30 Suppl 4:13-8.

30. Elliott DB, Chapman GJ. Adaptive gait changes due to spectacle magnification and dioptric blur in older people. Invest Ophthalmol Vis Sci. 2010 Feb;51(2):718-22.

31. Helbostad JL, Vereijken B, Hesseberg K, Sletvold O. Altered vision destabilizes gait in older persons. Gait Posture. 2009 Aug;30(2):233-8.

32. Roll R, Kavounoudias A, Roll JP. Cutaneous afferents from human plantar sole contribute to body posture awareness. Neuroreport. 2002 Oct 28;13(15):1957-61.

33. Kars HJ, Hijmans JM, Geertzen JH, Zijlstra W. The effect of reduced somatosensation on standing balance: a systematic review. J Diabetes Sci Technol. 2009 Jul 1;3(4):931-43.

34. Burke D, Dickson HG, Skuse NF. Task-dependent changes in the responses to low-threshold cutaneous afferent volleys in the human lower limb. J Physiol. 1991 Jan;432:445-58.

35. Proske U, Gandevia SC.The kinaesthetic senses. J Physiol. 2009 Sep 1;587(Pt 17):4139-46.

36. Windhorst U. Muscle spindles are multi-functional. Brain Res Bull. 2008 Mar 28;75(5):507-8.

37. Proske U. Kinesthesia: the role of muscle receptors. Muscle Nerve. 2006 Nov;34(5):545-58.

38. Windhorst U. Muscle spindles are multi-functional. Brain Res Bull. 2008 Mar 28;75(5):507-8.

39. Denslow JS, Korr IM, Krems AD. Quantitative studies of chronic facilitation in human motoneuron pools. Am J Physiol. 1947 Aug;150(2):229-238.

40. Patterson MM, Wurster RD. Somatic Dysfunction, Spinal Facilitation, and Viscerosomatic Integration. Chapt. 9. In: Chila AG. ed. Foundations of Osteopathic Medicine. 3rd ed. Philadelphia: Wolters Kluwer/Lippincott Williams and Wilkins; 2011:1106.

41. Zimny ML. Mechanoreceptors in articular tissues. Am J Anat. 1988 May;182(1):16-32.

42. Proske U, Gandevia SC. The kinaesthetic senses. J Physiol. 2009 Sep 1;587(Pt 17):4139-46.

43. Shaffer SW, Harrison AL. Aging of the somatosensory system: a translational perspective. Phys Ther. 2007 Feb;87(2):193-207.

44. Kenshalo DR Sr. Somesthetic sensitivity in young and elderly humans. J Gerontol. 1986 Nov;41(6):732-42.

45. Lin YH, Hsieh SC, Chao CC, Chang YC, Hsieh ST. Influence of aging on thermal and vibratory thresholds of quantitative sensory testing. J Peripher Nerv Syst. 2005 Sep;10(3):269-81.

46. Kaplan FS, Nixon JE, Reitz M, Rindfleish L, Tucker J. Age-related changes in proprioception and sensation of joint position. Acta Orthop Scand. 1985 Feb;56(1):72-4.

47. Petrella RJ, Lattanzio PJ, Nelson MG. Effect of age and activity on knee joint proprioception. Am J Phys Med Rehabil. 1997 May-Jun;76(3):235-41.

48. Low Choy NL, Brauer SG, Nitz JC. Age-related changes in strength and somatosensation during midlife: rationale for targeted preventive intervention programs. Ann N Y Acad Sci. 2007 Oct;1114:180-93.

49. Carmeli E, Reznick AZ. The physiology and biochemistry of skeletal muscle atrophy as a function of age. Proc Soc Exp Biol Med. 1994 Jun;206(2):103-13.

50. Lindle RS, Metter EJ, Lynch NA, Fleg JL, Fozard JL, Tobin J, Roy TA, Hurley BF. Age and gender comparisons of muscle strength in 654 women and men aged 20-93 yr. J Appl Physiol. 1997 Nov;83(5):1581-7.

51. Carmeli E, Reznick AZ. The physiology and biochemistry of skeletal muscle atrophy as a function of age. Proc Soc Exp Biol Med. 1994 Jun;206(2):103-13.

52. McCarter RJ. Age-related changes in skeletal muscle function. Aging (Milano). 1990 Mar;2(1):27-38.

53. Carmeli E, Reznick AZ. The physiology and biochemistry of skeletal muscle atrophy as a function of age. Proc Soc Exp Biol Med. 1994 Jun;206(2):103-13.

54. Janda, V. Muscles and motor control in low back pain: Assessment and management. In: Physical therapy of the low back, Twomey LT ed. New York NY: Churchill Livingstone, 1987.

55. Häkkinen K, Häkkinen A. Muscle cross-sectional area, force production and relaxation characteristics in women at different ages. Eur J Appl Physiol Occup Physiol. 1991;62(6):410-4.

56. Lord SR, Rogers MW, Howland A, Fitzpatrick R. Lateral stability, sensorimotor function and falls in older people. J Am Geriatr Soc. 1999 Sep;47(9):1077-81.

57. Johnson ME, Mille ML, Martinez KM, Crombie G, Rogers MW. Age-related changes in hip abductor and adductor joint torques. Arch Phys Med Rehabil. 2004 Apr;85(4):593-7.

58. Nitz JC, Choy NL, Isles RC. Medial-lateral postural stability in community-dwelling women over 40 years of age. Clin Rehabil. 2003 Nov;17(7):765-7.

59. Maki BE, Edmondstone MA, McIlroy WE. Age-related differences in laterally directed compensatory stepping behavior. J Gerontol A Biol Sci Med Sci. 2000 May;55(5):M270-7.

60. Brauer SG, Burns YR, Galley P. A prospective study of laboratory and clinical measures of postural stability to predict community-dwelling fallers. J Gerontol A Biol Sci Med Sci. 2000 Aug;55(8):M469-76.

61. Felson DT, Naimark A, Anderson J, Kazis L, Castelli W, Meenan RF. The prevalence of knee osteoarthritis in the elderly. The Framingham Osteoarthritis Study. Arthritis Rheum. 1987 Aug;30(8):914-8.

62. Hassan BS, Mockett S, Doherty M. Static postural sway, proprioception, and maximal voluntary quadriceps contraction in patients with knee osteoarthritis and normal control subjects. Ann Rheum Dis. 2001 Jun;60(6):612-8.

63. Johansson H, Sjölander P, Sojka P. A sensory role for the cruciate ligaments. Clin Orthop Relat Res. 1991 Jul;(268):161-78.

64. Assimakopoulos AP, Katonis PG, Agapitos MV, Exarchou EI. The innervation of the human meniscus. Clin Orthop Relat Res. 1992 Feb;(275):232-6.

65. Hassan BS, Mockett S, Doherty M. Static postural sway, proprioception, and maximal voluntary quadriceps contraction in patients with knee osteoarthritis and normal control subjects. Ann Rheum Dis. 2001 Jun;60(6):612-8.

66. Hall MC, Mockett SP, Doherty M. Relative impact of radiographic osteoarthritis and pain on quadriceps strength, proprioception, static postural sway and lower limb function. Dis. 2006 Jul;65(7):865-70.

67. Hassan BS, Doherty SA, Mockett S, Doherty M. Effect of pain reduction on postural sway, proprioception, and quadriceps strength in subjects with knee osteoarthritis. Ann Rheum Dis. 2002 May;61(5):422-8.

68. Grubb BD. Activation of sensory neurons in the arthritic joint. Novartis Found Symp. 2004;260:28-36; discussion 36-48, 100-4, 277-9.

69. Bennell KL, Hunt MA, Wrigley TV, Lim BW, Hinman RS. Role of muscle in the genesis and management of knee osteoarthritis. Rheum Dis Clin North Am. 2008 Aug;34(3):731-54.

70. Kroenke K, Mangelsdorff AD. Common symptoms in ambulatory care: incidence, evaluation, therapy, and outcome. Am J Med. 1989 Mar;86(3):262-6.

71. Tusa RJ. Dizziness. Med Clin North Am. 2009 Mar;93(2):263-71, vii.

72. Fife TD. Benign paroxysmal positional vertigo. Semin Neurol. 2009 Nov;29(5):500-8.

73. Riga M, Bibas A, Xenellis J, Korres S. Inner ear disease and benign paroxysmal positional vertigo: a critical review of incidence, clinical characteristics, and management. Int J Otolaryngol. 2011;2011:709469.

74. Kuether TA, Nesbit GM, Clark WM, Barnwell SL. Rotational vertebral artery occlusion: a mechanism of vertebrobasilar insufficiency. Neurosurgery. 1997 Aug;41(2):427-32; discussion 432-3.

75. Korres S, Balatsouras DG, Kaberos A, Economou C, Kandiloros D, Ferekidis E. Occurrence of semicircular canal involvement in benign paroxysmal positional vertigo. Otol Neurotol. 2002 Nov;23(6):926-32.

76. Dix MR, Hallpike CS. The pathology symptomatology and diagnosis of certain common disorders of the vestibular system. Proc R Soc Med. 1952 Jun;45(6):341-54.

77. Balatsouras DG, Koukoutsis G, Ganelis P, Korres GS, Kaberos A. Diagnosis of Single- or Multiple-Canal Benign Paroxysmal Positional Vertigo according to the Type of Nystagmus. Int J Otolaryngol. 2011;2011:483965.

78. Epley JM. The canalith repositioning procedure: for treatment of benign paroxysmal positional vertigo. Otolaryngol Head Neck Surg. 1992 Sep;107(3):399-404.

79. Fife TD. Benign paroxysmal positional vertigo. Semin Neurol. 2009 Nov;29(5):500-8.

80. De Stefano A, Dispenza F, Citraro L, Petrucci AG, Di Giovanni P, Kulamarva G, Mathur N, Croce A. Are postural restrictions necessary for management of posterior canal benign paroxysmal positional vertigo? Ann Otol Rhinol Laryngol. 2011 Jul;120(7):460-4.

81. Haynes DS, Resser JR, Labadie RF, Girasole CR, Kovach BT, Scheker LE, Walker DC. Treatment of benign positional vertigo using the semont maneuver: efficacy in patients presenting without nystagmus. Laryngoscope. 2002 May;112(5):796-801.

82. Menière P. Maladies de l'oreille interne offrant les symptômes de la congestion cérébrale apoplectiforme. Gaz Med de Paris 1861; 16: 88-9.

83. Arweiler DJ, Jahnke K, Grosse-Wilde H. Menière disease as an autosome dominant hereditary disease. Laryngorhinootologie. 1995 Aug;74(8):512-5.

84. Meniere's disease: overview, epidemiology, and natural history. da Costa SS, de Sousa LC, Piza MR. Otolaryngol Clin North Am. 2002 Jun;35(3):455-95.

85. Committee on Hearing and Equilibrium guidelines for the diagnosis and evaluation of therapy in Menière's disease. American Academy of Otolaryngology-Head and Neck Foundation, Inc. No authors listed. Otolaryngol Head Neck Surg. 1995 Sep;113(3):181-5.

86. Derebery MJ. Allergic and immunologic features of Ménière's disease. Otolaryngol Clin North Am. 2011 Jun;44(3):655-66, ix.

87. Arenberg IK, Lemke C, Shambaugh GE Jr. Viral theory for Ménière's disease and endolymphatic hydrops: overview and new therapeutic options for viral labyrinthitis. Ann N Y Acad Sci. 1997 Dec 29;830:306-13.

88. Gacek RR. Evidence for a viral neuropathy in recurrent vertigo. ORL J Otorhinolaryngol Relat Spec. 2008;70(1):6-14; discussion 14-5.

89. Pérez López L, Belinchón de Diego A, Bermell Carrión A, Pérez Garrigues H, Morera Pérez C. Ménière's disease and migraine. Acta Otorrinolaringol Esp. 2006 Mar;57(3):126-9.

90. Shulman A, Goldstein B. Brain and inner-ear fluid homeostasis, cochleovestibular-type tinnitus, and secondary endolymphatic hydrops. Int Tinnitus J. 2006;12(1):75-81.

91. Couloigner V, Teixeira M, Sterkers O, Rask-Andersen H, Ferrary E. Le sac endolymphatique: ses fonctions au sein de l'oreille interne. Med Sci (Paris). 2004 Mar;20(3):304-10.

92. Shulman A, Goldstein B. Brain and inner-ear fluid homeostasis, cochleovestibular-type tinnitus, and secondary endolymphatic hydrops. Int Tinnitus J. 2006;12(1):75-81.

93. Nakashima T, Sone M, Teranishi M, Yoshida T, Terasaki H, Kondo M. et al. A perspective from magnetic resonance imaging findings of the inner ear: Relationships among cerebrospinal, ocular and inner ear fluids. Auris Nasus Larynx. 2012 Aug;39(4):345-55.

94. Shulman A, Goldstein B. Brain and inner-ear fluid homeostasis, cochleovestibular-type tinnitus, and secondary endolymphatic hydrops. Int Tinnitus J. 2006;12(1):75-81.

95. Magoun HI. Osteopathy in the cranial field. 2nd ed. Kirksville, MO: The Journal Printing Company; 1966. p. 151.

96. Meniere's disease: overview, epidemiology, and natural history. da Costa SS, de Sousa LC, Piza MR. Otolaryngol Clin North Am. 2002 Jun;35(3):455-95.

97. Paparella MM, Sajjadi H.Endolymphatic sac enhancement. Otolaryngol Clin North Am. 1994 Apr;27(2):381-402.

98. Sajjadi H, Paparella MM. Meniere's disease. Lancet. 2008 Aug 2;372(9636):406-14.

99. Peck D, Buxton DF, Nitz A.. A comparison of spindle concentrations in large and small muscles acting in parallel combinations. J Morphol. 1984 Jun;180(3):243-52.

100. Kulkarni V, Chandy MJ, Babu KS. Quantitative study of muscle spindles in suboccipital muscles of human foetuses. Neurol India. 2001 Dec;49(4):355-9.

101. Corneil BD, Olivier E, Munoz DP. Neck muscle responses to stimulation of monkey superior colliculus. II. Gaze shift initiation and volitional head movements. J Neurophysiol. 2002 Oct;88(4):2000-18.

102. Kristjansson E, Treleaven J. Sensorimotor function and dizziness in neck pain: implications for assessment and management. J Orthop Sports Phys Ther. 2009 May;39(5):364-77.

103. Nolan M, Nitz J, Choy NL, Illing S. Age-related changes in musculoskeletal function, balance and mobility measures in men aged 30-80 years. Aging Male. 2010 Sep;13(3):194-201.

104. Field S, Treleaven J, Jull G. Standing balance: a comparison between idiopathic and whiplash-induced neck pain. Man Ther. 2008 Jun;13(3):183-91.

105. Sterling M, Jull G, Vicenzino B, Kenardy J, Darnell R. Development of motor system dysfunction following whiplash injury. Pain. 2003 May;103(1-2):65-73.

106. Treleaven J. Sensorimotor disturbances in neck disorders affecting postural stability, head and eye movement control. Man Ther. 2008 Feb;13(1):2-11.

107. Sterling M, Jull G, Vicenzino B, Kenardy J, Darnell R. Development of motor system dysfunction following whiplash injury. Pain. 2003 May;103(1-2):65-73.

108. Sterling M, Jull G, Vicenzino B, Kenardy J, Darnell R. Physical and psychological factors predict outcome following whiplash injury. Pain. 2005 Mar;114(1-2):141-8.

109. Treleaven J, Clamaron-Cheers C, Jull G. Does the region of pain influence the presence

of sensorimotor disturbances in neck pain disorders? Man Ther. 2011 Dec;16(6):636-40.

110. McPartland JM, Brodeur RR, Hallgren RC. Chronic neck pain, standing balance, and suboccipital muscle atrophy--a pilot study. J Manipulative Physiol Ther. 1997 Jan;20(1):24-9.

111. Glossary of Osteopathic Terminology. In: Chila AG. editor. Foundations of Osteopathic Medicine. 3rd ed. Philadelphia: Wolters Kluwer/Lippincott Williams and Wilkins; 2011:1106.

112. Kristjansson E, Treleaven J. Sensorimotor function and dizziness in neck pain: implications for assessment and management. J Orthop Sports Phys Ther. 2009 May;39(5):364-77.

113. Schweigart G, Chien RD, Mergner T. Neck proprioception compensates for age-related deterioration of vestibular self-motion perception. Exp Brain Res. 2002 Nov;147(1):89-97.

114. Kelders WP, Kleinrensink GJ, van der Geest JN, Feenstra L, de Zeeuw CI, Frens MA. Compensatory increase of the cervico-ocular reflex with age in healthy humans. J Physiol. 2003 Nov 15;553(Pt 1):311-7.

115. Denslow JS, Korr IM, Krems AD. Quantitative studies of chronic facilitation in human motoneuron pools. Am J Physiol. 1947 Aug;150(2):229-238.

116. Buzzell KA. The Potential Disruptive Influence of Somatic Input. In: The Physiological Basis of Osteopathic Medicine. Kugelmass IN editor. The Postgraduate Institute of Osteopathic Medicine and Surgery. New York NY. 1970:39-51.

117. Cuccia A, Caradonna C. The relationship between the stomatognathic system and body posture. Clinics (Sao Paulo). 2009;64(1):61-6.

118. Hiiemae KM, Palmer JB. Tongue movements in feeding and speech. Crit Rev Oral Biol Med. 2003;14(6):413-29.

119. Trulsson M. Sensory-motor function of human periodontal mechanoreceptors. J Oral Rehabil. 2006 Apr;33(4):262-73.

120. Klineberg I, Murray G. Osseoperception: sensory function and proprioception. Adv Dent Res. 1999 Jun;13:120-9.

121. Klineberg I, Murray G. Osseoperception: sensory function and proprioception. Adv Dent Res. 1999 Jun;13:120-9.

122. Yoshida M, Kikutani T, Okada G, Kawamura T, Kimura M, Akagawa Y. The effect of tooth loss on body balance control among community-dwelling elderly persons. Int J Prosthodont. 2009 Mar-Apr;22(2):136-9.

123. Yamaga T, Yoshihara A, Ando Y, Yoshitake Y, Kimura Y, Shimada M, Nishimuta M, Miyazaki H. Relationship between dental occlusion and physical fitness in an elderly population. J Gerontol A Biol Sci Med Sci. 2002 Sep;57(9):M616-20.

124. Ries LG, Bérzin F. Analysis of the postural stability in individuals with or without signs and symptoms of temporomandibular disorder. Braz Oral Res. 2008 Oct-Dec;22(4):378-83.

125. Matheus RA, Ramos-Perez FM, Menezes AV, Ambrosano GM, Haiter-Neto F, Bóscolo FN, de Almeida SM. The relationship between temporomandibular dysfunction and head

and cervical posture. J Appl Oral Sci. 2009 May-Jun;17(3):204-8.

126. Cuccia A, Caradonna C. The relationship between the stomatognathic system and body posture. Clinics (Sao Paulo). 2009;64(1):61-6.

127. de Farias Neto JP, de Santana JM, de Santana-Filho VJ, Quintans-Junior LJ, de Lima Ferreira AP, Bonjardim LR. Radiographic measurement of the cervical spine in patients with temporomandibular dysfunction. Arch Oral Biol. 2010 Sep;55(9):670-8.

128. Valentino B, Fabozzo A, Melito F. The functional relationship between the occlusal plane and the plantar arches. An EMG study. Surg Radiol Anat. 1991;13(3):171-4.

129. Darling DW, Kraus S, Glasheen-Wray MB. Relationship of head posture and the rest position of the mandible. J Prosthet Dent. 1984 Jul;52(1):111-5.

130. Milani RS, De Perière DD, Lapeyre L, Pourreyron L. Relationship between dental occlusion and posture. Cranio. 2000 Apr;18(2):127-34.

131. Marfurt CF, Rajchert DM. Trigeminal primary afferent projections to 'non-trigeminal' areas of the rat central nervous system. J Comp Neurol. 1991 Jan 15;303(3):489-511.

132. Stack B, Sims A. The relationship between posture and equilibrium and the auriculo-temporal nerve in patients with disturbed gait and balance. Cranio. 2009 Oct;27(4):248-60.

133. Gangloff P, Perrin PP. Unilateral trigeminal anaesthesia modifies postural control in human subjects. Neurosci Lett. 2002 Sep 20;330(2):179-82.

134. .Sergueef N, Nelson KE, Glonek T. Palpatory diagnosis of plagiocephaly Complement Ther Clin Pract. 2006 May;12(2):101-10.

135. Mitchell FL. The balanced pelvis and its relationship to reflexes. Year Book of the Academy of Applied Osteopathy. American Academy of Osteopathy. Indianapolis, IN. 1948:146-51.

136. Sergueef N. L'Odyssée de l'iliaque. Paris: Spek; 1985.

137. Sergueef N. L'Odyssée de l'iliaque. Paris: Spek; 1985.

138. Knutson GA. Anatomic and functional leg-length inequality: a review and recommendation for clinical decision-making. Part I, anatomic leg-length inequality: prevalence, magnitude, effects and clinical significance. Chiropr Osteopat. 2005 Jul 20;13:11.

139. Denslow JS, Chace JA. Mechanical stresses in the human lumbar spine and pelvis. J Am Osteopath Assoc. 1962 May;61:705-12.

140. Knutson GA. Anatomic and functional leg-length inequality: a review and recommendation for clinical decision-making. Part I, anatomic leg-length inequality: prevalence, magnitude, effects and clinical significance. Chiropr Osteopat. 2005 Jul 20;13:11.

141. Knutson GA. Anatomic and functional leg-length inequality: a review and recommendation for clinical decision-making. Part II. The functional or unloaded leg-length asymmetry. Chiropr Osteopat. 2005 Jul 20;13:12.

142. Nelson KE, Mnabhi A. The patient with back pain: Short leg syndrome and postural balance, Chapt. 26. In: Nelson, Glonek, eds., Somatic Dysfunction in Osteopathic

Family Medicine. Baltimore, MD: Lippincott, Williams & Wilkins; 2007;408-33.

143. Magoun HI Jr. Chronic psoas syndrome caused by the inappropriate use of a heel lift. J Am Osteopath Assoc. 2008 Nov;108(11):629-30; discussion 630.

144. Betsch M, Schneppendahl J, Dor L, Jungbluth P, Grassmann JP, Windolf J, Thelen S, Hakimi M, Rapp W, Wild M Influence of foot positions on the spine and pelvis. Arthritis Care Res (Hoboken). 2011 Dec;63(12):1758-65.

145. Cummings G, Scholz JP, Barnes K. The effect of imposed leg length difference on pelvic bone symmetry. Spine (Phila Pa 1976). 1993 Mar 1;18(3):368-73.

146. Cooperstein R, Lew M. The relationship between pelvic torsion and anatomical leg length inequality: a review of the literature. J Chiropr Med. 2009 Sep;8(3):107-18.

147. Young RS, Andrew PD, Cummings GS. Effect of simulating leg length inequality on pelvic torsion and trunk mobility. Gait Posture. 2000 Jun;11(3):217-23.

148. Denslow JS, Chace JA. Mechanical stresses in the human lumbar spine and pelvis. J Am Osteopath Assoc. 1962 May;61:705-12.

149. Beal MC. The short leg problem. J Am Osteopath Assoc. 1977 Jun;76(10):745-51.

150. Mitchell FL Sr. Structural pelvic function. In: Academy of Applied Osteopathy 1965 Yearbook. Indianapolis, IN: American Academy of Osteopathy; 1965;v2:178–199.

151. Strachan W.E., Beckwith C.G., Larson N.J., Grant J.H.: A Study of the Mechanics of the Sacroiliac Joint. J Am Osteopath Assoc. 1938; 37(12):575-8.

152. Beilke M.C. Simple Mechanics of the Sacrolumbar Group. J Am Osteopath Assoc. 1939;39:165-7.

153. Nichols PJ, Bailey NT. The accuracy of measuring leg-length differences; an observer error experiment. Br Med J. 1955 Nov 19;2(4950):1247-8.

154. Knutson GA. Anatomic and functional leg-length inequality: a review and recommendation for clinical decision-making. Part II. The functional or unloaded leg-length asymmetry. Chiropr Osteopat. 2005 Jul 20;13:12.

155. Sabharwal S, Kumar A. Methods for assessing leg length discrepancy. Clin Orthop Relat Res. 2008 Dec;466(12):2910-22.

156. Sabharwal S, Kumar A. Methods for assessing leg length discrepancy. Clin Orthop Relat Res. 2008 Dec;466(12):2910-22.

157. Hoskins ER. The Development of Posture and Its Importance. J Am Osteopath Assoc. 1933:529; 1934:72,125,175.

158. Beilke M. Roentgenological spinal analysis and the technic for taking standing X-ray plates. J Am Osteopath Assoc. 1936;35:414–418.

159. Denslow JS, Chace JA, Gutensohn OR, Kumm MG. Methods in taking and interpreting weight-bearing X-ray films. J Am Osteopath Assoc. 1955 Jul;54(11):663-70.

160. Willman MK. Radiographic technical aspects of the postural study. J Am Osteopath Assoc. 1977 Jun;76(10):739-44.

161. Kuchera ML. Postural Considerations in Osteopathic Diagnosis and Treatment.

Chapt. 36 in: Chila AG. ed. Foundations of Osteopathic Medicine. 3rd ed. Philadelphia, PA: Lippincott Williams and Wilkins; 2011:452-9.

162. Knutson GA. Anatomic and functional leg-length inequality: a review and recommendation for clinical decision-making. Part II. The functional or unloaded leg-length asymmetry. Chiropr Osteopat. 2005 Jul 20;13:12.

163. Nelson KE, Habenicht AL, Sergueef N. The Geriatric Patient. Chapt. 12 in: Nelson, Glonek, eds., Somatic Dysfunction in Osteopathic Family Medicine. Baltimore, MD: Lippincott, Williams & Wilkins; 2007;159-80.

164. Nelson KE, Mnabhi A. The patient with back pain: Short leg syndrome and postural balance, Chapt. 26. In: Nelson, Glonek, eds., Somatic Dysfunction in Osteopathic Family Medicine. Baltimore, MD: Lippincott, Williams & Wilkins; 2007;408-33.

165. Magoun HI Jr. Chronic psoas syndrome caused by the inappropriate use of a heel lift. J Am Osteopath Assoc. 2008 Nov;108(11):629-30; discussion 630.

166. Wright WG, Ivanenko YP, Gurfinkel VS. Foot anatomy specialization for postural sensation and control. J Neurophysiol. 2011 Dec 7.

167. Menz HB, Tiedemann A, Kwan MM, Plumb K, Lord SR. Foot pain in community-dwelling older people: an evaluation of the Manchester Foot Pain and Disability Index. Rheumatology (Oxford). 2006 Jul;45(7):863-7.

168. Thomas E, Peat G, Harris L, Wilkie R, Croft PR. The prevalence of pain and pain interference in a general population of older adults: cross-sectional findings from the North Staffordshire Osteoarthritis Project (NorStOP). Pain. 2004 Jul;110(1-2):361-8.

169. Roddy E, Muller S, Thomas E. Onset and persistence of disabling foot pain in community-dwelling older adults over a 3-year period: a prospective cohort study. J Gerontol A Biol Sci Med Sci. 2011 Apr;66(4):474-80.

170. Menz HB, Tiedemann A, Kwan MM, Plumb K, Lord SR. Foot pain in community-dwelling older people: an evaluation of the Manchester Foot Pain and Disability Index. Rheumatology (Oxford). 2006 Jul;45(7):863-7.

171. Scott G, Menz HB, Newcombe L. Age-related differences in foot structure and function. Gait Posture. 2007 Jun;26(1):68-75.

172. Menz HB, Morris ME, Lord SR. Foot and ankle risk factors for falls in older people: a prospective study. J Gerontol A Biol Sci Med Sci. 2006 Aug;61(8):866-70.

173. Menz HB, Tiedemann A, Kwan MM, Plumb K, Lord SR. Foot pain in community-dwelling older people: an evaluation of the Manchester Foot Pain and Disability Index. Rheumatology (Oxford). 2006 Jul;45(7):863-7.

174. Perera AM, Mason L, Stephens MM. The pathogenesis of hallux valgus. J Bone Joint Surg Am. 2011 Sep 7;93(17):1650-61.

175. Ferrari J, Malone-Lee J. The shape of the metatarsal head as a cause of hallux abductovalgus. Foot Ankle Int. 2002 Mar;23(3):236-42.

176. Nguyen US, Hillstrom HJ, Li W, Dufour AB, Kiel DP, Procter-Gray E. et al. Factors associated with hallux valgus in a population-based

study of older women and men: the MOBILIZE Boston Study. Osteoarthritis Cartilage. 2010 Jan;18(1):41-6.

177. Perera AM, Mason L, Stephens MM. The pathogenesis of hallux valgus. J Bone Joint Surg Am. 2011 Sep 7;93(17):1650-61.

178. Ward ED, Phillips RD, Patterson PE, Werkhoven GJ. 1998 William J. Stickel Gold Award. The effects of extrinsic muscle forces on the forefoot-to-rearfoot loading relationship in vitro. Tibia and Achilles tendon. J Am Podiatr Med Assoc. 1998 Oct;88(10):471-82.

179. Schwab F, Lafage V, Boyce R, Skalli W, Farcy JP. Gravity line analysis in adult volunteers: age-related correlation with spinal parameters, pelvic parameters, and foot position. Spine (Phila Pa 1976). 2006 Dec 1;31(25):E959-67.

180. Strachan WF. Applied anatomy of the pelvis and lower extremities. J Am Osteopath Assoc. 1940;40(2):59-60.

181. Roussouly P, Gollogly S, Berthonnaud E, Dimnet J. Classification of the normal variation in the sagittal alignment of the human lumbar spine and pelvis in the standing position. Spine (Phila Pa 1976). 2005 Feb 1;30(3):346-53.

182. Fryette HH. Physiologic movements of the spine. J Am Osteopath Assoc. 1918;18:1-2.

183. Fryette HH. Principles of Osteopathic Technic. Indianapolis, IN: American Academy of Osteopathy; 1954.

184. Glossary of Osteopathic Terminology. In: Chila AG. ed. Foundations of Osteopathic Medicine. 3nd ed. Philadelphia: Wolters Kluwer/Lippincott Williams and Wilkins; 2011:1099.

185. Fryette HH. Principles of Osteopathic Technic. Indianapolis, IN: American Academy of Osteopathy; 1980:29.

186. Gelb DE, Lenke LG, Bridwell KH, Blanke K, McEnery KW. An analysis of sagittal spinal alignment in 100 asymptomatic middle and older aged volunteers. Spine (Phila Pa 1976). 1995 Jun 15;20(12):1351-8.

187. Roussouly P, Gollogly S, Berthonnaud E, Dimnet J. Classification of the normal variation in the sagittal alignment of the human lumbar spine and pelvis in the standing position. Spine (Phila Pa 1976). 2005 Feb 1;30(3):346-53.

188. Gelb DE, Lenke LG, Bridwell KH, Blanke K, McEnery KW. An analysis of sagittal spinal alignment in 100 asymptomatic middle and older aged volunteers. Spine (Phila Pa 1976). 1995 Jun 15;20(12):1351-8.

189. Evcik D, Yücel A. Lumbar lordosis in acute and chronic low back pain patients. Rheumatol Int. 2003 Jul;23(4):163-5.

190. Obeid I, Hauger O, Aunoble S, Bourghli A, Pellet N, Vital JM. Global analysis of sagittal spinal alignment in major deformities: correlation between lack of lumbar lordosis and flexion of the knee. Eur Spine J. 2011 Sep;20 Suppl 5:681-5.

191. O'Brien K, Culham E, Pickles B. Balance and skeletal alignment in a group of elderly female fallers and nonfallers. J Gerontol A Biol Sci Med Sci. 1997 Jul;52(4):B221-6.

192. Regev GJ, Kim CW, Tomiya A, Lee YP, Ghofrani H, Garfin SR, Lieber RL, Ward SR.

Psoas Muscle Architectural Design, In Vivo Sarcomere Length Range, and Passive Tensile Properties Support Its Role as a Lumbar Spine Stabilizer. Spine (Phila Pa 1976). 2011 Dec 15;36(26):E1666-E1674.

193. Nelson KE, Rottmen J. The female patient. Chapt. 9. In: Somatic Dysfunction in Osteopathic Family Medicine. Nelson KE, Glonek T, eds., Baltimore, MD: Lippincott, Williams & Wilkins; 2007;105-26.

194. Häkkinen K, Häkkinen A. Muscle cross-sectional area, force production and relaxation characteristics in women at different ages. Eur J Appl Physiol Occup Physiol. 1991;62(6):410-4.

195. Takahashi K, Takahashi HE, Nakadaira H, Yamamoto M. Different changes of quantity due to aging in the psoas major and quadriceps femoris muscles in women. J Musculoskelet Neuronal Interact. 2006 Apr-Jun;6(2):201-5.

196. Lee LW, Zavarei K, Evans J, Lelas JJ, Riley PO, Kerrigan DC. Reduced hip extension in the elderly: dynamic or postural? Arch Phys Med Rehabil. 2005 Sep;86(9):1851-4.

197. Sinaki M, Itoi E, Rogers JW, Bergstralh EJ, Wahner HW. Correlation of back extensor strength with thoracic kyphosis and lumbar lordosis in estrogen-deficient women. Am J Phys Med Rehabil. 1996 Sep-Oct;75(5):370-4.

198. Fon GT, Pitt MJ, Thies AC Jr. Thoracic kyphosis: range in normal subjects. AJR Am J Roentgenol. 1980 May;134(5):979-83.

199. Kang KB, Kim YJ, Muzaffar N, Yang JH, Kim YB, Yeo ED. Changes of Sagittal Spinopelvic Parameters in Normal Koreans with Age over 50. Asian Spine J. 2010 Dec;4(2):96-101.

200. Ensrud KE, Black DM, Harris F, Ettinger B, Cummings SR Correlates of kyphosis in older women. The Fracture Intervention Trial Research Group. J Am Geriatr Soc. 1997 Jun;45(6):682-7.

201. Balzini L, Vannucchi L, Benvenuti F, Benucci M, Monni M, Cappozzo A, Stanhope SJ. Clinical characteristics of flexed posture in elderly women. J Am Geriatr Soc. 2003 Oct;51(10):1419-26.

202. Kado DM, Huang MH, Karlamangla AS, Barrett-Connor E, Greendale GA. Hyperkyphotic posture predicts mortality in older community-dwelling men and women: a prospective study. J Am Geriatr Soc. 2004 Oct;52(10):1662-7.

203. Katzman WB, Wanek L, Shepherd JA, Sellmeyer DE. Age-related hyperkyphosis: its causes, consequences, and management. J Orthop Sports Phys Ther. 2010 Jun;40(6):352-60.

204. Kado DM, Lui LY, Ensrud KE, Fink HA, Karlamangla AS, Cummings SR; Study of Osteoporotic Fractures. Hyperkyphosis predicts mortality independent of vertebral osteoporosis in older women. Ann Intern Med. 2009 May 19;150(10):681-7.

205. Schwab F, Lafage V, Boyce R, Skalli W, Farcy JP. Gravity line analysis in adult volunteers: age-related correlation with spinal parameters, pelvic parameters, and foot position. Spine (Phila Pa 1976). 2006 Dec 1;31(25):E959-67.

206. El Fegoun AB, Schwab F, Gamez L, Champain N, Skalli W, Farcy JP. Center of gravity and radiographic posture analysis: a preliminary review of adult volunteers and adult patients affected by scoliosis. Spine (Phila Pa 1976). 2005 Jul 1;30(13):1535-40.

207. Schwab F, Lafage V, Boyce R, Skalli W, Farcy JP. Gravity line analysis in adult volunteers: age-related correlation with spinal parameters, pelvic parameters, and foot position. Spine (Phila Pa 1976). 2006 Dec 1;31(25):E959-67.

208. Kappler RE. Postural balance and motion patterns. J Am Osteopath Assoc. May 1982;81(9):598-606.

209. Honaker JA, Boismier TE, Shepard NP, Shepard NT. Fukuda stepping test: sensitivity and specificity. J Am Acad Audiol. 2009 May;20(5):311-4.

210. Zhang YB, Wang WQ. Reliability of the Fukuda stepping test to determine the side of vestibular dysfunction. J Int Med Res. 2011;39(4):1432-7.

211. Larson NJ. Personal communication. Chicago College of Osteopathic Medicine. Chicago, Il. 1972.

212. Magoun HI. Entrapment neuropathy of the central nervous system. II. Cranial nerves I-IV, VI-VIII, XII. J Am Osteopath Assoc. 1968 Mar;67(7):779-87.

213. Gauchard GC, Gangloff P, Jeandel C, Perrin PP. Influence of regular proprioceptive and bioenergetic physical activities on balance control in elderly women. J Gerontol A Biol Sci Med Sci. 2003 Sep;58(9):M846-50.

214. Sergueef N, Nelson KE, Glonek T. The effect of light exercise upon blood flow velocity determined by laser-Doppler flowmetry. J Med Eng Technol. 2004 Jul-Aug;28(4):143-50.

215. Maki BE, McIlroy WE. The role of limb movements in maintaining upright stance: the 'change-in-support' strategy. Phys Ther. 1997 May;77(5):488-507.

# Chapter 3

# Cardiovascular conditions

*An Osteopath must know the shape and position of every bone in the body, as well as that part to which every ligament and muscle is attached. He must know the blood and the nerve supply. He must comprehend the human system as an anatomist, and also from a physiological standpoint.*

—A. T. Still[1]

Osteopathic principles have been applied to the treatment of cardiovascular disease and dysfunction since Still, who stated: "The osteopath of practice and skill knows and has demonstrated to his own satisfaction that when he adjusts the spine and ribs, the heart acts normally. To him this is not theory but a truth of his own demonstration."[2] Since that time, increased evidence has become available allowing us to discuss how osteopathic principles relate to cardiovascular dysfunctions, such as hypertension and congestive heart failure (CHF), and how patients with these conditions can benefit from osteopathic manipulative treatment (OMT).

It should be remembered nevertheless, that OMT is not specific treatment for organic pathology. It is appropriately employed as an integrative therapy within a holistic approach to the treatment of organic pathology. The elimination or reduction of the influence of somatic and visceral dysfunctions increases the patient's comfort and functional capacity, and augments their inherent ability for self-healing from a mechanical, neurophysiological, and circulatory perspective. Osteopathic manipulative treatment, therefore, may be used for its contribution to the treatment of cardiovascular dysfunction and disease. It should, however, never be employed without a complete medical diagnosis or as an alternative to accepted standards of medical practice.

## Hypertension

Hypertension (HTN) is a condition in which arterial blood pressure (BP) is chronically elevated. It is one of the most common clinical conditions affecting older individuals. In the United States, its prevalence is about 30% of the adult population[3]. Worldwide, it is estimated to be around 40%, and to be the cause of about 12.8% of total deaths.[4] The incidence of HTN is higher in older individuals and women, while it decreases with higher education and income levels. Typically, until age 45, a higher percentage of men than women have abnormally elevated BP. From age 45–55 the percentage of hypertensive men and women is comparable, while after age 55 a much higher percentage of women have HTN.[5]

According to the Seventh Report of the Joint National Committee on Prevention, Detection, Evaluation, and Treatment of High Blood Pressure of the American Heart Association (AHA), the criteria for HTN, in adults aged 18 years or older, are defined as follows:[6]

- Normal: systolic lower than 120 mm Hg, diastolic lower than 80 mm Hg.
- Prehypertension: systolic 120–139 mm Hg, diastolic 80–89 mm Hg.
- Stage 1: systolic 140–159 mm Hg, diastolic 90–99 mm Hg.
- Stage 2: systolic 160 mm Hg or greater, diastolic 100 mm Hg or greater.

Significant comorbidities exist, and worldwide, HTN increases the risk for coronary heart disease and stroke. Further possible complications include: heart failure, peripheral vascular disease, renal impairment, retinal hemorrhage, and visual impairment. Indeed, in 2011, heart disease and stroke were, respectively, the first and fourth leading causes of death in the United States.[7]

# Control of arterial pressure

Arterial BP results from a combination of cardiac output and systemic vascular resistance. In order to maintain normal BP and to provide adequate perfusion of all the different organ and tissue systems, a regulatory mechanism exists. This mechanism consists of several local and systemic hormonal and neural factors interacting closely, in response to any acute or chronic change in BP as monitored through baroreceptors. The baroreceptors constantly inform the central nervous system (CNS) about the status of BP. In response, rapid changes in the activity of the autonomic nervous system adjust the heart and vasculature to acutely regulate BP.

Over longer periods, hours or days, the release of hormones contributes to this regulation, influencing arterial pressure through their effect upon cardiovascular physiology and by modifying blood volume through their actions on renal function. Noradrenaline (norepinepherine) and adrenaline (epinephrine) are released by the adrenal medullae. Renin released by the kidneys activates the formation of angiotensin II. Aldosterone is released from the adrenal cortex, and vasopressin, the antidiuretic hormone, by the posterior pituitary gland. All participate in BP regulation.

## *The baroreflex*

The baroreflex is part of the nervous mechanism that controls arterial BP. It is triggered by stimulation of baroreceptors located in multiple areas of the cardiovascular system. When arterial BP increases, the arterial walls are stretched, which induces the baroreceptors to transmit afferent impulses to the CNS, resulting in feedback signals that maintain circulatory homeostasis.

Baroreceptors are highly specialized stretch-sensitive nerve endings found in the walls of a number of large systemic arteries including almost every large artery of the thoracic and neck regions. These receptors are particularly abundant in the carotid sinus, the slight dilation of the common carotid artery at its bifurcation into external and internal carotids, and in the wall of the aortic arch. Thus, it should be remembered during palpation of the neck that the carotid sinus is located anterior to the sternocleidomastoid muscle in the transverse plane connecting the upper edge of the thyroid cartilage to the lower edge of C4. Stimulation of its baroreceptors causes increased parasympathetic stimulation of the heart, which may induce bradycardia and syncope.

The carotid sinus baroreceptors send signals through Hering's nerves, which are branches of the glossopharyngeal nerves (CN IX), to the nucleus tractus solitarius (NTS) in the medulla of the brainstem. The aortic baroreceptors send signals to the NTS through Cyon's nerves, which are branches of the vagus nerves (CN X). Arterial baroreceptors offer significant moment-to-moment control of arterial BP. Their role in long-term BP regulation is still debated, however.

Baroreceptor input is integrated in the medulla resulting in feedback through the autonomic nervous system (ANS) to the circulation to balance arterial pressure toward the normal level. When systemic BP is increased, efferent sympathetic outflow is inhibited, reducing vascular tone, heart rate, and cardiac muscle contraction, while parasympathetic outflow is increased, reducing heart rate. This reduces arterial BP through both a decrease in peripheral resistance and a decrease in cardiac output. With a decrease in systemic BP, the opposite occurs. This alternating output results in the Traube-Hering waves observed in BP and blood flow velocity that have been clearly linked to the cranial rhythmic impulse and shown to be affected by cranial OMT.[8 9 10]

Besides the baroreceptors, BP also is controlled by chemoreceptors located in the bifurcation of each common carotid artery and along the aortic arch. When the BP drops under a critical level the diminished blood flow results in decreased oxygen

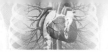

and increased carbon dioxide and hydrogen ion concentrations. This triggers a chemoreceptor reflex through Hering's nerves and Cyon's nerves that signals the vasomotor center of the brain stem to raise the arterial pressure back to normal.

## The autonomic nervous system

The neural control of the BP depends mainly upon the ANS. The sympathetic division of the ANS supplies the vasculature of almost all tissues. Sympathetic stimulation of the small arteries and arterioles augments resistance to blood flow while stimulation of the large vessels decreases their volume driving blood into the heart, thereby affecting heart pumping.

The sympathetic division of the ANS also provides fibers to the heart. When stimulated, these fibers increase both the heart rate and its force and output volume. Sympathetic stimulation also affects venous and lymphatic return. The low frequency oscillation of baroreflex activity increases the tone of resistance vessels, which in combination with the valves in the veins and lymphatic vessels, increases blood flow back to the heart. Conversely, the parasympathetic division of the ANS through the vagus nerve (CN X) slows the heart rate but has no direct effect upon peripheral vascular tone.

Sympathetic innervation to the heart arises from the preganglionic neurons that have their cell bodies in the intermediolateral horn of the spinal cord between T1–T5. Paradoxically, the ventricles are supplied by the higher thoracic segments, while the lower segments innervate the atria. These preganglionic fibers course through the white rami communicantes to synapse in a ganglion at the same spinal cord level from which they arise, or they ascend along the paravertebral chain to synapse in the cervical ganglia. From these ganglia, postganglionic fibers form the sympathetic cardiac nerves. Somatic dysfunction involving spinal segments in the T1–T5 region, because of the associated segmental facilitation, can produce somatovisceral reflexes with increased sympathetic stimulation of the myocardium. Increased sympathetic tone can precipitate sinus tachycardia and ventricular irritability with premature ventricular contractions.

Parasympathetic innervation of the heart arises from neurons in both the dorsal vagal nucleus that lies under the floor of the fourth ventricle, and the nucleus ambiguus of the medulla. The vagus exits the skull through the jugular foramen, and some fibers form vagal cardiac branches that synapse in the cardiac plexuses and atrial walls. Dysfunction of the cranial base between the petrous part of the temporal bone and the occiput can compromise the vagus nerve as it exits the skull. High cervical spinal somatic dysfunction is also associated with vagal somatovisceral reflexes. Vagal hyperactivity is associated with bradycardia and skipped ventricular beats. Because of the above relationships, somatic dysfunction particularly affecting the upper thoracic spine, upper cervical vertebrae, and cranial base should be looked for and addressed in individuals with dysfunctional BP.

## The renin-angiotensin system

While the ANS provides mainly short-term control of BP, by constantly adjusting peripheral vascular resistance and capacitance, and cardiac pumping ability, the kidneys contribute to arterial BP control through changes in extracellular fluid volume and through the renin-angiotensin system for long-term BP control. When the arterial pressure falls too low, renin, a protein enzyme, is released by the kidneys. Renin acts enzymatically on globulin, (angiotensinogen that is produced in the liver), to release the peptide, angiotensin I. A conversion then occurs, activated by angiotensin converting enzyme that transforms angiotensin I to angiotensin II. This occurs largely in the lung, but also in other tissues such as the kidneys and blood vessels. Angiotensin II is a potent vasoconstrictor that can quickly produce vasoconstriction in many areas of the body. This happens much more in the arterioles than in the veins. As a consequence, total peripheral resistance is augmented, contributing to increased blood pressure.

Angiotensin II also stimulates the secretion of the hormone aldosterone from the adrenal glands. Aldosterone affects the kidneys, increasing the reabsorption of sodium and water into the blood and the release of potassium into the urine. This gradually increases the extracellular fluid volume, and augments BP. Thus, BP can be controlled by this long-term mechanism. Indeed, BP control is the result of various interactions between the renin-angiotensin-aldosterone system and the nervous system.

## The pathophysiology of hypertension

Hypertension may be essential or secondary. Essential HTN (also referred to as primary or idiopathic HTN) develops from uncertain cause and accounts for more than 90% of HTN cases.[11] Secondary HTN develops as the result of underlying conditions, such as renovascular disease, chronic renal disease, sleep apnea, and thyroid disease. Excessive liquorice consumption, certain herbal remedies, and illegal drugs may also contribute to the development of secondary HTN.

The cause of essential HTN seems to be a multifactorial interaction of genetic and epigenetic factors. The genetic influence upon BP has been confirmed through multiple studies.[12][13] Many genetic loci have been found, with each of them having potential effects on BP.[14]

Epigenetic factors are well known, and include obesity, insulin resistance, high alcohol intake (more than one drink per day for women and more than two drinks per day for men), high salt intake, aging, a sedentary lifestyle, and stress. On the other hand, lifestyle modification (weight loss, reduced sodium and alcohol intake, and increased physical activity) may ameliorate BP to varying degrees.[15]

Exposure to stress as a factor that contributes to the development of HTN is well documented.[16] Sympathetic nervous activation is acknowledged as a process for both initiating and sustaining BP elevation.[17] Hyperreactivity of the hypothalamic-pituitary-adrenal axis (HPA) may also be a risk factor for HTN through the release of cortisol in response to stress.[18]

The baroreflex is of paramount importance in the control of BP, and normally, after sufficient changes in BP, baroreflex signals are transmitted to the CNS in order to maintain circulatory homeostasis. In hypertensive patients, however, there is impairment in the baroreflex function and baroreceptors are reset to a higher pressure, with progressive reduction of arterial baroreflex sensitivity.

Hypertension can also result from dysfunction of the renin-angiotensin-aldosterone system that regulates extracellular fluid volume and peripheral resistance. Increased peripheral resistance, a recognized factor that contributes to HTN, is influenced by several mechanisms including the renin-angiotensin-aldosterone system. Normally vascular tone and the regulation of the vascular intimal proliferation are controlled by endothelium-derived nitric oxide (NO). Conversely, endothelial dysfunction results in increased inactivation or reduced synthesis of NO, or both, leading to vascular inflammation and vasospasm.[19] This occurs in HTN, and evidence suggests that oxidative stress plays a significant role in this endothelial alteration.[20]

Increased oxidative stress is involved in the development of multiple age-related diseases.[21] Indeed, HTN tends to increase in older individuals, where changes in baroreflex function affect BP control.[22] With aging, there is also a decrease in the elasticity of the common carotid artery compliance.[23] This stiffening may lessen the effects of stimuli applied to baroreceptors, contributing to baroreflex dysfunction that occurs with aging.[24] Atherosclerosis may also be a contributing factor that stiffens arteries. Furthermore, ANS regulation is altered with age; in particular, basal sympathetic nerve activity is increased, with significant decrease of nocturnal parasympathetic activity manifested through a constant decline of cardiac vagal modulation.[25]

Hypertension is a major risk factor for stroke, myocardial infarction, and heart failure, and can be associated with possible complications, such as hypertensive retinopathy and hypertensive nephropathy. Therefore, hypertensive patients should be followed medically, with OMT employed for its complementary contribution. From an osteopathic perspective, it is interesting to consider the importance of the ANS and the baroreflex in the development of HTN, and how somatic dysfunction, particularly involving the skull, upper cervical, and upper thoracic regions, may affect their physiology. Because the goal of an osteopathic approach is to eliminate or decrease the influence of dysfunction in order to support the body's inherent capacity for self-healing, OMT has been recommended as an integrative treatment in essential HTN.[26][27][28]

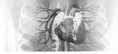
# Congestive heart failure

The Heart Failure Society of America gives the following definition of heart failure (HF):

"... a syndrome caused by cardiac dysfunction, generally resulting from myocardial muscle dysfunction or loss and characterized by either left ventricular (LV) dilation or hypertrophy or both. Whether the dysfunction is primarily systolic or diastolic or mixed, it leads to neurohormonal and circulatory abnormalities, usually resulting in characteristic symptoms such as fluid retention, shortness of breath, and fatigue, especially on exertion. In the absence of appropriate therapeutic intervention, HF is usually progressive at the level of both cardiac function and clinical symptoms. The severity of clinical symptoms may vary substantially during the course of the disease process and may not correlate with changes in underlying cardiac function. Although HF is progressive and often fatal, patients can be stabilized and myocardial dysfunction and remodeling may improve, either spontaneously or as a consequence of therapy. In physiological terms, HF is a syndrome characterized by either or both pulmonary and systemic venous congestion and/or inadequate peripheral oxygen delivery, at rest or during stress, caused by cardiac dysfunction."[29]

Heart failure is a clinical syndrome of increasing prevalence, having significant morbidity and mortality. Among individuals free of any cardiovascular disease (CVD) at 50 years of age, the likelihood of the occurrence of CVD during the remainder of their lives will be more than 50% for men and almost 40% for women.[30] According to the World Heart Failure Society, the average prevalence of heart failure is 2–2.5% in the western world, with a serious increase in this number as individuals age.[31] Congestive heart failure (CHF) is a pathophysiological condition wherein abnormal cardiac output results in the heart failing to sufficiently pump blood to meet the metabolic needs of the body. It is a secondary chronic condition, rather than a primary diagnosis, that typically develops from HF over time.

## The pathophysiology of congestive heart failure

Congestive heart failure may be classified as either systolic or diastolic. Systolic heart failure is the most common. It occurs when the heart does not contract well or peripheral resistance is too great, and the force necessary for blood circulation is insufficient. Diastolic heart failure occurs when the heart cannot relax properly, leading to fluid accumulation, especially in the lower extremities. Frequently, it is associated with high BP and a myocardial hypertrophy.

When the heart is damaged, as following a myocardial infarction, cardiac output can be seriously lowered. This triggers baroreceptor and chemoreceptor reflexes that, in turn, stimulate the sympathetic nervous system (SNS). As a result, sympathetic stimulation activates what is left of the ventricular musculature, and increases the tone of the blood vessels to augment venous return. Additionally, low cardiac output leads to renal fluid retention and increases in body fluid and blood volume, thereby increasing venous return. After several days to weeks, and with the return to nearly normal cardiac output and fluid retention, the patient will develop a compensated heart failure. Aging patients may ignore cardiac damage if the damage has occurred a little at a time, each time with compensation. During intense physical activities however, the heart is not capable of appropriately increasing its pumping capacity and the patient will experience the symptoms of cardiac failure.

In cases of serious heart damage with insufficient compensation, cardiac output is reduced and renal fluid retention is augmented. As a result, the amount of body fluid increases, and the patient develops edema. This is decompensated heart failure and can lead to death.

Aging is related to a decline in structure and function. As such, the aging heart develops some degree of left ventricular hypertrophy associated with an increase in the heart weight, even though there is no distinct source of increased afterload. Additionally, the heart demonstrates increased duration of contraction and some delay in relaxation that may contribute to the susceptibility of the aging patient to diastolic heart failure.[32] Aging vessels demonstrate physical changes as well, including vascular hypertrophy and stiffness, which may be considered as a prodromal phase of atherosclerotic disease, and may play a part in the increased systolic and pulse pressure.

Furthermore, with age, as already discussed, changes occur in baroreflex physiology. The baroreceptor heart rate reflex seems to be impaired, although control of blood pressure appears to be better preserved. Additionally, with age-related changes, cardiac vagal modulation consistently demonstrates age-related blunting.[33] These changes per se may contribute to the development of heart failure through a decrease of the sympathoinhibitory function of the arterial baroreceptor reflexes and an increase of the sympathoexcitatory cardiac sympathetic afferent and arterial chemoreceptor reflexes.

Heart failure is associated with a chronic reduction of tissue blood flow that may in turn influence the carotid body function, particularly the chemoreflex activation of sympathetic activity, thereby playing a role in the autonomic imbalance seen in CHF.[34] Dysfunction in central sympathetic regulation due to alterations in the renin-angiotensin-aldosterone axis and the cytokine system contributes to the dysregulation of the sympathetic division of the ANS as well.

Thus, with CHF patients, the initial activation of the SNS maintains the failing heart by stimulating the contractility of the muscular tissue, improving stroke volume and peripheral vasoconstriction to preserve arterial perfusion. Nevertheless with time, it contributes to cardiac decompensation and heart failure.[35]

Congestive heart failure is a complex syndrome with an ANS dysfunction component, including activation of the sympathetic division of the ANS and a decrease in vagal activity. Usually, the treatment of heart failure focuses upon the inhibition of the activated SNS through the use of beta-blockers or exercise training, or both. Several studies also suggest that chronic vagal stimulation might have important positive effects in the failing heart and in heart failure.[36 37] Indeed, it seems that the vagal dysfunction present in HF may be reversible.[38] Therefore, it has been suggested that it is possible to reset the autonomic tone for a better physiological balance[39] and that chronic vagal stimulation in patients with heart failure is a feasible treatment. Such treatment is conducted medically through the use of an implantable neurostimulator that delivers low current electrical pulses to stimulate the vagus nerve.[40]

# Cardiovascular function and somatic dysfunction

Normally, blood from the periphery flows into the thoracic cage and right atrium where it passes to the right ventricle that pumps the blood to the lungs. The oxygenated blood from the lungs then enters the left atrium, and flows into the left ventricle. The left ventricle pumps the blood to the aorta and then to all parts of the body. Blood from the periphery is returned to the heart by an interaction between alternating vasomotor tone, the appendicular action of the 'muscular pump,' and the central action of the thoracoabdominal 'two-chambered pump.' It is important to realize that this circulatory mechanism must function in a dynamic state of balance between its central and peripheral components. This balance can be compromised by the mechanical and neurophysiological impact of somatic dysfunction. Various aspects of the pathophysiology of HF, including increased beta adrenergic tone and altered baroreflex response are also associated with somatic dysfunction. Upper thoracic spinal facilitation results in increased myocardial sympathetic stimulation.[41 42] Thus the diagnosis and treatment of somatic dysfunction may be integrated into the treatment of HF patients to alleviate this source of stress upon the already compromised heart.

## The general systemic circulation

Cardiac output is the result of a complex interplay between the pumping capacity of the heart and the dynamics of peripheral circulation. The

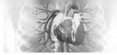

contractile force of the ventricles is a function of the end-diastolic length of cardiac muscle that is closely correlated to end-diastolic ventricular volume. Cardiac stroke volume corresponds directly with the volume of blood returning to the heart (preload) along with cardiac muscle fiber length, and inversely with arterial resistance (afterload). Ventricular stroke volume is consequently the result of the preload at the onset of ventricular contraction, the force-velocity-length relation, or inotropic state, of the muscle, and afterload, the tension that the muscle must develop for effective contraction. Diastolic heart failure is depression of the ejection fraction, the ratio between stroke volume and end diastolic volume that is normally 59-75%, and decreased cardiac output. Of interest here is that this may be present, even with normal cardiac function, as the result of decreased preload. Systolic heart failure occurs when either the heart is incapable of adequately contracting (decreased inotropic state), or when increased afterload exceeds myocardial contractile capacity, or as some combination of the two.

Cardiac performance is affected significantly, at any inotropic level or amount of afterload, by preload. The distribution of blood volume is among the major determinants of preload.[43] Distribution of blood volume between the intra- and extrathoracic compartments affects preload and is determined by multiple factors that can be impacted by the functional status of the musculoskeletal system. These factors include: 1) upright posture, 2) intrapericardial pressure, 3) the tonic oscillation of the baroreflex, 4) the muscular pump, and 5) negative mean intrathoracic pressure, a component of the two-chambered pump.

## Upright posture

Upright posture augments extrathoracic blood volume and decreases intrathoracic blood volume, thereby reducing preload and consequently stroke volume. In the upright position gravity tends to hold fluid in dependant, extrathoracic areas of the body. If factors 3), 4), and 5) are compromised, fluid tends to pool in dependant areas and it is not until the patient lies down that preload increases, stressing the limited capacity of the patient with HF.

## Intrapericardial pressure

Intrapericardial pressure physically defines the limits of ventricular end-diastolic volume. Pericardial tension (or effusion) limits ventricular capacity to accommodate preload or overcome afterload by physically limiting end-diastolic ventricular volume. Intrapericardial pressure is potentially affected by fascial dysfunction impacting the mediastinum. Of particular significance here is the impact of the functional state of the thoracic cage and thoracoabdominal diaphragm upon the fascia. The integrity of the body's entire fascial system means, however, that fascial dysfunction distal to the thorax could also impact the pericardium. (See further: 'Section 1: Osteopathy, fascia, fluid, and the primary respiratory mechanism,' p. 1.)

## The tonic oscillation of the baroreflex

The tonic oscillation of the baroreflex intermittently constricts smooth muscle in the walls of the peripheral vasculature. In the arterial system this creates the oscillation in blood pressure and blood flow velocity and modulates afterload. In the walls of veins, and larger lymphatic vessels this drives blood and lymph centrally, acting in harmony with factors 4 and 5, to counter the preload reduction and augment end-diastolic volume.

The pressure gradient for venous return is the mean systemic filling pressure. Although the rate of blood return to the heart is the result of both cardiac and peripheral factors, it is determined to a significant extent by the mean systemic filling pressure. Because the capacitance of the veins is as much as 20 times that of the arteries, the mean systemic filling pressure is predominantly a result of vascular tone within the venous system. If total peripheral resistance was increased by 20%, entirely from arterial vasoconstriction, venous return would be reduced approximately 6%. If that same 20% increase in peripheral resistance occurred as venous vasoconstriction, venous return would be reduced by a factor of nine to approximately 53%.[49]

Thus the functional capacitor within the peripheral circulatory system is predominantly venous. The lymphatic system also contributes to this peripheral capacitance. This capacitance, and its effect on preload, arterial tone, and afterload, is modulated by the low frequency oscillation in sympathetic tone of the baroreflex. The power of the baroreflex as manifest in peripheral blood flow velocity can be augmented by cranial OMT.[45]

### The 'muscular pump'

The muscular pump, i.e., appendicular muscular contractility, displaces venous blood and lymph centrally. The movement of the muscles dynamically changes fascial tensions compressing adjacent vessels and, because they possess valves preventing retrograde flow of venous blood and lymph, moves their contents centrally. This reduces extrathoracic blood volume while increasing intrathoracic blood volume and end-diastolic ventricular volume. The potentially compromising effect of somatic dysfunction, particularly affecting the lumbar spine, sacrum, pelvis, and lower extremities, can impair the efficacy of the muscular pump in the lower extremities.

### Negative mean intrathoracic pressure

Negative mean intrathoracic pressure, augmented further by the drop in intrathoracic pressure during inspiration, normally draws blood and lymph into the chest. This enhances preload and consequently ventricular end-diastolic volume.

The position of the thoracoabdominal diaphragm between the thoracic and abdominal cavities creates a 'two chambered pump' that draws blood and lymph centrally. The thoracic cage actively expands in all of its dimensions during inspiration. The diaphragm contracts and its dome descends. This decreases intrathoracic pressure while at the same time, the descent of the diaphragm compresses the abdominal contents, causing increased intra-abdominal pressure.[46] The thoracic cage then passively recoils against the air filled lungs during expiration, and the diaphragm relaxes and ascends back into the thorax, resulting in decreased intra-abdominal pressure and increased intrathoracic pressure. This alternating pressure gradient between the intrathoracic and intra-abdominal cavities, in association with the one-way valves of the veins and lymphatic vessels, pulls blood and lymph from the extremities.

Inhalation squeezes fluid from the abdomen at a time when negative intrathoracic pressure is sucking air and low pressure fluids into the thorax. During exhalation, air is pushed from the lungs, as blood and lymph is squeezed from the veins and thoracic duct, while the concomitant drop in intra-abdominal pressure sucks blood and lymph from the periphery into the abdomen in preparation for the next cycle. The driving mechanism of this two-chambered pump is dependent upon the efficient movement of the thoracic cage and diaphragm, and as such, dysfunctional mechanics of either can greatly reduce the pumping effect.

Neuromuscular compromise of the thoracoabdominal diaphragm and chest wall, as occurs with kyphoscoliosis, obesity and somatic dysfunction, can cause chronic hypoventilation that can, in turn, cause the heart to fail.[47] Motion restriction is one of the criteria for somatic dysfunction. Somatic dysfunction affecting the thoracic spine, ribs, thoracoabdominal diaphragm, accessory muscles of respiration, and intra- and extrathoracic fascia, with resultant decreased thoracic cage compliance is present to some extent in every adult, becoming progressively greater with age. As such, somatic dysfunction can reduce the return of venous blood and lymph centrally, decreasing preload, causing a predisposition to, or further aggravating, HF.

## The pulmonary circulation

The pulmonary circulation not only perfuses the lungs, it also acts as a blood volume reservoir and consequently, in a manner similar to the peripheral veins discussed above, as a capacitor for the left side of the heart. At any time, the pulmonary circulation contains approximately 10% of the total circulating blood volume. High distensibility of the pulmonary vasculature provides accommodation for significant changes in blood flow.[48] The pressure within the pulmonary vasculature is low. The mean pressure in the pulmonary artery (15 mm Hg) is about one sixth that of mean aortic pressure (100 mm Hg).

Because the pulmonary capillaries receive little support from the surrounding lung, they collapse, or distend, in response to pressures within and surrounding them. Intra-alveolar pressure

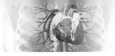 

determines the pressure surrounding the pulmonary capillaries, and when it exceeds the pressure within the capillaries, they collapse. The pulmonary parenchyma acts in a tensegrital fashion with the pulmonary arteries and veins. During inspiration, as the lungs expand, the larger pulmonary vessels are actually pulled open by radial traction from the surrounding lungs. Pulmonary vascular resistance is the result of the pulmonary pressure gradient (about 10 mm Hg) divided by pulmonary blood flow.

Lung volume is an additional determinant of pulmonary vascular resistance, and because of the tensegrital effect of the pulmonary parenchyma upon the caliber of extra alveolar vessels, pulmonary resistance is lower during inhalation even though inhalation tends to compress pulmonary capillaries with resultant increased vascular resistance. Thus, during inspiration, as blood and lymph

is drawn from the extrathoracic compartment into the intrathoracic compartment, blood is also drawn more readily into the pulmonary arterial system. At the same time, because of the collapse of the pulmonary capillaries from increased intra-alveolar pressure in association with decreased intrathoracic pressure, the pulmonary veins distend, increasing left heart preload. When the respiratory rate drops to approximately six breaths per minute, it entrains with the baroreflex, greatly enhancing the power in the entire mechanism, in both the pulmonary and systemic circulation.[50][51]

Dysfunction of the peripheral muscular pump, the thoracoabdominal diaphragm, and the musculoskeletal mechanics of the thoracic cage results in increased peripheral venous resistance and decreased right-sided cardiac preload. Pulmonary circulation is similarly impacted by thoracic cage dysfunction with reduced left-sided preload.

## The osteopathic contribution to the physical examination and treatment

According to Arthur D. Becker, in cardiac therapy: "Any discussion of the application of osteopathic principles must deal primarily with the autonomic nervous system."[52]

When treating patients with cardiovascular symptoms, a complete medical diagnosis should always be obtained. Because patients can present with cardiovascular symptoms that are not necessarily the result of primary cardiovascular pathology, potentially reversible non-cardiac causes must be considered. Even if the cause of the cardiovascular condition is irreversible, the treatment of somatic dysfunction with OMT as an integrative therapy can alleviate concomitant musculoskeletal, autonomic, and circulatory dysfunction, enabling the body's self-healing mechanism, and potentially improving the patient's functional capacity and quality of life.

Following the principles of osteopathic medicine, a holistic approach to the patient includes the consideration of the status of body, mind, and spirit. Cardiovascular dysfunctions affect these three components and during the examination and

treatment, the patient must feel safe: "If neuroception identifies a person as safe, then a neural circuit actively inhibits areas in the brain that organize the defensive strategies of fight, flight, and freeze."[53]

In both HTN and CHF, the distinctly osteopathic treatment objective is to reduce or eliminate the physical restrictions of somatic dysfunction and to optimize ANS function, and therefore to address any dysfunction that might interfere with the sympathetic and parasympathetic divisions of the ANS. As stated by Cathie: "Disturbances of autonomic function may be initiated centrally, terminally, or along the course or pathway of nerve impulses. Efforts to locate the primary source of the disturbance must take into consideration central representation, pathways, and the area of final response. In addition, the possibility of reflex pathways playing a part must be kept continually in mind...Fixed tensions are by no means limited to the somatic structures. They are found as visceral, vascular, and even mental disturbances."[54]

Start your assessment for somatic dysfunction with observation of the global posture of your patient. Kyphoscoliosis can have cardiopulmonary and respiratory effects. With aging, the progressive loss of muscle mass and associated weakness of the thoracic paravertebral extensor muscles contribute to increased kyphosis, resulting in rounded shoulders and a protracted head forward posture. In particular, the upper thoracic region undergoes significant changes, with marked flexion of the upper thoracic spine, sometimes referred to as Dowager's hump, a compensatory increase of the cervical lordosis. The cervicothoracic junction is an important transitional area of the spine and of major consideration in cardiovascular disorders because of its relationship with the inferior cervical sympathetic ganglia. The presence of an increased thoracic kyphosis tends to move the ribs into the position of expiration, increasing the amount of work necessary for inspiration and reducing the respiratory intrathoracic pressure gradient. Other deformities of the chest, such as pectus carinatum and pectus excavatum also reduce thoracic cage compliance.

With the patient seated, palpate the thoracic vertebrae and ribs paying particular attention to the upper thoracic area. Most osteopathic evaluations of patients with cardiovascular disease demonstrate somatic dysfunction in the T1–T4 area.[55][56] This area is important diagnostically for cardiac viscerosomatic reflexes, while treatment of dysfunction in the area can decrease sympathetic somatovisceral influence. An association between somatic dysfunction at levels C6, T2, and T6 and HTN has also been demonstrated.[57][58] Look for tissue texture change and restriction of mobility. Any thoracic dysfunction can be addressed at this time.

The progression of HF is associated with an increased activation of the SNS, a decreased activation of the parasympathetic nervous system (PNS), and a chronic inflammatory process that may be attenuated by regulation of ANS function through vagal stimulation. The spinal facilitation associated with upper thoracic somatic dysfunctions results in increased sympathetic tone to the heart and lungs. Similarly, thoracolumbar somatic dysfunction increases systemic vasomotor tone and cardiac afterload.[59] Appropriately applied OMT results in peripheral vasodilatation and as such can reduce afterload stresses placed upon the failing heart. Appropriately applied OMT should therefore contribute to the treatment of CHF.

Complete the exam with the patient supine. Observe the breathing pattern, which must be unencumbered; note any asymmetry between both sides of the thoracic cage, or decreased movement in some part of the thorax that can be related to dysfunctional ribs. Because of the relationship between the pericardium, which continues below to blend with the central tendon of the thoracic diaphragm via the pericardiacophrenic ligament and the diaphragm, any fascial mediastinal or diaphragmatic dysfunction must be addressed.

Note any edema in the legs, ankles, feet, and abdomen associated with CHF. Assess the clavicles and sternoclavicular and acromioclavicular joints and associated soft tissues, including myofascial structures and their related vascular, lymphatic, and neural elements. The venous and lymphatic vasculature is susceptible to compression from dysfunctional musculoskeletal structures. Venous and lymphatic return may be enhanced by treating somatic dysfunction to: 1) reduce local myofascial tensions that compress peripheral vessels, 2) improve mechanical efficiency of the thoracoabdominal two-chambered pump, and 3) reduce the effects of facilitation and increased sympathetic tone upon peripheral vasculature.

Congestive heart failure is the result of decompensation between cardiac function and peripheral circulation. A significant non-cardiac factor in the development of CHF is the functional compromise of the thoracoabdominal two-chambered pump. Disorders of the respiratory neuromusculoskeletal system will increase the workload on the myocardium through impairment of pulmonary and systemic circulation. The normal aging process is accompanied by progressive loss of mobility, with resultant functional impairment. This is encountered in the extreme with kyphoscoliosis, but similar musculoskeletal mechanics, although of lesser degree, are present in all aged individuals. Somatic dysfunction affecting the thoracic spine, ribs, and thoracoabdominal diaphragm decreases

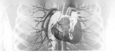

thoracic cage compliance with diminished intrathoracic inspiratory and expiratory pressure gradient. This decreases cardiac preload, ventricular filling, and cardiac output thereby inducing, or increasing cardiac failure. The effective use of OMT to enhance thoracic cage mechanics can potentially increase preload and, if the myocardium is physically capable of responding, increase cardiac output, reducing the debilitating symptoms of diastolic dysfunction.

Next, palpate the cervical spine for function with particular attention to C6–C7 as it applies to the identified hypertensive pattern.[60][61] Examine the anterior cervical structures and check the hyoid bone. The fibrous pericardium blends above with the pretracheal fascia, which is fixed to the hyoid bone. Indirect procedures are by far the treatment of choice in this delicate area.

Evaluation of the craniocervical junction follows due to its relation with CN X. Vagal somatovisceral reflexes can induce or aggravate dysrhythmias like bradycardia and dropped ventricular beats. Next, assess the cranial base that can also be associated with vagal dysfunction because of vagus nerve entrapment in the jugular foramen. It is also the site of insertion of the cervical fascia and potentially the origin of dysfunction affecting the cervical spine, the thoracic inlet, or both.

With the patient supine, using a vault hold, examine the skull. Evaluate the quality of the primary respiratory mechanism (PRM), and its palpable sensation, the cranial rhythmic impulse (CRI). Assess the power of the PRM and the frequency of the CRI. Evaluate the membranous patterns of the craniosacral area, paying close attention to the hypothalamic-pituitary-adrenal axis. Address any dysfunctional pattern and balance the PRM oscillation, associated with baroreflex and vagal physiology for its influence upon cardiac function and vasomotor tone.

Cranial osteopathy, in particular a gentle rocking of the temporal bones, is suggested to have a more or less immediate beneficial influence on blood pressure.[62] According to Magoun, a bilateral rotation of the temporal bones is indicated in hypotension, while a more repressant procedure, such as an alternating rotation of the temporal bones, applied with a very slow rhythmic motion, is indicated in the management of HTN.[63]

## Advice to the patient

In addition to appropriate medications integrated with the treatment of somatic dysfunction, the management of cardiovascular diseases includes dietary changes, weight loss, and appropriate physical exercise and training to reduce psychological stress. Additionally, the same advice can be given as prevention, in particular for patients with prehypertension who are at risk for progression.

Encourage your patient to maintain normal body weight. Increased body mass index and waist circumference are risk factors for conditions such as HTN and left ventricular hypertrophy. Epicardial adipose tissue in particular has been demonstrated to be a cardiometabolic risk factor.[64]

Explain the need for a balanced diet. Cholesterol levels should be monitored and controlled. Sodium sensitivity increases with age as well,[65] and dietary sodium intake should be reduced (<1.5 g of sodium per day). Consumption of alcohol should be limited and the diet must be rich in nuts, fruits, vegetables, and protein.

Regular exercise is associated with preservation of cardiovagal baroreflex function in older individuals, and should be encouraged.[66] For patients with heart failure, a supervised cardiac rehabilitation program is indicated. Walking for 30 minutes per day, several days a week is a simple option.

Methods to reduce stress such as biofeedback, relaxation, yoga, or meditation should be supported. In cardiovascular diseases, there is an increased activation of the SNS[67] and a reduced activation of the PNS. Biofeedback training has the potential to promote parasympathetic activity, which tends to decline in aging individuals.[68]

Slow, deep respiration, at a rate of six breaths per minute, has been demonstrated to be calming, lowering blood pressure and having a beneficial effect upon baroreflex physiology.[69] Also, pranayama, the yogic breathing technique, has the potential to increase parasympathetic activity while decreasing sympathetic activity.[70]

# References

1.  Still AT. Autobiography of Andrew T, Still. Kirskville, MO: A.T. Still; 1908. Reprinted, Colorado Springs, CO: American Academy of Osteopathy; 1981:277.
2.  Still AT. Chapt. Thoracic region, Pneumonia. In: Osteopathy. Research and Practice. Kirksville, MO: Published by the author, 1910:154.
3.  Yoon SS, Ostchega Y, Louis T. Recent trends in the prevalence of high blood pressure and its treatment and control, 1999-2008. NCHS Data Brief. 2010 Oct;(48):1-8.
4.  Raised blood pressure. World Health Organization. Available at http://www.who.int/gho/ncd/risk_factors/blood_pressure_prevalence_text/en/index.html#. Accessed Jan 26, 2013.
5.  High Blood Pressure. Statistical Fact Sheet: 2013 Update. American Heart Association. Availble at https://www.heart.org/idc/groups/heart-public/@wcm/@sop/@smd/documents/downloadable/ucm_319587.pdf. Accessed April 14, 2013.
6.  Chobanian AV, Bakris GL, Black HR, Cushman WC, Green LA, Izzo JL Jr, et al. Seventh report of the Joint National Committee on Prevention, Detection, Evaluation, and Treatment of High Blood Pressure. Hypertension. 2003 Dec;42(6):1206-52.
7.  Hoyert DL, Xu. Deaths:Preliminary Data for 2011. National Vital Statistics Report. Center for Disease Control. October 10, 2012; 61(6):1-51. Available at http://www.cdc.gov/nchs/fastats/lcod.htm. Accessed April 14, 2013.
8.  Nelson KE, Sergueef N, Lipinski CM, Chapman AR, Glonek T. Cranial rhythmic impulse related to the Traube-Hering-Mayer oscillation: comparing laser-Doppler flowmetry and palpation. J Am Osteopath Assoc. 2001 Mar;101(3):163-73.
9.  Sergueef N, Nelson KE, Glonek T. The effect of cranial manipulation on the Traube-Hering-Mayer oscillation as measured by laser-Doppler flowmetry. Altern Ther Health Med. 2002 Nov-Dec;8(6):74-6.
10. Nelson KE. The 2010Northup Memorial Lecture : Low Frequency Oscillations in Human Physiology and Cranial Osteopathy. AAO Journal March 2011, 21(1):12-23.
11. Oparil S, Zaman MA, Calhoun DA. Pathogenesis of hypertension. Ann Intern Med. 2003 Nov 4;139(9):761-76
12. Matsubara M. Genetic determination of human essential hypertension. Tohoku J Exp Med. 2000 Sep;192(1):19-33.
13. Hunt SC, Ellison RC, Atwood LD, Pankow JS, Province MA, Leppert MF. Genome scans for blood pressure and hypertension: the National Heart, Lung, and Blood Institute Family Heart Study. Hypertension. 2002 Jul;40(1):1-6.
14. Wain LV, Verwoert GC, O'Reilly PF, Shi G, Johnson T, Johnson AD, et al. Genome-wide association study identifies six new loci influencing pulse pressure and mean arterial pressure. Nat Genet. 2011 Sep 11;43(10):1005-11.
15. Funk KL, Elmer PJ, Stevens VJ, Harsha DW, Craddick SR, Lin PH, et al. PREMIER--a trial of lifestyle interventions for blood pressure control: intervention design and rationale. Health Promot Pract. 2008 Jul;9(3):271-80.
16. Šarenac O, Lozić M, Drakulić S, Bajić D, Paton JF, Murphy D, Japundžić-Žigon N. Autonomic mechanisms underpinning the stress response in borderline hypertensive rats. Exp Physiol. 2011 Jun;96(6):574-89.
17. Esler M. The sympathetic system and hypertension. Am J Hypertens. 2000 Jun;13(6 Pt 2):99S-105S.
18. Hamer M, Steptoe A. Cortisol responses to mental stress and incident hypertension in healthy men and women. J Clin Endocrinol Metab. 2012 Jan;97(1):E29-34.
19. Förstermann U. Nitric oxide and oxidative stress in vascular disease. Pflugers Arch. 2010 May;459(6):923-39. doi: 10.1007/s00424-010-0808-2.
20. Cai H, Harrison DG. Endothelial dysfunction in cardiovascular diseases: the role of oxidant stress. Circ Res. 2000 Nov 10;87(10):840-4.
21. Chung HY, Lee EK, Choi YJ, Kim JM, Kim DH, Zou Y, et al. Molecular inflammation as an underlying mechanism of the aging process and age-related diseases. J Dent Res. 2011 Jul;90(7):830-40.
22. Jones PP, Christou DD, Jordan J, Seals DR. Baroreflex buffering is reduced with age in healthy men. Circulation. 2003 Apr 8;107(13):1770-4.
23. Van Bortel LM, Spek JJ. Influence of aging on arterial compliance. J Hum Hypertens. 1998 Sep;12(9):583-6.
24. Monahan KD. Effect of aging on baroreflex function in humans. Am J Physiol Regul Integr Comp Physiol. 2007 Jul;293(1):R3-R12.
25. Furlan R, Colombo S, Perego F, Atzeni F, Diana A, Barbic F, et al. Abnormalities of cardiovascular neural control and reduced orthostatic tolerance in patients with primary fibromyalgia. J Rheumatol. 2005 Sep;32(9):1787-93.
26. Northup TL. Osteopathic cranial technic and its influence on hypertension. Year Book of the Academy of Applied Osteopathy. American Academy of Osteopathy. Indianapolis, IN. 1948:70-7.
27. Magoun HI. Osteopathy in the cranial field. 2nd ed. Kirksville, MO: The Journal Printing Company; 1966:87.
28. Driscoll DM. The Patient with Hypertension. Chapt.18. In: Somatic Dysfunction in Osteopathic Family Medicine. Nelson K, Glonek T. ed. Lippincott, Williams and Wilkins, 2007:262-78.
29. Heart Failure Society of America, Lindenfeld J, Albert NM, Boehmer JP, Collins SP, Ezekowitz JA, et al. HFSA 2010 Comprehensive Heart Failure Practice Guideline. J Card Fail. 2010 Jun;16(6):e1-194.
30. Lloyd-Jones DM, Leip EP, Larson MG, D'Agostino RB, Beiser A, Wilson PW, et al. Prediction of lifetime risk for cardiovascular disease by risk factor burden at 50 years of age. Circulation. 2006 Feb 14;113(6):791-8.
31. World Heart Failure Society. Heart Failure Worldwide - Facts and Figures. Available at http://www.worldheartfailure.org/index.php?item=75. Accessed Feb 8, 2013.
32. Ferrari AU, Radaelli A, Centola M. Invited review: aging and the cardiovascular system. J Appl Physiol. 2003 Dec;95(6):2591-7.
33. Ferrari AU, Radaelli A, Centola M. Invited review: aging and the cardiovascular system. J Appl Physiol. 2003 Dec;95(6):2591-7.
34. Ding Y, Li YL, Schultz HD. Role of blood flow in carotid body chemoreflex function in heart failure. J Physiol. 2011 Jan 1;589(Pt 1):245-58.
35. Triposkiadis F, Karayannis G, Giamouzis G, Skoularigis J, Louridas G, Butler J. The sympathetic nervous system in heart failure physiology, pathophysiology, and clinical implications. J Am Coll Cardiol. 2009 Nov 3;54(19):1747-62.
36. Kishi T. Heart failure as an autonomic nervous system dysfunction. J Cardiol. 2012 Mar;59(2):117-22.
37. Schwartz PJ. Vagal stimulation for heart diseases: from animals to men. An example of translational cardiology. Neth Heart J. 2013 Feb;21(2):82-4.
38. Bibevski S, Dunlap ME. Prevention of diminished parasympathetic control of the heart in experimental heart failure. Am J Physiol Heart Circ Physiol. 2004 Oct;287(4):H1780-5.
39. Bibevski S, Dunlap ME. Evidence for impaired vagus nerve activity in heart failure. Heart Fail Rev. 2011 Mar;16(2):129-35.
40. Schwartz PJ. Vagal stimulation for heart failure. Curr Opin Cardiol. 2011 Jan;26(1):51-4.
41. Korr IM, Wright HM, Chace JA. Cutaneous patterns of sympathetic activity in clinical abnormalities of the musculoskeletal system. Acta Neuroveg (Wien). 1964;25:589-606.
42. Beal MC, ed. Louisa Burns, DO, Memorial. Year Book of the American Academy of Osteopathy. Indianapolis, IN. 1994.
43. Braunwald E. Normal and abnormal myocardial function. In: Fauci AS, ed. Harrison's Principles of Internal Medicine. 14th ed. New York, NY: McGraw Hill; 1998:1278-82.
44. Ross J Jr, Covell JW, Frameworks for analysis of ventricular and circulatory function: Integrated responses. In: West JB ed. Best and Taylor's Physiologic Basis of Medical Practice. 12th ed. Baltamore MD: Williams and Wilkins; 1990:296-9.
45. Glonek T, Sergueef N, Nelson KE. Physiological Rhythms/Oscillations. Chapt 11. In: Chila AG. ed. Foundations of Osteopathic Medicine. 3rd ed. Philadelphia: Wolters Kluwer/Lippincott Williams and Wilkins. 2011:162-90.
46. Miller CE. The mechanics of lymphatic circulation: lymph hearts. J Amer Osteopath Assoc. 1923;22:397–8, 415-6.

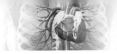 

47. Braunwald E. Cor pulmonale. In: Fauci AS, ed. Harrison's Principles of Internal Medicine. 14th ed. New York, NY: McGraw Hill; 1998:1327.

48. Ross J Jr, Introduction to the cardiovascular system. In: West JB, ed. Best and Taylor's Physiologic Basis of Medical Practice. 12th ed. Baltimore MD: Williams and Wilkins; 1990:112.

49. West JB. Pulmonary blood flow and metabolism. In: West JB, ed. Best and Taylor's Physiological Basis of Medical Practice. 12th ed. Baltimore, MD: Williams and Wilkins; 1990:529-31.

50. Barman SM, Gebber GL. Basis for synchronization of sympathetic and phrenic nerve discharges. Am J Physiol. 1976 Nov;231(5 Pt. 1):1601-7.

51. Ahmed AK, Harness JB, Mearns AJ. Respiratory control of heart rate. Euro J Appl Physiol Occupation Physiol 1982;50:95-104.

52. Becker AD. Manipulative osteopathy in cardiac therapy. J Am Osteopath Assoc. 1939;38(7).

53. Porges SW. The Polyvagal Theory: Neurophysiological Foundations of Emotions, Attachment, Communication, and Self-regulation. New York:WW Norton and Company; 2011.

54. Cathie AG. Some anatomicophysiologic aspects of vascular and visceral disturbances with special reference to cardiac disease. Year Book of the Academy of Applied Osteopathy. American Academy of Osteopathy. Indianapolis, IN. 1959:43-6.

55. Korr IM. Skin resistance patterns associated with visceral disease. Fed Proc. Mar 1949;8:87-88.

56. Beal MC. Palpatory testing for somatic dysfunction in patients with cardiovascular disease. J Am Osteopath Assoc. 1983 Jul;82(11):822-31.

57. Johnston WL, Kelso AF, Babcock HB. Changes in presence of a segmental dysfunction pattern associated with hypertension: Part 1. A short-term longitudinal study. J Am Osteopath Assoc. 1995 Apr;95(4):243-8, 253-5.

58. Johnston WL, Kelso AF. Changes in presence of a segmental dysfunction pattern associated with hypertension: Part 2. A long-term longitudinal study. J Am Osteopath Assoc. 1995 May;95(5):315-8.

59. McKee MG, Moravec CS. Biofeedback in the treatment of heart failure. Cleve Clin J Med. 2010 Jul;77 Suppl 3:S56-9.

60. Johnston WL, Kelso AF, Babcock HB. Changes in presence of a segmental dysfunction pattern associated with hypertension: Part 1. A short-term longitudinal study. J Am Osteopath Assoc. 1995 Apr;95(4):243-8, 253-5.

61. Johnston WL, Kelso AF. Changes in presence of a segmental dysfunction pattern associated with hypertension: Part 2. A long-term longitudinal study. J Am Osteopath Assoc. 1995 May;95(5):315-8.

62. Northup TL. Osteopathic cranial technic and its influence on hypertension. Year Book of the Academy of Applied Osteopathy. American Academy of Osteopathy. Indianapolis, IN. 1948:70-7.

63. Magoun HI. Osteopathy in the cranial field. Kirksville, MO: The Journal Printing Company; 1951:86-7.

64. Pierdomenico SD, Pierdomenico AM, Cuccurullo F, Iacobellis G. Meta-analysis of the relation of echocardiographic epicardial adipose tissue thickness and the metabolic syndrome. Am J Cardiol. 2013 Jan 1;111(1):73-8.

65. Weinberger MH, Miller JZ, Luft FC, Grim CE, Fineberg NS. Definitions and characteristics of sodium sensitivity and blood pressure resistance. Hypertension. 1986 Jun;8(6 Pt 2):II127-34.

66. Hunt BE, Farquhar WB, Taylor JA. Does reduced vascular stiffening fully explain preserved cardiovagal baroreflex function in older, physically active men? Circulation. 2001 May 22;103(20):2424-7.

67. Kalil GZ, Haynes WG. Sympathetic nervous system in obesity-related hypertension: mechanisms and clinical implications. Hypertens Res. 2012 Jan;35(1):4-16.

68. McKee MG, Moravec CS. Biofeedback in the treatment of heart failure. Cleve Clin J Med. 2010 Jul;77 Suppl 3:S56-9.

69. Bernardi L, Sleight P, Bandinelli G, Cencetti S, Fattorini L, Wdowczyc-Szulc J, Lagi A. Effect of rosary prayer and yoga mantras on autonomic cardiovascular rhythms: comparative study. BMJ. 2001 Dec 22-29;323(7327):1446-9.

70. Bhavanani AB, Madanmohan, Sanjay Z. Immediate effect of chandra nadi pranayama (left unilateral forced nostril breathing) on cardiovascular parameters in hypertensive patients. Int J Yoga. 2012 Jul;5(2):108-11

# Chapter 4

# Respiratory dysfunctions

Still recommended osteopathic manipulative treatment (OMT) for patients with respiratory disorders.[1] OMT is not a specific treatment for organic pulmonary pathology, however. The elimination or reduction of the influence of somatic dysfunction from a mechanical, neurophysiological, and circulatory perspective facilitates the body's inherent capacity for self-healing. OMT, therefore, may be used for its complementary contribution in the treatment of respiratory disorders. It should, however, never be employed without a complete medical diagnosis or as an alternative to accepted standards of medical practice.

Understanding the basic anatomic and physiological principles of respiration is necessary to recognize when OMT may enhance the inherent capacities of the patient's body to improve their condition. After reviewing basic pulmonary anatomy, we will discuss particular disorders such as chronic obstructive pulmonary disease (COPD), pneumonia, and sleep apnea.

## Lungs

During pulmonary ventilation, air inflow and outflow between the atmosphere and lung alveoli make oxygen available for the tissues while removing carbon dioxide from the blood. Airflow involves the lungs and the conducting airways.

The lungs, the essential organs of respiration, are located within the walls of the thoracic cage on both sides of the heart and mediastinal contents. Each lung is covered by a serous membrane (the pleura). The parietal pleura coats the thoracic wall and diaphragm, and reflects onto the lung to form the visceral pleura. Between the two pleurae exists a potential space, the pleural cavity, filled with a thin layer of pleural fluid secreted by the parietal layer. Thus, the facing surfaces of the parietal and visceral pleurae slide smoothly against each other during all phases of respiration. In addition to its continual drainage into the lymphatic channels, the pleural fluid is reabsorbed by the visceral layer. Normally, the inward elastic recoil of the lung and the outward pull of the chest wall maintain a negative pressure in the pleural cavity.

The parietal pleura has costovertebral, mediastinal, diaphragmatic, and cervical parts. The costovertebral part covers the internal surface of the thoracic wall and the vertebral bodies. The mediastinal pleura lines the structures between the lungs, while the diaphragmatic pleura lies on the thoracic surface of the diaphragm. The cervical pleura, also referred to as the dome of the pleura, coats the pulmonary apices. A fascial suprapleural membrane, Sibson's fascia, reinforces the cervical pleura. It attaches to the internal border of the first rib and the transverse processes of the seventh cervical vertebra, and its summit is 2.5 cm above the junction of the medial and middle thirds of the clavicle. Because the scalenus minimus muscle spreads into the pleural dome, placing tension upon it, it has been proposed that the suprapleural membrane is the tendon of the scalenus medius.[2] Fibers from the cervical fasciae also blend into the dome of the pleura. Because of these relationships, somatic dysfunction of the cervical spine, thoracic spine, ribs, diaphragm, and related myofascial structures must be addressed to provide complete motility and optimal function of the lungs.

During a normal inspiration, the expansion of the thoracic cage and the descent of the diaphragm pull outward and downward upon the lungs and result in augmentation of the negative pleural cavity pressure, thereby, holding the lungs to the thoracic wall. Normally, after having been stretched by inspiration, the elastic recoil of the lungs and the relaxation of the diaphragm results in expiration. With aging, however, physiological changes occur, with a decrease in the elastic recoil of the lung, in the compliance of the thoracic wall, and in the strength of respiratory muscles. Although these changes are irreversible, additional somatic dysfunction of the spine, ribs, or diaphragm will contribute to a dysfunctional respiratory mechanism, and this is reversible with OMT. Mid-cervical dysfunctions may also affect the phrenic nerve and consequently the function of the diaphragm. Restriction of diaphragmatic movement will increase venous and lymphatic stasis in the lungs and in the rest of the body, as well. Therefore, by alleviating somatic dysfunction in the cervical spine, thoracic cage, and respiratory muscles (the diaphragm in particular), OMT can improve pulmonary function.

## Conducting airways

The conducting airways between the trachea and the alveoli display a branching structure forming the respiratory tree. From the nasal cavities (or oral cavity), the air pathway consists of the pharynx and the trachea that divides into the left and right main bronchi at the level of the sternal angle and fifth thoracic vertebra. The main bronchi branch into lobar bronchi that divide into segmental bronchi, and then into multiple primary bronchioles. The primary bronchioles then divide into terminal bronchioles, each of which gives rise to several respiratory bronchioles that continue to form alveolar ducts. Gas exchange between the air in the lungs and the blood in the capillaries occurs in the five or six alveolar sacs associated with the alveolar duct where thin alveolar walls and a squamous epithelium allow a rapid diffusion of oxygen and carbon dioxide.

Inhaled air passes from the restricted capacity of the nose, pharynx, and trachea to expand to a surface area of 70 m$^2$ (about 800 square feet) at the level of the alveoli.[3] During that progression, the air is in direct contact with the respiratory mucosa that lines the airways. The epithelium of the mucosa rests on a fine connective tissue lamina propria, with a submucosa, containing glands, airway smooth muscle, blood vessels, lymphoid tissue, and nerves. Additionally, some cartilaginous plates are present from the level of the trachea to that of the smallest bronchi.

One of the functions of the epithelium that lines the airways is to protect the lung against infectious and noxious agents. This is accomplished with the presence of tight junctions that unite the epithelial cells providing a physical barrier between tissue and airspace. Lymphocytes, mostly T-cells originating in mucosa-associated lymphoid tissue located in the walls of the airways, and immunoglobulins from B cells, contribute to the immune protection of the airways. Additionally, the predominantly ciliated, pseudostratified epithelium contains interspersed mucus-secreting goblet cells, with serous glands lying beneath them. In combination they produce a bilayered secretion. The sticky outer mucous layer entraps particulate matter. When particles are inhaled and entrapped, they are eliminated by the mucociliary current in the fluid serous layer beneath the outer mucous layer. Ciliated columnar cells play a significant role in producing a mucociliary rejection current all along the surface of bronchioles, bronchi, and trachea upwards. Indeed, all the conducting airways from the nose to the bronchioles are lined with a ciliated epithelium with approximately 200 cilia on every epithelial cell. [4] Most of the inhaled particles entrapped in the viscous fluid are propelled by the beating of cilia at a rate of 10–20 times per second, and eliminated at a rhythm of 1 cm/min. [5] Small particles are phagocytized. Mucociliary clearance is assisted by airway reflexes such as coughing and sneezing. The cough reflex and the sneeze reflex result from irritative substances brought into contact with, respectively, the very sensitive bronchi and trachea, or the nasal passageways. Impulses are conveyed from the airways mostly through the vagus nerves to the medulla of the brain where the reflexes are triggered.

The importance of mechanical epithelial clearance of mucus, as the primary innate airway defense mechanism, has, however, been challenged. Besides replacing the water lost from airway surfaces associated with the conditioning of inhaled air, another function of the epithelia in the proximal regions of the airway is to form a 'chemical shield' that protects the lung against inhaled bacteria. For this, the epithelia secrete into airway lumens salt-sensitive defensins and on airway surfaces a low-salt liquid that activates defensins.[6]

## Muscular wall and nervous control

All the walls of the trachea and bronchi, except portions occupied by cartilage plates, contain smooth muscle. The walls of the bronchioles, with the exception of the respiratory bronchioles where gas exchange occurs, are nearly exclusively smooth muscle. Dysfunctional contraction of these smooth muscles tightens the smaller bronchi and larger bronchioles of the lung as seen in obstructive diseases.

Smooth muscles of the bronchioles are under the control of the autonomic nervous system (ANS). Only a small number of sympathetic nerve fibers access the central portions of the lung. Therefore, sympathetic dilation of the bronchioles results primarily from the release of noradrenaline into the blood by sympathetic stimulation of the adrenal medullae.[7]

Parasympathetic efferent nerve fibers, derived from the vagus nerves, infiltrate the lung parenchyma and modulate bronchiole constriction preserving bronchial muscle tone. Normally, when stimulated they release acetylcholine that results in a moderate constriction of the bronchioles. In pathological conditions where bronchiolar constriction is present, parasympathetic influence can, however, exacerbate the constriction. Bronchoconstriction, then, further increases airway resistance, that can be critical in conditions such as asthma and COPD.

Several pulmonary reflexes can stimulate parasympathetic fibers. Some start in the lungs, where the epithelial membrane of the respiratory airways can be irritated by cigarette smoke, pollutants, or bronchial infection. Others may begin in the upper airways. These are the naso-pharyngo-bronchial reflexes involving the trigeminal and the vagus nerves. Inflammation stimulates the receptors in the nose and pharynx, and some of the afferent fibers from these receptors contribute to the trigeminal nerve that connects with the dorsal vagal nucleus in the brainstem through the reticular formation.

Several deep brain structures, additionally, are associated in the modulation of pulmonary autonomic balance. They include the amygdala, periaqueductal grey matter of the midbrain, dorsal pons, and medulla and may have an inhibitory effect upon the airway-related vagal preganglionic fibers, consequently attenuating their cholinergic bronchoconstrictive action.[8]

Besides controlling the bronchiolar musculature, the ANS affects the blood supply to the lungs and controls glandular secretion. Parasympathetic activity in the tracheobronchial subepithelial capillary network has a vasodilatory effect and increases the fluidity of mucosal secretions, while sympathetic activity produces a vasoconstriction and more viscous secretions.

Vascular processes, such as vasodilatation, vasoconstriction, plasma extravasation, and exudation are responses to the condition of inspired air, as perceived by sensory nerves. Furthermore, after stimulation of unmyelinated, or lightly myelinated, nociceptive C fibers that results in an axon local reflex with antidromic conduction, sensory neuropeptides can be released.[9] This can affect the mucosal vasculature and produce vasodilatation.

The sympathetic innervation of the lungs arises in spinal cord segments T2–T7.[10] Preganglionic fibers synapse in the cervical cord and the first four paravertebral ganglia to reach the pulmonary plexus with parasympathetic fibers from the vagus nerves. Since the sympathetic fibers to the lungs carry vasoconstrictor fibers, any somatic dysfunction from T2–T7 may affect the blood supply to the lungs through somatovisceral reflexes, and must be addressed.[11] Additionally, the occipital and upper cervical areas, potential sites for somatic dysfunction with somatovisceral reflexes through the vagus nerve, should be evaluated and treated, as appropriate, to optimize parasympathetic function.

# Age-related changes

With aging, several major structural changes take place in the respiratory system. Lung elasticity declines, stiffness of the chest wall intensifies, respiratory muscles weaken, and, because of gradual postural modification associated with age, the position of the upper respiratory tract is modified. As a result, respiratory functions, such as vital capacity and gas exchange, decline. Understanding the effects of aging upon the lung is important to distinguish between pathologic changes and changes that are part of the normal aging process, and to understand how OMT may contribute to the treatment of respiratory disorders in the elderly.

In healthy subjects, rib cage compliance decreases with increasing age, starting as soon as the fourth decade, far before any radiologically detectable sign of joint degeneration is present.[12] Increased kyphotic curvature of the spine begins after 40 years of age, and progresses more quickly in women than men.[13 14] This produces an increased anteroposterior diameter of the chest and a decreased diaphragmatic dome, resulting in increased respiratory effort. Indeed, although dynamic lung compliance increases with age,[15] respiratory system compliance decreases by 20%

between the ages of 20 and 60.[16] Besides fatigue and ventilatory failure resulting from increasing ventilatory load, decreased strength of the respiratory muscles with resultant inefficient cough can impair mucociliary clearance assistance.

Maturation of the lungs occurs at approximately 20 years in females and 25 years in males.[17] After that, lung function starts to weaken at around 35 years, with a marked reduction in ventilatory responses to hypoxia and hypercapnia.

In the development of age-related diseases, proinflammatory physiology and increased oxidative stress seem to be of paramount importance.[18 19] In fact, oxidative stress, defined as a disruption of redox signaling and control,[20] can intensify inflammation processes and aging at the cellular level. The ends of chromosomes are protected by telomeres that prevent them from fusing between themselves, or reorganizing. Although there is a decline in cellular division as the individual ages, the telomere ends become shorter eventually because of every cell division. Indeed, oxidative stress has a strong effect on telomere shortening,[21] which seems to be correlated with decreased lung function and increased risk of COPD.[22]

# Obstructive pulmonary disease

Chronic obstructive pulmonary disease is presently defined as: "a common preventable and treatable disease...characterized by persistent airflow limitation that is usually progressive and associated with an enhanced chronic inflammatory response in the airways and the lung to noxious particles or gases. Exacerbations and comorbidities contribute to the overall severity in individual patients."[23]

Obstruction of small airways, as occurs in chronic obstructive bronchiolitis, chronic asthmatic bronchitis, and emphysema, characterizes COPD. Chronic bronchitis, however, defined by a productive cough lasting more than three months, in more than two consecutive years, does not display airflow limitation.

Chronic obstructive pulmonary disease is also described as a disease of accelerated lung aging, and because it develops slowly over years, its prevalence is age-dependent.[24] The occurrence of COPD is increasing, with more than 10% of individuals affected worldwide among adults 40 years and older.[25] Chronic obstructive pulmonary disease, with the necessity to medically manage the increasing number of people living longer with this disease, is considered to be one of the major health challenges of the next few decades.[26]

Genetic factors may be part of the etiology of COPD.[27] Epigenetic factors also play a significant part in the development of COPD. These include environmental stimuli such as tobacco smoke, exposure to second-hand smoke, occupational exposure to dusts and chemicals, outdoor and indoor air pollution, and allergens.

## The pathophysiology of chronic obstructive pulmonary disease

Although not totally understood, the recognized pathogenesis of COPD is an innate and adaptive inflammatory immune response to the inhalation of toxic particles and gases.[28] Normally, mucociliary clearance eliminates infectious and noxious particles, and tight epithelial intercellular junctions form a protective barrier. When the epithelium is exposed to irritants, in particular cigarette smoke, this barrier is broken. As a result, inflammatory cells infiltrate the mucosa, submucosa, and glandular tissue with proliferation of mucus, epithelial cell hyperplasia, inflammatory edema of the bronchiolar epithelium, and disturbed tissue repair. Chronic inflammation is characterized by greater than normal numbers of alveolar macrophages, neutrophils, and cytotoxic T-lymphocytes, and the release of numerous inflammatory mediators such as lipids, chemokines, cytokines, and growth factors.[29] Chronic inflammation leads to obstruction of the smaller airways. Greater expiratory difficulty follows, causing entrapment of air in the alveoli, overstretching them, which combined with lung infection has the potential to destroy the alveolar walls. Additionally, the destruction of alveolar walls decreases blood oxygenation and carbon dioxide removal.

Many similarities have been described between the aged lung and COPD, although lung function declines quicker in COPD than in the aging patient.[30] One of the main similarities in both aging patients and patients with COPD is the increase in size of the alveolar spaces.[31] This can lead to emphysema—the abnormal enlargement of airspaces distal to the terminal bronchiole, alveolar wall damage, and destruction of the gas-exchanging surface of the lung, as occurs in COPD patients.

### Inflammation and infections

Pro-inflammatory physiology and increased oxidative stress plays a major role in many of the pathogenic mechanisms in COPD.[32] Oxidative stress has a strong effect on telomere shortening,[33] associated with decreased lung function and increased risk of COPD.[34]

Viral and bacterial infections seem to play a role in COPD exacerbations, in particular influenza and respiratory syncytial virus.[35] Additionally, exposure to direct and passive tobacco smoking has a significant impact on oropharyngeal bacterial flora, increasing pathogenic microorganisms and decreasing the normal flora that would otherwise interfere with the growth of pathogens.[36] In these patients, the protection against silent aspiration of pharyngeal secretions that occurs frequently during sleep is less efficient, with the resultant possibility of inflammation and respiratory infection.

Once an innate and adaptive inflammatory immune response occurs in COPD patients, progression of the disease and severity of airflow limitation is linked to the degree and gravity of the tissue response. Changes take place in the small conducting airways that become the major sites of obstruction in COPD. These include: increase of bronchial mucus glands, thickened airways walls, and the accumulation of inflammatory exudates, leading to airway occlusion. Indeed, the progression of COPD is strongly correlated with the thickening of the airway wall by this remodeling process.[37] Furthermore, the emphysematous alveolar wall damage and destruction of the gas-exchanging surface of the lung lower the elastic recoil pressure necessary to push air out of the lung during forced expiration.[38]

### Dyspnea

Dyspnea (shortness of breath; difficulty or distress in breathing) is one of the primary symptoms of COPD. It is associated with reduced exercise tolerance and plays a significant role in decreasing quality of life. Causes of dyspnea and diminished exercise tolerance are complex and multifactorial. Among them, abnormal dynamic ventilatory mechanics and lung hyperinflation are key features. During expiration, lung emptying is restricted due to the emphysematous alveolar wall damage and loss of elastic recoil pressure combined with the increased airway resistance as a result of exudate accumulation and narrowing of the small airways.

Narrowed airways may result in expiratory wheezing, typical in asthma. In severe cases, lung emptying is impaired. Consequently, during activities, ventilatory abnormalities produce higher ventilatory demand, with a fairly rapid and shallow breathing pattern. As the disease progresses, exercise intolerance increases.

Further, stiffness of the rib cage associated with extension dysfunction of the thoracic vertebrae, inspiratory rib dysfunctions, or the latter two together will reduce the thoracic cage contraction normally occurring during exhalation. Thus, an osteopathic treatment that reduces somatic dysfunction impacting the process of breathing will optimize the patient's own resources.

# Pneumonia

Osteopathic manipulative treatment has long been advocated for patients with pneumonia. Indeed, Still stated: "I have successfully treated many cases of pneumonia, both lobar and pleuritic, by correcting the ribs at their spinal articulations."[39]

Pneumonia is still an important cause of morbidity and mortality worldwide, and antibiotic treatment is recommended in most of the consensus guidelines on the management of community-acquired pneumonia (CAP) in adults.[40][41] As an adjunct therapy, however, OMT has demonstrated its ability to optimize the body's self-healing mechanism to defend against infection. The great influenza and pneumonia epidemic of 1918 is a classic example, when a major drop in morbidity and mortality was demonstrated among patients treated by an osteopathic physician.[42][43] More recently, the use of OMT for hospitalized elderly patients with pneumonia has been shown to significantly decrease the duration of intravenous antibiotic treatment needed, as well as the length of hospital stay.[44]

Community-acquired pneumonia is the most common type of pneumonia, and is caught outside of hospitals and other healthcare settings, while hospital-acquired pneumonia is caught during a hospital stay for another illness. Pneumonia is the sixth leading cause of death in the United States and the most frequent cause of death from infectious disease.[45] Pneumonia is an inflammation of the parenchymal structures of one or both of the lungs, where some or all of the alveoli are filled with fluid and blood cells. Typical classification is based upon the anatomic and radiologic patterns. As such, a lobar pneumonia involves part or all of a lung lobe, whereas a bronchopneumonia is

irregular and affects more than one lobe. Adults 65 years of age or older, and subjects who have a chronic illness or a weak immune system are most at risk.

## Pathophysiology of pneumonia

Usually caused by an infection, pneumonia is often a complication of another condition, such as influenza. *Streptococcus pneumoniae*, or pneumococcus, is the most common cause of bacterial CAP. Viruses and, to a much lesser extent, fungi and parasites, can also cause pneumonia. Infection can occur from the inhalation of microorganisms released into the air when an infected person sneezes, coughs, or talks. Other cases exist from aerosolized water originating in contaminated air conditioners, showerheads, or respiratory therapy equipment.

Under normal conditions Waldeyer's tonsillar ring, located at the entry of the upper respiratory and alimentary tract, forms the primary defense against pathogens. Waldeyer's tonsillar ring is a significant collection of lymphoid tissue, organized in a circular fashion in the internal mucous layer lining the nasal cavities and pharynx. It includes the nasopharyngeal, palatine, tubal, and lingual tonsils, plus lymphoid tissue in the intertonsillar intervals. This defensive ring is at a strategic point where many antigens, both food supported and airborne, come into contact with the body. Therefore, its role in the immune system as a site of antigen recognition and synthesis of antibodies is significant. The nasopharyngeal and palatine tonsils are major sources of T-lymphocytes that participate in cell-mediated immunity and B-lymphocytes producing immunoglobulins.[46]

Infectious processes can, however, overcome this first line of defense, and spread into the lower respiratory tracts. Indeed, a strong relationship exists between the upper and lower respiratory airways, referred to as the united airways theory.[47] The upper and lower respiratory tracts are connected without interruption to allow the passage of air into and out of the lungs. They form a functional unit completely covered by a ciliate epithelium with mucinous glands and a rich vasculature and innervation. The post-nasal drip of mucus and inflammatory cells can disseminate an infection down the respiratory tract into the lungs. Also, according to the concept of the united airways theory, another possible route of spread is from the migration of inflammatory cells to the lungs through the vasculature.

Infection from bacteria or viruses in the upper respiratory tract may therefore spread to the alveoli. After the infection reaches the alveoli, inflammation follows, with exudation of fluid, including red and white blood cells, into the air-filled spaces of the alveoli. The alveoli gradually fill with fluid and cells and the infection disseminates by spreading from alveolus to alveolus, to ultimately contaminate greater areas of the lungs, lobes, or sometimes in severe cases, a whole lung. As a result, alveolar ventilation is reduced, thereby decreasing the ventilation-perfusion ratio and, because blood flow throughout the lung remains normal, hypoxemia and hypercapnia result.

The onset of pneumonia is often sudden, with symptoms such as high fever, nausea and vomiting, hypothermia, shaking chills, tachypnea, tachycardia, and malaise. Next, cough appears, with expectoration of sputum and the presence of auscultable crepitance, rales, and rhonchi. With progression of the disease, the sputum becomes purulent, blood-tinged, or rust-colored and the patient may describe chest pain.

Complications of pneumonia may occur, in particular in older patients, smokers, and individuals with pre-existent heart failure or pulmonary disease. Infection can spread through the bloodstream, potentially causing septic shock and failure of multiple organs. Pneumonia may also result in pleurisy and acute respiratory distress syndrome.

The rational for OMT in the treatment of patients with pneumonia is based upon anatomophysiological principles, and directed at optimizing the patient's self-healing capacities. Since Still, mobilization of the thoracic cage, with paraspinal muscle stretching, articulation of the thoracic spine, and rib raising has been recommended. Further, any dysfunction in the cervical spine, thoracic cage, diaphragm, intercostal muscles and accessory muscles of respiration must be addressed. The treatment of the upper thoracic spine and upper cervical spine should be included for somatovisceral (sympathetic and parasympathetic respectfully) influence as well. Besides improving thoracic cage compliance, respiratory efficiency, and blood and lymphatic circulation, the goal of treatment is aimed at reducing sympathetic activity, increasing parasympathetic activity, and assisting bronchial ciliary clearance.

# Obstructive sleep apnea

Prevalence numbers for obstructive sleep apnea (OSA) differ because of variability in definitions of the disease, its process of evaluation, and differences in sampling methods. In the general population, the occurrence of OSA, associated with daytime sleepiness, is approximately 3–7% for adult men and 2–5% for adult women. Numbers are higher for overweight or obese people, and older individuals.[48] However, it should be stressed that as many as 93% of women and 82% of men may have a moderate to severe sleep apnea syndrome that is not clinically diagnosed.[49]

## Definition

The classical description of an individual presenting with OSA syndrome was provided by Charles Dickens, in 'The Posthumous Papers of the Pickwick Club,' published in 1837.[50] His character "Joe" snored forcefully, was obese, and always sleepy. Thus, in 1956, the term 'Pickwickian' was adopted to describe obese patients with somnolence attributed to hypercapnia.[51] The terms 'sleep apnea syndrome' and 'obstructive sleep apnea syndrome,' however, appeared later in 1976, coined by Guilleminault et al. to stress the occurrence of this syndrome in non-obese patients as well.[52]

An apnea is defined as the total cessation of airflow for at least ten seconds. When an episode of shallow breathing occurs that causes oxygen desaturation, it is referred to as a hypopnea. In contrast, 'upper airway resistance syndrome' describes abnormal respiratory efforts during sleep without apneas.[53] Besides these breathing abnormalities, there are other possible etiologies of apneic occurrence not associated with inspiratory effort and suggesting a reduced central respiratory drive, referred to as central apneas. This characterizes Cheyne-Stokes breathing that can result from conditions impairing the brain's ability to regulate respiration including: hyperventilation with decreased partial carbon dioxide pressure, congestive heart failure, stroke, pulmonary hypertension, and agonal respiration from many other causes.

Classically, diagnosis of OSA is done overnight with a polysomnogram in a sleep laboratory, although now, portable polysomnograms to diagnose OSA are also available.[54] This technology measures: sleep time, sleep stages, respiratory effort, airflow, cardiac rhythm, nocturnal hypoxemia (e.g., average oxyhemoglobin desaturation), and the frequency of apneic and hypopneic events. This procedure generates a numeric measurement—the apnea-hypopnea index (AHI) —which is the average number of apneas and hypopneas per hour of sleep. An AHI of five or greater with associated symptoms, such as excessive daytime sleepiness, fatigue, or impaired cognition, or an AHI of 15 or greater, regardless of associated symptoms identifies an OSA syndrome.[55]

# Pathophysiology of obstructive sleep apnea

Several predisposing factors are recognized in OSA. A possible genetic factor has been suggested, [56] [57] along with a hypothesis suggesting changes in neural activation mechanisms intrinsic to sleep.[58] Other predisposing factors include anatomical characteristics that allow for a narrowing of the upper airway. Because reversible somatic dysfunction may be responsible for such narrowing, a review of the evolution, and function, of the anatomy of the upper airway, and the potential effect of somatic dysfunction, may help the understanding, and consequently treatment, of OSA.

## Phylogenetic and ontogenetic evolution

The upper airway is a very complex area, which contributes to physiological functions as diverse as deglutition, respiration, and vocalization. It is also a site where changes associated with phylogenetic and ontogenetic evolution are considerable. Indeed, comparative anatomic studies between non-human primates and modern humans provide an appreciation of the development of the functions, and the potential for dysfunctions, of the upper airway. Throughout the first two months of life, the larynx is positioned high in the pharynx, and throughout both deglutition and respiration, the epiglottis contacts the soft palate, providing a continuous airway from the nose through the larynx into the trachea. Progressively, this contact disappears and at about six months of age, it is present only during deglutition. Then, the larynx descends from its high position in the neck, at the level of C1–C3 during the first two and a half to three years of life, to a lower position in the adult, between the upper border of C4 and the upper border of C7.[59]

Thus, ontogeny repeats phylogeny. In all animals, including non-human primates, the larynx is positioned high in the neck. With the acquisition of upright posture, the larynx descends and the soft palate shortens, opening the space between the epiglottis and the soft palate. Now, laryngeal sounds can escape from the oral cavity, and produce human speech vowel sounds and consonants in the increased supralaryngeal region of the pharynx. These evolutionary modifications in the human upper respiratory tract to facilitate speech have been referred to as 'The Great Leap Forward' in human evolution.[60] They are also considered as the anatomic basis for the acquisition of OSA.[61]

In addition to the descent of the larynx, other changes have occurred in the phylogenetic and ontogenetic evolution of bipedal posture that contribute to the development of OSA. One of the significant differences between humans and other primates is the increased flexion of the cranial base along the midline in humans. Note here, that most of the basilar flexion occurs at the sphenobasilar synchondrosis, located on the superoposterior wall of the nasopharynx. As a consequence of this increased flexion, the angle between the pharynx and nasal cavity tends to flex as well, reducing the respiratory efficiency of the upper airways.

Concomitantly to the basilar flexion, the facial block rotates anteriorly in relation to the posterior cranial base. As a result, space for the teeth is much reduced and the mandible, maxillae, ethmoid, and palate are shortened. The tongue moves backward as well, from being completely located in the oral cavity in non-human primates, to being partially in the pharynx in humans.

Taking all of these changes into account it is interesting to note that a significant correlation exists between the AHI and laryngeal descent, cranial base angulation, and anterior rotation of the viscerocranium, in male individuals suffering OSA.[62]

## Anatomic specificities of obstructive sleep apnea

Additional anatomical characteristics have been demonstrated in multiple studies of OSA patients. Indeed, OSA perfectly illustrates the osteopathic principle of the relationship between structure and function. Narrowing of the upper airway, as present in OSA, can be associated with a dysfunction of any of the structures related to the upper airway, including the pharynx, larynx, hyoid bone, cranial base, maxilla, mandible, soft palate, tongue, and cervical spine. As such any somatic dysfunction affecting these structures must be addressed when treating OSA.

*The pharynx*: Cephalically, the pharynx is attached to the cranial base: on the posterior borders of the medial plates of the pterygoid processes of the sphenoid bone, on the petrous parts and styloid processes of the temporal bones, and on the pharyngeal tubercle of the occipital bone.

Posteriorly the pharynx is attached to the cervical spine and prevertebral fascia. It also connects with the pterygomandibular raphe, the mandible, the tongue, the hyoid bone, and the thyroid and cricoid cartilages.

The pharynx consists of two groups of muscles: three paired constrictor and two paired longitudinal muscles. These muscles are innervated by the vagus nerve (CN X), except for the stylopharyngeus muscles that are innervated by the glossopharyngeal nerve (CN IX). The role of the vagus nerve is of paramount importance in the preservation of pharyngeal airway patency. For this reason, any dysfunction of the cranial base—in particular at the level of the jugular foramen—and cervical spine must be addressed when airway patency is functionally compromised. The position of the cervical spine also affects oropharyngeal size: it is reduced in cervical flexion and increased in cervical extension. [63] Hence, improvement of cervical dysfunction can be valuable for patients with OSA, who typically demonstrate a neck flexion associated with a narrower pharynx.[64] Cervical anteroposterior mechanics are often a reflection of thoracic spinal mechanics. Thus, when problem-solving dysfunction of the cervical spine it is always appropriate to look for and treat contributory thoracic dysfunction.

Several studies demonstrate a narrowing in the anteroposterior dimension of the airway at all levels associated with the severity of OSA. Usually, the oropharynx is the narrowest place when the hypopharynx is positioned in extension.[65]

*The soft palate*: Another significant structure in the establishment of the breathing route and the process of snoring is the soft palate. Often compared to a curtain hanging from the posterior border of the hard palate, i.e., the posterior borders of the two palatine bones, the soft palate extends downwards and backwards between the mouth and pharynx. When positioned more horizontally, it separates the nasopharynx from the oropharynx and facilitates the oral route of breathing. When depressed against the base of the tongue, it closes the oropharyngeal isthmus, opening the nasal breathing route. The soft palate consists of the palatal aponeurosis, fat, lymphoid tissue, and five pairs of muscles: levator veli palatini (LVP), tensor veli palatini (TVP), musculus uvulae, palatopharyngeus, and palatoglossus. Both LVP and TVP arise from the base of the skull. The LVP arises from the apex of the petrous part of the temporal bone and from the cartilage of the pharyngotympanic tube. The TVP arises from the scaphoid fossa of the medial pterygoid plate, from the spina angularis of the sphenoid, and from the lateral wall of the cartilage of the pharyngotympanic tube, and then descends vertically, turning around the pterygoid hamulus. The musculus uvulae form the uvula. The palatopharyngeus arises from the pharynx and the palatoglossus from the tongue. All of these muscles are innervated by the pharyngeal plexus (CN IX and CN X) with the exception of the TVP that is innervated by the mandibular nerve (CN $V_3$).

Because of the location of the insertions of the soft palate muscles, it follows that dysfunction of the cranial base can affect the soft palate's mechanics and strategic position between the base of the skull and the tongue and pharynx. The position and surface area of the soft palate affects OSA. The retropalatal surface area is significantly smaller in OSA patients.[66] Soft palate length also affects snoring. An enlarged uvula is associated with OSA.[67] It must, however, be recognized that the mucosa of the soft palate can become edematous and consequently enlarged as a result of the mechanical stress caused by the vibrations of snoring.[68][69]

### Additional risk factors

*Sleep posture*: The position in which one sleeps has also been studied, and it has been found that more severe apneic events occur in the supine position than in the lateral position.[70] Gravity is partly responsible, as in the supine position the tongue and soft palate move posteriorly, reducing the oropharyngeal space.[71] In fact the lateral position preserves the passive pharyngeal airway, and in this position, patients with obstructive OSA demonstrate less nocturnal obstructive events.[72]

*The protrusive action of the tongue*: Lingual position depends upon the bilateral genioglossi muscles. They play an important role in keeping the tongue from falling backward against the pharyngeal wall, thus keeping the air passage open in the oropharyngeal region. However, during REM sleep, genioglossal motor units may become inactive for periods of up to 90 seconds.[73] This leads some authors to consider hypoglossal nerve (CN XII) stimulation as a possible alternative therapy for OSA.[74] Cranial nerve XII exits the skull through the hypoglossal canal of the cranial base, close to the jugular foramen, and, as such, this area should be part of the osteopathic assessment and treatment of the cranial base.

*The hyoid bone*: The genioglossi and hyoglossi muscles attach to the hyoid bone. Consequently, these muscles can affect, and be affected by, hyoid position. Several studies demonstrate that in individuals with OSA the hyoid bone is lower and more posterior than in controls.[75][76] Additionally, the position of the hyoid bone tends to become more inferior with aging,[77] and aging is associated with a greater prevalence of OSA.[78]

While the hyoid bone has no direct articulation with other skeletal structures, it is a link between the head and neck; an interface between the mandible and tongue above and the upper thoracic area below. As such, its position and motion are influenced by changes occurring at the level of the mandible or anywhere in the thorax. Indeed, the position of the hyoid bone depends upon the maxillomandibular anteroposterior relationship,[79] and retroposition of the mandible is found in OSA.[80] Mandibular advancement devices are sometimes used in subjects with OSA to increase the lateral and anteroposterior dimension of the pharyngeal lumen, particularly in the retroglossal level.[81]

*Gender*: Males have a greater prevalence of OSA than females. One possible explanation for this is that although the pharyngeal air spaces display similar dimensions in men and women, in women they are surrounded by smaller structures and because of this, it may require less effort to maintain airway patency.[82]

Differences in fat distribution between men and women may also account, in part, for gender differences in the prevalence of OSA. Two sites are specifically associated with this in the pathogenesis of OSA: 1) fat deposition in the neck around the pharyngeal airway that may increase tissue pressure and affect pharyngeal airway narrowing; 2) intra-abdominal fat that may decrease lung volumes.[83]

### Associated features

Daytime sleepiness is a common complaint among patients with OSA. It can have serious negative effects on a person's quality of life. Besides sleepiness, fragmentation of sleep is associated with decreased cognitive performance, reduced physical activity, and eventually weight gain. Decreased sleep continuity and sleep time increases sympathetic nerve activation with potential systemic consequences that affect vascular tone, inflammatory mediators, and hormonal balance. The development of hypertension, coronary artery disease, congestive heart failure, arrhythmias, stroke, glucose intolerance, and diabetes may follow.[84 85 86 87 88]

It should be stressed that in OSA patients, functional anatomic factors that have been identified as part of the OSA pathophysiology are the most likely areas of possible somatic dysfunction. Thus, treatment of OSA patients consists of assessing these potentially dysfunctional sites and treating any identified somatic dysfunction.

# The osteopathic contribution to the physical examination and treatment

Osteopathic practitioners use their knowledge of anatomy and physiology to develop a rationale for treatment. In cases of respiratory disorders, the osteopathic treatment is directed at optimizing the mechanics of respiration, enhancing the arterial, venous, and lymphatic circulation of the respiratory tract, balancing autonomic function by addressing somatovisceral influences and through these mechanisms, when appropriate, augmenting the body's defenses against infection.

Diagnosis should begin with observation. Patients' postures are influenced by pulmonary disorders. To facilitate respiration, patients may take a position in which they support their torso by leaning upon their arms in order to fix their shoulder and neck muscles to help respiration.

Look at the pectoral girdle, often protracted in patients with respiratory disorders. Examine and palpate the clavicles and subclavian fossae that may be retracted, with apparent tension of the myofascial structures. Study the cervicothoracic junction, as well as the cervical spine and its relationship to the skull for lack of mobility. Patients may demonstrate a shrugged shoulder posture, with the appearance of a shortened and stiff neck. There is often an increase in the kyphotic curve of the upper thoracic spine with increased cervical lordosis. When observed from the side, the head seems to be thrust forward, with increased tension on the anterior cervical soft tissues. Palpate the spine and cranial base for structure and function. The viscerosomatic reflexes from the respiratory tract are to be found at the level of T1–T4. Conditions involving both lungs result in bilateral reflex findings. Conditions involving one lung result in a reflex on the same side as the involved lung. The parasympathetic reflex is vagal, occiput, C1, and C2.

Continue with an overall inspection of the thorax, its shape, and dynamics. With aging, there is a tendency to develop a 'barrel chest' configuration, where the anteroposterior diameter approximates the lateral diameter. The ribs that are normally oblique tend to become more horizontal, as well. This pattern is increased in respiratory disorders, in particular with COPD.

With the patient supine, evaluate their breathing pattern and the ease of thoracoabdominal respiration. Usually, throughout quiet breathing, the rib cage movements are of small amplitude, with displacements of the costal margin outwards and upwards, and expansion of the upper rib cage, during inspiration, almost imperceptible. Diaphragmatic respiration should be unencumbered, with a coordinated alternation between the rise and fall of the abdomen and thoracic cage mechanics during inspiration and expiration. Normal expiration is passive. Note any asymmetry, predominance of respiratory movement, or both between the abdomen and thoracic cage. Look also for the possible use of the accessory muscles of respiration and check for hypertrophy of these muscles. Look for any area of rib dysfunction that may be painful leading the patient to avoid respiratory motion at this level. With respiratory disorders abnormal breathing patterns are often observed. Frequently, there is asynchronicity between thoracic and abdominal motion—referred to as the abdominal paradox, a sign of diaphragmatic dysfunction—where the abdominal wall goes inward as the rib cage inflates. Look for somatic dysfunction by palpating global chest motion for function. Movement of the thorax is restricted on the side of the lung involved. It may also be restricted on the side of the concavity of a thoracic spinal group curve. Next, palpate the diaphragm, intercostal spaces, ribs, and sternum. Impaired musculoskeletal mechanics can predispose the older individual to pulmonary dysfunction and disease, but they can also result from, and in a circular fashion increase, pulmonary pathology.

While palpating the thoracic cage it is appropriate to palpate for tactile fremitus, the vibration perceived by palpation when the patient speaks. During palpation, place the palmar surfaces of your hands upon the thorax and instruct the patient to repeat numbers, such as "ninety nine," that produce good vibration. Compare the two sides and different portions: anterior, lateral, and posterior, of the chest. Tactile fremitus provides information regarding the density of the underlying lung tissue and chest. It is decreased with air or fluid in the pleural space and with distension of the lung. It is increased in conditions, like pneumonia, where there is increased density of lung tissue.

Look at the submandibular spaces, and observe the position and motion of the mandible, hyoid bone, and trachea. Palpation of the trachea may be done by placing two fingers on either side of the trachea just above the jugular notch of the sternum, medial to the sternocleidomastoid muscles. This should be done with the lightest possible touch to avoid inducing a cough reflex. Note any lateral deviation, and motion during inspiration, when the trachea normally descends about 1–2 cm.

Next, examine the patient's head with particular attention to the face. Check the patency of the nares, the presence of nasal flaring i.e., the outward inspiratory motion of the nares, normally barely visible. Study the position of the lips; patients with severe COPD and emphysema tend to spontaneously purse their lips during expiration, an action that increases pressure within the bronchial tree, maintaining patency of the smaller airways. Ask the patient to open their mouth and observe the relationship between their tongue and teeth. To evaluate the genioglossi muscle for OSA patients, ask them to stick their tongue out forward and laterally, noting any asymmetry. To further assess the tone of these muscles, ask the patient to push their tongue laterally against the inside of their cheek while palpating the movement with your fingers on the outside of the cheek.

Using indirect principles treat any identified dysfunction in the:
- cranial base, jugular foramen for CN X, and hypoglossal canal for CN XII;
- orofacial area, mandible, hyoid bone, and tongue (particularly in OSA patients);
- cervical spine, C1, C2 for CN X, and C3–C5 for their relation with the phrenic nerve and diaphragm;
- thoracic spine, ribs, sternum, and clavicles;
- diaphragm;
- lungs, liver, and spleen.

Correction of the somatic dysfunction, with release of myofascial tension, will improve arterial blood supply, and venous and lymphatic drainage of the tissues. Procedures such as the thoracic pump and release of the thoracic inlet will also improve lymphatic drainage and bronchial ciliary clearance. Additionally, the thoracic pump will increase negative intrathoracic pressure, clearing secretions from the tracheobronchial tree. Rib raising and soft tissue release in the thoracic region will relax the muscles along the thoracic spine and reduce sympathetic activity. Lung dysfunction through viscerosomatic reflexes contributes to the muscular contraction, which in turn stimulates the sympathetic nervous system. Inhibitory pressures may be used to reduce sympathetic activity, while parasympathetic activity may be increased with suboccipital myofascial release and compression of the fourth ventricle (CV4). Increasing parasympathetic activity will assist bronchial ciliary clearance. Diaphragmatic redoming and diaphragmatic function improvement will reduce the need to use accessory respiratory muscles.

Osteopathic manipulative treatment procedures must be specifically directed to enhance the inherent capacities of the patient's body as dictated by specific respiratory disorders. In patients who have chronic decreased respiratory capacity, as in COPD, OMT is aimed at allowing them to function at the highest level they can possibly function in the light of their pulmonary pathology. The practitioner should exercise extreme care not to overdose the patient. Patients with respiratory disorders can very easily develop respiratory distress if treated too aggressively. For the greatest impact the patient should be relaxed and to do so they must trust the practitioner. (See further description of procedures in 'Section 3: Treatment of the patient,' p. 84.)

"I have successfully treated many cases of pneumonia, both lobar and pleuritic, by correcting the ribs at their spinal articulations. If I find much cutting pain in lung and pleura, I carefully palpate over the upper ribs of the side on which the pain is located. I usually find the sixth, seventh, and eighth ribs pushed above or below or twisted upon the transverse processes thus closing up the intercostal veins by pressure and disturbing the vaso motors (sic) to the lungs. I carefully adjust the misplaced ribs and if a cough continues to annoy the patient, explore higher up for a displaced first, second, third, or fourth rib and correct any variations found. Such variations may cause a tightening of the clavicle pressing down on branches of the pneumogastric nerve as they pass under it. Carefully adjust ribs and clavicle and the cough will cease, if taken in time. When the ribs are adjusted and the blood and nerve supply freed from pressure, the fever generally goes down and ease will follow."[89]

## Advice to the patient

Improvement of the body's inherent capacity for self-healing is enhanced with basic principles of good living. Every patient suffering respiratory disorders should try to get seven to nine hours of sleep on a regular basis, in order to balance the ANS and promote homeostasis.

Diet is an important consideration, as well. Daily intake of protein, fresh fruits, and vegetables should be recommended to provide the essential vitamins, minerals, and amino acids needed to repair and restore body functions. Processed sugars and foods that increase gastric acidity should be restricted and, since they increase mucus production, should be consumed early, preferably before 5pm, to make gastric emptying before bedtime possible. Encourage the patient to drink plenty of liquids, such as water, juice, or weak tea, and to drink at least six to ten cups of liquid a day, and to avoid alcohol.

Help your patient to recognize their limits and not to exceed them. Exercise, as tolerated, is essential to maintain and improve well-being. The sensation of suffocation that patients experience during breathing is quite stressful and respiratory exercises may empower them, by giving them some control over their respiration. When a patient begins to experience dyspnea, their first reaction is typically anxiety. This is extremely counterproductive since it increases the rate and effort of respiration, adding to the sensation of dyspnea. Rather, they should consciously slow their respiration, taking slow deep breaths. Start by making them aware of their breathing pattern. Teach them to use their diaphragm for better breathing. Ask the patient to place one hand on their upper chest and the other just below the rib cage.

Instruct them to breathe in slowly through the nose and to feel as their stomach moves out against their hand. During exhalation they should tighten their abdominal muscles and exhale through pursed lips. During this exercise, the neck and shoulders should be relaxed. You can further teach them to clear their airways with forceful expiration also known as 'huffing.' Instruct the patient to inhale deeply, filling their lungs as much as possible and to then exhale through their open mouth in forceful bursts while saying "huh." This process may be repeated as many times as necessary to loosen and clear the mucus from the airway.

Insist on the importance of nasal breathing, and advise the patient to practice vocal activities such as singing or humming to help control and enhance their breathing pattern. Gentle stretches of the neck, shoulder, and thoracic cage such as spinal flexion/extension, sidebending right/left, and rotation right/left will facilitate respiration. Good posture must be encouraged, with special attention on improving a protracted pectoral girdle, thoracic kyphosis, and cervical lordosis.

Additional advice may be given specific to particular disorders.

## Chronic obstructive pulmonary disease

Encourage your patient to quit smoking, explaining that it is the best way to influence the disease progression. Counseling should be proposed. Encourage your patient to avoid occupational, indoor, and outdoor air pollution, as well. Allergens should be sought out, identified, and eliminated as much as possible. They most often include pollens, foods, molds, dusts, and animal dander.

Chronic obstructive pulmonary disease patients should, as much as possible, maintain regular activity adapted to their level of respiratory tolerance. Rehabilitation with training programs, where patients are taught how to improve exercise tolerance, and how to manage their symptoms of dyspnea and fatigue, may be indicated. Encourage them to relieve shortness of breath with pursed-lip breathing, in particular when taking a long walk or doing more demanding activities. Pa-

tients will also benefit from relaxation techniques, guided imagery, progressive muscle relaxation, or meditation.

## Pneumonia prevention

Encourage your patient to respect strict sanitary precautions, in particular washing their hands often with soap and water such as before eating and when preparing foods. They should drink plenty of fluids and maintain a warm and humified environment to help liquify sticky mucus.

## Obstructive sleep apnea

Weight loss and the abstinence from alcohol and sedatives are important to reduce OSA. Encourage your patient to avoid a supine sleeping position as well. Continuous positive airway pressure is regarded as a good treatment, but patients often do not comply. Other classical options are: oral device therapy that repositions the mandibular forward, or surgery. As such, OMT offers a good alternative for a conservative approach. Postural dysfunction must be taken into consideration, with particular focus upon the cranial, cervical, and upper thoracic areas.

Teach your patient exercises that strengthen and tone the soft palate and tongue. The tongue, particularly the genioglossi muscles, can be strengthened by having the patient stick their tongue out, forward, and alternately to the right and left. Increased strengthening may be obtained by instructing the patient to place their fingers against the cheek, and to push the tongue laterally against the inside of the cheek while resisting with the fingers. Singing brings relaxation. It is an excellent breathing exercise that also tones the soft palate and orofacial muscles.

# References

1.  Still AT. Philosophy of Osteopathy. Kirksville, MO: A.T. Still; 1899. Reprinted, Indianapolis, IN: American Academy of Osteopathy; 1971.
2.  Standring S, ed. Gray's Anatomy: The anatomical basis of clinical practice. 40th ed. Edinburgh: Churchill Livingstone; 2008.
3.  Knowles MR, Boucher RC. Mucus clearance as a primary innate defense mechanism for mammalian airways. J Clin Invest. 2002 Mar;109(5):571-7.
4.  Hall JE. Chapt 37, Pulmonary Ventilation. In: Guyton and Hall textbook of medical physiology, 12th ed. Philadelphia: Saunders, 2010.
5.  Standring S, ed. Gray's Anatomy: The anatomical basis of clinical practice. 40th ed. Edinburgh: Churchill Livingstone; 2008.
6.  Knowles MR, Boucher RC. Mucus clearance as a primary innate defense mechanism for mammalian airways. J Clin Invest. 2002 Mar;109(5):571-7.

7. Hall JE. Chapt 37, Pulmonary Ventilation. In: Guyton and Hall textbook of medical physiology, 12th ed. Philadelphia: Saunders, 2010.

8. Hyam JA, Brittain JS, Paterson DJ, Davies RJ, Aziz TZ, Green AL. Controlling the lungs via the brain: a novel neurosurgical method to improve lung function in humans. Neurosurgery. 2012 Feb;70(2):469-77; discussion 477-8.

9. Pisi G, Olivieri D, Chetta A. The airway neurogenic inflammation: clinical and pharmacological implications. Inflamm Allergy Drug Targets. 2009 Jul;8(3):176-81.

10. Litton HE. Manipulative treatment of pneumonia. Year Book of the Academy of Applied Osteopathy. American Academy of Osteopathy. Indianapolis, IN. 1965:136-8.

11. Litton HE. Manipulative treatment of pneumonia. Year Book of the Academy of Applied Osteopathy. American Academy of Osteopathy. Indianapolis, IN. 1965:136-8.

12. Estenne M, Yernault JC, De Troyer A. Rib cage and diaphragm-abdomen compliance in humans: effects of age and posture. J Appl Physiol. 1985 Dec;59(6):1842-8.

13. Fon GT, Pitt MJ, Thies AC Jr. Thoracic kyphosis: range in normal subjects. AJR Am J Roentgenol. 1980 May;134(5):979-83.

14. Kang KB, Kim YJ, Muzaffar N, Yang JH, Kim YB, Yeo ED. Changes of Sagittal Spinopelvic Parameters in Normal Koreans with Age over 50. Asian Spine J. 2010 Dec;4(2):96-101.

15. Dyer C. The interaction of ageing and lung disease. Chron Respir Dis. 2012 Feb;9(1):63-7.

16. Janssens JP. Aging of the respiratory system: impact on pulmonary function tests and adaptation to exertion. Clin Chest Med. 2005 Sep;26(3):469-84, vi-vii.

17. Sharma G, Goodwin J. Effect of aging on respiratory system physiology and immunology. Clin Interv Aging. 2006;1(3):253-60.

18. Chung HY, Lee EK, Choi YJ, Kim JM, Kim DH, Zou Y, Kim CH, Lee J, Kim HS, Kim ND, Jung JH, Yu BP. Molecular inflammation as an underlying mechanism of the aging process and age-related diseases. J Dent Res. 2011 Jul;90(7):830-40.

19. Rahman I, MacNee W. Antioxidant pharmacological therapies for COPD. Curr Opin Pharmacol. 2012 Jun;12(3):256-65.

20. Jones DP. Redefining oxidative stress. Antioxid Redox Signal. 2006 Sep-Oct;8(9-10):1865-79.

21. von Zglinicki T. Oxidative stress shortens telomeres. Trends Biochem Sci. 2002 Jul;27(7):339-44.

22. Rode L, Bojesen SE, Weischer M, Vestbo J, Nordestgaard BG. Short telomere length, lung function and chronic obstructive pulmonary disease in 46 396 individuals. Thorax. 2013 May;68(5):429-35.

23. Global Initiative for Chronic Obstructive Lung Disease. Pocket guide to COPD diagnosis, management, and prevention. Revised 2011. Available at http://www.goldcopd.org/uploads/users/files/GOLD_Pocket_May2512.pdf. Accessed Jan 3, 2013.

24. Papaioannou AI, Rossios C, Kostikas K, Ito K. Can we Delay the Accelerated Lung Aging in COPD? Anti-Aging Molecules and Interventions. Curr Drug Targets. 2013 Feb;14(2):149-57.

25. Gershon AS, Wang C, Wilton AS, Raut R, To T. Trends in chronic obstructive pulmonary disease prevalence, incidence, and mortality in ontario, Canada, 1996 to 2007: a population-based study. Arch Intern Med. 2010 Mar 22;170(6):560-5.

26. Decramer M, Janssens W, Miravitlles M. Chronic obstructive pulmonary disease. Lancet. 2012 Apr 7;379(9823):1341-51.

27. Boezen HM. Genome-wide association studies: what do they teach us about asthma and chronic obstructive pulmonary disease? Proc Am Thorac Soc. 2009 Dec;6(8):701-3.

28. Hogg JC, Timens W. The pathology of chronic obstructive pulmonary disease. Annu Rev Pathol. 2009;4:435-59.

29. Barnes PJ, Shapiro SD, Pauwels RA. Chronic obstructive pulmonary disease: molecular and cellular mechanisms. Eur Respir J. 2003 Oct;22(4):672-88.

30. Ito K, Barnes PJ. COPD as a disease of accelerated lung aging. Chest. 2009 Jan;135(1):173-80.

31. Gillooly M, Lamb D. Airspace size in lungs of lifelong non-smokers: effect of age and sex. Thorax. 1993 Jan;48(1):39-43.

32. Rahman I, MacNee W. Antioxidant pharmacological therapies for COPD. Curr Opin Pharmacol. 2012 Jun;12(3):256-65.

33. von Zglinicki T. Oxidative stress shortens telomeres. Trends Biochem Sci. 2002 Jul;27(7):339-44.

34. Rode L, Bojesen SE, Weischer M, Vestbo J, Nordestgaard BG. Short telomere length, lung function and chronic obstructive pulmonary disease in 46 396 individuals. Thorax. 2013 May;68(5):429-35.

35. De Serres G, Lampron N, La Forge J, Rouleau I, Bourbeau J, Weiss K, Barret B, Boivin G. Importance of viral and bacterial infections in chronic obstructive pulmonary disease exacerbations. J Clin Virol. 2009 Oct;46(2):129-33.

36. Brook I. The impact of smoking on oral and nasopharyngeal bacterial flora. J Dent Res. 2011 Jun;90(6):704-10.

37. Hogg JC, Chu F, Utokaparch S, Woods R, Elliott WM, Buzatu L, Cherniack RM, Rogers RM, Sciurba FC, Coxson HO, Paré PD. The nature of small-airway obstruction in chronic obstructive pulmonary disease. N Engl J Med. 2004 Jun 24;350(26):2645-53.

38. Hogg JC. Lung structure and function in COPD. Int J Tuberc Lung Dis. 2008 May;12(5):467-79.

39. Still AT. Chapt. Thoracic region, Pneumonia. In: Osteopathy. Research and Practice. Kirksville, MO: Published by the author, 1910:156-165.

40. Mandell LA, Wunderink RG, Anzueto A, Bartlett JG, Campbell GD, Dean NC. et al. Infectious Diseases Society of America/American Thoracic Society consensus guidelines on the management of community-acquired pneumonia in adults. Clin Infect Dis. 2007 Mar 1;44 Suppl 2:S27-72.

41. Postma DF, van Werkhoven CH, Huijts SM, Bolkenbaas M, Oosterheert JJ, Bonten MJ. New trends in the prevention and management of community-acquired pneumonia. Neth J Med. 2012 Oct;70(8):337-48.

42. Magoun HI Jr. More about the use of OMT during influenza epidemics. J Am Osteopath Assoc. 2004 Oct;104(10):406-7.

43. Smith RK. One hundred thousand cases of influenza with a death rate of one-fortieth of that officially reported under conventional medical treatment. 1919. J Am Osteopath Assoc. 2000 May;100(5):320-3.

44. Noll DR, Shores JH, Gamber RG, Herron KM, Swift J Jr. Benefits of osteopathic manipulative treatment for hospitalized elderly patients with pneumonia. J Am Osteopath Assoc. 2000 Dec;100(12):776-82.

45. Heron M. National Vital Statistics Reports. Deaths: Leading Causes for 2009. 61(7). Available at http://www.cdc.gov/nchs/data/nvsr/nvsr61/nvsr61_07.pdf. Accessed Jan 13, 2013.

46. Bourges D, Wang CH, Chevaleyre C, Salmon H. T and IgA B lymphocytes of the pharyngeal and palatine tonsils: differential expression of adhesion molecules and chemokines. Scand J Immunol 2004;60(4):338−50.

47. Ciprandi G, Caimmi D, Miraglia Del Giudice M, La Rosa M, Salpietro C, Marseglia GL. Recent developments in United airways disease. Allergy Asthma Immunol Res. 2012 Jul;4(4):171-7.

48. Punjabi NM. The epidemiology of adult obstructive sleep apnea. Proc Am Thorac Soc. 2008 Feb 15;5(2):136-43.

49. Young T, Evans L, Finn L, Palta M. Estimation of the clinically diagnosed proportion of sleep apnea syndrome in middle-aged men and women. Sleep. 1997 Sep;20(9):705-6.

50. Dickens C. The posthumous papers of the pickwick club. London: Chapman and Hall; 1837.

51. Bickelmann AG, Burwell CS, Robin ED, Whaley RD. Extreme obesity associated with alveolar hypoventilation; a Pickwickian syndrome. Am J Med. 1956 Nov;21(5):811-8.

52. Guilleminault C, Tilkian A, Dement WC. The sleep apnea syndromes. Annu Rev Med. 1976;27:465-84.

53. Guilleminault C, Abad VC. Obstructive sleep apnea syndromes. Med Clin North Am. 2004 May;88(3):611-30, viii.

54. LCD for Positive Airway Pressure (PAP) Devices for the Treatment of Obstructive Sleep Apnea (L27230). Available at http://www.nationwidemedical.com/wp-content/uploads/2010/06/LCD-for-Positive-Airway-Pressure-doc-region-b.pdf. Accessed Jan 21, 2013.

55. Park JG, Ramar K, Olson EJ. Updates on definition, consequences, and management of obstructive sleep apnea. Mayo Clin Proc. 2011 Jun;86(6):549-54.

56. Schwab RJ. Genetic determinants of upper airway structures that predispose to obstructive sleep apnea. Respir Physiol Neurobiol. 2005 Jul 28;147(2-3):289-98.

57. Song CM, Lee CH, Rhee CS, Min YG, Kim JW. Analysis of genetic expression in the soft palate of patients with obstructive sleep apnea. Acta Otolaryngol. 2012 Jun;132 Suppl 1:S63-8.

58. Ayappa I, Rapoport DM. The upper airway in sleep: physiology of the pharynx. Sleep Med Rev. 2003 Feb;7(1):9-33.

59. Laitman JT, Crelin ES. Developmental change in the upper respiratory system of human infants. Perinatol Neonatol 1980;4:15–22.

60. Diamond J. The Third Chimpanzee: the evolution and future of the human animal. New York: HarperCollins: 1992.

61. Davidson TM, Sedgh J, Tran D, Stepnowsky CJ Jr. The anatomic basis for the acquisition of speech and obstructive sleep apnea: evidence from cephalometric analysis supports The Great Leap Forward hypothesis. Sleep Med. 2005 Nov;6(6):497-505.

62. Davidson TM, Sedgh J, Tran D, Stepnowsky CJ Jr. The anatomic basis for the acquisition of speech and obstructive sleep apnea: evidence from cephalometric analysis supports The Great Leap Forward hypothesis. Sleep Med. 2005 Nov;6(6):497-505.

63. Isono S, Tanaka A, Tagaito Y, Ishikawa T, Nishino T. Influences of head positions and bite opening on collapsibility of the passive pharynx. J Appl Physiol 2004;97(1):339-46.

64. Isono S, Remmers JE, Tanaka A, Sho Y, Sato J, Nishino T. Anatomy of pharynx in patients with obstructive sleep apnea and in normal subjects. J. Appl Physiol. 1997 Apr;82(4):1319-26.

65. Svaza J, Skagers A, Cakarne D, Jankovska I. Upper airway sagittal dimensions in obstructive sleep apnea (OSA) patients and severity of the disease. Stomatologija. 2011;13(4):123-7.

66. Tanyeri H, Serin GM, Polat S, Aksoy E, Cuhadaroglu C. Quantification of retropalatal region in obstructive sleep apnea. J Craniofac Surg. 2012 Sep;23(5):1410-3.

67. Schellenberg JB, Maislin G, Schwab RJ. Physical findings and the risk for obstructive sleep apnea. The importance of oropharyngeal structures. Am J Respir Crit Care Med. 2000 Aug;162(2 Pt 1):740-8.

68. Strollo PJ Jr, Rogers RM. Obstructive sleep apnea. N Engl J Med. 1996 Jan 11;334(2): 99-104.

69. Mariën S, Schmelzer B. Velopharyngeal anatomy in snorers and patients with obstructive sleep apnea. Acta Otorhinolaryngol Belg. 2002;56(2):93-9.

70. Oksenberg A, Khamaysi I, Silverberg DS, Tarasiuk A. Association of body position with severity of apneic events in patients with severe nonpositional obstructive sleep apnea. Chest. 2000 Oct;118(4):1018-24.

71. Fouke JM, Strohl KP. Effect of position and lung volume on upper airway geometry. J Appl Physiol. 1987 Jul;63(1):375-80.

72. Isono S, Tanaka A, Nishino T. Lateral position decreases collapsibility of the passive pharynx in patients with obstructive sleep apnea. Anesthesiology. 2002 Oct;97(4):780-5.

73. Sauerland EK, Harper RM. The human tongue during sleep: electromyographic activity of the genioglossus muscle. Exp Neurol. 1976 Apr;51(1):160-70.

74. Zaidi FN, Meadows P, Jacobowitz O, Davidson TM. Tongue Anatomy and Physiology, the Scientific Basis for a Novel Targeted Neurostimulation System Designed for the Treatment of Obstructive Sleep Apnea. Neuromodulation. 2012 Aug 31. doi: 10.1111/j.1525-1403.2012.00514.x.

75. Bucchieri A, Mastrangelo C, Stella R, Poladas EG. Cephalometric evaluation of hyoid bone position in patients with obstructive sleep apnea. Minerva Stomatol. 2004 Jan-Feb;53(1-2):33-9.

76. Fusco G, Macina F, Macarini L, Garribba AP, Ettorre GC. Magnetic resonance imaging in simple snoring and obstructive sleep apnea-hypopnea syndrome. Radiol Med. 2004 Sep;108(3):238-54.

77. Kollias I, Krogstad O. Adult craniocervical and pharyngeal changes--a longitudinal cephalometric study between 22 and 42 years of age. Part I: Morphological craniocervical and hyoid bone changes. Eur J Orthod. 1999 Aug;21(4):333-44.

78. Edwards BA, O'Driscoll DM, Ali A, Jordan AS, Trinder J, Malhotra A. Aging and sleep: physiology and pathophysiology. Semin Respir Crit Care Med. 2010 Oct;31(5):618-33.

79. Deljo E, Filipovic M, Babacic R, Grabus J. Correlation analysis of the hyoid bone position in relation to the cranial base, mandible and cervical part of vertebra with particular reference to bimaxillary relations / teleroentgenogram analysis. Acta Inform Med. 2012 Mar;20(1):25-31.

80. Jamieson A, Guilleminault C, Partinen M, Quera-Salva MA. Obstructive sleep apneic patients have craniomandibular abnormalities. Sleep. 1986 Dec;9(4):469-77.

81. Kaur A, Chand P, Singh RD, Siddhartha R, Tripathi A, Tripathi S, Singh R, Mishra A. Computed tomographic evaluation of the effects of mandibular advancement devices on pharyngeal dimension changes in patients with obstructive sleep apnea. Int J Prosthodont. 2012 Sep-Oct;25(5):497-505.

82. Daniel MM, Lorenzi MC, da Costa Leite C, Lorenzi-Filho G. Pharyngeal dimensions in healthy men and women. Clinics (Sao Paulo). 2007 Jun;62(1):5-10.

83. Isono S. Obesity and obstructive sleep apnoea: mechanisms for increased collapsibility of the passive pharyngeal airway. Respirology. 2012 Jan;17(1):32-42.

84. Strollo PJ Jr, Rogers RM. Obstructive sleep apnea. N Engl J Med. 1996 Jan 11;334(2):99-104.

85. Narkiewicz K, Somers VK. The sympathetic nervous system and obstructive sleep apnea: implications for hypertension. J Hypertens. 1997 Dec;15(12 Pt 2):1613-9.

86. Narkiewicz K, Somers VK. Sympathetic nerve activity in obstructive sleep apnoea. Acta Physiol Scand. 2003 Mar;177(3):385-90.

87. Parish JM, Somers VK. Obstructive sleep apnea and cardiovascular disease. Mayo Clin Proc. 2004 Aug;79(8):1036-46.

88. Thorpy M. Obstructive sleep apnea syndrome is a risk factor for stroke. Curr Neurol Neurosci Rep. 2006 Mar;6(2):147-8.

89. Still AT. Chapt. Thoracic region, Pneumonia. In: Osteopathy. Research and Practice. Kirksville, MO: Published by the author, 1910:156-165.

# Chapter 5

# Gastrointestinal dysfunctions

*I will say, after forty years' observation and practice, that no good can come to the patient by pulling, pushing, and gouging in the sacred territory of the abdominal organs; but much harm can and does follow bruising the solar plexus, from which a branch of nerves goes to each organ of the abdomen. Upon that center depends all the elaborate work of the functioning of the abdomen. I say, 'Hands off.' Go to the spine and ribs only. If you do not know the power of the spinal nerves on the liver to restore health, you must learn or quit, because you are only an owl of hoots, more work than brains. I want the man who wishes to know the work that is done by the organs or contents of the abdomen also to know the danger of ignorance, and that wild force in treating the abdomen cannot be tolerated as any part of this sacred philosophy.*

—A. T. Still[1]

Healthy gastrointestinal (GI) function is essential for comfortable aging. It allows the aged individual to preserve independence. Nevertheless, throughout aging, histological and physiological modifications take place in the GI tract that may be associated with multiple disorders. Any portion of the GI tract may be affected. The upper portion of the GI tract consists of the mouth cavity, the pharynx, the esophagus, the stomach, and the duodenum. Dysphagia and gastroesophageal reflux (GER) are among the most frequent disorders of this portion. The lower portion includes most of the small intestine and all of the large intestine. Irritable bowel syndrome (IBS), flatus, and constipation are the common complaints of this area.

The fundamental osteopathic association between structure and function has never been greater than it is in the consideration of GI function and dysfunction. The GI tract is connected with the rest of the body by the lymphatic and vascular systems. Through its nervous supply it influences and is under the influence of the ribs and the spine by way of viscerosomatic, somatovisceral, and viscerovisceral reflexes.[2] Knowledge of these structures is necessary to understand function and dysfunction of the GI tract and to be able to let healthy function prevail.

## Dysphagia

Dysphagia, or difficulty swallowing, is one of the problems encountered with aging that frequently leads to ingested material entering the trachea. This can result in lower respiratory tract infections, and can also be a major problem in the maintenance of sufficient nutrition. It can result from a wide variety of conditions, disorders, and diseases such as functional or structural deficits of the oral cavity, pharynx, larynx, esophagus, or esophageal sphincters. Organic pathologies necessitating definitive medical treatment should first, and always, be ruled out. Osteophytes on the anterior aspect of the cervical vertebrae are common with aging and may interfere with the easy passage of food. Nearly 22% of healthy, independent-living seniors report dysphagia.[3] Multiple etiologies, from neural dysfunction to functional changes in the larynx, or dysfunction of the muscles involved in the process of swallowing can result in functional dysphagia. Osteopathic principles may be applied to address these issues and improve the function of swallowing.

Swallowing is, usually, subdivided into three phases: oral, pharyngeal, and esophageal. The smooth passage of a bolus of food from the mouth to the stomach involves multiple sensorimotor functions with the participation of the orofacial, lingual, laryngeal, pharyngeal, and esophageal musculature, and the involvement of diverse levels of the central nervous system (CNS) from the cerebral cortex to the medulla oblongata and the cranial nerves that innervate the striated muscles.

## Oral phase of swallowing

Typically, the oral phase of swallowing is considered to be voluntary and its duration depends upon the functional status of the subject's dentition, the quality and taste of the food and, particularly for the aged patient, the environment. Orofacial structural aspects also have to be considered. Longer duration for swallowing has been identified in association with "increased gonial angles, increased mandibular body and ramus lengths, raised anterior lower facial heights, lingually inclined mandibular incisors, and increased arch lengths."[4]

One of the major participants in the oral phase of swallowing is the tongue. As food is masticated and transformed into a bolus it is pressed against the hard palate by the tongue. The tongue then propels the bolus toward the back of the mouth and into the pharynx, where the swallowing reflex is initiated.

The tongue is a muscular structure. It is comprised of both intrinsic and extrinsic muscles.

The intrinsic muscles are the superior longitudinal, inferior longitudinal, transverse, and vertical muscles. They alter the shape of the tongue, permitting the precise movements of sucking, swallowing, and speech.

There are four pairs of extrinsic muscles that symmetrically attach the tongue to the skull and to the hyoid bone. They are the genioglossus, hyoglossus, styloglossus, and palatoglossus muscles. A midline fibrous sagittal septum divides the tongue into two halves, and attaches to the body of the hyoid bone. These muscular pairs work in concert, symmetrically or asymmetrically to cause the

tongue to protrude, retract, and move laterally left or right.

The genioglossus muscles originate bilaterally from the mandible and insert upon the hyoid bone. They blend with the intrinsic muscles of the tongue and are the main muscles of protrusion.

The hyoglossus muscles originate from the hyoid bone and insert into the tongue. They retract the tongue.

The styloglossus muscles originate from the styloid processes of the temporal bones. Their insertion is incorporated into the lateral aspect of the tongue. They also retract the tongue.

The palatoglossus muscles originate from the aponeurosis of the soft palate. They insert into the lateral aspect of the tongue. They act to elevate the posterior part of the tongue, closing the oropharyngeal isthmus.

The complexity of the above motions is further added to by the participation of the suprahyoid muscles: the digastric, stylohyoid, geniohyoid, and mylohyoid muscles. They work to elevate the tongue from the floor of the mouth. Additionally, the contraction of the muscles of the lips and cheeks (the orbicularis oris and buccinator muscles) is essential to avoid the escape of food or liquid from the oral cavity.

Normally, the tongue demonstrates large movements in all three planes of space.[5] It adjusts its shape and form in order to assist in the mixing of food during mastication and to propel the resultant food bolus posteriorly into the oropharynx. However, the structures upon which the tongue attaches, the mandible, hyoid bone, styloid processes of the temporal bones, and the posterior border of the soft palate and its aponeurosis, must be free of somatic dysfunction in order to allow the most effective expression of these lingual motions. During eating and speech, the position of the tongue is normally coordinated with changes in the position of the hyoid bone and mandible.[6] Even if the hyoid bone has no direct articulation with other skeletal structures, it is, nevertheless, an important interface between the mandible and tongue above, and the upper thoracic area below. As a result, its position and motion are influenced by the function and position of the mandible or

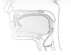

any part of the thorax that in turn will affect the function of the tongue.

Posture, and the function of the tongue during swallowing, is also significantly linked to dentofacial morphology. The relationship between lingual movement and the palatal vault and arch length, but not arch width, illustrates the association between structure and function in the stomatognathic system. Studies reveal that the intermaxillary vertical dimension is significantly and positively associated with the magnitude of motion of the tongue.[7] Increased palatal arch length is also associated with prolonged duration of swallowing. Therefore aging patients, with artificial replacement for one or more of their natural teeth, such as dentures, may experience difficulties. This is especially true if the dental prosthesis is not perfectly adapted to the individual. The resultant malocclusion, where the teeth and jaws are misaligned from the habitual bite, causes lower efficiency of mastication, with larger particle volume of the triturated food bolus making it more difficult to swallow. Temporomandibular joint dysfunction may also be present, with associated pain that may decrease coordination of orofacial muscles.

When the food bolus reaches the back of the tongue, the swallowing reflex is elicited. Multiple receptors around the opening of the oropharynx are stimulated by the bolus. Sensory impulses are conducted to the swallowing center in the brainstem via the maxillary branch of the trigeminal nerve (CN V), the glossopharyngeal nerve (CN IX), and the vagus nerve (CN X), especially its superior laryngeal branch. These nerves innervate the dorsum of the tongue, the epiglottis, the pillar of the fauces, and the walls of the pharynx. At the brainstem level, the afferent fibers implicated in instigating swallowing travelling with CNs V, IX, and X join the solitary tract and end in the nucleus tractus solitarius. Swallowing may also depend on regions above the brainstem and studies show that healthy older subjects display activity in more regions of the cortex than young participants when swallowing. One reason may be that with aging, more effort is necessary to swallow, resulting in more neural activation.[8]

## Pharyngeal phase of swallowing

During the pharyngeal stage, boluses of food and liquids are transferred from the oral cavity toward the stomach through the esophagus. While the tongue propels the bolus posteriorly, the hyoid bone moves anteriorly, the larynx superiorly and anteriorly toward the base of the tongue, and the epiglottis covers the superior opening of the larynx. The displacement of the epiglottis and the

**Figure 4.5.1:** The pharynx

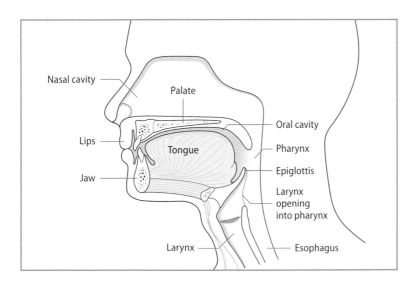

approximation of the vocal cords in the larynx combine to avoid the passage of food into the trachea. Thus, the bolus passes into the pharynx, dividing around the epiglottis while the soft palate moves against the posterior pharyngeal wall to close the nasopharyngeal entrance. The muscles attached to the hyoid bone pull the larynx superiorly and anteriorly. This stretches the opening of the esophagus, and the bolus, always under the influence of gravity and contractions of the pharyngeal constrictors, enters into the esophagus. During this phase, inadequate velopharyngeal closure may produce nasal regurgitation and decrease the pharyngeal pressure necessary for swallowing.

The pharynx is a musculomembranous half-cylinder that connects the nasal and oral cavities with the larynx and esophagus. It extends from the base of the skull to the level of the sixth cervical vertebra where it joins the esophagus. Three layers form the pharyngeal wall: an internal mucous layer, an intermediate fibrous layer, and an external layer. The thickest portion of the intermediate fibrous layer of the superior part of the pharyngeal wall forms the pharyngobasilar fascia, which is tightly attached to the base of the skull in an irregular U-shaped line. Anteriorly, the fascia inserts upon the posterior margin of the medial plate of the sphenoidal pterygoid process. It then curves under the cartilaginous part of the pharyngotympanic tube and inserts onto the petrous part of the temporal bone, and expands to the pharyngeal tubercle of the occipital basilar part to meet the attachment from the other side.

The anterior border of the pharyngeal wall is not continuous. Rather, it has multiple areas of attachment: the medial pterygoid plate, the pterygomandibular raphe, the mandible, the tongue, the hyoid bone, and the thyroid and cricoid cartilages.

Six muscles participate in the formation the pharyngeal wall. On each side, the superior, middle, and inferior constrictor muscles constrict the pharyngeal cavity, and three longitudinal muscles (the stylopharyngeus, salpingopharyngeus, and palatopharyngeus) elevate the pharyngeal wall and contribute to swallowing. The fibers of the three constrictor muscles fan out posteriorly into the median pharyngeal raphe, a fibrous band that is attached above to the pharyngeal tubercle of the occipital basilar part. The pharyngeal raphe descends to the level of the sixth cervical vertebra where it blends into the posterior wall of the esophagus. A thin retropharyngeal space, filled with loose areolar tissue, unites the pharynx with the cervical portion of the vertebral column and the prevertebral fascia covering the longus colli and longus capitis muscles.

The pharynx consists of three portions: the nasopharynx positioned above and behind the hard palate; the oropharynx that extends from the nasopharynx to the base of the epiglottis; and the laryngopharynx, which extends from the base of the tongue to the larynx. The pharynx provides a channel for two functions: the passage of boluses of food and liquids from the oral cavity in the direction of the stomach through the esophagus; and the passage of air to and from the lungs. The pharynx must coordinate respiration and swallowing in order to prevent the passage of food into the lungs. Secure bolus passage through the pharynx without the aspiration of food is critical. Airway security against retrograde aspiration is multifactorial and engages subtle interaction between upper airway and upper GI tracts.[9] First, vocal cord adduction closes the space between the vocal folds (the glottis) that forms the upper part of the larynx. Additionally, the laryngeal arytenoid cartilages, upon which the vocal cords are attached, tilt forward to join the epiglottic base. The larynx is pushed under the base of the tongue and the epiglottis inclines backward to seal the laryngeal vestibule. The displacement of the hyoid bone and the larynx superiorly and anteriorly, added to the pressure of the descending bolus, results in the opening of the upper esophageal sphincter that allows the bolus to enter into the esophagus.

Normally, with healthy aging, the processes involved in the elevation of the larynx, particularly the initiation of maximal hyolaryngeal excursion, are generally slower compared to that of younger adults.[10] This may be because older individuals have subdued oral sensations as compared to young adults.[11] The pharyngeal swallow reflex is a response to the stimulation of the oropharyngeal sensory receptors by the various properties of the bolus such as volume, viscosity, and temperature.[12] As a result of longer delays in initiation of the pharyngeal swallow, more residues may be left within the oral and pharyngeal cavities.

From an osteopathic perspective, keeping in mind the relationship between structure and function, muscular activities of the pharynx may be influenced by its zones of attachment. They should be free of any somatic dysfunction in order to allow the muscles to optimize their function with the best leverage possible. Consequently, dysfunctions of the cranial base, cervical spine, hyoid bone, and mandible should be considered when evaluating dysfunctional swallowing. Furthermore because CN IX and CN X trigger the motor activity of swallowing, the relationship between the occipital bone and temporal bones should be assessed for its effect upon the jugular foramina.

## Esophageal phase of swallowing

The third stage of the mechanism of swallowing is the esophageal phase. The esophagus is a tubular structure with muscular sphincters (the upper and lower esophageal sphincters) connecting the pharynx and stomach.

The upper portion of the esophagus, the upper one third, is the cervical esophagus and consists mainly of skeletal muscle. The remainder, the lower two thirds, the thoracic part, consists of smooth muscle. After swallowing, the bolus of food passes through the pharynx and the upper esophageal sphincter (UES) to enter the esophagus. A primary wave of contraction starts in the pharynx and goes along the whole length of the esophagus, reinforced by secondary waves in the body of the esophagus. These peristaltic waves assist gravity to propel the bolus through the esophagus, and into the stomach. In the thoracic part of the esophagus, the motion of the bolus is different from that of the pharynx and is totally under the influence of the autonomic nervous system via the vagus nerves and the cervical and thoracic sympathetics. This results in a true peristalsis.

The functional definition of the UES is the intraluminal high-pressure zone that lies in between the pharynx and the cervical esophagus.[13] It consists of the inferior pharyngeal constrictor muscles, the cricopharyngeus muscle, and the most proximal part of the esophagus. At rest it is closed by tonic muscular contraction. Therefore, during inspiration, it stops air from entering the digestive tract and by preventing esophageal matter from refluxing into the hypopharynx the UES shields the airways from aspiration.

During swallowing, in order for the bolus to pass into the esophagus, the UES relaxes transiently. Several factors are combined in this process. The cricopharyngeus muscle must relax, the hyoid bone must be pulled anteriorly, and the larynx superiorly and anteriorly through the contraction of the suprahyoid and thyrohyoid muscles. Pressure from the descending bolus adds to these muscular activities, contributing to the opening of the UES. Stiffness of the UES can produce inadequate UES opening and may be caused by fibrosis or inflammation.[14] Somatic dysfunction of the cranial base, the cervical spine, the thoracic spine, or a combination of dysfunction in the latter two, may prevent the UES musculature from relaxing properly.

At the gastroesophageal junction (GEJ) is the lower esophageal sphincter (LES). Usually under tension at rest, it prevents regurgitation from the stomach, while it relaxes during swallowing to allow the bolus of liquid or food to pass into the stomach.

# Gastroesophageal reflux

Between the esophagus and the stomach, a specific region (the gastroesophageal junction) consists of the LES and its contiguous anatomic structures: the gastric sling and the crura of the diaphragm. Normally these structures operate together to maintain competence in static circumstances and throughout the dynamics of increased intra-abdominal pressure or swallowing. They, therefore, prevent reflux of gastric contents through the GEJ and yet, they must also allow the

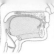

passage of ingested food into the stomach during swallowing.

Dysfunction at the GEJ barrier is the primary etiology of GER.[15] In the presence of GER, acidic gastric contents reflux into the esophagus and may ascend as high as the level of the upper esophagus, the pharynx, and larynx, with potential aspiration into the trachea. Stimulation of the mid- or upper esophageal mucosa chemoreceptors may be the source of reflex respiratory inhibition, hypertension, and bradycardia. Furthermore, excessive exposure of the esophageal mucosa to acidic gastric contents subsequent to reflux can produce serious erosions of the esophagus, leading to complications, such as esophagitis, peptic strictures, Barrett's esophagus (change in mucosal cell type), and eventually metaplasia and esophageal cancer. Usually, the majority of patients have mild to moderately severe complaints. Still, pain related to GER affects quality of life despite the presence or absence of esophageal erosions.[16]

Symptoms of this dysfunction include recurrent heartburn, acid regurgitation, and possible chronic irritative cough. The estimated prevalence of GER, with the occurrence of symptoms such as heartburn, regurgitation, or retrosternal pain at least once a week, is 10–20% in the Western world, while in Asia it is less than 5%.[17] Significant association exists between the incidence of GER and having an immediate relative with the disease. An association also exists with having a spouse with GER that may call into question the role of shared environmental factors, such as diet.[18] In addition, higher body mass and smoking seems to be significantly associated with the incidence of GER.[19] However, no significant association is found between gender and GER.[20] Because structure and function are linked, understanding the anatomy and function of the GEJ may help the understanding and treatment of GER.

## Esophageal hiatus

A little above the gastroesophageal junction, the esophagus passes between the thorax and abdomen through an opening, most often in the right diaphragmatic crus (the esophageal hiatus) located between the central tendon of the diaphragm and the hiatus aorticus. The two vagus nerves (CN X) also traverse the diaphragm through the esophageal hiatus. At this hiatus, frequently the medial part of the right crus, surrounds the esophagus forming an

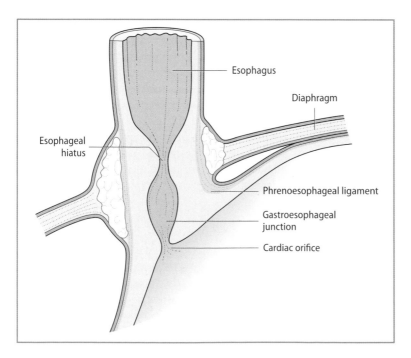

Figure 4.5.2: Esophageal hiatus

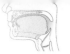

external sphincter, yet the fibers from the crus are not directly connected to the esophageal wall. To be more precise, some fibers appear from the transversalis fascia and continue to form a fascia under the diaphragm, and then pass into the esophageal hiatus, enveloping the esophagus to blend into its walls 2–3 cm above the GEJ. Some of the elastic fibers of the fascia extend into the esophageal submucosa.[21] This connection between the diaphragm and esophagus is named the phrenoesophageal ligament. At the same time, this ligament permits GEJ mobility, allowing some displacement during respiration and swallowing, while restricting an upward displacement of the esophagus. Furthermore, during pulmonary inspiration, the diaphragmatic esophageal hiatus contracts in response to increased intra-abdominal pressure.[22]

Part of a vast layer of fascia lying between the peritoneum and the abdominal walls (the transversalis fascia) extends below with the pelvic fasciae, behind with the thoracolumbar fascia, and above with the fascial sheet coating the inferior surface of the diaphragm. Fibers expanding from this layer form the phrenoesophageal ligament shaped as a conc enveloping the GEJ. Additionally, the portion of the greater omentum that extends from the greater curvature of the stomach to the inferior surface of the diaphragm (the gastrophrenic ligament) bonds the stomach to the diaphragm.

From an osteopathic point of view, following the principles of relationship between structure and function, the fascial relationships between the esophagus and the diaphragm must be balanced when addressing dysfunction of the GEJ.

After the vagus nerves descend through the esophageal hiatus of the diaphragm, they give rise to the gastric nerves. The drainage from the lower esophageal venous plexus also descends through the hiatus to join the portal vein. From below the diaphragm, the esophageal branches of the left gastric arteries and some lymphatic vessels ascend along the esophagus through this orifice.

## Cardiac orifice

The opening from the esophagus into the stomach is the cardiac orifice. This is situated below, and anatomically separate from the esophageal hiatus of the diaphragm. Because there is no particular sphincter associated with the cardiac orifice, the relationship between the esophageal hiatus and the lower esophagus is functionally extremely important.

The esophagus is not straight and below the diaphragm its small abdominal part curves to the left where it opens into the stomach at the cardiac orifice. The right side of the abdominal esophagus is continuous with the lesser curvature of the stomach, whereas the left side is continuous with the greater curvature. The left lateral border of the esophagus and the curvature of the fundus of the stomach come together at the incisura cardiac (angle of His).

Normally, the cardiac orifice is located to the left of the midline, posteriorly at the level of the eleventh thoracic vertebra, and anteriorly at the level of the left seventh costal cartilage. It is anterior and higher than the aortic orifice, and a little to the left of it.

## Motion of the stomach

Embryologically, both the esophagus and stomach mature from the foregut. At four weeks of gestation, the dilatation of the foregut for the future stomach begins in the sagittal plane. Several spatial changes take place before the stomach reaches its final position. Growth is greater along the dorsal border of the stomach, resulting in the development of the

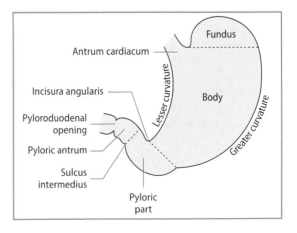

Figure 4.5.3: The stomach

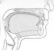

greater curvature dorsally and the lesser curvature ventrally. Next, the foregut rotates in such a fashion so that the greater curvature migrates to the left and the lesser curvature migrates to the right. The two vagus nerves follow this rotation. Consequently, the right vagus turns out to be posterior where it supplies the dorsal part of the stomach, while the left vagus becomes anterior to supply the ventral part of the stomach. Some torsion of the stomach takes place between the lower part of the esophagus and the pyloric canal, which are therefore no longer in the same plane. This is considered to be risk factor for the GER. Remember also that the upper part of the esophagus (the pharynx) is attached to the cranial base and that because of their tensegrital relationship, dysfunction of this cranial area may contribute to dysfunction of the gastroesophageal complex.

When a test of listening is employed to palpate the stomach for motion, in order to feel the spontaneous motions of the stomach, the practitioner may visualize motions occurring in the same directions as occur during the developmental process. Motion can be described in the context of the three cardinal planes, with a major motion occurring in the coronal (frontal) plane and two minor components taking place in the transverse (horizontal) and sagittal planes. In the coronal plane, the apex of the fundus of the stomach moves inferiorly and to the right when the inferior portion of the stomach moves superiorly and to the right. This results in a more concave lesser curvature. In the transverse plane, the greater curvature moves anteriorly and medially producing a rotation of the stomach to the right, with its anterior face directed to the right. In the sagittal plane the apex of the fundus of the stomach moves anteriorly, with minimal motion at the inferior portion.

The identification of restriction of mobility or a strong torsional sensation in this region may be an indication for osteopathic treatment that should be directed at the alleviation of the identified dysfunction.

## Lower esophageal sphincter

For histological and endoscopic purposes, the internal transition between esophagus and stomach is frequently identified as the gastroesophageal junction. The precise location of this junction is difficult to delineate since mucosa of gastric fundal type continues some distance up into the abdominal esophagus.[23]

Internally, at the lower end of the esophagus, the LES consists of smooth muscle that generates a tonic pressure at the GEJ. This constitutes the major barrier for reflux of gastric contents into the esophagus. Externally, surrounding the esophagus, the gastric sling and the crura of the diaphragm contribute to the function of the LES. Normally, these two sphincters relax quickly and at the same time allow the passage of a bolus of food into the stomach.

Because there is a pressure gradient between the abdomen and the thorax, intragastric contents tend to be driven towards the esophagus. Approximately 90% of basal pressure at the GEJ is produced by the smooth muscle of the distal esophagus at the LES. Additionally, when abdominal pressure is augmented, for instance during inspiration and when exercising, the crura of the diaphragm (the external portion of the LES) contract to participate in the defense against GER. Conversely, immediately after swallowing, expiration relaxes the crura of the diaphragm to allow the passage of the esophageal contents into the stomach by peristaltic movement.

Classically, GER has been considered multifactorial, involving different mechanisms: a temporary increase in intra-abdominal pressure; a dysfunctional diaphragmatic crus; disorders in esophageal acid clearance; gastric acid secretion; and gastric emptying or a spontaneous free reflux, related to a low resting pressure of the LES, or both. However, some studies challenge the traditional concept that most reflux episodes are the consequence of a weak steady state LES tone, but rather the result of transient complete relaxation of the LES.[24 25] The incisura cardiac, (angle of His) formed by the junction of the greater curvature of the stomach and the esophagus is also considered to have some influence; GER seems to occur more frequently when this angle is less acute.[26]

As the result of a brainstem-mediated vagovagal pathway, a transient LES relaxation (TLESR), producing a complete relaxation of the LES without pharyngeal swallowing, appears to be associated frequently with GER.[27][28] This reflex is initiated by stimulation of mechanoreceptors or mucosal receptors, with activation of sensory afferents from the pharyngeal area (superior laryngeal and glossopharyngeal nerves). This information is sent centrally to the hindbrain, where the motor output to the LES is modulated. Sensory fibers from the LES are carried with either the sympathetic or vagal innervation.[29] The sympathetic nerves have their cell bodies in the dorsal root ganglia at T1 to L3–4. They terminate in the thoracic and lumbar spinal cord, and are believed to transmit mainly nociceptive stimuli. Vagal afferents have their cell bodies in the nodose ganglion and terminate centrally in the nucleus of the solitary tract and the adjoining reticular formation. Usually, they transport non-painful stimuli. The neurons of the nucleus tractus solitarius are closely related to the dorsal motor nucleus of the vagal nerve. Additionally, the vagal nerve supplies the motor innervation to the LES and contains the efferent neurons that can increase or decrease LES tone by stimulation of inhibitory or excitatory motor neurons in the myenteric plexus of the LES.[30] Excitatory myenteric neurons in the LES are cholinergic and stimulate muscarinic receptors on the smooth muscle, whereas inhibitory motor neurons get powerful cholinergic nicotinic inputs from the vagal efferent nerves. Experimentally however, even though the vagus innervates both inhibitory and excitatory myenteric motor neurons, vagal stimulation usually produces LES relaxation.[31] Although LES motor innervation is provided essentially by the

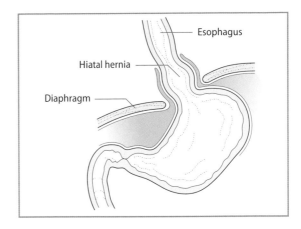

Figure 4.5.4: Hiatal hernia

vagus, it has been reported that stimulation of the splanchnic sympathetic nerves causes LES relaxation through adrenoreceptor activation.

Normally, TLESR permits belching, venting gas trapped above the gastric contents. At this time, a small amount of gastric acid may reflux normally, without consequence for the esophageal mucosa. Non-deglutitive TLESR is influenced by posture, and happens more often in the upright than in the supine position.[32] Also, a high-fat diet can contribute to increase the occurrences of TLESR.[33] Additionally, impairment of proximal gastric motor function and increased gastric sensitivity contribute to a tendency for GER.[34] Proximal stomach dysfunction may be part of the process of delayed gastric emptying, and a strong relationship between TLESR and GER.

# Hiatal hernia

Hiatal hernia occurs when structures within the abdomen are herniated through the esophageal hiatus of the diaphragm. As a consequence, LES competence is weakened and the function of the GEJ is impaired, resulting in impaired esophageal acid clearance with greater esophageal acid exposure. Although hiatal hernia is associated with GER, it does not have to be present for reflux to occur.

Hiatal hernia is commonly associated with an enlarged muscular hiatal aperture of the diaphragm and laxity of the phrenoesophageal ligament. As a result, the gastric cardia can slide upwards and in critical cases, other organs (spleen or pancreas) herniate.[35]

The cone shaped phrenoesophageal ligament enveloping the GEJ has also been described as a fascial tube (the phrenoesophageal fascial tube[36]) permitting some gliding motion of the esophagus, while at the same time avoiding the development of a hiatal hernia. Nevertheless with aging, typically

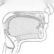

after the age of 50 years, the phrenoesophageal ligament is apt to become stretched in its vertical dimension. At the lower portion of the ligament the elastic tissue is lost and loose areolar tissue fills the space between the ligament and the esophagus allowing for greater mobility of the esophagus. Hiatal hernia is also, in fact, more frequent with an increased BMI and among men.[37]

# Irritable bowel syndrome

From the pyloric orifice of the stomach to the ileocecal junction, the small intestine forms the longest part of the GI tract. Nearly 6–7 m long, it includes the duodenum, the jejunum, and the ileum. The ileum opens into the large intestine where the cecum and ascending colon unite together at the ileocecal junction. From the ileum two flaps extend into the lumen to form a valve. Into each flap, musculature from the ileum outlines a sphincter that encircles the opening. Closed at rest, it opens during each terminal ileal contraction to release ileal contents into the cecum. This structure may prevent reflux of chyme from the cecum into the ileum.

Nearly 1.5 m long, the large intestine extends from the distal end of the ileum to the anus. It includes the cecum, appendix, colon, rectum, and anal canal and absorbs fluids and salts from the gut contents, thus forming feces.

Irritable bowel syndrome is very common and is also identified as functional bowel syndrome, irritable colon, spastic bowel, and spastic colon. It should, however, be differentiated from inflammatory bowel diseases like ulcerative colitis and Crohn's disease.[38]

Irritable bowel syndrome is more common in women, with symptoms typically appearing at around age 20. They range from experiencing bloating and gas to feeling a powerful desire to have a bowel movement, presenting either as diarrhea, in particular after eating or first thing in the morning, or constipation and occasionally with mucus in the stool.

Although the etiology is unknown, several factors may play a role in the pathophysiology and clinical presentation of IBS symptoms. Variations in the microbiota—bacteria that live in the gut (see below)—disrupt the balance of the internal GI environment. Facilitation of segmentally related spinal segments that provide innervation of the affected GI tract can result in increased sensitivity of the intestine to distension and other general visceral afferent signaling. Viscerovisceral reflexes from segmentally related viscera and central facilitation as the result of emotional stress can further augment IBS symptoms.

## Gut microbiota

Four main layers form the gut wall; they are the mucosa, submucosa, muscularis externa, and serosa. The deepest layer, the mucosa, consists of a lining of epithelium with an underlying lamina propria and a layer of smooth muscle, the muscularis mucosa. Functioning as a protective barrier, the epithelium is also a location where secretion and absorption takes place. Multiple mucosal folds, pits, crypts, villi, and glands augment the area for secretion or absorption. Furthermore, each absorptive cell displays microvilli on its surface that further increases the area for secretion or absorption. Neuroendocrine cells, i.e., enteroendocrine cells, distributed within the epithelium secrete various regulatory molecules that control physiological and homeostatic functions. Supporting the surface epithelium, a layer of loose connective tissue (the lamina propria) also supplies nutrient vessels and lymphatics. Over the entire epithelium, tight junctions where the membranes of adjacent cells are in contact function as a barrier against pathogenic dietary and enteric flora found in the intestinal lumen, although, at the same time, they allow the selective absorption of nutrients.

The strongest layer of the gut wall is the submucosa. Nevertheless, this layer demonstrates a capacity to adapt to volume changes of the gut. It is the location of the major arterial network of the intestinal wall, distributed to the mucosa and the muscularis externa.

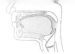

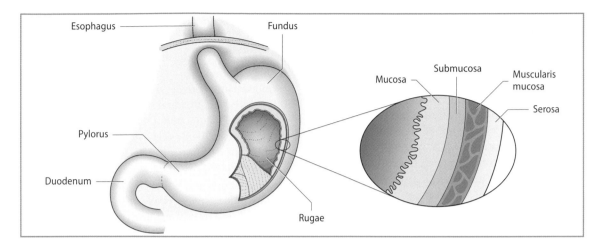

Figure 4.5.5: The stomach layers

The layer of smooth muscle of the mucosa (the muscularis mucosa) allows adjustments of the structure of the mucosa in order to adapt to the contents of the gut. Cells from the muscularis mucosae are also present inside the mucosal villi that extend into the intestinal lumen. By its contraction, the muscularis mucosa augments vascular exchange and lymphatic drainage.

Surrounding the muscularis externa, an external layer of connective tissue, rich in adipose tissue, forms the serosa. This outermost layer of the intestinal wall is covered by visceral peritoneum. In other places the serosa forms the adventitia and combines with the surrounding fasciae.

Approximately 200–300 m² in surface area, the mucosal surface of the human GI tract is colonized by 1014 bacteria of greater than 1,000 different species and subspecies as detected by ordinary culture methods.[39] Several factors seem to have an effect on their number. Among them are: the portion of the GI tract considered, mucin secretion, pH, peristalsis, bacterial adhesion sites, and nutrient availability. Decreased peristalsis and low oxidation-reduction potentials explain probably why the colon is the principal site of microbial colonization. Conversely gastric, bile, and pancreatic secretions inhibit the colonization of the stomach and proximal small intestine by most bacteria.

The bacterial colonization of the sterile GI tract of neonates starts quickly upon delivery. By the age of about two, the child's gut microflora resembles that of the adult. Any individual's population of microflora is affected by: mode of delivery, diet, hygiene levels, and exposure to medications. Breastfed infants' bacterial flora is composed typically of bifidobacteria whereas in bottle-fed infants anaerobic bacteria, as well as aerobic species, are present.[40] In addition, breastfed infants' flora includes far fewer species that are liable to be pathogenic.[41]

Following the first connection between early colonizers and epithelial cells, the host organism may react to the bacterial signals. Alteration of gene expression in the host may follow, producing an appropriate environment for beneficial bacteria that prevents the possible growth of other bacteria afterward. It is generally accepted that the equilibrium of the microbiota barrier ecosystem is of paramount importance in the maintenance of homeostasis and intestinal immune responses throughout an individual's life. Thus, the colonization of the gut early in life can impact the individual's health well into old age. In fact, damage and injury to the intestinal surface barrier is detected in a variety of diseases including IBS, Crohn's disease, and ulcerative colitis.[42]

Once the equilibrium of the microbiota barrier ecosystem is unbalanced, penetration and absorption of toxic and immunogenic factors into the body may increase. Pathogenic bacteria from the gut

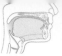

infiltrate the arteriovenous circulation or the lymphatics with the potential for the release of endotoxins, such as lipopolysaccharides, that stimulate macrophages to produce excess cytokines, such as tumor necrosis factor (TNF) and interleukin.[43]

Some patients may be genetically predisposed to develop IBS, but environmental factors that the patient is exposed to should also be considered. When environmental factors are involved, an imbalance between commensal bacteria with pathogenic potential and commensal bacteria with beneficial potential can develop and contribute to pathogenesis.[44] Additionally, in aging patients, decreased blood flow, resulting in potential ischemia, and an intensified use of medications, like non-steroidal anti-inflammatory drugs (NSAIDs) participate in the damage of the intestinal epithelial barrier.[45]

## Gut sensitivity

The innervation of the gut consists of intrinsic and extrinsic nerves from the enteric nervous system (ENS) and autonomic nervous system, respectively. The ENS consists of ganglionated and non-ganglionated plexi, whereas the vagus, splanchnic, and pelvic nerves form the extrinsic innervation.

### Intrinsic innervation

Intrinsic innervation of the gut comes from neurons of the ENS that are located within the gut wall in intramural ganglionated plexuses. Between the circular and longitudinal layers of the muscularis externa, a mesh of delicate axons and tiny ganglia constitutes the myenteric plexus, or Auerbach's plexus. In the submucosal layer lie several plexuses; among them, the Meissner's plexus is the most superficial. Additionally, non-ganglionated nerve plexuses are dispersed throughout the gut wall. They are found in the lamina propria, between the submucosa and muscularis externa, within the muscularis externa, and the serosa. Cell bodies of the ENS provide the intrinsic sensory and motor supply of the gut wall. They join the extrinsic sensory, motor, and sensorimotor nerves of cranial and spinal origin, to regulate gut motility and mucosal transport.

### Extrinsic innervation

Extrinsic innervation of the gut comes from neurons located outside the gut. It consists of functional parts from the sympathetic, parasympathetic, and visceral sensory divisions of the peripheral nervous system. Visceral sensory endings respond to any extreme muscular activity of the gut, either contraction or distension. Vagal sensory neurons have their cell bodies in the nodose and jugular ganglia of the vagus nerve (CN X). The spinal sensory input takes place through perivascular nerves passing through the prevertebral ganglia to the dorsal horn of the spinal cord; these neurons have their cell bodies in the dorsal root ganglia situated immediately peripheral to the spinal cord. Parasympathetic efferent axons have their cell bodies in the vagal dorsal motor nucleus in the medulla oblongata. Sympathetic efferent neurons originate in the thoracic and lumbar spinal cord and synapse in prevertebral sympathetic ganglia i.e., the coeliac, mesenteric, and pelvic ganglia.

Cranial nerve X contains up to 80% afferent fibers. Integration of GI sensation appears to be in the medulla oblongata and the nucleus of the tractus solitarius, from where impulses pass to the thalamus and cortex.[46] Normally, the hypothalamus integrates GI and environmental information, and these processes, with the exception of hunger, satiety, the need to defecate, and gastric and rectal distension, do not reach conscious perception.

A constant interaction, either through somatic or autonomic neurons and referred to as the brain-gut axis, exists between the gut and the CNS. As a result, the CNS modulates gut motor activity through the autonomic nervous system (sympathetic and parasympathetic) preserving the normal rhythm of activity in the GI tract as well as adjusting autonomic output to accommodate any external challenge. Acetylcholine released by the parasympathetic fibers increases gut motility, whereas noradrenaline, somatostatin, and neuropeptide Y released by sympathetic fibers diminishes the motility. Furthermore, communication occurs between the different areas of the GI tract through myogenic and neurogenic signals along the gut, and through reflex arcs transmitted via autonomic neurons.

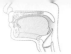

Individual differences are present in CNS physiology. In patients with functional GI disorders, an increased sensitivity to stimuli, such as distension of the gut, is encountered.[47] Genetic susceptibility to functional GI disorders may exist. Additionally, because visceral afferents are responsible for initiating GI reflexes, intestinal hypersensitivity may change the motility of the GI tract by increasing intestinal afferent/efferent (viscerosomatic, somatovisceral, and viscerovisceral) reflexes.

### Sensitization

Normally, the sensory innervation of the gut is responsible for the regulation of visceral motility and secretory activity, and conduction of visceral sensations, like pain. However, stimuli affecting sensory neurons may alter their sensitivity. This can often occur rapidly, but when it occurs slowly the resultant sensitization is more often persistent. When neurons become sensitized, a decrease of neurotrophic factors with alteration of gene expression in the sensory neurons may follow. This can, in turn, result in pathophysiological conditions such as IBS.[48]

The sensitization of GI afferent neurons through the summation of peripheral and central processes may contribute to the pathogenesis of visceral hypersensitivity to luminal distension of the gut, abdominal pain, and discomfort experienced by IBS patients. It should be noted here, however, that all IBS patients do not necessarily demonstrate this latter manifestation because a multifactorial model, with intrinsic and environmental factors frequently appears to be present.

A phenomenon of spatial summation may be activated in the GI tract. When significant distension is produced at multiple sites, at the same time, the perception of distension is more intense than if it was produced by distension in only one location. Therefore spatial summation should be considered with patients presenting excessive intestinal gas, confined at different sites of the GI tract. It should be noted that rapid phasic distention stimulates splanchnic afferent neurons. This suggests that sensitization in patients with IBS occurs in the splanchnic lumbar afferent nerves.[49] From an osteopathic point of view this justifies the normalization of the lumbar spine and lumbar soft tissues surrounding the vertebrae.

### Pain perception

Pain perception is thought to be essentially mediated by spinal innervation.[50] The visceral afferents found in the thoracolumbar dorsal root ganglia are mainly high threshold afferent and nociceptor fibers from the GI tract. They are able to encode noxious events. Chemicals, released during inflammation and injury, stimulate spinal nociceptors which may activate the processes of sensitization and increased nociceptive activity.[51] Conversely, the neurons of the nodose ganglia and the caudal dorsal root ganglia of the parasympathetic division of the autonomic nervous system supply generally low-threshold mechanoreceptors from the proximal GI tract and chemoreceptors from the large intestine.[52]

The abdominal pain experienced by IBS patients has been associated with the occurrence of abnormal intestinal contractions. With aging, visceral afferents demonstrate dystrophic and regressive structural remodeling that seems to be associated with diminished trophic support.[53] Afferent feedback from the gut and GI viscerovisceral reflexes, as well as viscerosomatic reflexes, may result.

## Exposure to stress

Multiple factors are involved in IBS, many of them being the result of complex neural and muscular interactions that take place at several levels, under the influence of neurotransmitters and hormones.[54] Altered bowel habits result from dysfunction of the autonomic nervous system and persistent alteration of autonomic responsiveness. Irritable bowel syndrome patients, typically, demonstrate increased stress responsiveness. It should be emphasized that stress, defined as an acute threat to the homeostasis of an organism, may come from the external or the internal environment. In order to maintain the stability of the internal environment and to ensure the survival of the organism, an adaptive response occurs.[55] Both psychological and environmental stress has been shown to increase GI permeability. The resultant weakening of the intestinal mucosal barrier

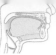

permits the exposure of the mucosal immune system to the intestinal contents, predisposing the individual to chronic intestinal inflammation and increasing the symptoms of IBS.[56] Emotions, nervousness, fasting or eating, visceral hypersensitivity, lactose or gluten intolerance, enteric infections, surgery, or somatic dysfunction can all be considered as stress triggers, and activate an enhanced response of the autonomic system.

## Homeostasis

In the mid-nineteenth century Claude Bernard developed the concept of the milieu intérieur. His theory stated that the body tries to maintain constancy of the various internal functions. About 75 years later Walter Cannon developed the theory of homeostasis based on the same principles, to which he added the roles of behavior and emotion as factors affecting the various internal functions. Modern theories embrace the concept of homeostasis in a broader sense, and emphasize that the normal resting function of the internal environment is not physiologically static, but rather that it is continuously readjusting itself to maintain a state of functional balance.[57]

In order to maintain this subtle balance, reciprocity is constantly in action. There is continuous sensory input to the CNS from the cardiovascular, digestive, respiratory, genitourinary, and endocrine systems, as well as from chemical, osmotic, and volume changes, cognitive functions, and emotion. Reciprocally, the brain exerts influence upon all of the bodily functions.

## Interoception

About a century ago, Charles Scott Sherrington employed the word 'interoceptor' to describe sensory nerve receptors originating inside the body. These general visceral afferent (GVA) neurons return to the CNS via the peripheral nerves of the autonomic (parasympathetic and sympathetic) nervous system. Interoceptive GVA neurons that provide input from the GI tract synapse at the level of the spinal cord and brainstem before reaching the higher levels of the CNS. The anatomic reliability of GVA input from the viscera results in diagnostically useful GI viscerosomatic reflexes. The

GVA neurons that travel with the parasympathetic, vagus, and pelvic splanchnic nerves result in palpable paraspinal reflexes in the cervico-occipital and sacral regions respectively. The GI GVA neurons that travel with the sympathetic nerves result in viscerosomatic reflexes in the thoracolumbar region.[58] (See boxed text: 'Viscerosomatic reflexes' in 'Section 4: Clinical considerations, Chapter 1: Musculoskeletal dysfunctions, Part 1: Axial system,' p. 184.)

The peripheral nerve with possibly the greatest number of GVA neurons is the vagus, CN X. It is highly involved in interoception, the perception of internal sensory states, containing up to 80% GVA fibers. These afferent neurons of the parasympathetic CN X, as well as those from the parasympathetic facial and glossopharyngeal cranial nerves (CN VII and CN IX) synapse in the brainstem, on the nucleus of the tractus solitarius (NTS), an area located along the length of the medulla and with a small portion extending into the lower pons. Interconnecting neurons from the NTS project to the parabrachial nucleus of the pons, the locus coeruleus, the nucleus ambiguus, and then to higher centers at the hypothalamic and cortical levels. It is of interest to note that the NTS receives input from baroreceptors located in the carotid bodies, the arch of the aorta, and elsewhere, and is, in turn, responsible for the baroreflex activity that has been shown to be associated with the cranial rhythmic impulse (CRI).[59 60 61 62 63 64 65 66 67 68]

Considered as an integrator, the hypothalamus receives input from multiple areas of the CNS and the periphery, including information from the viscera and the sensory (olfactory, gustatory, visual), and limbic systems. It also receives input from the hormonal, psychoemotional, and immune systems, thermoregulation, and biorhythms of the body.

Under the cortex, several structures together form the limbic system; they are the fornix, the stria terminalis, the amygdalae, and the dentate, cingulate, and hippocampal gyri. It is generally acknowledged that these structures are engaged in emotional-motivational behavior. The amygdalae perform a major role in the processing and memory of emotional reactions. The frontal cortex

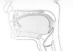

is also implicated in emotional functions, in addition to its commonly accepted role in the mediation of the highest brain functions such as thought and judgment. Therefore the frontal cortex may be considered as part of the visceral sensory processing system.[69]

Variations exist among individuals regarding their awareness of visceral sensations that have different effects upon thought, emotion, and behavior. Visceral sensations are known to contribute to the consciousness of the 'self'.[70] In subjects with functional GI disorders, studies reveal a visceral hypersensitivity. When monitored with anorectal manometry, rectal distension results in IBS patients experiencing increased sensitivity, not only at the level of the rectum, but over the entire extent of the gut. Visceral hypersensitivity is considered as a key pathogenetic factor underlying the emotional state demonstrated by patients with functional GI disorders.[71]

Predisposed individuals may experience symptom exacerbation because of sensitized feedback between the brain and the GI tract developed in infancy. Studies reveal that, in fact, stress experienced early in life, during a vulnerable period in the developing nervous system, can cause long-term changes in the brain-gut axis.[72][73] Altered pain pathways and visceral hyperalgesia may result in a predisposition to develop functional and affective disorders later in life. During exposure to sensory stimulation such as rectal distension, IBS patients demonstrate increased activation of the anterior cingulate cortices, insula, and ventral medial prefrontal regions. This suggests amplified affective responses to painful visceral stimuli.[74] Additionally, about 40% of IBS patients show evidence for increased anxiety.[75]

## Constipation

Aging is associated with a multiplicity of GI disorders. Functional GI disorders have been described and classified by a committee of multinational expert reviewers, who have defined the Rome diagnostic criteria for functional bowel disorders and functional abdominal pain.[76] To meet these criteria, symptoms must be present for at least 12 weeks during the preceding 12 months in the absence of a structural or biochemical explanation.[77] Patients with constipation must report less than three defecations a week. In at least 25% of these defecations there must be straining, lumpy, or hard stools, and the experience of incomplete evacuation or of anorectal obstruction or blockade, potentially requiring the use of manual maneuvers, such as digital evacuation, to facilitate defecation. Additionally, loose stools cannot be present and consequently there are insufficient criteria for the diagnosis of IBS.

In this context, functional constipation includes functional disorders described as "persistent, difficult, infrequent, or seemingly incomplete defecation."[78] However, physicians and patients may have a different definition. Most physicians define constipation as a bowel movement every three or four days or less, sometimes in combination with hard stool. In contrast, 27% of patients identify constipation as defecation every two days or less and 25% as hard stool alone.[79]

Constipation occurs in up to 27% of individuals, depending on the definition used and demographic factors.[80] Although a common complaint among older individuals, it seems that, related to age, there is actually no increase in the percentage of individuals reporting infrequent bowel movements. However, with advancing age, more individuals self-report constipation, with a greater prevalence among women. Commonly, older subjects' reports of constipation are combined with feelings of poor health, anxiety, social isolation, and depression.[81] Low income and low education level, as well as low calorie intake and inactivity are factors typically linked to constipation.[82] Concomitant with aging is a greater use of laxatives,[83] and the number of medications being taken, some of them resulting in constipation as a side effect. Among non-prescription drugs most commonly associated with constipation are antacids, calcium and iron supplements, antidiarrheal agents, and NSAIDs.[84]

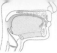

In any patient presenting with constipation, a careful history and thorough physical examination must be performed because increased large bowel transit time and impaired motility is not necessarily a consequence of aging. Studies, in fact, show that sigmoidal, rectosigmoidal, and rectal motility are not influenced by age or gender.[85]

## Colonic motility

Constipation is multifactorial, potentially involving abnormal colonic motility, epithelial, neural, and muscular changes, including dysfunction of the pelvic floor. Normally, the colon demonstrates a motility with high-amplitude contractions that is thought to be the mechanism for the movement of colonic contents. Constipated patients demonstrate some colonic inertia. Decreased peristalsis increases the transit time through the ascending and transverse colons. Additional slower transit through the rectosigmoidal part of the colon, acting as a resistance to normal transit, creates a delay in evacuation of fecal content.[86][87]

There are four main layers that form the gut wall: the mucosa, submucosa, muscularis externa, and serosa. The muscularis externa consists mainly of smooth muscle. It is made up of two muscular layers: an inner circular layer and outer longitudinal layer. Peristalsis is the result of the coordinated muscular activities of these two layers causing colonic motility that propels stool into the rectum.

The interstitial cells of Cajal (ICC) are pacemaker cells that are located at a number of sites within the gut wall. They are found within the myenteric plexus, at the myenteric edge between the circular and longitudinal smooth muscle cell layers, and at the interface between the circular muscle and the submucosa. Changes in membrane potential in ICC produce slow waves of rhythmic electrical activity that extend throughout the muscularis externa. Additionally, ICC, through input from the ENS and from the extrinsic innervation of the gut, modulate enteric neural activity. They display a close relationship with the intramuscular terminals of vagal afferent neurons and, in that way, may have a role in afferent signaling.[88] Studies show a decrease in their number with patients presenting with slow-transit constipation.[89]

## Pelvic floor dysfunction

Failure of rectal evacuation may also be associated with pelvic floor dysfunction. When stool reaches the rectum, it results in the perception of rectal fullness, most likely from activation of stretch receptors in the mesentery or pelvic floor muscles. This triggers the anorectal inhibitory, or rectosphincteric, reflex that produces a relaxation of the internal anal sphincter and contraction of the external sphincter. Then, if the environment is conducive, defecation can follow. If an individual habitually postpones defecation, changes in colonic function can develop, with increased transit times in the rectosigmoid and right hemicolon. This may explain some cases of functional anorectal outlet obstruction with constipation.[90]

### Anal canal

As the fecal mass moves, the pelvic floor muscles relax in order to allow alignment of the rectum with the anal canal. The rectum measures 15–20 cm long, and extends from the rectosigmoid junction at the level of third sacral vertebra to the anal orifice. Distal to the rectum is the anal canal, directed in an anteroposterior direction, its lateral walls are in close contact.

Normally, the anal canal is occluded by the internal and external anal sphincters. The internal anal sphincter is the thick lower end of the inner circular smooth muscle layer of the gut. As such, ICC are found within the circular layer of the internal anal sphincter. The external sphincter consists of three portions: superficial, subcutaneous, and deep. The puborectalis muscle, the medial portion of the levator ani, combines with the deep portion of the external sphincter of the anal canal and, as such, contributes to the ring encircling the anorectal junction. Further, fibers of the levator ani muscle mix with the outer longitudinal muscular layer of the muscularis externa that envelops the anal canal. Posterior to the rectum, the pubococcygeal fibers of the levator ani muscles attach to the anterior surface of the coccyx.

### Anorectal junction

Typically, the anorectal junction, between the rectum and the anal canal, forms an angle of

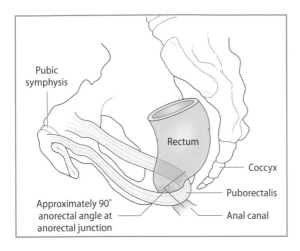

Figure 4.5.6: The anorectal junction

approximately 90° that is open posteriorly. Constant contraction of the puborectalis muscles maintains this angulation between the rectum and the anal canal. Consequently, the puborectalis plays an important role in anal continence. Defecation is initiated by an increase in intra-abdominal pressure produced by bilateral muscular contraction of the quadratus lumborum, the rectus abdominis, the external and internal oblique, and the transversus abdominis muscles. Then, relaxation of the puborectalis and external anal sphincter muscles results in the opening of the anal canal allowing defecation. Throughout the passage of feces, the anorectal junction moves down and back, and the anorectal angle increases to about 130–140°. Normally, contractions of the circular muscles of the rectum contribute to the movement of feces toward the anus. At the same time, the pelvic floor moves slightly downward. After the feces pass from the anus, the anus and rectum return to their normal positions.

Squatting during defecation allows for better alignment of the rectum and anal canal than can occur when seated on common toilets. In studies, subjects describe more expulsive effort in order to get a sensation of satisfactory bowel emptying in the sitting position compared to the squatting posture.[91] As such, squatting may prevent excessive straining with possible damage to the anorectal region.[92]

### Perineal influence

Dysfunction of the puborectalis and external anal sphincter muscles may contribute to delayed or reduced opening of the anal canal. The innervation of these muscles comes from the pudendal nerve—the ventral rami of roots of S2, S3, S4, and less regularly S1 and S5. The structures upon which the puborectalis muscles attach, and the structures surrounding the pudendal nerve should be assessed when treating somatic dysfunction that may impede their function.

In general, anal sphincter pressures, particularly in females, are lower with aging.[93] In these patients, thinning of the external anal sphincter and thickening of the internal anal sphincter is often present.[94] Initiating defecation, therefore, requires more effort and produces descent of the perineum. Furthermore, the rectum may empty incompletely. Aging may also contribute to excessive perineal descent because of slowed pudendal nerve conduction.[95] Another situation that may contribute to excessive perineal descent and constipation in females is damage to the nerve supply of the pelvic floor experienced during childbirth. Neuropathic weakness of the external anal sphincter may be explained by the vulnerability of the pudendal nerve along its path (see below: 'Anal sphincter innervation'). During vaginal birth, as the fetal head descends, the pudendal nerve may be compressed and stretched, in particular as it winds around the ischial spine.

## Anal sphincter innervation

Both sympathetic and parasympathetic autonomic nerves, as well as somatic nerves supply the pelvic floor and anorectum. The rectum and internal anal sphincter are innervated by the inferior hypogastric plexus that gets neural projections from spinal roots T10–L1 via the superior hypogastric plexus and from S2–4 via branches of the sacral plexus. The smooth muscle of the rectum and internal anal sphincter receives innervation from the autonomic nervous system via the inferior hypogastric plexus, whereas the external anal sphincter and levator muscles are generally under the control of the somatic nervous system via the sacral nerves (S2–4).

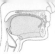

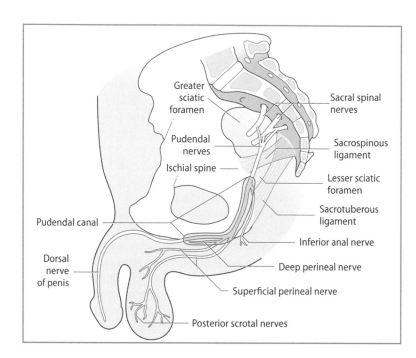

**Figure 4.5.7:** The pudendal nerve

- Greater sciatic foramen
- Sacral spinal nerves
- Pudendal nerves
- Sacrospinous ligament
- Ischial spine
- Lesser sciatic foramen
- Sacrotuberous ligament
- Pudendal canal
- Inferior anal nerve
- Dorsal nerve of penis
- Deep perineal nerve
- Superficial perineal nerve
- Posterior scrotal nerves

Sacral parasympathetic innervation of the colon has both excitatory and inhibitory constituents. Colonic propulsive activity during defecation is under the influence of excitatory pathways, while adaptation of colonic volume and colonic relaxation is, conversely, under the control of inhibitory pathways.

The somatic motor fibers leave the spinal cord through the spinal nerves. After the intervertebral foramen, the spinal nerves divide into dorsal and ventral rami. The pudendal nerve is derived from the ventral rami of roots of S2, S3, and S4, and less regularly S1 and S5. Positioned medially and caudally to the trunk of the sciatic nerve, it passes into the infrapiriform canal and continues through the greater sciatic foramen to enter in a lateral direction into the ischiorectal fossa. The pudendal nerve lies in close contact with the sacrospinous ligament. Nearby the attachment of the ligament to the ischial spine and between the sacrospinous ligament ventrally and the sacrotuberous ligament dorsally, the pudendal nerve winds around the ischial spine. It then passes through the lesser sciatic foramen to penetrate the perineal region, where it enters within a duplication of the fascia of the obturator internus muscle that constitutes the Alcock's, or pudendal, canal.[96]

Typically the three branches of the pudendal nerve, as they appear inside the Alcock's canal, are the inferior rectal nerve, the perineal nerve, and the dorsal nerve of the clitoris. The inferior rectal nerve supplies the integument around the anus. It provides sensory innervation to the distal portion of the anal canal and to the perianal skin, and motor innervation to the external anal sphincter. The perineal nerve innervates the ischiocavernosus, bulbocavernosus, superficial transverse, and urethral sphincter muscles of the pelvic floor. The dorsal nerve of the clitoris, at the level of the symphysis pubis, provides sensory innervation from the clitoris.

Considering the anatomical and physiological relationships between the pelvic floor muscles and nerves, it is of paramount importance to address any somatic dysfunction of the pelvic floor and associated spinal segments. Afferent stimuli from viscera affect somatic tissues innervated by the same spinal segments producing viscerosomatic reflexes. Visceral receptors transmit afferent impulses through the dorsal horn of the spinal cord where they synapse with interconnecting

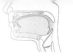

neurons. These neurons transmit impulses to the sympathetic, parasympathetic, and peripheral motor efferent nerves, the source of sensory and motor changes in somatic structures i.e., muscle, fascia, and skin of the pelvic floor. Constant muscle contraction of the pelvic floor associated with noxious visceral stimulation can result in pelvic floor dysfunction. Somatic dysfunction that is reticent to manipulative treatment should raise the possibility of a viscerosomatic etiology. It is therefore of the greatest importance that, when addressing somatic dysfunction, visceral pathology is sought out and appropriately treated.

## Visceroptosis

Visceroptosis refers to prolapse of any abdominal viscus. Originally described by Frantz Glénard as "entéroptose," it is an imbalance of GI posture ("statique intestinale") associated with ptosis of any portion of the GI tract.[97] This results in a dysfunctional influence upon digestion and the global health of the individual. Its symptoms include abdominal distention and pain, nausea, vomiting, constipation, diarrhea, headache, backache, tachycardia, vasomotor disorders, fatigue, and anxiety. Because visceroptosis can produce such a broad spectrum of GI symptoms, as well as symptoms across many other systems, it is imperative that organic pathology be ruled out. Visceroptosis has been identified as a causative factor in potentially severe conditions such as superior mesenteric artery syndrome.[98]

Diagnosis using Glénard's test is performed as follows: Standing behind the patient, the practitioner's arms are placed around the patient's abdomen. With their hands clasped together, the practitioner lifts the anterior abdominal wall in a posterior and superior direction. The patient is then allowed to slump forward against the practitioner's hold. In the presence of visceroptosis, this will result in a decrease of the patient's abdominal discomfort, followed by reoccurrence of the symptoms when holding pressure is released.

A modification of this procedure, as demonstrated by Martin C. Beilke, may be performed while standing in front of the patient with one hand lifting the abdomen while auscultating the heart rate. The alleviation of visceroptosis is associated with slowing of the heart rate.[99]

Treatment consists of osteopathic procedures to balance the components of the abdominal GI tract, the thoracoabdominal diaphragm, and the lumbar spine with attention to psoas mechanics. Postural issues, including the identification and treatment of leg length inequality, which can contribute to increased intra-abdominal pressure, should be addressed. Stabilization and visceral repositioning exercises may be employed. If necessary an abdominal wall support, in the form of a properly fitted truss, may also be employed. In extreme cases, surgical repair may be necessary.

## The osteopathic contribution to the physical examination and treatment

In the context of a patient with a GI complaint, the physical examination for dysfunction should begin with an examination of the area of the patient's complaint—in this case the thoracoabdominal area. Aside from being a logical way to begin a holistic structural examination, it is psychologically important to demonstrate to the patient that their complaint has been understood. Following which, the examination can extend to include the reminder of the body for associated somatic dysfunction i.e., the vertebral column, cranium, pelvis, and musculature including but not limited to the thoracoabdominal diaphragm, abdominal prevertebral musculature, and pelvic diaphragm.

If at all possible, begin the musculoskeletal portion of the examination with the patient standing. Observe them from the front, side, and back. Usually, patients with abdominal dysfunction have a

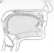

typical posture, with a prominent abdomen and an increased upper thoracic kyphosis. Observe the contour of the abdomen (prominent, flat, or symmetrical) and the tone of the abdominal musculature. Decreased anterior abdominal wall tone, often found in association with an increased lumbar lordosis, can be responsible GI visceroptosis.[100] Examine the spine for dysfunctional anterior/posterior and lateral curvatures, for positional asymmetries, and for alterations in paravertebral muscular tension. If paravertebral tissue texture change is identified, consider the viscera that could be responsible for viscerosomatic reflex somatic dysfunction at the identified spinal level(s).

Postural asymmetry from unequal leg length, sometimes as minor as 3 mm, can be a source of chronic somatic dysfunction with resultant somatovisceral GI reflexes. Note the presence of a pelvic sideshift that may be the result of an asymmetric contraction of the psoas major muscle on the opposite side of the sideshift. Psoas contraction is frequent with IBS, as a viscerosomatic reflex of irritation of the ileocolic junction.

Then examine the abdomen with the patient lying down. Inspect the abdomen, noting its shape, contour, and movement with respiration. Is there good motion with respiration in the thoracic cage as well as in the abdomen? Observe for abdominal asymmetry; note if the abdominal wall is tense, with bowel distension from flatulence; note areas that seem more filled, with subcutaneous tissue texture change that could reveal some underlying dysfunction. IBS patients demonstrate a distended abdomen with subcutaneous tissue texture change in the periumbilical and hypogastric areas. Note any tension under the inferior border of the thoracic cage, in particular under the xiphoid process that may be present with GER. Note if the umbilicus is centered or displaced.

Observe the thoracic inlet. Note any tension in the cervical spine. Evaluate the position of the hyoid bone and the mandible: are they centered? Monitor swallowing for ease or discomfort. Observe the inside of the mouth to note the condition of the teeth, and, if present, of dentures. Have the patient clench their teeth and observe the dental occlusion: the upper and lower midlines between the incisors should be in alignment and the upper incisors should slightly override the lower incisors. The upper molars should rest upon the lower molars. Note the potential association with dysfunctional mastication. Having performed diagnostic palpation for structure and motion, proceed to treatment.

In general, manipulative treatment should, preferably, follow indirect principles. Manipulation should be specifically directed at clearly identified somatic dysfunction. Reflexly, somatic dysfunction also affects the autonomic nervous system. The resulting state of facilitation, in turn, increases the response to either mechanical or chemical intestinal stimuli. Visceral hypersensitivity and dysfunction follows. Somatic dysfunction can involve and affect any osseous, articular, ligamentous, membranous, fascial, muscular, visceral, and vascular structures anatomically associated with the GI tract. Vagal sensory neurons have their cell bodies in the nodose and jugular ganglia located near the jugular foramen. Spinal sensory input takes place via perivascular nerves passing through the prevertebral ganglia to the dorsal horn of the spinal cord. The cell bodies of these neurons are located in the dorsal root ganglia. The perception of visceral pain is, essentially, thought to be mediated by the spinal innervation.[101] The craniocervical junction and sacropelvic region (parasympathetic) and the thoracic and thoracolumbar spine (sympathetic) may be sites of somatic dysfunction resulting from viscerosomatic input, which produces somatovisceral dysfunction. The recognition of somatic dysfunction in these areas can be diagnostically useful, and treating them may contribute to the reestablishment of balance in gut function.

Somatic dysfunction involving the thoracic spine, ribs, and thoracoabdominal diaphragm should be identified and treated to address its impact upon the lymphatic and venous drainage of the contents of the abdomen. Diaphragmatic, abdominal wall, and pelvic dysfunction should be identified and treated to reduce the impact of dysfunctional fascial tensions upon the GI tract. The function of the mesenteric plexus is affected by dysfunction of the thoracoabdominal

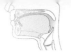

diaphragm. In every treatment procedure it is very important to pay attention to the inherent motility of the primary respiratory mechanism (PRM) as it is manifest throughout the body. Treating this physiological rhythm affects the autonomic nervous system and its impact upon tissue perfusion, reducing congestion.[102]

## Dysphagia

When evaluating dysphagia, consider dysfunction of the cranial base, cervical spine, and cervical soft tissues, larynx, hyoid bone, mandible, and temporomandibular joints. The relationship between the occiput and temporal bones should also be evaluated for its potential affect upon the jugular foramina and CN IX and X. Viscerosomatic reflex tissue texture change may be present in the upper thoracic region (T2–T6 right) from the esophagus, and C0, C1, C2 from the vagus. Primary somatic dysfunction in these same areas can influence the esophagus through somatovisceral influences.[103] The recognition of somatic dysfunction in these spinal areas should lead to further evaluation of the segmentally related areas. Its treatment can affect the esophagus through somatovisceral influence.

## The gastroesophageal junction

To evaluate and treat GEJ, palpate the epigastric and sternal regions. Assess and treat the diaphragm and its relationships with the GEJ. The thoracoabdominal diaphragm should demonstrate freedom and symmetry of its excursion. Its attachment at the xiphoid process and its anterior costal attachments should be free of dysfunction. Check and balance the cervical area (C3, C4, and C5) because of the phrenic nerve and its action upon the diaphragm. Examine and treat identified somatic dysfunction affecting the thoracolumbar junction because of its potential to affect the crura of the diaphragm.

Palpate the left hypochondriac region and using tests of listening, observe the inherent motion of the stomach. The inherent motion of the stomach demonstrates a curling and uncurling action in a pattern that is similar to the embryologic developmental process that created its curvatures. There should be a palpable balance between the curling and uncurling phases of this gastric motion. A predominance of one phase may be treated using an indirect approach. This may be further enhanced by balancing the fascial connections between the stomach and diaphragm and the torsional relationship between the stomach and the esophagus if present.

To improve the condition of patients with GER, hiatal hernia or both, any dysfunction of the lumbar vertebrae (L1, L2, L3, and sometimes L4) should be treated because of their potential to affect the crura of the diaphragm. The costal insertions of the diaphragm, ribs 7–12, the associated costal cartilages, and thoracic vertebrae should be examined and treated if necessary, as well.

Because compression of the jugular foramen can impact the exit of the parasympathetic vagus nerve, examine and treat the craniocervical junction with specific attention to the relationship between the occiput and temporal bones. Also examine and balance any high cervical dysfunction (C0, C1, and C2) associated with the high cervical, vagal, and viscerosomatic/somatovisceral reflexes. Further, address the phrenic nerve and its action upon the diaphragm, and check and balance the mid cervical area (C3, C4, and C5).

## Irritable bowel syndrome

When considering the patient with IBS, viscerosomatic reflex somatic dysfunction from, and areas of somatovisceral influence upon, the small intestine can be identified in the regions of spinal levels T8–T10 (sympathetic) and C0, C1, and C2 (vagal, parasympathetic). Reflex dysfunction associated with the proximal colon can be found from T12–L1 on the right (sympathetic) and C0, C1, and C2 (vagal, parasympathetic). The sympathetic reflexes, for the distal colon are L1–L2 left and the parasympathetic reflexes are S2–S4. The identification of somatic dysfunction in these areas will assist in diagnosis, and its treatment can result in somatovisceral influence.[104]

To further evaluate and treat IBS, palpate and, following indirect principles, treat identified dysfunction in the periumbilical and hypogastric

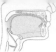

areas. Examine and treat the thoracolumbar spine for primary somatic dysfunction and somatovisceral affect. Examine the iliopsoas muscle. Balance any identified dysfunction of this muscle group very gently to avoid stimulating the sympathetic ganglia located between the muscles fibers. Dysfunction of the iliopsoas can be the result of primary somatic dysfunction of the thoracolumbar spine; the lumbosacral spine; the sacroiliac joints, hip joints, or both. The resultant iliopsoas dysfunction can mimic disorders of the abdominal and pelvic organs. Dysfunction from T12–L4 affects the lumbar plexus and femoral nerve and therefore the iliopsoas innervated through these nerves. Also, the iliopsoas may spasm as a consequence of a viscerosomatic reflex from visceral structures innervated from T12–L4 nerve roots. A psoas sign—a limited right hip extension in a patient with acute abdominal pain—is a diagnostic clue for acute appendicitis. It is thought to occur when an inflamed retrocecal appendix lies directly upon the psoas major. Although this is certainly feasible, it is also quite possible to have increased psoas tension as a result of the right-sided T12 viscerosomatic reflex from an inflamed appendix in any position.

Quite often there is deep tissue texture change palpable in the area of the cecum and ascending colon where they unite together at the ileocecal junction. Using tests of listening, observe the inherent motion in the area. Release any dysfunction using the gentlest form of indirect principles.

Examine and treat the cervical spine and the craniocervical junction, with particular attention to the relationship between the occiput and temporal bones, because compression of the jugular foramen can affect the vagus and high cervical parasympathetic viscerosomatic/somatovisceral reflexes. Similarly, examine the sacrum and treat any identified somatic dysfunction to address pelvic splanchnic (S2, S3, and S4) parasympathetic viscerosomatic/somatovisceral reflexes.

Cranial assessment and treatment is of value because empirical observation has shown that individuals with IBS generally feel better after cranial osteopathy, particularly following normalization of the frontal area. Also if the patient is under stress, the application of compression of the fourth ventricle (CV4) to balance their autonomic nervous system may prove salutary.

## Constipation

To evaluate and treat the patient with constipation, palpate the left iliac region. Assess the motility of the colon. Address any dysfunction of the pelvis, i.e., the sacrum, the coccyx, and the innominates, for their relation with the pelvic floor musculature and pelvic parasympathetic somatovisceral reflexes. Balance the innominates with the sacrum to release any myofascial stress affecting the pudendal nerve. Address any dysfunction of the thoracolumbar junction for the somatovisceral relation with the inferior hypogastric plexus and innervations of the rectum and internal anal sphincter.[105] [106]

# Advice to the patient

The effective treatment of patients with GI dysfunction, as well as those with organic disease always necessitates that they become actively involved in the therapeutic protocol. For any problem related to the GI tract, it is always beneficial to improve diet, increase exercise, and decrease stress and fatigue.

## For dysphagia

Instruct patients to create a non-stressful, pleasant environment for their meals. It is important

to foster their awareness of the qualities of food and oral sensations. Patients should eat at regular times, and try to have a variety of foods with different flavors. Patients should be instructed to chew their food thoroughly, and make every effort not to swallow air, since aerophagia is responsible for postprandial gastric distension and belching. Chewing gum or drinking through a straw can also result in aerophagia. They should be encouraged to 'sit straight,' particularly when eating. It appears that erect posture tends to straighten the path of

the esophagus through the thorax to the stomach, thereby providing easier passage as the food bolus descends the esophagus. Finally, patients should be counseled about how to reduce stressful responses to psychological or social stressors. Activities like meditation that will induce relaxation are often beneficial and should be encouraged.

## For gastroesophageal reflux

It is known that certain foods and beverages promote acid reflux. As such, dietary restrictions can benefit the GER patient. Foods to avoid include: chocolate, cruciferous vegetables (such as cauliflower, spinach, onions, cabbage, Brussels sprouts, and broccoli), and acidic foods (such as tomatoes and citrus fruits and juices). Fatty foods delay gastric emptying and tend to reduce the competence of the LES, facilitating reflux. Beverages to avoid include: carbonated soft drinks, coffee, and alcohol. Alcohol not only increases gastric acid secretion, it also decreases LES tone. Additionally, everyone has different sensitivities to certain foods and beverages, or both. Patients should be instructed to identify those foods and beverages that are likely to cause GER and to avoid them. If this proves difficult they may find it useful to keep a food diary in which they record the contents of their diet along with the status (none, mild, moderate, severe) of their symptoms for several weeks, or longer. If they identify a food or beverage that appears to aggravate their symptoms, they should avoid it for several days, and if their symptoms subside, they should try the offending item again. If it again aggravates their symptoms they will know that this is a food or beverage to be avoided. Finally, they should avoid eating large meals that, by sheer volume, promote acid reflux and prolong gastric emptying.[107]

Patients should avoid lying down for up to three hours after eating. When they do go to bed they may benefit from elevating the head of their bed 6-8 inches with blocks. They may also find that they have less reflux if they sleep lying on their left side.[108]

Smoking is so harmful that it should not be tolerated under any circumstances. For the GER patient specifically, nicotine is harmful to the LES.

Additionally, smoking reduces the body's ability to replace damaged esophageal mucosal cells and retards gastric emptying.

Many over the counter medications and dietary supplements may cause direct esophageal mucosal injury. They include NSAIDs including aspirin, ascorbic acid, ferrous sulfate, and low sodium salt substitutes containing potassium chloride.[109]

The use of calcium carbonate antacids may paradoxically result in a rebound gastric acid production. In addition, antacids, in general, must be used with caution in the elderly because of the potential risk of salt overload, constipation, diarrhea, and the possible interference with the absorption of other drugs.

Anticholinergic drugs that impede esophageal function and retard gastric emptying should be avoided whenever possible. Many herbal supplements are anticholinergic and should also be avoided. Powerful herbal anticholinergics include belladonna and jimson weed. Milder, more commonly encountered anticholinergic herbs include: chamomile, fennel, lobelia, motherwort, valerian, evening primrose, and members of the mint family.

Posture and exercise are important. Patients should be encouraged to 'sit straight.' It appears that erect posture tends to straighten the path of the esophagus through the thorax to the stomach, augmenting tone in the cardioesophageal sphincter, while sitting in a slumped position tends to compress the stomach between the abdominal contents and the diaphragm, increasing intra-abdominal pressure and aggravating reflux. Similarly, they should avoid wearing clothes that fit tightly around the abdomen. Patients should be encouraged to lose excess weight. This can be accomplished with a combination of caloric restriction and physical activity.

## For irritable bowel syndrome

Emotional and physical stresses are major contributors to IBS. As such, activities like meditation that will induce relaxation are often beneficial. Physical exercise often works to dissipate tension and relieve depression and stress, allowing

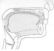

patients to feel better about themselves. Exercise also stimulates normal peristalsis of the intestines. Patients should be encouraged to select a form of physical exercise that they find enjoyable and to exercise with a regular schedule. Inactive individuals should be encouraged to start slowly. They should decide how much they think they can do, and then to begin with half that amount. It is easier and more gratifying to begin slowly and to gradually increase the amount of time for exercise than to exceed tolerance and suffer for this and to then have to start all over again from the beginning. To further address physical stress patients should also adopt a regular daily schedule and they should sleep at least eight hours a night.

It is also extremely important that patients maintain optimal dietary habits. The symptoms of IBS (alternating cramping, abdominal pain, bloating, gas, diarrhea, and constipation) necessitate that various approaches may need to be employed depending upon which symptoms are present. To help regulate bowel function, meals should be eaten at about the same time each day and should not be skipped. If diarrhea is prominent, eating small, frequent meals may be desirable. If, however, constipation is a dominant symptom, eating larger amounts of high-fiber foods may help stimulate colonic transit time. Patients must, however, keep themselves well hydrated. Water is best. Drinking eight cups (approximately 1½ liters) daily is a minimum amount for the average adult. Alcohol and beverages that contain caffeine stimulate the intestines and aggravate diarrhea. Carbonated beverages can produce gas, adding to abdominal bloating.

Food and beverages that aggravate the patient's symptoms should be avoided. These include, but are not limited to, alcohol, chocolate, coffee, and soda pop (as well as over-the-counter medications), that contain caffeine. Sugar substitutes containing sorbitol or mannitol can act as osmotic laxatives in the large intestine. Fatty foods may also be a problem for some individuals. If bloating and flatus is a problem, high fiber foods like beans, cabbage, cauliflower, and broccoli that commonly increase these symptoms should be avoided. Chewing gum or drinking through a straw can lead to aerophagia, further aggravating abdominal bloating.

Dietary fiber may or may not prove to be beneficial. It is beneficial to address constipation, but, as mentioned above, too much fiber can aggravate abdominal bloating, flatus, and cramping. Because the symptoms of IBS are volatile, it is best to gradually increase dietary fiber over a period of weeks. Foods high in fiber include fruits, vegetables, legumes, and whole grains. If the patient is gluten intolerant, caution must be exercised with whole grains (see below). Some individuals find a supplemental fiber product, like psyllium fiber, to be more acceptable. If so, it should still be initiated gradually, and with adequate water as discussed above. If dietary fiber proves beneficial it should be consumed consistently on a daily basis.

Consider lactose and gluten intolerance that may make IBS symptoms worse. Some individuals are only partially lactase deficient. That is, their body produces some lactase, but once it is used up, they are deficient until they produce more of the enzyme. These individuals may be able to consume small amounts of milk products infrequently. They may get relief using lactase containing products to help digest lactose. Or they can completely eliminate cow's milk products substituting with sheep or goat's milk or soy products. In any case, they must be sure to get enough protein, calcium, and B vitamins from other sources.[110]

Gluten is found in most commonly available grains. An inability to tolerate gluten results in abdominal pain and cramping, bloating, gas, and diarrhea. As such patients with IBS can find their symptoms greatly aggravated and anything containing these grains must be avoided. Gluten free sources include: amaranth, buckwheat, corn, montina (Indian rice grass), quinoa, rice, sorghum, teff, and wild rice.

The diet must contain a variety of healthy foods, and foods that aggravate symptoms should be avoided. If this proves difficult, patients may find it useful to keep a food diary in which they record the contents of their diet along with the status (none, mild, moderate, severe) of their symptoms for several weeks, or longer. If they identify a food that appears to aggravate their symptoms, they should

avoid it for several days and if their symptoms subside, they should try the offending food again. If it again aggravates their symptoms they will know that this is a food to be avoided.

It is also appropriate to consider a diet high in probiotics that promote the growth of beneficial bacteria (*Bifidobacterium*, *Lactobacillus*, and *Bacteroides*). This includes prebiotic carbohydrates such as inulin and oligofructose—plant carbohydrates that are not digestible in the small intestine, but rather are fermented by bacteria in the colon.[111]

## For constipation

Individuals often become constipated because of insufficient hydration, inadequate dietary fiber, and lack of physical activity.

Patients must maintain hydration. Water is best. Drinking eight cups (approximately 1½ liters) daily is a minimum amount for the average adult.

Eating high-fiber foods can decrease colonic transit time. Dietary fiber is the portion of plants in the diet that passes through the GI tract undigested. It is categorized as either soluble or insoluble. Both types of dietary fiber are important for health.

Soluble fiber attracts water, forming a gel that, although potentially constipating, helps to keep water in the stool. It also helps to lower serum low-density lipoprotein (LDL) cholesterol by interfering with the absorption of dietary cholesterol. Dietary sources of soluble fiber include: blueberries, apples, oranges, pears, strawberries, cucumbers, celery, carrots, lentils, beans, dried peas, oatmeal, oat bran, flaxseeds, and nuts. Some individuals find a supplemental fiber product, like psyllium fiber, to be acceptable.

Insoluble fiber is the fiber that most helps prevent constipation by adding bulk to the stool. It does not dissolve in water. It therefore passes through the GI tract relatively intact, reducing colonic transit time. Dietary sources of insoluble fiber include: whole grains, barley, bulgur, couscous, brown rice, seeds, nuts, wheat bran, corn bran, broccoli, cabbage, carrots, celery, cucumbers, dark leafy vegetables, green beans, onions, tomatoes, zucchini, raisins, grapes, and fruit and root vegetable skins. If the patient is gluten intolerant caution must be exercised with most whole grains (see above).

The average American consumes approximately 11 grams of fiber daily. The recommended amount of dietary fiber to be consumed daily is 21 to 25 grams for women and 30 to 38 grams for men.[112]

Increased fiber (dietary or supplemental) consumption is of great benefit when managing chronic constipation. It can be a source of bloating and flatus, however, and if consumed excessively, particularly without concomitant adequate water intake, it can actually be constipating. If the use of dietary fiber proves to be beneficial, it should be initiated gradually, slowly increasing the amount consumed daily, in conjunction with adequate water intake. Once this has been satisfactorily titrated, the determined amount of fiber should be consumed consistently on a daily basis.

Low fiber foods including fats, meats, and dairy products should be consumed in moderation, and then only as part of a balanced diet. Other low fiber foods, including processed foods, refined grains, snack foods, and candy are best avoided.

Patients should try to establish and maintain regularity in their daily schedule. To help regulate bowel function, meals should be eaten at about the same time each day and should not be skipped. It is important that patients learn to recognize, and respond to, the urge to have a bowel movement. Consciously holding back a bowel movement blocks normal colonic motility. When attempting to defecate, evacuation can be initiated by stimulating the gastrocolic reflex. This can often be accomplished by drinking a glass of hot water while seated on the toilet.

Physical activity mechanically stimulates peristalsis. Patients should be regularly and consistently active. This can be as simple as walking. For individuals who are unable to effectively move about, gentle transabdominal manipulative procedures can be self administered, or performed by a family member.

The use of medicinal laxatives should be avoided. They ultimately cause dependence and irritate the GI tract.

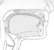

# References

1. Still AT. The philosophy and mechanical principles of osteopathy. Kirksville, MO: Osteopathic Enterprise; 1986:146.

2. Nelson KE. Viscerosomatic and somatovisceral reflexes. Chapt. 5. In: Nelson, Glonek, eds., Somatic Dysfunction in Osteopathic Family Medicine. Baltimore, MD: Lippincott, Williams & Wilkins; 2007;33-55.

3. Wilkins T, Gillies RA, Thomas AM, Wagner PJ. The prevalence of dysphagia in primary care patients: a HamesNet Research Network study. J Am Board Fam Med. 2007 Mar-Apr;20(2):144-50.

4. Cheng CF, Peng CL, Chiou HY, Tsai CY. Dentofacial morphology and tongue function during swallowing. Am J Orthod Dentofacial Orthop. 2002 Nov;122(5):491-9.

5. Abd-el-Malek S. The part played by the tongue in mastication and deglutition. J Anat. 1955 Apr;89(2):250-4.

6. Matsuo K, Palmer JB. Kinematic linkage of the tongue, jaw, and hyoid during eating and speech. Arch Oral Biol. 2010 Apr;55(4):325-31.

7. Cheng CF, Peng CL, Chiou HY, Tsai CY. Dentofacial morphology and tongue function during swallowing. Am J Orthod Dentofacial Orthop. 2002 Nov;122(5):491-9.

8. Humbert IA, Fitzgerald ME, McLaren DG, Johnson S, Porcaro E, Kosmatka K. et al. J. Neurophysiology of swallowing: effects of age and bolus type. Neuroimage. 2009 Feb 1;44(3):982-91.

9. Shaker R, Hogan WJ. Reflex-mediated enhancement of airway protective mechanisms. Am J Med. 2000 Mar 6;108 Suppl 4a:8S-14S.

10. Robbins J, Hamilton JW, Lof GL, Kempster GB. Oropharyngeal swallowing in normal adults of different ages. Gastroenterology. 1992 Sep;103(3):823-9.

11. Ostreicher HJ, Hawk AM. Patterns of performance for two age groups of normal adults on a test of oral form discrimination. J Commun Disord. 1982 Jul;15(4):329-35.

12. Miller AJ. Oral and pharyngeal reflexes in the mammalian nervous system: their diverse range in complexity and the pivotal role of the tongue. Crit Rev Oral Biol Med. 2002;13(5):409-25.

13. Sivarao DV, Goyal RK. Functional anatomy and physiology of the upper esophageal sphincter. Am J Med. 2000 Mar 6;108 Suppl 4a:27S-37S.

14. Matsuo K, Palmer JB. Anatomy and physiology of feeding and swallowing: normal and abnormal. Phys Med Rehabil Clin N Am. 2008 Nov;19(4):691-707, vii.

15. Blackshaw LA. New insights in the neural regulation of the lower oesophageal sphincter. Eur Rev Med Pharmacol Sci. 2008 Aug;12 Suppl 1:33-9.

16. Blackshaw LA. New insights in the neural regulation of the lower oesophageal sphincter. Eur Rev Med Pharmacol Sci. 2008 Aug;12 Suppl 1:33-9.

17. Dent J, El-Serag HB, Wallander MA, Johansson S. Epidemiology of gastro-oesophageal reflux disease: a systematic review. Gut. 2005 May;54(5):710-7.

18. Diaz-Rubio M, Moreno-Elola-Olaso C, Rey E, Locke GR 3rd, Rodriguez-Artalejo F. Symptoms of gastro-oesophageal reflux: prevalence, severity, duration and associated factors in a Spanish population. Aliment Pharmacol Ther. 2004 Jan 1;19(1):95-105.

19. Dent J, El-Serag HB, Wallander MA, Johansson S. Epidemiology of gastro-oesophageal reflux disease: a systematic review. Gut. 2005 May;54(5):710-7.

20. Locke GR 3rd, Talley NJ, Fett SL, Zinsmeister AR, Melton LJ 3rd. Prevalence and clinical spectrum of gastroesophageal reflux: a population-based study in Olmsted County, Minnesota. Gastroenterology. 1997 May;112(5):1448-56.

21. Williams PL, editor. Gray's anatomy. 38th ed. Edinburgh: Churchill Livingstone; 1995.

22. Williams PL, editor. Gray's anatomy. 38th ed. Edinburgh: Churchill Livingstone; 1995.

23. Standring S . Ed. Gray's Anatomy : The anatomical basis of clinical practice . 39th ed . Edinburgh : Churchill Livingstone ; 2004.

24. Schoeman MN, Tippett MD, Akkermans LM, Dent J, Holloway RH. Mechanisms of gastroesophageal reflux in ambulant healthy human subjects. Gastroenterology. 1995 Jan;108(1):83-91.

25. Dent J. Patterns of lower esophageal sphincter function associated with gastroesophageal reflux. Am J Med. 1997 Nov 24;103(5A):29S-32S.

26. Fujiwara Y, Nakagawa K, Kusunoki M, Tanaka T, Yamamura T, Utsunomiya J. Gastroesophageal reflux after distal gastrectomy: possible significance of the angle of His. Am J Gastroenterol. 1998 Jan;93(1):11-5.

27. Mittal RK, Holloway RH, Penagini R, Blackshaw LA, Dent J. Transient lower esophageal sphincter relaxation. Gastroenterology. 1995 Aug;109(2):601-10.

28. Orlando RC. Overview of the mechanisms of gastroesophageal reflux. Am J Med. 2001 Dec 3;111 Suppl 8A:174S-177S.

29. Hornby PJ, Abrahams TP, Partosoedarso ER. Central mechanisms of lower esophageal sphincter control. Gastroenterol Clin North Am. 2002 Dec;31(4 Suppl):S11-20, v-vi.

30. Boeckxstaens GE. The lower oesophageal sphincter. Neurogastroenterol Motil. 2005 Jun;17 Suppl 1:13-21.

31. Boeckxstaens GE. The lower oesophageal sphincter. Neurogastroenterol Motil. 2005 Jun;17 Suppl 1:13-21.

32. Wyman JB, Dent J, Heddle R, Dodds WJ, Toouli J, Downton J. Control of belching by the lower oesophageal sphincter. Gut. 1990 Jun;31(6):639-46.

33. Osatakul S. The natural course of infantile reflux regurgitation: a non-Western perspective. Pediatrics. 2005 Apr;115(4):1110-1; author reply 1111.

34. Penagini R, Hebbard G, Horowitz M, Dent J, Bermingham H, Jones K, Holloway RH. Motor function of the proximal stomach and visceral perception in gastro-oesophageal reflux disease. Gut. 1998 Feb;42(2):251-7.

35. Dodds WJ. 1976 Walter B. Cannon Lecture: current concepts of esophageal motor func-

tion: clinical implications for radiology. AJR Am J Roentgenol. 1977 Apr;128(4):549-61.

36. Friedland GW. Progress in radiology: historical review of the changing concepts of lower esophageal anatomy: 430 B.C.--1977. AJR Am J Roentgenol. 1978 Sep;131(3):373-8.

37. Menon S, Trudgill N. Risk factors in the aetiology of hiatus hernia: a meta-analysis. Eur J Gastroenterol Hepatol. 2011 Feb;23(2):133-8.

38. Information from your family doctor. Irritable bowel syndrome: controlling your symptoms. Am Fam Physician. 2010 Dec 15;82(12):1449-51.

39. Cucchiara S, Iebba V, Conte MP, Schippa S.The microbiota in inflammatory bowel disease in different age groups. Dig Dis. 2009;27(3):252-8.

40. Fanaro S, Chierici R, Guerrini P, Vigi V. Intestinal microflora in early infancy: composition and development. Acta Paediatr Suppl. 2003 Sep;91(441):48-55.

41. Bourlioux P, Koletzko B, Guarner F, Braesco V. The intestine and its microflora are partners for the protection of the host: report on the Danone Symposium 'The Intelligent Intestine,' held in Paris, June 14, 2002. Am J Clin Nutr. 2003 Oct;78(4):675-83.

42. O'Hara AM, Shanahan F. The gut flora as a forgotten organ. EMBO Rep. 2006 Jul;7(7):688-93.

43. Pirlich M, Norman K, Lochs H, Bauditz J. Role of intestinal function in cachexia. Curr Opin Clin Nutr Metab Care. 2006 Sep;9(5):603-6.

44. Cucchiara S, Iebba V, Conte MP, Schippa S.The microbiota in inflammatory bowel disease in different age groups. Dig Dis. 2009;27(3):252-8.

45. Meier J, Sturm A. The intestinal epithelial barrier: does it become impaired with age? Dig Dis. 2009;27(3):240-5.

46. Delvaux M. Role of visceral sensitivity in the pathophysiology of irritable bowel syndrome. Gut. 2002 Jul;51 Suppl 1:i67-71.

47. Kellow JE, Delvaux M, Azpiroz F, Camilleri M, Quigley EM, Thompson DG. Principles of applied neurogastroenterology: physiology/motility-sensation. Gut. 1999 Sep;45 Suppl 2:II17-24.

48. McMahon SB. Sensitisation of gastrointestinal tract afferents. Gut. 2004 Mar;53 Suppl 2:ii13-5.

49. Lembo T, Munakata J, Mertz H, Niazi N, Kodner A, Nikas V, Mayer EA. Evidence for the hypersensitivity of lumbar splanchnic afferents in irritable bowel syndrome. Gastroenterology. 1994 Dec;107(6):1686-96.

50. Boeckxstaens GE. Understanding and controlling the enteric nervous system. Best Pract Res Clin Gastroenterol. 2002 Dec;16(6):1013-23.

51. Grundy D. Neuroanatomy of visceral nociception: vagal and splanchnic afferent. Gut. 2002 Jul;51 Suppl 1:i2-5.

52. Phillips RJ, Walter GC, Powley TL. Age-related changes in vagal afferents innervating the gastrointestinal tract. Auton Neurosci. 2010 Feb 16;153(1-2):90-8.

53. Phillips RJ, Walter GC, Powley TL. Age-related changes in vagal afferents innervating the gastrointestinal tract. Auton Neurosci. 2010 Feb 16;153(1-2):90-8.

54. Hansen MB. Neurohumoral control of gastro-intestinal motility. Physiol Res. 2003;52(1):1-30.

55. Mayer EA, Naliboff BD, Chang L, Coutinho SV. V. Stress and irritable bowel syndrome. Am J Physiol Gastrointest Liver Physiol. 2001 pr;280(4):G519-24.

56. Meddings JB, Swain MG. Environmental stress-induced gastrointestinal permeability is mediated by endogenous glucocorticoids in the rat. Gastroenterology. 2000 Oct;119(4):1019-28.

57. Cameron OG. Visceral sensory neuroscience: interoception. New York, NY; Oxford University Press, Inc. 2002.

58. Nelson KE. Viscerosomatic and somatovisceral reflexes, chapt. 5. In: Nelson, Glonek, eds., Somatic Dysfunction in Osteopathic Family Medicine. Baltimore, MD: Lippincott, Williams & Wilkins; 2007;33-55.

59. Nelson KE, Sergueef N, Lipinski CM, Chapman AR, Glonek T. Cranial rhythmic impulse related to the Traube-Hering-Mayer oscillation: comparing laser-Doppler flowmetry and palpation. J Am Osteopath Assoc. 2001 Mar;101(3):163-73.

60. Sergueef N, Nelson KE, Glonek T. The effect of cranial manipulation on the Traube-Hering-Mayer oscillation as measured by laser-Doppler flowmetry. Altern Ther Health Med. 2002 Nov-Dec;8(6):74-6.

61. Nelson KE. The primary respiratory mechanism. AAO Journal. Winter 2002;12(4): 25–34.

62. Sergueef N, Nelson KE, Glonek T. The effect of light exercise upon blood flow velocity determined by laser-Doppler flowmetry. J Med Eng Technol. 2004 Jul-Aug;28(4):143-50.

63. Nelson KE, Sergueef N, Glonek T. Cranial Manipulation Induces Sequential Changes in Blood Flow Velocity on Demand. AAO Journal. September 2004:14(3):15-17.

64. Nelson KE, Sergueef N, Glonek T. Letter to the editor; Commentary on 'The effect of cranial manipulation upon intracranial fluid dynamics.' AAO Journal September 2004;14(3):11-12.

65. Sergueef N, Glonek T, Nelson KE. The Cranial Rhythmic Impulse and the Traube-Hering-Mayer Oscillation. Proceedings of the International Research Conference in Celebrating the 20th Anniversary of the Osteopathic Center for Children, Feb. 6-10, 2002, San Diego, California, King HH, ed. Indianapolis, IN: American Academy of Osteopathy; 2005:39-51.

66. Nelson KE, Sergueef N, Glonek T. Recording the Rate of the Cranial Rhythmic Impulse. J Am Osteopath Assoc. 2006 Jun;106(6):337-41.

67. Nelson KE, Sergueef N, Glonek T. The effect of an alternative medical procedure upon low-frequency oscillations in cutaneous blood flow velocity. J Manipulative Physiol Ther. 2006 Oct;29(8):626-36.

68. Glonek T, Sergueef N, Nelson KE. Physiological Rhythms/Oscillations. Chapt 11. In: Chila AG. ed. Foundations of Osteopathic Medicine. 3rd ed. Philadelphia: Wolters Kluwer/Lippincott Williams and Wilkins. 2011:162-190.

69. Cameron OG. Interoception: the inside story--a model for psychosomatic processes. Psychosom Med. 2001 Sep-Oct;63(5):697-710.

70. Cameron OG. Interoception: the inside story--a model for psychosomatic processes. Psychosom Med. 2001 Sep-Oct;63(5):697-710.

71. Van Oudenhove L, Demyttenaere K, Tack J, Aziz Q. Central nervous system involvement in functional gastrointestinal disorders. Best Pract Res Clin Gastroenterol. 2004 Aug;18(4):663-80.

72. Helmuth L. Neuroscience. Early insult rewires pain circuits. Science. 2000 Jul 28;289(5479):521-2.

73. Miranda A, Sood M. Treatment options for chronic abdominal pain in children and adolescents. Curr Treat Options Gastroenterol. 2006 Sep;9(5):409-15.

74. Hall GB, Kamath MV, Collins S, Ganguli S, Spaziani R, Miranda KL, Bayati A, Bienenstock J. Heightened central affective response to visceral sensations of pain and discomfort in IBS. Neurogastroenterol Motil. 2010 Mar;22(3):276-e80.

75. Mayer EA, Naliboff BD, Chang L, Coutinho SV. V. Stress and irritable bowel syndrome. Am J Physiol Gastrointest Liver Physiol. 2001 Apr;280(4):G519-24.

76. Thompson WG, Longstreth GF, Drossman DA, Heaton KW, Irvine EJ, Müller-Lissner SA. Functional bowel disorders and functional abdominal pain. Gut. 1999 Sep;45 Suppl 2:II43-7.

77. Drossman DA. The functional gastrointestinal disorders and the Rome III process. Gastroenterology. 2006 Apr;130(5):1377-90.

78. Thompson WG, Longstreth GF, Drossman DA, Heaton KW, Irvine EJ, Müller-Lissner SA. Functional bowel disorders and functional abdominal pain. Gut. 1999 Sep;45 Suppl 2:II43-7.

79. Herz MJ, Kahan E, Zalevski S, Aframian R, Kuznitz D, Reichman S. Constipation: a different entity for patients and doctors. Fam Pract. 1996 Apr;13(2):156-9.

80. Longstreth GF, Thompson WG, Chey WD, Houghton LA, Mearin F, Spiller RC. Functional bowel disorders. Gastroenterology. 2006 Apr;130(5):1480-91.

81. Whitehead WE, Drinkwater D, Cheskin LJ, Heller BR, Schuster MM. Constipation in the elderly living at home: definition, prevalence and relationship to lifestyle and health status. J Am Geriatr Soc. 1989;37:423-429.

82. Locke GR 3rd, Pemberton JH, Phillips SF. AGA technical review on constipation. American Gastroenterological Association. Gastroenterology. 2000 Dec;119(6):1766-78.

83. Harari D, Gurwitz JH, Avorn J, Bohn R, Minaker KL. Bowel habit in relation to age and gender. Findings from the National Health Interview Survey and clinical implications. Arch Intern Med. 1996 Feb 12;156(3):315-20.

84. Locke GR 3rd, Pemberton JH, Phillips SF. AGA technical review on constipation. American Gastroenterological Association. Gastroenterology. 2000 Dec;119(6):1766-78.

85. Loening-Baucke V, Anuras S. Sigmoidal and rectal motility in healthy elderly. J Am Geriatr Soc. 1984 Dec;32(12):887-91.

86. Melkersson M, Andersson H, Bosaeus I, Falkheden T. Intestinal transit time in constipated and non-constipated geriatric patients. Scand J Gastroenterol. 1983 Jul;18(5):593-7.

87. Stivland T, Camilleri M, Vassallo M, Proano M, Rath D, Brown M, et al. Scintigraphic measurement of regional gut transit in idiopathic constipation. Gastroenterology. 1991 Jul;101(1):107-15.

88. Quigley EM. What we have learned about colonic motility: normal and disturbed. Curr Opin Gastroenterol. 2010 Jan;26(1):53-60.

89. Quigley EM. What we have learned about colonic motility: normal and disturbed. Curr Opin Gastroenterol. 2010 Jan;26(1):53-60.

90. Klauser AG, Voderholzer WA, Heinrich CA, Schindlbeck NE, Müller-Lissner SA. Behavioral modification of colonic function. Can constipation be learned? Dig Dis Sci. 1990 Oct;35(10):1271-5.

91. Sikirov D. Comparison of straining during defecation in three positions: results and implications for human health. Dig Dis Sci. 2003 Jul;48(7):1201-5.

92. Sikirov BA. Primary constipation: an underlying mechanism. Med Hypotheses. 1989 Feb;28(2):71-3.

93. Bannister JJ, Abouzekry L, Read NW. Effect of aging on anorectal function. Gut. 1987 Mar;28(3):353-7.

94. O'Mahony D, O'Leary P, Quigley EM. Aging and intestinal motility: a review of factors that affect intestinal motility in the aged. Drugs Aging. 2002;19(7):515-27.

95. Jameson JS, Chia YW, Kamm MA, Speakman CT, Chye YH, Henry MM. Effect of age, sex and parity on anorectal function. Br J Surg. 1994 Nov;81(11):1689-92.

96. Stav K, Dwyer PL, Roberts L. Pudendal neuralgia. Fact or fiction? Obstet Gynecol Surv. 2009 Mar;64(3):190-9.

97. Glénard F. Application de la méthode naturelle à l'analyse de la dyspepsie nerveuse. - détermination d'une espèce. Lyon médical. Société de médecine de Lyon. Lyon, France. 1885;49:8-30.

98. Lo CM, Lau HK, Kei SK. Superior Mesenteric Artery Syndrome: An uncommon cause of abdominal pain mimicking gastroenteritis. Hong Kong J Em Med. 2008; 15(4):235-239.

99. Beilke MC. Personal communication with the author, Nelson KE. Chicago, Il. 1972.

100. McCallum HA. A Clinical Lecture on Visceroptosis: Its Symptoms and Treatment. Brit Med J Feb 18, 1905:345-347.

101. Boeckxstaens GE. Understanding and controlling the enteric nervous system. Best Pract Res Clin Gastroenterol. 2002 Dec;16(6): 1013-23.

102. Nelson KE. The primary respiratory mechanism. AAO Journal. Winter 2002;12(4):25–34.

103. Nelson KE. Viscerosomatic and somatovisceral reflexes. Chapt. 5. In: Nelson, Glonek, eds., Somatic Dysfunction in Osteopathic Family Medicine. Baltimore, MD: Lippincott, Williams & Wilkins; 2007:33-55.

104. Nelson KE. Viscerosomatic and somatovisceral reflexes. Chapt. 5. In: Nelson, Glonek, eds., Somatic Dysfunction in Osteopathic Family Medicine. Baltimore, MD: Lippincott, Williams & Wilkins; 2007:33-55.

105. Van Buskirk RL, Nelson KE. Osteopathic family practice: An application of the primary care model. In: Ward RC, ed. Foundations for Osteopathic Medicine. 2nd ed. Philadelphia, PA: Lippincott Williams and Wilkins; 2002:289–297.

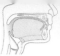

106. Nelson KE. Viscerosomatic and somatovisceral reflexes. Chapt. 5. In: Nelson, Glonek, eds., Somatic Dysfunction in Osteopathic Family Medicine. Baltimore, MD: Lippincott, Williams & Wilkins; 2007:33-55.

107. Middlemiss C. Gastroesophageal reflux disease: a common condition in the elderly. Nurse Pract. 997 Nov;22(11):51-2, 55-9.

108. Kaltenbach T, Crockett S, Gerson LB. Are lifestyle measures effective in patients with gastroesophageal reflux disease? An evidence-based approach. Arch Intern Med. 2006 May 8;166(9):965-71.

109. Poh CH, Navarro-Rodriguez T, Fass R. Review: treatment of gastroesophageal reflux disease in the elderly. Am J Med. 2010 Jun;123(6): 496-501.

110. Mayo Clinic staff. Lifestyle and home remedies. Available at http://www.mayoclinic.com/ health/irritable-bowel-syndrome. Accessed June 30, 2011.

111. Cherbut C. Inulin and oligofructose in the dietary fibre concept. Br J Nutr. 2002 May;87 Suppl 2:S159-62.

112. Position of the American Dietetic Association: Health Implications of Dietary Fiber. Journal of the American Dietetic Association (October 2008) 108(10):1716-31.

# Chapter 6

# Urogenital dysfunctions

In this chapter we will discuss pelvic floor disorders, including pelvic organ prolapse, lower urinary tract dysfunctions (LUTD) and benign prostate disorders.

## Pelvic floor disorders

Pelvic floor disorders are common among women, associated most often with childbirth and aging. Several interrelated clinical entities may be present: pelvic organ prolapse, urinary or anal incontinence, or both, overactive bladder, and dysfunctional defecation. Up to 67.7% of women experience some form of pelvic floor dysfunction of at least one major type in their lifetime.[1] These can be incapacitating conditions, often resulting in shame, isolation, loss of independence, and reduced quality of life. All of these conditions have dysfunction of the constituents of the pelvic floor in common. In the extreme pelvic organ prolapsed, cystocele and rectocele require surgical repair. Once a thorough evaluation for organic colorectal, gynecologic, and urologic pathology has been performed and the appropriate treatment of any identified pathologies initiated, the treatment of identified somatic dysfunction with osteopathic manipulative treatment (OMT) is appropriate.

### Pelvic floor

The pelvic floor consists of a bilaterally symmetrical network of striated muscles, ligaments, and tissues that unite in the midline, acting like a hammock

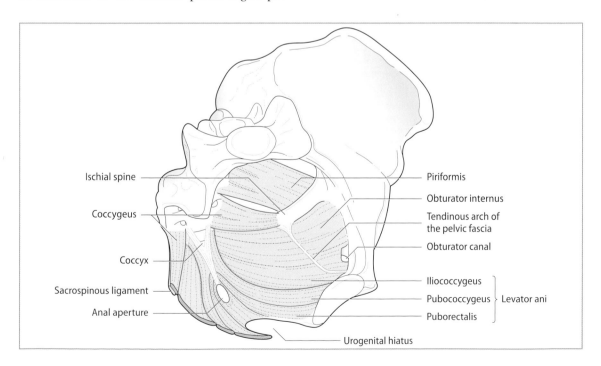

Figure 4.6.1: The pelvic floor

| Ischial spine | Piriformis |
| Coccygeus | Obturator internus |
| Coccyx | Tendinous arch of the pelvic fascia |
| Sacrospinous ligament | Obturator canal |
| Anal aperture | Iliococcygeus |
| | Pubococcygeus |
| | Puborectalis |
| | Levator ani |
| | Urogenital hiatus |

that supports the organs of the pelvis, i.e., from front to back, bladder, urethra, uterus, vagina, and rectum. The pelvic floor is, typically, described as a diaphragm formed by the paired levator ani muscles and, in the anterior portion, the perineal membrane (urogenital diaphragm) and the paired muscles located in the deep perineal pouch. On each side of the pelvis, the levator ani muscles constitute a significant portion of the pelvic diaphragm. They each consist of several muscular portions that, in close contact to one another, form a large muscular sheet. Each portion, the iliococcygeus, ischiococcygeus, and pubococcygeus, is named according to its origin and insertion within the pelvis. In close relation with the pelvis where it attaches with the pelvic fascia, the pelvic diaphragm resists the downward forces that normally result from increases in intra-abdominal pressure.

## Levator ani

Although described separately, the different portions of the levator ani muscle, iliococcygeus, ischiococcygeus, and pubococcygeus are in close contact and difficult to separate.

## Iliococcygeus

The iliococcygeus is the thin lateral part of the levator ani. It spreads from the inner surface of the ischial spine and the obturator fascia to the inferior lateral margin of the last two segments of the coccyx. Medially, the fibers of the iliococcygeus muscles from both sides of the pelvis unite to form a raphe that is continuous with the fibroelastic anococcygeal ligament. Located between the anus and the coccyx, this raphe provides additional strength to the pelvic floor posteriorly, where the pelvic organs rest.

## Ischiococcygeus

The ischiococcygeal part of the levator ani is sometimes described as a separate muscle from the levator ani—the coccygeus muscle. Triangular in shape, with its apex directed laterally, it extends from the ischial spine to the lateral margins of the coccyx and the fifth sacral segment. As such, it forms the posterior part of the pelvic diaphragm and covers the inner surface of the sacrospinous ligament.

## Pubococcygeus

The pubococcygeus is the third constituent of the levator ani. Also named the pubovisceral muscle, it is subdivided into several portions according to the pelvic viscera associated with each portion, i.e., pubourethralis and puborectalis in the male, pubovaginalis and puborectalis in the female. Arising on either side from the inner surface of the body of the pubic bone and the anterior portion of the arcus tendineus, a linear thickening in the fascia covering the obturator internus muscle, the pubococcygeus is directed posteriorly, and almost horizontally, behind the rectum. Bilaterally, its most medial fibers form the lateral borders of the levator hiatus, also named the urogenital hiatus. On each side, they pass lateral to the urethra, vagina, and anorectum. It is through this opening that genital prolapse occurs, therefore the baseline muscular activity of the paired pubococcygeus muscles is of paramount importance in keeping the urogenital hiatus closed. In males, the pubococcygeus muscles attach to periurethral supporting tissues to form the pubourethralis, coursing laterally and inferiorly to the prostate. In females, the same fibers continue posteriorly to encircle the posterior wall of the vagina to form the pubovaginalis. In both sexes, some of the medial fibers join the perineal body and the anorectal junction, where some mingle with the muscular fibers of the external anal sphincter. Posterior to the rectum, the puborectalis muscles form a thick muscular sling around the anorectal junction. Some fibers of the pubococcygeus muscles also join the medial raphe at this location.

## Innervation of the levator ani

The innervation of the levator ani comes mostly from the second, third, and fourth sacral spinal segments. Different components of the pubococcygeus, i.e., pubourethralis, puborectalis, and pubovaginalis are supplied by the second and third sacral spinal segments passing through the pudendal nerve. The ischiococcygeus and iliococcygeus are innervated by direct branches of the sacral plexus from the third and fourth sacral spinal segments.

The pudendal nerve has frequently been described as supplying part of the levator ani

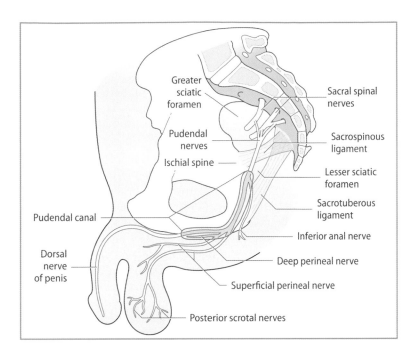

Figure 4.6.2: The pudendal nerve

Greater sciatic foramen

Sacral spinal nerves

Pudendal nerves

Sacrospinous ligament

Ischial spine

Lesser sciatic foramen

Sacrotuberous ligament

Pudendal canal

Inferior anal nerve

Dorsal nerve of penis

Deep perineal nerve

Superficial perineal nerve

Posterior scrotal nerves

muscles. Recent studies, however, challenge this description and indicate that the pudendal nerve does not contribute to levator muscle innervation.[2] The levator ani nerve comes from S3, S4, and S5, supplying the coccygeus and the components of the levator ani muscle. Once it leaves the sacral foramina, it runs medially, for 2–3 cm, to the ischial spine and arcus tendineus, and then on across the coccygeus, iliococcygeus, pubococcygeus, and puborectalis muscles.

## Function of the levator ani

The pubococcygeus globally compresses the visceral canals that traverse the pelvic floor. It also lifts the vagina, perineal body, and anus. When in spasm, it contributes to low abdominal pain, back pain, and dyspareunia. Besides reinforcing the external anal sphincter, the contractile action of the puborectalis keeps the urogenital hiatus tight and pulls the distal parts of the urethra, vagina, and rectum toward the pubic bones. In women, therefore, it functions as a vaginal sphincter. It also helps to maintain the anorectal angle, of about 90°, between the rectum and the anal canal, obstructing the rectal outlet and restraining rectal evacuation. Its role in anal and urinary

continence is primordial, and is helped, in this function, by the iliococcygeus and the ischiococcygeus muscles. Relaxation of the puborectalis and external anal sphincter muscles, conversely, increases the anorectal angle to about 130–140° and opens the anal canal to permit defecation. After defecation, the ischiococcygeal muscles pull the coccyx forward.

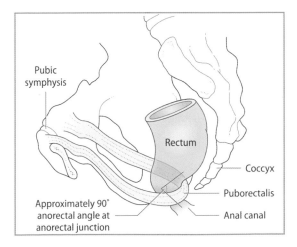

Pubic symphysis

Rectum

Coccyx

Puborectalis

Approximately 90° anorectal angle at anorectal junction

Anal canal

Figure 4.6.3: The anorectal junction

During the inspiratory phase of quiet respiration, the levator ani works in a synergistic way with the abdominothoracic diaphragm.[3] Through the rhythmic motion of respiration, the pelvic diaphragm contributes to the drainage of fluids away from the pelvis and perineal tissues and to the pumping of fluids from lower extremities into the abdominal cavity.

The assessment of the function of and synergy between the three diaphragms, i.e., cranial, abdominothoracic, and pelvic is part of an osteopathic total-body examination.[4] Any restriction in the motion of one or more of these diaphragms indicates somatic dysfunction of the structures upon which they attach, the viscera related to the diaphragm, or the diaphragm itself. As an integral part of the reciprocal tension membrane (RTM), restriction at the level of the cranial diaphragm, formed by the tentorium cerebellum and related structures, may be the result of cranial dysfunction or, through the RTM, pelvic dysfunction. Restriction at the level of the abdominothoracic diaphragm may be the result of lumbar or thoracic cage dysfunction, or both. Restriction at the level of the pelvic diaphragm may be the result of pelvic dysfunction or, again through the RTM, cranial dysfunction.

### Perineal membrane

The perineal membrane, in the anterior portion of the pelvic floor, consists of a thick fascial arrangement lying in the transverse (horizontal) plane and connecting the midline to the pelvic side walls. In 1873, Jacob Henle described this portion of the pelvic floor as the urogenital diaphragm,[5] a name that has been given up because of its inaccuracy. The perineal membrane is a thick sheet of connective tissue and not a muscular diaphragm, as suggested with the denomination urogenital diaphragm.

Triangular in shape, the perineal membrane's posterior base is anchored in the midline by the perineal body. Anteriorly, a small space separates the membrane from the inferior pubic ligament. On each side, the borders of the perineal membrane fix the pelvic organs laterally to the pubic arch. The perineal membrane is divided into two portions: the ventral portion, that consists of combined tissue from surrounding elements, continuous with the insertion of the arcus tendineus, and the dorsal portion that consists of a separate dense fibrous sheet.[6]

### Perineal pouch

Above the perineal membrane is the deep perineal pouch. It consists of skeletal muscle and various neurovascular elements. The perineal membrane and deep perineal pouch take part in the constitution of the pelvic floor and support structures for the urogenital system within the pelvic cavity. Together they divide the pelvic cavity above from the

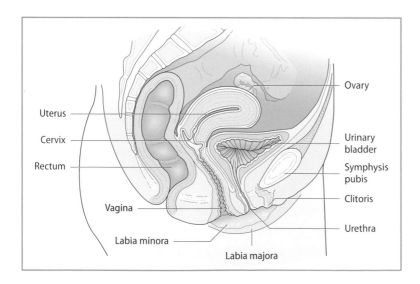

**Figure 4.6.4:** Organs of the female reproductive system

Uterus

Cervix

Rectum

Vagina

Labia minora

Labia majora

Ovary

Urinary bladder

Symphysis pubis

Clitoris

Urethra

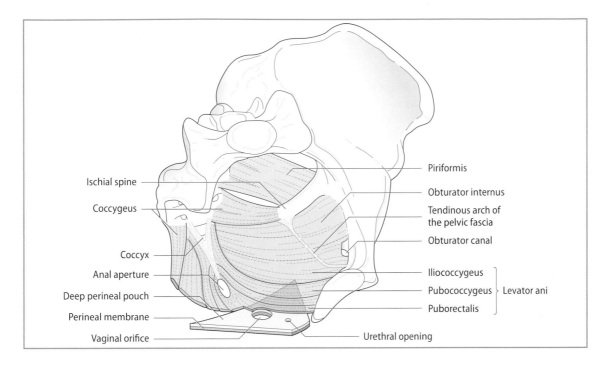

Figure 4.6.5: The perineal membrane and the deep perineal pouch

perineum below. Centrally, a circular hiatus allows the distal urethra to exit. In women, another hiatus, posterior to the urethral hiatus, provides an opening for the distal vagina into the vulval vestibule.

Anteriorly, the external genitalia and related muscles attach to the perineal membrane and adjacent bony pelvis. Superiorly, the perineal membrane is associated with the anterior levator ani muscles that fuse with the paraurethral and paravaginal connective tissues. This relationship between the perineal membrane and the levator ani muscles means that the perineal membrane contributes to support the vagina and urethra.

Several muscles enclosed in the deep perineal pouch act as sphincters, principally for the urethra. The external urethral sphincter muscle encircles the membranous part of the urethra. On each side of the urethra, a deep transverse perineal muscle runs from the medial aspect of the ischial ramus, along the free border of the perineal membrane, and blends with the muscle of the opposite side, stabilizing the position of the perineal body and further reinforcing the external urethral sphincter. In women, there is also the urethrovaginalis sphincter muscle, previously called the deep transverse perineal muscle. It runs anteriorly from the perineal body, lateral to the vagina, to combine anteriorly to the urethra with its fellow from the other side. Additionally, there is also, in women, the compressor urethrae muscle. It passes bilaterally from the ischiopubic ramus blending together anterior to the urethra.

Below the perineal membrane is the superficial perineal space that encloses the superficial ischiocavernosus, bulbospongiosus, and superficial transverse perineal muscles. In men, it also encloses the erectile tissue of the penis and the corpus spongiosum and in women the clitoris, the vestibular bulbs, and Bartholin's glands.

The perineal body is formed from the convergence of several structures at the center of the pelvic floor. It is located roughly midway between the two ischial tuberosities, along the posterior edge of the perineal membrane, to which it is fixed. The perineal body, although not, per se, a distinct anatomic structure, is of great importance in the function of the pelvic floor. Positioned posterior to the distal third of the posterior vaginal wall and anterior to the anterior anal wall, to which it attaches directly, the perineal body consists of the fibromuscular gathering of the levator ani muscles of the pelvic diaphragm, the deep transverse perineal muscles, the external anal sphincter, the superficial transverse perineal muscles, and the bulbospongiosus muscles of the perineum. In women, the sphincter urethrovaginalis also attaches to the perineal body. Support of the distal vagina and healthy anorectal function are greatly influenced by the condition of the perineal body.

During childbirth, the maternal coccyx is pushed posteriorly by the descent of the fetal head. This increases tension in the pelvic floor, and normally results in a greater amount of resistance posteriorly where the perineal body may be stretched and torn. To prevent such a possibility, in some cases the obstetrician may perform an episiotomy, making a midline incision through the skin and the perineal body, to facilitate the passage of the fetal head through the vagina. Some episiotomies are performed in a posterolateral direction thus avoiding the perineal body and more effectively maintaining the functional integrity of the pelvic floor.

Note although the area between the vagina and anus is often referred to, clinically, as the 'perineum,' it is more appropriately named the perineal body. The term perineum should be limited to the anatomical description of the entirety of the pelvic outlet.[7] Vascular and nerve supply to the perineum comes from the pudendal neurovascular bundle. (See further above: 'Levator ani,' and 'Anal canal' in 'Section 4: Clinical considerations, Chapter 5: Gastrointestinal dysfunctions,' p. 302.)

## Pelvic organ prolapse

Patients with pelvic floor somatic dysfunction may present with pelvic organ prolapse, symptoms of fecal or urinary incontinence, or both. In many cases, these conditions are associated. Pelvic organ prolapse refers to the downward displacement of pelvic organs with a protrusion of the vagina and, in the extreme, uterus, through the vulval vestibule. As many as 41% of women between 50–79 years of age demonstrate some degree of pelvic organ pro-

lapse.[8] For women 55 years old, or older, pelvic organ prolapse is the leading cause for hysterectomy in the United States.[9] The etiology of pelvic floor prolapse is complex, resulting from a combination of factors. The loss of support from the muscles or connective tissue that constitute the pelvic floor, or both, is most often involved. Vaginal delivery is commonly thought to be the main etiology that weakens or stretches supporting structures within the pelvis. Increased pelvic organ descent following delivery has been demonstrated.[10] Neuromuscular dysfunction of levator ani and external anal sphincter muscles in women with pelvic floor dysfunction, as compared to nulliparous women, seems to be consistent with a neuropathic mechanism of injury.[11] With each delivery the risk increases and parity shows the strongest relation to pelvic organ prolapse. In one study, women with two vaginal deliveries had significantly more probability of having surgery for prolapse than women who had no vaginal deliveries.[12]

The physiology of aging also appears to decrease the integrity of pelvic support structures, thereby contributing to pelvic floor disorders. Statistically, the prevalence of pelvic organ prolapse increases with advancing age.[13,14] Additional factors, such as a genetic predisposition[15] or some acquired and congenital factors, or both, may also play a role. In fact, up to 30% of the cases of pelvic organ prolapse in young women appear to be familial.[16] Other factors such as obesity, chronic coughing, frequent and excessive straining during bowel movements, deficient connective tissues with a previous history of varicose veins, hernia, hemorrhoids, and heavy lifting may also be factors contributing to pelvic floor disorders.[17] However, even though multiple factors have been identified in association with pelvic organ prolapse, its etiology remains poorly understood. It is here that a thorough appreciation of pelvic anatomy and the effect of pelvic somatic dysfunction on the bones of the pelvis and any of the structures that form the pelvic floor becomes extremely valuable.

### The levator plate

In 1907, Halban and Tandler coined the name levator plate as follows: "... in the posterior segment where (the levator muscles) unite with the similar

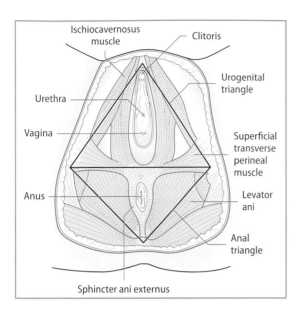

Figure 4.6.6: The urogenital and anal triangles

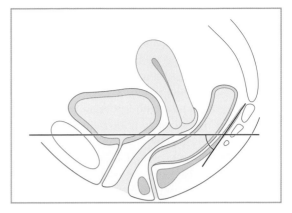

Figure 4.6.7: The levator plate angle

muscle of the other side, intertwined with each other. Thereby the posterior part of the diaphragm in the back of the rectum is considerably strengthened. We want to designate this part as the levator plate."[18]

Anatomically, the levator plate refers to the region between the anus and the coccyx, where the iliococcygeus fibers and the posterior fibers of the pubococcygeus muscle blend and form a raphe continuous with the fibroelastic anococcygeal ligament. This solid addition to the posterior pelvic floor provides support for the rectum and upper two thirds of the vagina above.

Initially, the levator plate was described as being in a transverse plane, if the subject was in a standing position. Therefore the theory was that any weakness of the levator ani muscle would slacken the sling behind the anorectum and produce sagging of the levator plate, resulting in an increased urogenital hiatus and leading to pelvic organ prolapse. More recent descriptions of the orientation of the levator plate are, however, different. When considering the pelvis, a line joining the ischial tuberosities separates the perineum into two triangles, anteriorly, the urogenital triangle, and posteriorly, the anal triangle, where the levator plate is found.

Normally, in the standing position, the urogenital triangle is situated in the transverse plane, whereas the anal triangle is inclined such that its deep endopelvic side is facing anteriorly.

In women with normal pelvic floors, dynamic MRI studies, with the subject in the supine position, demonstrated that, relative to an anteroposterior reference line, the levator plate has a mean angle of 44.3°, opened anteriorly.[19] Women with pelvic organ prolapse had a significantly greater levator plate angle as compared with the control group. In addition, these women demonstrated inferior displacement of the perineal body.

### Levator ani syndrome

Levator ani syndrome is not associated with any specific organic pathology. Rather it is a collection of symptoms and findings. Although not all patients have all of the symptoms, the levator ani syndrome can manifest as dyspareunia, irritative voiding symptoms, constipation, vaginal, vulvar and anorectal pain, levator ani spasm, low abdominal pain and low back pain.

It has been proposed that neuromuscular damage to the levator muscles may contribute to sagging of the levator plate, increasing the urogenital hiatus. Morphologic changes in the levator ani have been demonstrated with MRI studies and some authors propose a subclassification for pelvic organ prolapse on this basis.[20]

Normally, the levator ani muscle complex sustains a constant state of contraction. This results in an active pelvic floor that resists the downward forces from increased intra-abdominal pressure. These muscles consist of a mixture of slow contraction time fibers (type I) and fast contraction time fibers (type II). The levator ani muscles, in women, consist of 66% slow fibers, a higher percentage than the 48% found in other human female muscles.[21] These type I, slow contraction time fibers provide a baseline activity of the levator ani muscles that maintains closure of the urogenital hiatus and pulls the distal urethra, vagina, and rectum toward the pubic bones. Type II, fast contraction time fibers activate in response to rapid increases in abdominal pressure or may be used voluntarily as in pelvic floor rehabilitation exercises such as Kegel exercises.[22] In association with the striated muscular components of the urethral and anal sphincters, the levator ani fibers are able to contract rapidly in critical situations, as during coughing or sneezing, to maintain continence. Conversely, throughout voiding, defecation, and parturition the levator ani fibers relax.

Each component of the levator ani muscles: iliococcygeus, ischiococcygeus, and pubococcygeus (further subdivided into pubourethralis, pubovaginalis, and puborectalis) may be visualized with MRI.[23] By recognizing the origin and insertion of each of these components, their function becomes comprehensible and the identification of damage to a particular portion allows understanding of the precise functional and dysfunctional patterns of pelvic floor disorders.

The pubococcygeus muscular complex, with attachments to the urethra, vagina, and anorectum, compresses the visceral canals that pierce the pelvic floor. It also elevates the vagina, perineal body, and anus. In pelvic floor disorders, MRI studies of these muscles demonstrate that pubococcygeal muscle defects are more frequently encountered than iliococcygeal muscle defects.[24] Deficiency in the muscular attachments may be at the muscular origin, at the inner surface of the body of the pubic bone. They may also be found at the pubococcygeal insertions into the lateral vaginal wall, the perineal body, and the intersphincteric gap.[25] Because of the function of the pubococcygeus muscle, defect of this muscle explains why women with pelvic or-

gan prolapse demonstrate a larger urogenital hiatus. Levator muscular volume, shape, and integrity are different between groups of asymptomatic and prolapse subjects.[26]

In MRI studies after a vaginal delivery, 20% of primiparous women demonstrated perceptible defects in the pubococcygeal and iliococcygeal portions of the levator ani muscle complex, whereas none of the control group had such findings.[27] This implies that vaginal delivery contributes to the development of pelvic organ prolapse through levator ani muscle injury. The mechanism of injury may be the stretch of the pelvic floor associated with tears at the muscular attachment sites at the time of vaginal birth. Fetal head size seems to influence tissue stretch ratios with the greatest degree of stretch applied to the pubococcygeal portion of the levator ani, more often at the end of the second stage of labor. Difficult vaginal delivery, prolonged second stage of labor, large infant birth weight, shoulder or occiput posterior presentation and forceps delivery are often associated with increased incidence of prolapse.

Besides direct trauma to the levator ani muscle complex, vaginal delivery may also be responsible for neuropathic injury. The component parts of the pubococcygeus muscles, i.e., pubourethralis, puborectalis, and pubovaginalis, are supplied by second and third sacral spinal segments via the pudendal nerve. Compression or ischemic damage to this nerve, as may occur during the descent of the fetal head, has to be considered. Excessive straining and related perineal descent also can cause stretch and compression injury to the pudendal nerve. This is particularly true at the point where it curves around the ischial spine and passes through Alcock's canal (the pudendal canal), a tight fibrous sheath within a duplication of the fascia of the internal obturator muscle. Additional areas of possible compression of the pudendal nerve lie at the level of the piriformis, and between the sacrotuberous and the sacrospinous ligaments. A 3D computer model of vaginal delivery demonstrates that during the second stage of labor, the main inferior rectal nerve is stretched beyond the 15% strain threshold known to cause permanent damage in appendicular nerves.[28] Considering the clinical and neurophysiological data, these injuries present a very real cause for the postpartum development of the chronic pelvic pain of levator ani syndrome.

To some extent this may be addressed with pelvic floor muscle training before and throughout pregnancy. Such training may improve muscle control and flexibility during delivery, without affecting labor and birth outcomes or complication rates.[29] However pelvic floor muscle activation during vaginal delivery is correlated with more resistance to the progression of the fetus that may be an obstacle to fetal descent and lengthen labor.[30]

### Vaginal prolapse

During pregnancy, hormones affect the biochemical composition of the pelvic floor tissues and thus the viscoelastic properties of the vaginal wall, pubovisceral muscles, and perineal body. As a result, the response to the stretch that is applied to these structures during delivery may vary from one individual to another.

Each of the organs of the pelvis is surrounded by a network of dense, fibrous connective tissue—the endopelvic fascia, or parietal pelvic fascia—which interconnects with the pelvic viscera and fixes them to the pelvic walls. As such, the vagina is enveloped by the endopelvic fascia, and attached on each side to the arcus tendineus, that is fixed anteriorly to the pubic bone and posteriorly to the ischial spine. The vagina and uterus are, therefore, secured within the pelvis, while permitting, at the same time, a certain amount of movement in response to the actions of micturition, defecation, coitus, and parturition. Although several component parts of the endopelvic fascia have been given specific names, according to the organs that they cover, it is actually one uninterrupted entity, consisting of collagen, elastin, and non-vascular smooth muscle fibers surrounding blood and lymph vessels and nerves.

On each side of the uterus, the parametrium consists to a large extent of venous connective tissue with a flexible morphology that adapts to the uterine position.[31] It is organized to form the cardinal and uterosacral ligaments. The cardinal ligaments contain the vessels supplying the uterus and vagina and attach to the pelvic walls posterolaterally. The uterosacral ligaments are mainly the combination of connective tissue and smooth muscle fibers surrounding some of the pelvic autonomic nerves. Posteriorly, they consist of slight filaments of tissue fixed to the presacral fascia in front of the lower portion of the sacroiliac articulation.[32] The covering peritoneum is continuous with that overlying the rectum, and because of the normal left-sided entry of the sigmoid colon into the pelvis, the right uterosacral ligament seems

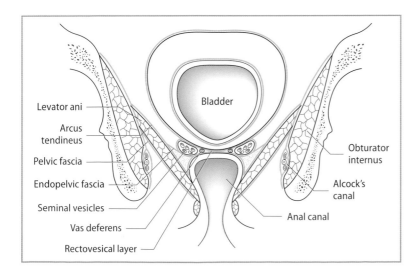

Figure 4.6.8: The pelvic fascia

more anterior. Somatic dysfunction of the sacrum, such as torsions, as well as sacroiliac and ilioilial dysfunctions can affect the position of the utero-sacral ligaments and consequently of the uterus.

Inferiorly, the parametrial border approximates the insertion of the levator ani muscle, at the junction of the middle and inferior thirds of the vagina. Anteriorly, the fascia surrounding the vagina blends with that of the urethra. Laterally it is fixed, on either side, to the pubovaginalis muscles and perineal membrane, and posteriorly to the perineal body. These attachments provide the strongest vaginal support, and when weakened, they are believed to predispose to the development of distal rectoceles and perineal descent.[33] Also, it is known that stretching or avulsion of these attachments may occur during vaginal delivery, with chronic straining, and as the result of the normal aging process.

Because the endopelvic fascia consists of connective tissue, patients with prolapse may have altered collagen metabolism, and in fact, the quantity of total collagen in the vagina was found to be increased in women with prolapse as compared to that of women without prolapse.[34] Although there is ongoing debate as to whether this alteration is a cause or a consequence of pelvic organ prolapse, the fact that the changes observed are essentially an augmented expression of collagen III implies that this increase may be a consequence of the stress applied on the fascia instead of a host predisposition to prolapse.[35] In fact, collagen III expression prevails in tissues where flexibility and distensibility are required in response to stress.

## Pelvic bone dynamics

Prolapse of the pelvic floor is certainly multifactorial. Every woman experiences stretching of their pelvic floor during the birth process, but not all of them sustain damage. In order to fully comprehend the etiology of pelvic organ prolapse, the consequences of somatic dysfunction of the pelvic bones, attached ligaments, fascia, and viscera upon any structure that contributes to the structure of the pelvic floor should be considered. Somatic dysfunction results in impaired function of the "skeletal, arthrodial, and myofascial structures and related vascular, lymphatic, and neural element."[36]

Four main osseous components form the pelvis: the paired innominate bones, the sacrum, and the coccyx. The innominate bones consist of the ilium, ischium, and pubis, fused at the acetabulum. Posteriorly, the innominate articulates with the sacrum at the sacroiliac joint, and anteriorly, the pubic portion of the innominates articulate with each other at the symphysis pubis.

The pelvis is divided by an oblique plane into the greater, also called the 'false' pelvis,' and the lesser, or 'true' pelvis. This plane passes through the pelvic brim delineated posteriorly by the promontory of the sacrum, anteriorly by the upper margin of the symphysis pubis, and laterally by the iliopectineal lines. The pelvic organs lie in the true pelvis or pelvic cavity that is shaped like a curved canal. Its superior circumference is referred to as the pelvic inlet, whereas the inferior circumference is the pelvic outlet.

In quadrupeds, the sacrum is almost horizontal and continues along the roughly horizontal line of the vertebral column. As such, their pelvic viscera are supported in part by the abdominal musculature, and partially by the ventral portion of the pelvic cavity. With the establishment of erect posture, the human pelvis has rotated backward. In the standing position, when the posture of the individual is balanced, however, the pelvis is in a slightly anteverted position such that the anterior superior iliac spines and the anterior part of the pubic symphysis are situated in the same coronal plane, perpendicular to the floor. The anterior superior iliac spine and the posterior inferior iliac spine are located in the same transverse plane. Normally, in a standing position, the pressure exerted from the intra-abdominal contents is applied to the bony pelvis, i.e., the pubis, the anterior pelvic girdle, and the flared iliac bones. As a result, the stress put on the pelvic muscles, the endopelvic fascia, and the pelvic floor is decreased.

Changes in the orientation and shape of the bony pelvis have been linked with the development of pelvic organ prolapse. Platypelloid pelvic shape i.e., a pelvis with a wider transverse diameter, is significantly associated with pelvic floor disorders. Conversely, anthropoid pelvis, with a narrow transverse diameter may present the lowest risk.[37] Black women have narrower transverse diameters of the bony pelvis than white women;[38] they also have a lower prevalence of pelvic organ prolapse.[39]

The angle of the pelvic inlet refers to an angle measured between the intersection of a line drawn from the sacral promontory to the top of the pubic bone and a vertical line.

In women without prolapse, this angle is about 29.5°, whereas in women with advanced pelvic organ prolapse, this angle is about 37.5°.[40] This is consistent with a diminution of the lumbar lordosis or a posterior displacement of the sacral base. As such, a greater proportion of the pressure from the intra-abdominal content is directed toward the pelvic viscera, their connective tissue, and muscular supports, and may contribute to pelvic organ prolapse. Aging is associated

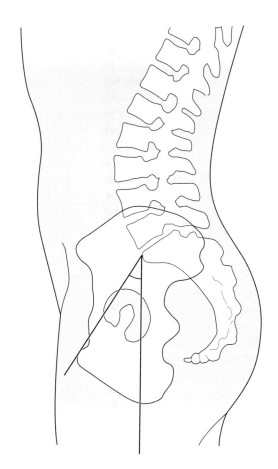

Figure 4.6.9: The angle of the pelvic inlet

with a decrease of the lumbar lordosis; however a common cause for this decrease is dysfunction of the psoas muscles that may be addressed using OMT. Dysfunction of the sacrum in cranial flexion-anatomic extension may be correlated, as well, with a decrease of the lumbar lordosis. This may follow a fall on the buttocks, with displacement of the coccyx anteriorly. Because several of the muscles that are part of the levator ani attach to the coccyx, any coccygeal somatic dysfunction may affect their function and should also be considered.

Normal spinal curvatures protect the pelvis from direct intra-abdominal forces. Still, as a woman ages, postural changes contribute to diminish the protective effects of the spinal column and the bony pelvis. Increased thoracic kyphosis is found to be correlated to pelvic organ prolapse. In this case, the position of the rib cage over the abdomen changes in such a way that intra-abdominal pressure is augmented.[41]

Evidently, every part of the pelvic complex—bones, nerves, muscles, and connective tissues—interacts constantly with the spinal column and its surrounding structures. Therefore, pelvic floor disorders may result from any somatic dysfunction of one or several of these structures.

### Symptoms of pelvic organ prolapse

Pelvic organ prolapse refers to the downward descent of the pelvic organs that results in the extreme in a protrusion of the vagina, uterus, or both, through the vulval vestibule. Pelvic organ prolapse is different from rectal prolapse, where the rectum projects through the anus. Although pelvic organ prolapse affects only women, rectal prolapse may affect both women and men.

Typically, the anterior vaginal wall is the segment of the vagina that protrudes. It is often associated with a descent of the bladder, which is a cystocele.[42] Other parts of the pelvic organs can prolapse such as the posterior vaginal wall and the apex of the vagina or the uterus, or both. Posterior vaginal wall prolapse may be associated with a descent of the rectum, which is a rectocele; it can also involve the small or large bowel.

Many women with pelvic organ prolapse are asymptomatic.[43] Patients with symptoms evoca-

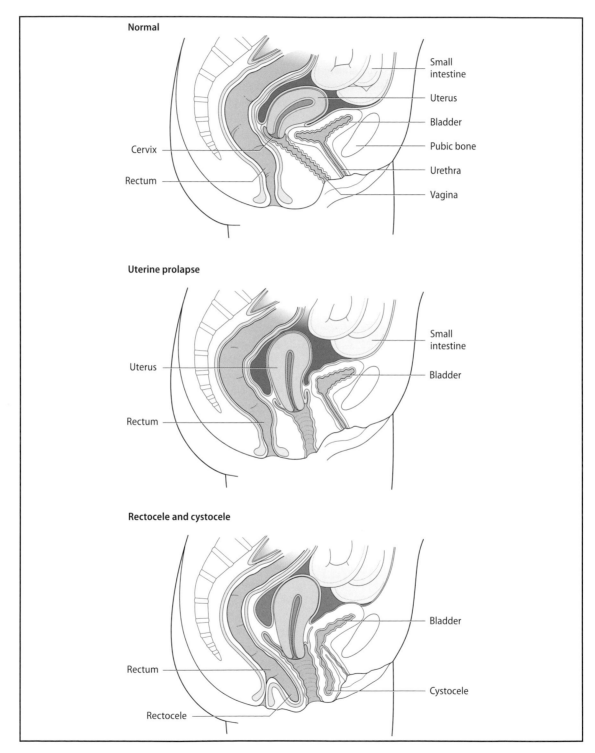

**Figure 4.6.10:** Prolapse of uterus and vagina; rectocele and cystocele

tive of prolapse should seek medical advice. Most commonly, these women will describe a sensation of heaviness or pressure in the area of the vagina and a feeling that the uterus, bladder, or rectum is dropping out. In advanced pelvic organ prolapse, a vaginal bulge can be felt or seen in the vulval vestibule. All of the symptoms are aggravated in the standing position or during straining or coughing. They diminish in the supine position. Difficulty having a bowel movement, with a feeling of incomplete emptying, or difficulty urinating, with signs of incontinence may be associated with uterine prolapse. These symptoms are, however, overlapping with other pelvic floor disorders such as conditions involving the bladder or lower gastrointestinal tract.

Pelvic organ prolapse is associated with dysfunction of the levator ani. Clinically, dyspareunia and lower abdominal pain are found in association with dysfunction of the pubococcygeus, iliococcygeus, and coccygeus, whereas painful defecation and constipation are found with dysfunction of the puborectalis. Additionally, dysfunction of the obturator internus may contribute to urinary symptoms, dyspareunia, and hip pain.[44]

## Lower urinary tract dysfunctions

Lower urinary tract dysfunctions include urinary incontinence, overactive bladder, and nocturia. Urinary incontinence, more common in women than men, is frequent in women with pelvic organ prolapse. However, urinary incontinence and overactive bladder are seen in both men and women. Various percentages of incidences have been reported for the prevalence of LUTD, depending upon the definition proposed for the condition, the different populations studied, and the population sampling procedures employed. As such, the reported incidence of urinary incontinence in women ranges from 5–69%, although a large number of studies reporting a prevalence of any type of urinary incontinence describe a range of 25–45%.[45] About 25% of men 40 years of age and older had some LUTD, but because most of these men are not terribly disturbed by their symptoms, only 5%–10% of them think that their symptoms

are sufficiently severe to necessitate some intervention.[46] In order to understand these conditions in the context of somatic dysfunction, a review of the relationships between the structures of the pelvic floor and their function and the bladder is de rigueur.

### Bladder

Located completely within the pelvic cavity when empty, the bladder varies in size and position according to its content, and when full, it swells anterosuperiorly into the abdominal cavity. It is the most anterior viscus of the pelvic cavity and its position is also influenced by the situation and repletion of other viscera. Classically, the bladder is described as consisting of a superior surface, an apex, two inferolateral surfaces, a base, and a neck.

The superior surface of the bladder is triangular, with its vertex, the apex of the bladder, directed anteriorly. On each side, a border runs from the apex to the upper corner of the base where the ureter enters the bladder. The posterior border connects the two ureteric openings. In females, the superior surface is mostly coated by peritoneum that continues posteriorly onto the junction of the uterine body and cervix, forming the vesicouterine pouch. Fibroareolar tissue fills the space between the most posterior part of the superior surface of the bladder and the supravaginal cervix. In males, the superior surface is totally covered by peritoneum, prolonged posteriorly into the rectovesical pouch and anteriorly into the median umbilical fold. When the bladder fills, the vesical superior surface becomes more convex.

The apex of the bladder points in the direction of the upper part of the symphysis pubis. From the apex, the median umbilical ligament, the urachus, rises to the umbilicus, behind the anterior abdominal wall.

On each side of the bladder, the inferolateral surface is located between the levator ani muscle of the pelvic diaphragm and the adjacent obturator internus muscle. It is not covered by peritoneum.

The base of the bladder, also named the fundus, is directed posteroinferiorly, shaped like an invert-

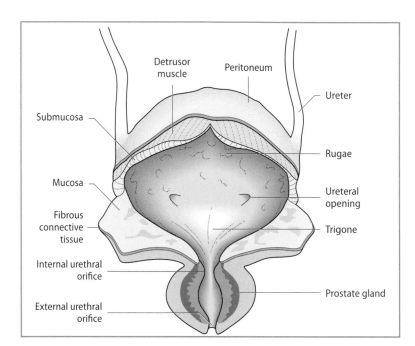

**Figure 4.6.11:** The urinary bladder

ed triangle. In females, it is located in front of the anterior vaginal wall, and lies somewhat upon it. In males, the base of the bladder is in front of the rectum between the rectovesical pouch above and the seminal vesicles and vas deferens on either side below.

The bladder neck is the most inferior and the most inflexible part of the urinary bladder. Located about 3–4 cm behind the inferior part of the symphysis pubis, it is contiguous with the internal urethral orifice and is sometimes referred to as the posterior urethra. It measures 2–3 cm. In females, the neck of the bladder is in relation with the pelvic fascia and in males, it lies immediately above the prostate. On each side, a strong fibromuscular band secures the position of the vesical neck and fixes it, as the pelvic part of the urethra, to the posteroinferior surface of the pubic bone. In combination with the fibrous capsule of the prostate that encircles the neck of the bladder and the contiguous part of the urethra, this fibromuscular band forms the puboprostatic ligaments. In women, the two fibromuscular bands form the pubovesical ligaments that, in association with the perineal membrane, its related muscles, and

the levator ani muscles, contribute to the support of the bladder.

Smooth muscle contributes to the formation of the bladder neck. Different from the detrusor muscle that forms the wall of the bladder, the bladder neck represents a distinct functional unit. The muscle in this portion is called the internal sphincter. In females, it is a distinct smooth muscle that consists of small diameter fasciculi spreading obliquely or longitudinally into the urethral wall. As a rule, the bladder neck is above the pelvic floor with the pubovesical ligaments, the endopelvic fascia, and the levator ani muscle maintaining it in this position. In response to an increase in intra-abdominal pressure, the levator ani contract, raising urethral closure pressure and maintaining continence. In males, the bladder neck is entirely encircled by a collar of smooth muscle that continues to envelop the preprostatic portion of the urethra and is referred to as the preprostatic sphincter.

Inferiorly, the bladder is fixed to the pubis, the lateral pelvic walls, and the rectum by the pelvic fascia. On each side, some dense fibromuscular slips connect the vesical neck to the inferior part of the pubic bones, forming the pubovesical ligaments. In females they are extensions of the pubourethral ligaments and, in males, the puboprostatic ligaments. Laterally, the peritoneum covering the bladder extends to the pelvic walls to form the lateral ligaments and posteriorly, the sacrogenital folds.

When the bladder fills, it becomes more ovoid in shape. Anteriorly, it lifts the parietal peritoneum from the suprapubic region of the abdominal wall. Its inferolateral surfaces move anteriorly and lean against the abdominal wall for about 5–7 cm above the symphysis pubis.

Externally, the wall of the bladder consists of the serosa covering the smooth muscle fibers of the detrusor muscle and an extracellular matrix. Under this layer are the lamina propria, and the urothelium. The fibers of the detrusor muscle extend in all directions. Throughout the storage phase of the micturition cycle, bladder compliance is ensured by a thinning of the lamina propria, a flattening of the urothelium, and a reorientation of the detrusor muscle fibers and connective tissue so that they are parallel to the lumen.[47] During the voiding phase, the contraction of the detrusor muscle is of paramount importance in emptying the bladder.

Detrusor muscle fibers run into the inferior part of the bladder, its apex, and its base. During the voiding phase of the micturition cycle, the detrusor muscle contracts to expel urine from the bladder using the extracellular matrix as a scaffold to generate tension. In fact, the significant viscoelastic properties of the detrusor smooth muscle that can influence the time-course of a contraction depend in part upon the extracellular matrix.[48] Another peculiarity of the detrusor muscle is that the fusion between its cells allows some low-resistance electrical activity to spread from one muscle cell to the other. As a consequence, an action potential can reach every cell at once producing a simultaneous contraction of the entire bladder. During the filling phase of the bladder, it relaxes to allow urine to accumulate in the bladder. Simultaneously to the actions of the detrusor muscle, the urethra acts in a reciprocal fashion by contracting during storage and relaxing during evacuation.

## Urethra

Inferiorly, the bladder neck is continuous with the urethra. In women, the urethra is only about 4 cm in length, whereas in men it measures about 20 cm. Also in men, just under the bladder, the prostate encircles the urethra. In both sexes, below the bladder neck, the urethra traverses the urogenital diaphragm, encircled by a striated muscle named the external sphincter of the bladder. Differing from the smooth muscle of the bladder, this muscle is under control of the voluntary nervous system and can be consciously activated to put off urination when involuntary controls are trying to void the bladder.

Significant to urethral function, the pubococcygeal portion of the levator ani muscle is part of the urogenital diaphragm. It runs, almost horizontally, anteriorly from the body of the pubic bone to the dorsal part of the rectum posteriorly, with its most medial fibers passing just lateral to the urethra, vagina, and anorectum. Here the pubococcygeus bonds with the periurethral support to form the pubourethralis, running inferolaterally in males to the prostate. In females, it surrounds the dorsal wall of the vagina posteriorly, to form the pubovaginalis. In both sexes some pubourethralis fibers unite with the perineal body. As such, sufficient levator ani muscle tone is necessary for maintenance of the position of the bladder neck. During micturition, as during defecation, the levator ani must relax; when the levator ani is dysfunctional, the position of the urethra may change, which modifies intraurethral pressure and continence.

## Innervation

Normal lower urinary tract function includes the retention of urine without leakage. From time to time, this function is appropriately interrupted by the voluntary expulsion of urine. In order to accomplish this, there must be a balance between the peripheral autonomic, peripheral somatic, and central nervous systems (CNS).

The peripheral autonomic system consists of afferent and efferent nerve fibers. Afferent nerve fibers convey peripheral sensory information to the dorsal portion of the spinal cord and from there to the central processing centers of the CNS. Efferent

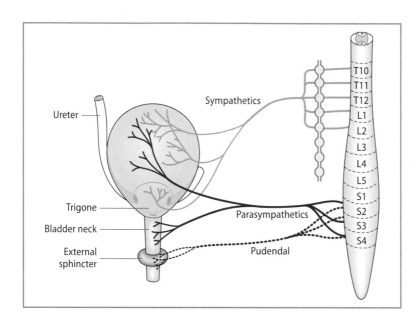

**Figure 4.6.12:** Urinary bladder innervation

motor axons exit from the ventral root of the spinal cord.

On each side of the pelvic floor, the pelvic plexus, a network of autonomic nerves and ganglia with sympathetic and parasympathetic components, derives from the superior hypogastric plexus and pelvic splanchnic nerves respectively. The anterior portion of the pelvic plexus, situated closer to the bladder, constitutes the vesical plexus. Preganglionic sympathetic efferent fibers originate from the thoracolumbar segments of the spinal cord between T10 and L2. They travel to the pelvic plexus and then to the lower urinary tract within the pelvic nerves. Preganglionic parasympathetic efferent fibers come from the second, third, and fourth sacral segments of the spinal cord where their cell bodies are located. Their axons run in the anterior rami of the sacral spinal nerves as the pelvic splanchnic nerves to join branches of the sympathetic fibers in the pelvic plexus. They synapse with postganglionic parasympathetic neurons within the plexuses and within the wall of the bladder.

The sympathetic efferent nerves increase contraction of the urethral smooth muscle and bladder outlet and reflexly decrease the parasympathetic activity. The primary neurotransmitter for preganglionic sympathetic fibers is acetylcholine (ACh), and norepinephrine for postganglionic sympathetic fibers. Conversely, the parasympathetic efferent nerves cause contraction of the detrusor muscle and relaxation of the urethral smooth muscle and bladder outlet. The primary parasympathetic neurotransmitter is ACh for pre- and postganglionic parasympathetic fibers. Afferent axons in the pelvic nerves transmit information from the lower urinary tract to the lumbosacral spinal cord. The neck of the bladder and the initial portion of the urethra possess the thickest plexus of afferent nerves, whereas the lamina propria of the superior region of the bladder has no afferent innervation. These afferent nerves are found in the suburothelium, as a plexus that rests under the urothelial lining, with some nerve terminals stretching into the urothelium. Conversely, the afferent innervation of the musculature seems consistent all over the bladder.[49] The sensory fibers perceive the degree of stretch in the bladder wall. In particular, the stretch signals from the bladder neck are primarily responsible for initiating the reflexes that produce bladder voiding. These afferent nerves make use of numerous neurotransmitters, including: substance P, neurokinins, calcitonin gene-related polypeptide, and vasoactive intestinal polypeptide.

Two kinds of bladder afferent fibers exist in the pelvic nerves. They are the Aδ myelinated fibers that respond to bladder distension, and the C un-myelinated fibers that respond normally to cold or chemical irritation. In certain circumstances, the sensitivity of afferent endings may be affected by the release of mediators from diverse cell catego-ries, such as the urothelium, smooth muscle, mast cells, and other connective tissue cells.[50] Thus, the afferent endings become sensitized and produce pathologic voiding reflexes.

The peripheral somatic system consists of skel-etal motor fibers conveyed via the pudendal nerve (ventral rami of roots S2, S3, S4 and less regularly S1 and S5) to the external bladder sphincter. These are somatic nerve fibers under voluntary control of the nervous system that innervate the muscle of the sphincter and can be consciously solicited to stop urination.

## Normal micturition

Normal micturition is the storage and voiding of waste fluids from the body through the urinary tract. Continence is the ability to store urine, and to micturate when it is socially acceptable.

During the storage phase, the bladder is capable of storing about 600 ml of urine. Because of its vis-coelastic properties, the bladder can accumulate 250–350 ml of urine with little increase in internal pressure. With closure of the urethral sphincter, continence is maintained because the intraure-thral pressure is higher than the intravesical pres-sure. When the tension in the walls of the bladder increases above a threshold level, the micturition reflex is elicited. While the micturition reflex is essentially an autonomic spinal reflex, it can also be influenced by higher centers of control in the cerebral cortex or brainstem. Micturition can be prevented by repeated contraction of the external bladder sphincter. Once circumstances are ap-propriate to permit urination, the cortical cent-ers inhibit the external bladder sphincter so that voiding of the bladder can occur. Contraction of the abdominal muscles, at this time, contributes to the increased pressure in the bladder and further stimulates the stretch receptors.

## Urinary disorders

Urinary disorders should be differentiated from abnormalities of micturition caused by traumatic

or disease-associated interference with, or de-struction of, sensory nerve fibers. Such organic pathology is not directly considered in this text. Urinary disorders, sub-categories and defini-tions, based on patients' symptoms, have been reviewed by the International Continence Society in an effort to homogenize communication be-tween physicians, patients, and researchers. Most of these LUTD are classified in three categories. They are: storage, voiding, and post-micturition disorders.[51] Storage symptoms are "experienced during the storage phase of the bladder" and in-clude increased urinary incontinence, increased daytime frequency, and nocturia. Voiding symp-toms are "experienced during the voiding phase" and include slow stream, splitting or spraying of the urine stream, intermittent stream, and hesi-tancy. Post-micturition symptoms are "experi-enced immediately after micturition" such as dribbling.

## Urinary incontinence

Urinary incontinence, a storage disorder, is de-fined as the complaint of "any involuntary leakage of urine."[52] The prevalence of urinary incontinence is commonly considered to be multifactorial and several risk factors are recognized. They are: smok-ing, chronic bronchitis, asthma, ethnicity,[53] age,[54] parity, vaginal delivery,[55] hysterectomy, obesity,[56 57] collagen disorders,[58] chronic illness, constipation, and diabetes, as well as neurological illnesses.[59] In women, vaginal delivery is considered as a chief etiology. In a group of persons, with an age range of 15–86 years, urinary incontinence is found in up to 50.7% of the women although if only nulliparous subjects were considered, urinary incontinence decreases to 24.3%.[60] In another study, it was found that black women were less likely to have incon-tinence than white non-Hispanic women.[61] Inter-estingly, black women also display narrower trans-verse diameters of the pelvis than white women,[62] a 5.1% smaller total pelvic floor area,[63] and have a lower prevalence of pelvic organ prolapse.[64] These observations appear to stress the importance of the bony pelvis and supportive system of the pel-vic floor.

Urinary incontinence may be further subdivid-ed into three categories:[65]

1. Stress urinary incontinence (SUI), the complaint of "involuntary leakage on effort or exertion, or on sneezing or coughing."
2. Urge urinary incontinence (UUI), the complaint of "involuntary leakage accompanied by or immediately preceded by urgency."
3. Mixed urinary incontinence (MUI), the complaint of "involuntary leakage associated with urgency and also with exertion, effort, sneezing, or coughing."

In adult populations of women, the prevalence of any form of urinary incontinence is between 49.2 and 50.7%, whereas the prevalence of SUI is between 16.1 and 23.7%, UUI between 7.7 and 9.9%, and MUI between 14.5 and 26.9 %.[66][67]

The prevalence of SUI peaks during the fifth decade of life, and then declines, whereas prevalence of UUI shows a small peak in the fourth decade and then increases after the age of 50. The incidence of MUI occurs consistently throughout life.[68] Several factors may contribute to urinary incontinence with aging. Because the pubourethralis and pubovaginalis are supplied by the second and third sacral spinal segments passing through the pudendal nerve, decreased pudendal nerve conduction, associated with aging, may weaken the function of the levator ani muscles.[69] Additionally, in the ventral wall of the urethra, the sum of striated muscle fibers declines sevenfold as women mature from 15 to 80 years of age, with a mean loss of 2% per year.[70] The changes in muscle contractility result in a longer time needed for striated muscles to produce the same force as compared to young adults.[71] Nevertheless, although there is a decrease in the relative volume of striated muscle in the human female urethra, there is no change in the smooth muscle parts.[72] While the incidence of urinary incontinence generally increases with age, this may not be totally an age-related effect. Studies on the effects of aging on lower urinary tract and pelvic floor function in nulliparous women show that there is a decrease of the maximal urethral closure pressure when women age, but pelvic organ support, urethral support, and levator function are not affected.[73] Consequently, incontinence should not be considered as a normal result of aging. Alterations of the normal lower urinary tract and associated structures can play a part in the establishment of incontinence.

Normally, two systems interact to prevent urinary incontinence. They are a sphincteric system and a supportive system.[74] Frequently, the decrease in outflow resistance during urinary storage that results in SUI is due to weakness in one, or both, of these systems, i.e., the urethral sphincter mechanism and urethral musculature, possibly associated with weakness of the pelvic floor.[75]

Below the bladder neck, the urethra is surrounded by striated muscle—the urethral sphincter. After the urethra traverses the urogenital diaphragm, the urethral compressor and the urethrovaginal sphincter become continuations of the urethral sphincter. The urethral compressor surrounds the urethra, attaching anteriorly into the urogenital diaphragm near the pubic ramus. The urethrovaginal sphincter also encircles the urethra and the vagina. These periurethral muscles contribute to the maintenance of urinary continence.

Additionally, the urethra lies on a supportive floor, which consists of the anterior vaginal wall, secured on each side by its attachments to the tendinous arch of the pelvic fascia and the levator ani muscles. Anteriorly, the urethra is fixed to the pubic bones by the pubourethral ligaments.

In order to maintain urine in the bladder at rest, and during any increases in abdominal pressure, as occurs with coughing or laughing, urethral closure pressure must be superior to bladder pressure. At rest, this function is assumed by the urethral sphincter constriction that prevents leakage of urine. During a sudden increase in abdominal pressure, muscular contraction of the levator ani raises the resistance of the pelvic fascia and vagina, resulting in more pressure against the bladder neck and urethra, maintaining urethral closure. In 'hammock' theory of urethral closure, the anterior and posterior surfaces of the urethra are compressed between the abdominal and pelvic pressures. [76]

Any weakness or dysfunction of the levator ani muscle or in the integrity of the endopelvic fascia can consequently compromise urinary continence. Impairment of the levator ani muscle, its nerve supply, or any portion of the endopelvic fascia, weakens the stabilization of the urethra.[77] Vaginal delivery may cause such a dysfunction, in particular when women become pregnant later in life. There is for every year of delay in childbearing, in fact, an increase of nearly 10% in the probability of levator trauma.[78] When vaginal delivery alters the urethral support, the position of the bladder neck is lower, as compared to that of nulligravid women, or those who have had elective cesarean delivery. Post vaginal delivery, there is also more difficulty elevating the bladder neck with pelvic muscle contraction.[79] When the bladder neck remains beneath the pelvic floor, the stabilization of the urethra is unsuccessful, particularly when the intra-abdominal pressure rises, leading to stress incontinence as a result of urethral hypermobility.

Additionally, during vaginal childbirth, the pudendal nerve that supplies the external bladder sphincter is susceptible to injury. Stretch and compression of the nerve can result in ischemia that compromises nerve function. [80] This is most apt to occur where it passes between the sacrospinous and sacrotuberous ligaments or through Alcock's canal, before entering the ischiorectal fossa and innervating the external urethral sphincter.

Levator ani muscle weakness and dysfunction may lead to muscle atrophy, putting more stress on the endopelvic fascia for the support of the pelvic organs. Progressively, the connective tissues overstretch and consequently cannot completely fulfill their supportive function. Pelvic organ prolapse, incontinence, or both can follow.

After addressing any somatic dysfunction affecting the pelvis, pelvic floor exercises that may reduce urinary incontinence and increase pelvic floor strength should be encouraged. Coaching the patient to teach them when and how to use pelvic muscles is fundamental. When structural defects are present, surgery may be necessary.

## Increased urinary frequency

Besides urinary incontinence, storage symptoms experienced during the filling phase of the bladder include daytime frequency and nocturia. According to the International Continence Society, increased daytime frequency is the "complaint by the patient who considers that he/she voids too often by day," and nocturia is "the complaint that the individual has to wake at night one or more times to void."[81]

Normally, the bladder is compliant, allowing for an increase in volume with little increase in internal pressure. Nevertheless with aging, bladder compliance may decline and less filling is sufficient to augment the internal pressure leading to a threshold that initiates a reflex micturition. Smaller bladder capacity is frequently associated with premature contractions of the detrusor muscle. This is part of the overactive bladder syndrome defined by the International Continence Society as a "syndrome based on symptomatology, characterized by urgency, with or without urge incontinence." Usually frequency and nocturia are also part of the overactive bladder syndrome but no infection or other obvious etiology should be present.

The prevalence of overactive bladder is about 16% in men and women over 40 years of age and is typically more commonly encountered in women than in men.[82] Frequency is present in 85% of the subjects with overactive bladder, followed by urgency (54%), and urge incontinence (36%). Frequently, these symptoms have a major influence on quality of life and sleep, even in patients without incontinence. In the overactive bladder syndrome, the urge to urinate occurs at least eight times a day and two times a night. A sudden urge to go to the toilet to urinate, with no advance warning, may result in incontinence if the person is unable to get to the bathroom in time. Leakage of urine during the day, without being able to control it may also be present.

Nocturia—awakening at night to void—may have different etiologies including: nocturnal polyuria, where voided urine volume during the hours of sleep exceeds 35% of the 24-hour output;[83] bladder storage problems such as nocturnal detrusor overactivity, a primary sleep disorder; or a combination of these. Organic pathology associated with nocturnal polyuria may include:

neurological conditions, hypertension, and congestive heart failure.

Normally, the detrusor voiding function is "achieved by a voluntarily initiated continuous detrusor contraction that leads to complete bladder emptying within a normal time span, and in the absence of obstruction."[84] Abnormal detrusor activity can be observed on urodynamics studies and is classified either as detrusor underactivity or detrusor overactivity. Detrusor underactivity is defined as: "a contraction of reduced strength and/or duration, results in prolonged bladder emptying and/or a failure to achieve complete bladder emptying within a normal time span." Detrusor overactivity is: "involuntary detrusor contractions during the filling phase which may be spontaneous or provoked."[85] Furthermore, detrusor overactivity may be divided in two subcategories: 1) neurogenic detrusor overactivity when there is a relevant neurological condition, and 2) idiopathic detrusor overactivity when there is no distinct cause. Although somatic dysfunction can contribute to the presentation of any form of abnormal detrusor activity, the diagnosis of idiopathic detrusor overactivity should particularly lead one to search diligently for somatic dysfunction as an etiology.

A number of explanations have been proposed to describe the occurrence of detrusor overactivity. They include: possible alteration in the autonomic function; supersensitivity to acetylcholine; interruption of inhibitor pathways issued from cerebral regions; ultrastructural modifications of bladder urothelium; and an increase in nerve growth factor that may alter receptor expression in sensory fibers, lessening their threshold to react to natural stimuli. Increased sympathetic activity has also been associated with detrusor overactivity.[86] Increased sympathetic activity is a significant component of thoracic and thoracolumbar somatic dysfunction.[87]

In postmenopausal women, modifications in the urogenital system are associated with decreased levels of circulating estrogens. Subsequent atrophic alterations of the lower urogenital tract can contribute to disorders in urinary function such as incontinence.[88] Additionally, diminution of blood supply to the urogenital tissues impedes normal tissular trophicity.

## Voiding and post-micturition disorders

Voiding symptoms are experienced during the voiding phase of micturition. Normal voiding involves a reciprocal interaction between efficient contraction of the detrusor and total relaxation of the urethral sphincters, efficiently evacuating urine from the bladder.

In men, bladder neck obstruction secondary to prostate hyperplasia commonly occurs. Prostatic enlargement leads to a constriction of the bladder neck and posterior urethra. With an obstruction of bladder outflow, the subject may have trouble getting the stream started. He may also demonstrate a weak stream during urination and describe an intermittent stream where urinary flow stops and starts, one or several times, during micturition. After urinating, dribbling often prolongs the final part of micturition. Emptying of the bladder may not be complete, with residual urine that can promote infection.

Changes in the neurological and musculoskeletal systems frequently influence micturition. Dysfunctions in the musculoskeletal system include dysfunction of the lumbopelvic bones and joints, i.e., the lumbar vertebrae, the innominate bones, the sacrum and coccyx, and the lumbar, lumbosacral, sacroiliac, pubic symphysis, and the sacrococcygeal joints. It also includes dysfunction of the fascia and muscles of the pelvic floor, but also of the piriformis, the obturator internus on which the levator ani attach, and the psoas iliacus. Pelvic floor dysfunction is thought to cause congestion to the pelvic organs, therefore vascular and lymphatic drainage should be considered. Finally any dysfunction of the autonomic, somatic, and central nervous systems, often resulting from somatic dysfunction involving the thoracolumbar (sympathetic) and sacropelvic (parasympathetic) regions, should be addressed. Patients with primary complaints of urinary frequency have been improved following manual therapy treatment including a combination of direct myofascial release, joint mobilization, muscle energy techniques, strengthening, stretching, and neuromuscular re-education.[89]

# Benign prostate disorders

The prostate is a fibromuscular gland of the male reproductive system that surrounds the prostatic urethra and lies in the lesser pelvis, just inferior to the bladder, posterior to the inferior border of the pubic symphysis and pubic arch, and anterior to the rectum. Although a strong but thin connective tissue capsule encases the prostate, it may be readily palpated through the rectum.

Throughout childhood, the prostate gland stays rather small. Then, during puberty the prostate begins a maturation phase under the stimulus of testosterone and its size increases more than twofold. In the young adult, the anteroposterior prostate dimension is about 2 cm, whereas its vertical dimension is about 3 cm. At this time, its weight is approximately 8 g. After the age of 45–50 years, with the occurrence of benign prostatic hyperplasia (BPH), it very frequently increases in size up to 40 g, even reaching 150 g, after 50 years of age.[90]

The prostate is shaped, to some extent, like a flattened inverted pyramid. Superiorly, the pyramidal base of the prostate measures about 4 cm transversely and is continuous, above, with the neck of the bladder. The pyramidal apex of the prostate lies on the pelvic floor inferiorly. On each side, the inferolateral surface is bound by the anterior fibers of the levator ani muscle forming the pubourethralis muscle.

Located posterior to the arch of the pubis, the anterior surface of the prostate is transversely narrow and convex. Anterosuperiorly, the capsule of the prostate combines to mix with the puboprostatic ligaments that attach it to the pubic bones. The posterior surface of the prostate is transversely flat and vertically convex. It demonstrates a median sulcus that separates the two lateral lobes. During palpation of the prostate, the disappearance of this sulcus indicates an increase in the size of the gland. A prostatic capsule and a thick condensation of the pelvic fascia named the Denonvillier's fascia separate the prostate, the seminal vesicles, and the ampullae of the vasa deferentia from the rectum.

On each side of the prostate, the seminal vesicles drain into the prostatic ends of the ampullae of the vas deferens. The contents from the ampullae and the seminal vesicles go through the ejaculatory ducts, crossing the body of the prostate gland, to open into the prostatic urethra. The prostatic ducts also empty from the prostate into the ejaculatory duct, and from there into the prostatic urethra.

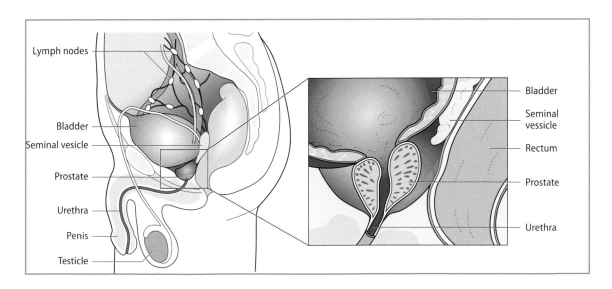

Figure 4.6.13: The prostate and the bladder

The urethra has multiple tiny urethral glands surrounding it, that produce mucus. The urethra and ejaculatory ducts pass through the prostate. The urethra enters the prostate near its anterior border and runs between the anterior and middle thirds of the gland. The ejaculatory ducts enter the prostate more posteriorly and course anteroinferiorly through its posterior region to empty into the prostatic urethra.

The prostate's glandular tissue is typically divided into three separate portions: a peripheral portion that is about 70% by volume; a central portion, 25% by volume; and a transitional portion, 5% by volume. Clinically, this differentiation is important. Nearly all carcinomas appear in the peripheral portion. Benign prostatic hyperplasia, on the other hand, develops in the transitional portion, around the distal part of the preprostatic urethra, proximal to the apex of the central portion and the ejaculatory ducts. Benign prostatic hyperplasia may expand the transitional portion to constitute the greater part of the prostate. Thus from above, and on either side of the urethra, the rounded prostatic lobes can end up compressing or twisting the preprostatic and prostatic parts of the urethra.

Benign prostatic hyperplasia is a disease of the prostate that develops in most men with age. If a man lives long enough, it is to be expected, even if it is not always symptomatic. Typically, the transitional portion of the prostate enlarges progressively, causing urinary obstruction. Other symptoms include: a weak urine stream, difficulty initiating micturition, interruption of urination, nocturia, difficulty emptying the bladder entirely, urinary tract infection, and kidney disorders. Many men with prostate gland enlargement, however, may only have minor urinary symptoms.

Any underlying pathology should be identified and appropriately addressed medically. On digital rectal examination, with BPH, the prostate feels 'bulky.' If any discrete mass is felt, when palpating the prostate, the patient should be further evaluated for possible neoplasia before manipulative treatment is employed. If BPH is found, any lumbopelvic somatic dysfunction should be specifically identified and treated. Lumbar, sacral, and pelvic dysfunction, including sacrococcygeal and hip joints, pelvic fascia, and ligaments should be considered. Particular attention should be given to the piriformis, obturator internus, levator ani, and other pelvic floor muscles, as well as the sacrospinous and sacrotuberous ligaments. Improvement of the motion of these structures can be expected to improve pelvic circulation and decrease stasis within the prostate. Using indirect principles to release any identified restriction of motion, practitioners, with the appropriate credentials, may balance the prostate and surrounding structures transrectally.

## The osteopathic contribution to the physical examination and treatment

Conducting a complete physical examination is indispensable for a good diagnosis of chronic pelvic pain and dysfunction. First, observe the patient's gait. Next, observe the patient in the standing position as described in 'Section 2: Osteopathic assessment,' p. 46. Assess global posture; any dysfunction in postural balance affects the distribution of pressure between the intrathoracic, intra-abdominal, and intrapelvic cavities and should be considered. Note any asymmetry in the lower extremities and lumbosacral spine that can interfere with normal function of the pelvic area.

Observe the patient sitting. They may sit unevenly in order to avoid pressure on the dysfunctional side. They may have difficulty staying immobile when seated, moving constantly to search for a comfortable position. This may result from a coccygeal, lumbosacral, or sacroiliac joint dysfunction.

Next, with the patient lying supine upon the treatment table, observe the pelvis for increased anterior or posterior tilt, possibly the result of craniosacral extension or flexion of the sacrum. Look also for modified lumbar lordosis, possibly the result of lumbar dysfunction. A common cause for a decrease of the lumbar lordosis is a dysfunction of the psoas muscle.

Visually observe for asymmetry in the position of the pelvis. Note any torsion of the pelvis, potentially indicative of a sacral torsion. In female patients, somatic dysfunction of the sacrum, such as sacral torsions, can alter tensions upon the uterosacral ligaments, therefore affecting the uterus. Pelvic positioning, such that one side of the pelvis is contacting the surface of the treatment table with more pressure than the other side can be the result of a sacroiliac joint dysfunction or lumbar dysfunction. Observe the pelvis for asymmetry and inequity of the heights of the greater trochanters and iliac crests.

Palpate the pelvic bones looking for any asymmetry of position and motion. Similarly, note any asymmetry at the pubic symphysis that may reveal a dysfunction of this joint affecting myofascial structures attached to it such as the pelvic floor muscles and the puboprostatic and pubovesical ligaments.

With the patient still in the supine position, palpate the soft tissues of the pelvis and the lower anterior abdominal wall including the inguinal area. Note any tension or difference in the quality of the soft tissues. Perform tests of listening upon the pelvic organs. Appreciate their inherent motion. See 'Section 3: Treatment of the patient,' p. 84. If dysfunctional motion is identified, decide whether it is the result of intrinsic organ dysfunction or a consequence of dysfunction of the surrounding bony and myofascial structures.

Proceed to palpate and evaluate the pelvic floor with particular attention to evaluation of the levator ani muscles. If necessary, perform an internal rectal or vaginal examination, or both, with particular attention to the pelvic floor muscles: the levator ani, puborectalis, iliococcygeus, and obturator internus muscles. In male patients check the bladder and prostate, in female patients check the bladder and uterus.

With the patient in the prone position, observe and note any asymmetry in the lumbar spinous processes, the depth and position of the sacroiliac joints, the position of the inferolateral angles of the sacrum, and the position of the coccyx. Palpate the lumbar spine, lumbosacral junction, sacrum, coccyx, and sacrospinous and sacrotuberous ligaments.

The palpation of these structures may be done in the supine position if you can slide your hands under the back and pelvis of the patient. The supine position is also recommended for this portion of the examination if the patient has difficulty moving comfortably on the examination table.

Perform tests of listening upon the pelvic bones, sacrum, coccyx, and lumbar spine to identify articular mobility and intraosseous motility. Because the innervation of the levator ani derives from fibers coming mostly from the second, third, and fourth sacral spinal segments, dysfunction affecting the intraosseous motility of the sacrum can result in fluid stasis and congestion at the level of the sacral foramina. This can in turn impact the function of the sacral nerves and consequently the levator ani muscles.

Once somatic dysfunction has been clearly delineated in any of the above areas proceed to treat it using indirect principles.

# Advice to the patient

Patients with pelvic floor disorders will often benefit from the use of specific exercises. All of these patients should strive to acquire better posture. Improved posture balances the distribution of pressure between the intrathoracic, intra-abdominal, and intrapelvic cavities. This, in turn, decreases the pressure applied upon the pelvic floor when posture is incorrect. Particular attention should be paid to: decreasing the kyphotic upper thoracic spine, stretching the psoas, piriformis, and obturator internus muscles, and toning of the gluteus muscle group. Exercises should feel easy and convenient to perform, without the need for big and costly equipments.

## Stretching the upper thoracic region

An easy way to stretch the upper thoracic region is for the patient to stand facing a wall, with their feet about a foot away from the wall. They should then place both the palms of both of their hands flat on the wall as high as possible, with their arms as straight as possible. The position of the hands and arms should be as comfortable as possible. From this position, if possible, they should gently bring their anterior chest forward to contact the wall. They should remain with their chest in contact with the wall and take three or four slow deep breaths. They then return to the initial position and repeat the complete routine four or five times.

## Stretching of the psoas muscle

The psoas muscle group may be stretched using a similar position to that employed to stretch the upper thoracic region. Facing the wall, as above, the patient places their hands against the wall at the level of their shoulders. Then, standing on one foot, they extend the other hip to stretch the hip flexors, particularly the psoas major muscle. They should keep their back straight, tightening their abdominal, lumbar paravertebral, and gluteus muscles. The stretch should be maintained for about 30 seconds and gently repeated about ten times. The process should then be repeated on the other side. This exercise may also be employed to strengthen the gluteal muscles.

## Piriformis and obturator internus muscle stretching

In order to stretch the piriformis or obturator internus muscles, the patient should lie in a supine position on the floor, or on a firm bed. One leg is kept straight on the floor, or on the bed throughout the procedure. The other leg—the one on the side that the muscles are going to be stretched—is then flexed at the hip and knee, while keeping the foot flat on the floor or bed. This is the starting position for the exercise. The patient then clasps their hands together and holds the flexed knee in such a manner that they can apply a medially-directed force to the lateral aspect of the knee. With gentle pressure, they try to bring the knee medially, introducing internal rotation to the hip by pulling that knee in the direction of their opposite shoulder. This internally rotated position of the hip is maintained for 30 seconds. During that time the patient should be instructed to breath slowly to increase muscular relaxation. They should then return the lower extremity slowly to the neutral starting position and repeat the process about ten times.

## For pelvic floor disorders

Typically, conservative treatments for pelvic floor disorders start with a program of strengthening of the pelvic floor with Kegel exercises during a period of two to three months. Results are more satisfactory if any pelvic dysfunction has been treated before starting the exercises. This will help the patient to have a better control of their musculature. In order for a muscle to work properly, the points of attachment must be balanced to facilitate the mechanism of levers. If prolapse is present a pessary may be used to support the pelvic organs, in particular if the patient cannot have surgery. In severe cases, surgery may be considered.

Kegel exercises are intended to strengthen the pelvic floor muscles. Arnold Kegel reported that Van Skolkvik was observing strong perinea among a tribe of natives in South Africa.[91] After childbirth, the midwives would check the perineal strength of the mother and several days post-partum the new mother would begin exercises consisting of contraction of vaginal muscles on distended fingers. This process was continued for some weeks, until the desired result was achieved.

In order to practice these exercises properly, the patient should be coached. Many women initially have some difficulty contracting their pelvic floor muscles correctly. They often, incorrectly, contract other muscles such as the outer pelvic muscles: the gluteals, hip adductors, and abdominal muscles. Some basic description of the anatomy and physiology of the pelvic floor organs and of the levator ani components, in particular the pubococcygeus muscles may help to create some awareness in order to allow the patient to identify the correct muscles and to contract them voluntarily during vaginal palpation. The practitioner must insist on the role of the pubococcygeus. It forms the lateral border of the levator hiatus, passing lateral to the urethra, vagina, and anorectum, and consequently, through its muscular activity, it is responsible for keeping the urogenital hiatus closed. If the practitioner has appropriate credentials, intravaginal palpation during the instruction for the performance of the exercise can help the patient to identify the pubococcygeus muscles and to contract them properly.

Before beginning the exercise the patient should empty their bladder. To properly perform the Kegel exercises they should tightly contract the pubococcygeus muscles for about five or six seconds, and then relax for about ten seconds. The exercise is to be repeated about ten times, and should be performed several times daily for the next three or four months. Progression of performance includes practicing the exercises in different postures, at the beginning lying down, then sitting, standing, and squatting, always trying to relax abdominal, gluteal, and hip abductor muscles.

In cases where the patient has difficulty identifying and contracting the proper muscles, cone-shaped devices, ranging from 20–70g, placed in the vagina may help the woman to concentrate on contracting the correct muscles. When she stands and walks with the cone in place, she must contract the pelvic floor muscles only, and not the abdominal and gluteal muscles. Initially, the patient should start with the smallest weight cone, and when she is able to keep it within the vagina for 20 minutes, two times successively during normal daily activities, she may progress to a cone of greater weight.[92]

Biofeedback techniques may be used as well. A probe can be inserted into the vagina that allows the patient to visualize the efficacy of her contractions on a video screen and to adjust them accordingly. Electrical stimulation can be produced by some of the probes so that the conduction of an electrical current stimulates the contraction of the correct muscles.

## For lower urinary tract dysfunctions

All the advices given above for pelvic floor disorders apply also for LUTD. Improvement of the contractility of the pelvic muscles is of paramount importance. Because the pubococcygeus muscle's fibers intermingle with the musculature surrounding the bladder neck, its function must be improved. Additionally, in reaction to a rise in intra-abdominal pressure, the levator ani must be able to contract in order to increase the urethral closure pressure, thus maintaining continence.

Active contraction of the pelvic floor muscles affects the micturition reflex. Detrusor pressure diminishes while urethral pressure rises. It appears that contraction of the pelvic floor muscles inhibits the relaxation of the internal sphincter generated by the micturition reflex that in turn, produces reflex detrusor relaxation.[93]

Attention should, additionally, be given to the urethral sphincters. Description of the anatomy and physiology of the bladder and urethral sphincters will help the patient to understand normal and abnormal bladder function and to contract their sphincters appropriately. To improve their awareness of the pelvic floor muscles, the patient can visualize trying to put off the passing of stool, paying attention not only to the posterior sphincters surrounding the anal canal but also to the anterior sphincters surrounding the urethra. Men can visualize moving the penis up and down. Patients may also try to interrupt the urinary stream flow when voiding to improve their perception of the urethral sphincters.

Once awareness of the urethral sphincters is established, the patient should be instructed to actively contract them, progressively increasing the length of the contraction for up to ten seconds, with an equal period of relaxation between contractions. This exercise can be repeated up to 15 times, three or four times a day. The patient should alternate rapid contractions to strengthen the urethral sphincters with slow contractions to gain endurance. After several days of doing the exercise, the patient should be encouraged to practice in different positions such as sitting and standing. Repetition of the contraction is key to the improvement of urinary continence and toward this end the exercises should be continued for at least two or three months.

Conscious contraction of the pelvic floor muscles just before and during the occurrence of the increased intra-abdominal pressure that occurs during stressful activities such as coughing is also advised to improve stress urinary incontinence. This "single, intentionally timed contraction," a technique called 'the knack' can be differentiated from 'Kegel exercises,' the repetitive exercises performed to strengthen the pelvic floor.[94]

Besides pelvic floor exercises, the patient should also learn techniques to control and suppress urgency in order to restore normal bladder function. Some patients have the habit of emptying their bladder on the 'never miss a chance' principle, to prevent the urinary leakage.[95] Conversely, others disregard the need to urinate, which leads to distension of the bladder and voiding disorders. Encourage the patient to urinate daily when getting up, in the morning, and before going to sleep at night. During the day, a timed voiding routine at regular intervals should be established. Normally, the bladder should be emptied every 3 to 4 hours. As the patient adjusts to this schedule the time between bladder voiding during the day may be progressively increased.

When urgency urinary incontinence is present, the patient should be encouraged to change the habit to rush immediately to the bathroom. Instead they should be encouraged to relax, and to distract their attention from their bladder, focusing, for instance, on their breathing instead, and, in a relaxed manner, walk quietly to the bathroom.

Straight forward lifestyle adjustments are also part of the therapy. Modification of the diet must be considered. Consumption of bladder irritants such as caffeine and carbonated drinks that produce a diuretic effect should be eliminated or at least reduced. Although it is recommended that the patient reduce liquid intake before bedtime, they should be encouraged to drink about 1500 ml, or roughly six 8 oz glasses, per day. Restricting fluid intake too much results in urinary concentration, which irritates the bladder mucosa and promotes urgency, frequency, and urinary tract infections.[96]

Weight management, smoking cessation, and the establishment of regular bowel habits are part of the program to restore normal bladder function.

Although beyond the scope of this discussion, the complete medical management of these patients should include the consideration of the addition of symptom modulating medications, or elimination of over-the-counter and prescription medications with undesirable urinary tract side effects. If this exercise program is not successful, it is appropriate to consider biofeedback techniques with or without pelvic floor electrical stimulation, as discussed above.

## For benign prostate disorders

Conservative measures may be undertaken, after a medical examination has been done to identify and appropriately address: neoplasia, recurrent urinary tract infections, gross or microscopic hematuria, and signs of obstruction, including elevated residual urine and hydronephrosis. The effects of medications upon the prostate must also be taken into consideration.

Lifestyle changes may be employed to help ease some of the symptoms of an enlarged prostate and reduce further aggravation of the condition. These, however, will not cure the disorder.

In addition to pelvic floor exercises, the patient must learn good urinary habits in order to assist in the restoration of normal bladder function. Urination at the first sensation of the urge is recommended. Delaying urination can overstretch the detrusor muscle, resulting in weakness. The patient should also, however, learn to control the urge to urinate, with the use of relaxation techniques, such as slow breathing or mental distraction, as described above for the management of LUTD.

A timed voiding schedule must be established, with regular intervals approximately every three to four hours to reset the bladder function. Double voiding, the act of urination followed by a second attempt at urination a few moments later, may help to reestablish and strengthen urethral sphincter control. If possible, after emptying of the bladder, the patient should stroll out of the toilet for a minute or two and then come back before attempting the second urination. This exercise can be useful for learning to empty the bladder more completely than just voiding one time, and it can also help to prevent overflow incontinence.

The patient should be encouraged to stay active, to prevent retention of urine. The consumption of liquids an hour or two before bedtime should be discouraged, to prevent nocturia. Caffeinated beverages and alcohol particularly act as diuretics and should be avoided. Dietary modifications, to include the restriction of spicy foods that can irritate the bladder and result in urinary frequency and night time voiding, should be considered.

The importance of staying warm should be explained to the patient. Colder environmental temperatures can cause contraction of the pelvic floor muscles, increasing urinary retention and making voiding of the bladder difficult. It is also important, wherever possible, to avoid direct pressure upon the pelvic floor and prostate gland such as occurs when performing such activities as bicycling.

# References

1. Kepenekci I, Keskinkilic B, Akinsu F, Cakir P, Elhan AH, Erkek AB, Kuzu MA. Prevalence of pelvic floor disorders in the female population and the impact of age, mode of delivery, and parity. Dis Colon Rectum. 2011 Jan;54(1):85-94.

2. Barber MD, Bremer RE, Thor KB, Dolber PC, Kuehl TJ, Coates KW. Innervation of the female levator ani muscles. Am J Obstet Gynecol. 2002 Jul;187(1):64-71.

3. Standring S, Ed. Gray's Anatomy: The anatomical basis of clinical practice. 39th ed. Edinburgh: Churchill Livingstone; 2004.

4. Frymann VM. The core-link and the three diaphragms - Unit for respiratory function. Year Book of the Academy of Applied Osteopathy. American Academy of Osteopathy. Indianapolis, IN. 1968:13-9.

5. Henle J. Handbusch der Systematischen Anatomie des Menschen. Bd II, Braunschweig: Druck und Verlag von Friedrich Vieweg und Sohn; 1873. In: Mirilas P, Skandalakis JE. Urogenital diaphragm: an erroneous concept casting its shadow over the sphincter urethrae and deep perineal space. J Am Coll Surg. 2004 Feb;198(2):279-90.

6. Brandon CJ, Lewicky-Gaupp C, Larson KA, Delancey JO. Anatomy of the perineal membrane as seen in magnetic resonance images of nulliparous women. Am J Obstet Gynecol. 2009 May;200(5):583.e1-6.

7. Barber MD. Contemporary views on female pelvic anatomy. Cleve Clin J Med. 2005 Dec;72 Suppl 4:S3-11.

8. Hendrix SL, Clark A, Nygaard I, Aragaki A, Barnabei V, McTiernan A. Pelvic organ prolapse in the Women's Health Initiative: gravity and gravidity. Am J Obstet Gynecol. 2002 Jun;186(6):1160-6.

9. Lepine LA, Hillis SD, Marchbanks PA, Koonin LM, Morrow B, Kieke BA, Wilcox LS. Hysterectomy surveillance--United States, 1980-1993. MMWR CDC Surveill Summ. 1997 Aug 8;46(4):1-15.

10. Dietz HP, Bennett MJ. The effect of childbirth on pelvic organ mobility. Obstet Gynecol. 2003 Aug;102(2):223-8.

11. Weidner AC, Barber MD, Visco AG, Bump RC, Sanders DB. Pelvic muscle electromyography of levator ani and external anal sphincter in nulliparous women and women with pelvic floor dysfunction. Am J Obstet Gynecol. 2000 Dec;183(6):1390-9; discussion 1399-401.

12. Mant J, Painter R, Vessey M. Epidemiology of genital prolapse: observations from the Oxford Family Planning Association Study. Br J Obstet Gynaecol. 1997 May;104(5):579-85.

13. Hunskaar S, Burgio KL, Clark A, et al: Epidemiology of urinary (UI) and fecal (FI) incontinence and pelvic organ prolapse. In: Abrams P, Cardozo L, Khoury S, Wein A, ed. Incontinence: 3rd International Consultation, Plymouth, UK: Health Publications; 2005:255-312.

14. Kepenekci I, Keskinkilic B, Akinsu F, Cakir P, Elhan AH, Erkek AB, Kuzu MA. Prevalence of pelvic floor disorders in the female population and the impact of age, mode of delivery, and parity. Dis Colon Rectum. 2011 Jan;54(1):85-94.

15. Visco AG, Yuan L. Differential gene expression in pubococcygeus muscle from patients with pelvic organ prolapse. Am J Obstet Gynecol. 2003 Jul;189(1):102-12.

16. Rinne KM, Kirkinen PP. What predisposes young women to genital prolapse? Eur J Obstet Gynecol Reprod Biol. 1999 May;84(1):23-5.

17. Miedel A, Tegerstedt G, Maehle-Schmidt M, Nyrén O, Hammarström M. Nonobstetric risk factors for symptomatic pelvic organ prolapse. Obstet Gynecol. 2009 May;113(5):1089-97.

18. Halban, J.; Tandler, J. Anatomie und atiologie der genitalprolapse beim weibe. Wilhelm Braumüller; Wien: 1907. In: Hsu Y, Summers A, Hussain HK, Guire KE, Delancey JO. Levator plate angle in women with pelvic organ prolapse compared to women with normal support using dynamic MR imaging. Am J Obstet Gynecol. 2006 May; 194(5):1427-33.

19. Hsu Y, Summers A, Hussain HK, Guire KE, Delancey JO. Levator plate angle in women with pelvic organ prolapse compared to women with normal support using dynamic MR imaging. Am J Obstet Gynecol. 2006 May;194(5):1427-33.

20. Singh K, Jakab M, Reid WM, Berger LA, Hoyte L. Three-dimensional magnetic resonance imaging assessment of levator ani morphologic features in different grades of prolapse. Am J Obstet Gynecol. 2003 Apr;188(4):910-5.

21. Helt M, Benson JT, Russell B, Brubaker L. Levator ani muscle in women with genitourinary prolapse: indirect assessment by muscle histopathology. Neurourol Urodyn. 1996;15(1):17-29.

22. Corton MM. Anatomy of pelvic floor dysfunction. Obstet Gynecol Clin North Am. 2009 Sep;36(3):401-19.

23. Margulies RU, Hsu Y, Kearney R, Stein T, Umek WH, DeLancey JO. Appearance of the levator ani muscle subdivisions in magnetic resonance images. Obstet Gynecol. 2006 May;107(5):1064-9.

24. Ashton-Miller JA, Delancey JO. On the biomechanics of vaginal birth and common sequelae. Annu Rev Biomed Eng. 2009;11:163-76.

25. Margulies RU, Huebner M, DeLancey JO. Origin and insertion points involved in levator ani muscle defects. Am J Obstet Gynecol. 2007 Mar;196(3):251.e1-5.

26. Hoyte L, Schierlitz L, Zou K, Flesh G, Fielding JR. Two- and 3-dimensional MRI comparison of levator ani structure, volume, and integrity in women with stress incontinence and prolapse. Am J Obstet Gynecol. 2001 Jul;185(1):11-9.

27. Ashton-Miller JA, Delancey JO. On the biomechanics of vaginal birth and common sequelae. Annu Rev Biomed Eng. 2009;11:163-76.

28. Lien KC, Morgan DM, Delancey JO, Ashton-Miller JA. Pudendal nerve stretch during vaginal birth: a 3D computer simulation. Am J Obstet Gynecol. 2005 May;192(5):1669-76.

29. Bo K, Fleten C, Nystad W. Effect of antenatal pelvic floor muscle training on labor and birth. Obstet Gynecol. 2009 Jun;113(6):1279-84.

30. Parente MP, Natal Jorge RM, Mascarenhas T, Silva-Filho AL. The influence of pelvic muscle activation during vaginal delivery. Obstet Gynecol. 2010 Apr;115(4):804-8.

31. Bazot M, Deligne L, Boudghène F, Buy JN, Truc JB, Lassau JP, Bigot JM. Anatomic approach to the parametrium: value of computed tomographic in vitro study compared to dissection. Surg Radiol Anat. 1998;20(2):123-7.

32. Campbell RM. The anatomy and histology of the sacrouterine ligaments. Am J Obstet Gynecol. 1950 Jan;59(1):1-12, illust.

33. Corton MM. Anatomy of pelvic floor dysfunction. Obstet Gynecol Clin North Am. 2009 Sep;36(3):401-19.

34. Moalli PA, Shand SH, Zyczynski HM, Gordy SC, Meyn LA. Remodeling of vaginal connective tissue in patients with prolapse. Obstet Gynecol. 2005 Nov;106(5 Pt 1):953-63.

35. Moalli PA, Shand SH, Zyczynski HM, Gordy SC, Meyn LA. Remodeling of vaginal connective

tissue in patients with prolapse. Obstet Gynecol. 2005 Nov;106(5 Pt 1):953-63.

36. Glossary of Osteopathic Terminology. In: Ward RC, ed. Foundations for Osteopathic Medicine. 2nd ed. Baltimore: Williams and Wilkins; 2003:1249.

37. Handa VL, Pannu HK, Siddique S, Gutman R, VanRooyen J, Cundiff G. Architectural differences in the bony pelvis of women with and without pelvic floor disorders. Obstet Gynecol. 2003 Dec;102(6):1283-90.

38. Handa VL, Lockhart ME, Fielding JR, Bradley CS, Brubaker L, Cundiff GW, Ye W, Richter HE; Pelvic Floor Disorders Network.Racial differences in pelvic anatomy by magnetic resonance imaging. Obstet Gynecol. 2008 Apr;111(4):914-20.

39. Whitcomb EL, Rortveit G, Brown JS, Creasman JM, Thom DH, Van Den Eeden SK, Subak LL. Racial differences in pelvic organ prolapse. Obstet Gynecol. 2009 Dec;114(6):1271-7.

40. Nguyen JK, Lind LR, Choe JY, McKindsey F, Sinow R, Bhatia NN. Lumbosacral spine and pelvic inlet changes associated with pelvic organ prolapse. Obstet Gynecol. 2000 Mar;95(3):332-6.

41. Lind LR, Lucente V, Kohn N. Thoracic kyphosis and the prevalence of advanced uterine prolapse. Obstet Gynecol. 1996 Apr;87(4):605-9.

42. Jelovsek JE, Maher C, Barber MD. Pelvic organ prolapse. Lancet. 2007 Mar 24;369(9566):1027-38.

43. Jelovsek JE, Maher C, Barber MD. Pelvic organ prolapse. Lancet. 2007 Mar 24;369(9566):1027-38.

44. Hull M, Corton MM. Evaluation of the levator ani and pelvic wall muscles in levator ani syndrome. Urol Nurs. 2009 Jul-Aug;29(4):225-31.

45. Milsom I. Lower urinary tract symptoms in women. Curr Opin Urol. 2009 Jul;19(4):337-41.

46. Albertsen PC. Estimating a population's needs for the treatment of lower urinary tract symptoms in men: what is the extent of unmet need? J Urol. 2002 Aug;168(2):878-9.

47. Clemens JQ. Basic bladder neurophysiology. Urol Clin North Am. 2010 Nov;37(4):487-94.

48. Wagg A, Fry CH. Visco-elastic properties of isolated detrusor smooth muscle. Scand J Urol Nephrol Suppl. 1999;201:12-8.

49. Birder L, de Groat W, Mills I, Morrison J, Thor K, Drake M. Neural control of the lower urinary tract: peripheral and spinal mechanisms. Neurourol Urodyn. 2010;29(1):128-39.

50. Birder L, de Groat W, Mills I, Morrison J, Thor K, Drake M. Neural control of the lower urinary tract: peripheral and spinal mechanisms. Neurourol Urodyn. 2010;29(1):128-39.

51. Abrams P, Cardozo L, Fall M, Griffiths D, Rosier P, Ulmsten U, et al. The standardisation of terminology in lower urinary tract function: report from the standardisation sub-committee of the International Continence Society. Urology. 2003 Jan;61(1):37-49.

52. Abrams P, Cardozo L, Fall M, Griffiths D, Rosier P, Ulmsten U, et al. The standardisation of terminology in lower urinary tract function: report from the standardisation sub-committee of the International Continence Society. Urology. 2003 Jan;61(1):37-49.

53. Thom DH, Brown JS, Schembri M, Ragins AI, Subak LL, Van Den Eeden SK. Incidence of and risk factors for change in urinary incontinence status in a prospective cohort of middle-aged and older women: the reproductive risk of incontinence study in Kaiser. J Urol. 2010 Oct;184(4):1394-401.

54. Kepenekci I, Keskinkilic B, Akinsu F, Cakir P, Elhan AH, Erkek AB, Kuzu MA. Prevalence of pelvic floor disorders in the female population and the impact of age, mode of delivery, and parity. Dis Colon Rectum. 2011 Jan;54(1):85-94.

55. Kepenekci I, Keskinkilic B, Akinsu F, Cakir P, Elhan AH, Erkek AB, Kuzu MA. Prevalence of pelvic floor disorders in the female population and the impact of age, mode of delivery, and parity. Dis Colon Rectum. 2011 Jan;54(1):85-94.

56. Buchsbaum GM, Chin M, Glantz C, Guzick D. Prevalence of urinary incontinence and associated risk factors in a cohort of nuns. Obstet Gynecol. 2002 Aug;100(2):226-9.

57. Thom DH, Brown JS, Schembri M, Ragins AI, Subak LL, Van Den Eeden SK. Incidence of and risk factors for change in urinary incontinence status in a prospective cohort of middle-aged and older women: the reproductive risk of incontinence study in Kaiser. J Urol. 2010 Oct;184(4):1394-401.

58. Landau EH, Jayanthi VR, Churchill BM, Shapiro E, Gilmour RF, Khoury AE, et al. Loss of elasticity in dysfunctional bladders: urodynamic and histochemical correlation. J Urol. 1994 Aug;152(2 Pt 2):702-5.

59. Milsom I. Lower urinary tract symptoms in women. Curr Opin Urol. 2009 Jul;19(4):337-41.

60. Kepenekci I, Keskinkilic B, Akinsu F, Cakir P, Elhan AH, Erkek AB, Kuzu MA. Prevalence of pelvic floor disorders in the female population and the impact of age, mode of delivery, and parity. Dis Colon Rectum. 2011 Jan;54(1):85-94.

61. Thom DH, Brown JS, Schembri M, Ragins AI, Subak LL, Van Den Eeden SK. Incidence of and risk factors for change in urinary incontinence status in a prospective cohort of middle-aged and older women: the reproductive risk of incontinence study in Kaiser. J Urol. 2010 Oct;184(4):1394-401.

62. Handa VL, Lockhart ME, Fielding JR, Bradley CS, Brubaker L, Cundiff GW, et al. Pelvic Floor Disorders Network.Racial differences in pelvic anatomy by magnetic resonance imaging. Obstet Gynecol. 2008 Apr;111(4):914-20.

63. Baragi RV, Delancey JO, Caspari R, Howard DH, Ashton-Miller JA. Differences in pelvic floor area between African American and European American women. Am J Obstet Gynecol. 2002 Jul;187(1):111-5.

64. Whitcomb EL, Rortveit G, Brown JS, Creasman JM, Thom DH, Van Den Eeden SK, Subak LL. Racial differences in pelvic organ prolapse. Obstet Gynecol. 2009 Dec;114(6):1271-7.

65. Abrams P, Cardozo L, Fall M, Griffiths D, Rosier P, Ulmsten U, et al. The standardisation of terminology in lower urinary tract function: report from the standardisation sub-committee of the International Continence Society. Urology. 2003 Jan;61(1):37-49.

66. Minassian VA, Stewart WF, Wood GC. Urinary incontinence in women: variation in prevalence estimates and risk factors. Obstet Gynecol. 2008 Feb;111(2 Pt 1):324-31.

67. Kepenekci I, Keskinkilic B, Akinsu F, Cakir P, Elhan AH, Erkek AB, Kuzu MA. Prevalence of pelvic floor disorders in the female population and the impact of age, mode of delivery, and parity. Dis Colon Rectum. 2011 Jan;54(1):85-94.

68. Minassian VA, Stewart WF, Wood GC. Urinary incontinence in women: variation in prevalence estimates and risk factors. Obstet Gynecol. 2008 Feb;111(2 Pt 1):324-31.

69. Jameson JS, Chia YW, Kamm MA, Speakman CT, Chye YH, Henry MM. Effect of age, sex and parity on anorectal function. Br J Surg. 1994 Nov;81(11):1689-92.

70. Perucchini D, DeLancey JO, Ashton-Miller JA, Peschers U, Kataria T.Age effects on urethral striated muscle. I. Changes in number and diameter of striated muscle fibers in the ventral urethra. Am J Obstet Gynecol. 2002 Mar;186(3):351-5.

71. Delancey JO, Ashton-Miller JA. Pathophysiology of adult urinary incontinence. Gastroenterology. 2004 Jan;126(1 Suppl 1):S23-32.

72. Carlile A, Davies I, Rigby A, Brocklehurst JC. Age changes in the human female urethra: a morphometric study. J Urol. 1988 Mar;139(3):532-5.

73. Trowbridge ER, Wei JT, Fenner DE, Ashton-Miller JA, Delancey JO. Effects of aging on lower urinary tract and pelvic floor function in nulliparous women. Obstet Gynecol. 2007 Mar;109(3):715-20.

74. Delancey JO, Ashton-Miller JA. Pathophysiology of adult urinary incontinence. Gastroenterology. 2004 Jan;126(1 Suppl 1):S23-32.

75. Tunn R, Goldammer K, Neymeyer J, Gauruder-Burmester A, Hamm B, Beyersdorff D. MRI morphology of the levator ani muscle, endopelvic fascia, and urethra in women with stress urinary incontinence. Eur J Obstet Gynecol Reprod Biol. 2006 Jun 1;126(2):239-45.

76. DeLancey JO. Structural support of the urethra as it relates to stress urinary incontinence: the hammock hypothesis. Am J Obstet Gynecol. 1994 Jun;170(6):1713-20; discussion 1720-3.

77. Howard D, Miller JM, Delancey JO, Ashton-Miller JA. Differential effects of cough, valsalva, and continence status on vesical neck movement. Obstet Gynecol. 2000 Apr;95(4):535-40.

78. Dietz HP, Simpson JM. Does delayed child-bearing increase the risk of levator injury in labour? Aust N Z J Obstet Gynaecol. 2007 Dec;47(6):491-5.

79. Peschers U, Schaer G, Anthuber C, Delancey JO, Schuessler B. Changes in vesical neck mobility following vaginal delivery. Obstet Gynecol. 1996 Dec;88(6):1001-6.

80. Sajadi KP, Gill BC, Damaser MS. Neurogenic aspects of stress urinary incontinence. Curr Opin Obstet Gynecol. 2010 Oct;22(5):425-9.

81. Abrams P, Cardozo L, Fall M, Griffiths D, Rosier P, Ulmsten U, et al. The standardisation of terminology in lower urinary tract function: report from the standardisation sub-commit-

tee of the International Continence Society. Urology. 2003 Jan;61(1):37-49.

82. Milsom I, Abrams P, Cardozo L, Roberts RG, Thüroff J, Wein AJ. How widespread are the symptoms of an overactive bladder and how are they managed? A population-based prevalence study. BJU Int. 2001 Jun;87(9):760-6.

83. Weiss JP, Blaivas JG, Stember DS, Brooks MM. Nocturia in adults: etiology and classification. Neurourol Urodyn. 1998;17(5): 467-72.

84. Abrams P, Cardozo L, Fall M, Griffiths D, Rosier P, Ulmsten U, et al. The standardisation of terminology in lower urinary tract function: report from the standardisation sub-committee of the International Continence Society. Urology. 2003 Jan;61(1):37-49.

85. Abrams P, Cardozo L, Fall M, Griffiths D, Rosier P, Ulmsten U, et al. The standardisation of terminology in lower urinary tract function: report from the standardisation sub-committee of the International Continence Society. Urology. 2003 Jan;61(1):37-49.

86. Kim JC, Joo KJ, Kim JT, Choi JB, Cho DS, Won YY. Alteration of autonomic function in female urinary incontinence.Int Neurourol J. 2010 Dec;14(4):232-7.

87. Korr IM. The spinal cord as organizer of disease processes: II. The peripheral autonomic nervous system. J Amer Osteopath Assoc, Oct. 1979; 79(2):82/57-90/65.

88. Lachowsky M, Nappi RE. The effects of oestrogen on urogenital health. Maturitas. 2009 Jun 20;63(2):149-51.

89. Lukban J, Whitmore K, Kellogg-Spadt S, Bologna R, Lesher A, Fletcher E. The effect of manual physical therapy in patients diagnosed with interstitial cystitis, high-tone pelvic floor dysfunction, and sacroiliac dysfunction. Urology. 2001 Jun;57(6 Suppl 1):121-2.

90. Standring S , Ed. Gray's Anatomy: The anatomical basis of clinical practice. 39th ed. Edinburgh: Churchill Livingstone; 2004.

91. Kegel AH. Progressive resistance exercise in the functional restoration of the perineal muscles. Am J Obstet Gynecol. 1948 Aug;56(2):238-48.

92. Bourcier A, Peyrat L. Prise en charge rééducative de l'incontinence urinaire chez la femme. Encycl Méd Chir [Elsevier Masson, Paris]. Urologie; 18-207-D-23. 2008.

93. Shafik A, Shafik IA. Overactive bladder inhibition in response to pelvic floor muscle exercises. World J Urol. 2003 May;20(6):374-7.

94. Miller JM, Ashton-Miller JA, DeLancey JO. A pelvic muscle precontraction can reduce cough-related urine loss in selected women with mild SUI. J Am Geriatr Soc. 1998 Jul;46(7):870-4.

95. Benvenuti F, Caputo GM, Bandinelli S, Mayer F, Biagini C, Sommavilla A. Reeducative treatment of female genuine stress incontinence. Am J Phys Med. 1987 Aug;66(4):155-68.

96. Wyman JF, Burgio KL, Newman DK. Practical aspects of lifestyle modifications and behavioural interventions in the treatment of overactive bladder and urgency urinary incontinence. Int J Clin Pract. 2009 Aug;63(8):1177-91.

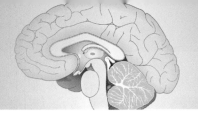

# Chapter 7

# Autonomic dysfunctions

*"...je me suis mis à être un peu gai, parce qu'on m'a dit que cela est bon pour la santé."*

—F. M. Arouet[1]

Also referred to as the vegetative nervous system, visceral nervous system, or involuntary nervous system, the autonomic nervous system (ANS) is involved in a myriad of clinical conditions. Because osteopathic procedures affect the ANS, a description of its organization and components is a prerequisite for understanding the effect of somatic dysfunction and the physiological basis of an osteopathic treatment. Then, it is appropriate to discuss the influence of the ANS upon several disorders affecting the aging individual: dysautonomia, chronic fatigue syndrome, fibromyalgia, and disorders associated with sleep and menopause.

The nervous system is usually described as consisting of two components: the sensory motor system, which controls functions in relation to the external environment and the ANS, which regulates the internal environment. These two components are, however, closely related by their embryological origins and physiological relationships. Rather than being two separate systems, they are often functionally overlapping.

All centers and nerves that belong to the ANS innervate smooth and cardiac muscles and glands, and regulate visceral processes including cardiovascular activity, digestion, metabolism, and thermoregulation. Essentially involuntary, this system consists of three parts: the sympathetic, parasympathetic, and enteric systems, which are in constant interaction with each other. A good number of structures innervated by the ANS receive both sympathetic and parasympathetic supply. The enteric nervous system is, on the other hand, an arrangement of neurons within the walls of the gastrointestinal (GI) tract. The peripheral activity of the ANS is further coordinated by neuronal networks in the forebrain, hypothalamus, midbrain, and medulla. In this chapter we will focus primarily upon the sympathetic and parasympathetic components of the ANS.

The ANS maintains the equilibrium of the internal environment. The need for consistency within the internal biological environment is a concept that has been recognized since Hippocrates proposed harmonic balance among the 'humors' of the body.[2] Later, in numerous publications from 1854 until his death in 1878, Claude Bernard described the '*milieu intérieur*,' and its steadiness.[3] In 1926, Walter Cannon reinforced this concept coining the term 'homeostasis.'[4] Although living creatures are repeatedly subjected to disrupting circumstances, Cannon emphasized that a constant internal environment must prevail to retain favorable living conditions. He was the first to propose that the parasympathetic and sympathetic systems have definitely different functions.[5] Cannon described how the parasympathetic component is involved in '*rest*' and '*digest*,' preserving basal heart rate, respiration, and metabolism under normal conditions, while the sympathetic regulates urgent situations with a '*fight*' or '*flight*' reaction that implies augmentation of output from the heart and other viscera, the peripheral vasculature, sweat glands, and the piloerector muscles.

The functions and relations between the parasympathetic and sympathetic systems are, nevertheless, not as straightforward as might initially

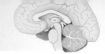

appear. Both are involved with each other, as well as with the somatic motor system, to form an inte-grated system that controls, modulates, and coordinates neural regulation of most of our activities.

# Organization and components

The ANS consists of neurons situated within the central and peripheral nervous systems. The ANS depends upon autonomic reflexes. Afferent inputs are transmitted from the periphery to the central nervous system (CNS) and efferent impulses from the CNS to peripheral organ systems.

Sensory information is usually sent via both cranial and spinal nerves to homeostatic control centers, such as those located in the hypothalamus and brainstem, with further control from higher centers in the limbic system and cerebral cortex. As a result, efferent fibers convey impulses from the CNS to the autonomic effectors that can modulate different functions such as glandular secretion, GI peristalsis, heart rate, blood pressure, thermoregulation, thirst, and hunger.

## General organization of the afferent autonomic nervous system

Visceral afferent pathways are very similar to somatic afferent pathways in morphology and function. Afferent neurons consist of:
- peripheral processes that convey sensory impulses from visceral organs or blood vessels to
- cell bodies situated in the dorsal root or cranial sensory ganglia that, in turn, connect with
- central processes travelling along with somatic afferent fibers through dorsal spinal roots or cranial nerves and ending in the CNS.

The central processes terminate in the CNS on interneurons that connect to autonomic effector neurons. These interneurons are located in the gray matter of the spinal cord or brainstem and form the preganglionic neurons of the efferent ANS. Although functionally part of both components, the visceral afferent neurons are not classified as either sympathetic or parasympathetic. Visceral afferent fibers may be categorized as:
- General visceral afferent (GVA) neurons that convey visceral information from the organs of the thorax, abdomen, and pelvis to the CNS, via spinal and cranial nerves.
- Special visceral afferent (SVA) neurons that convey impulses for smell and taste via cranial nerves. These are found in the olfactory nerve (CN I) for smell, and the facial (CN VII), glossopharyngeal (CN IX), and vagus (CN X) nerves for taste.

## General organization of the efferent autonomic nervous system

In the somatic nervous system there is only one neuron between the spinal cord and the effector organ, which is the skeletal muscle. In the ANS, in contrast, there are at least two neurons between the CNS and the effector organ or target tissue: the preganglionic and postganglionic neurons connected by an autonomic or relay ganglia. The somata (cell bodies) of preganglionic neurons are located in the visceral efferent nuclei of the brainstem or in the intermediolateral columns of the spinal cord. From there, most of the time, myelinated axons leave the CNS following cranial or spinal nerves in the direction

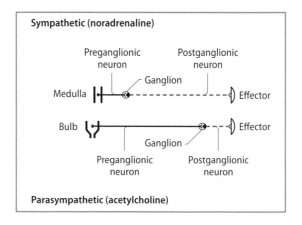

Figure 4.7.1: General organization of the efferent autonomic nervous system

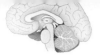

of the peripheral ganglia, where they synapse with typically, unmyelinated postganglionic neurons. These neurons then go on to innervate the effector organ or target tissue. Each preganglionic neuron can synapse with 15 to 20 postganglionic neurons, thereby broadening the distribution of the numerous autonomic effects.

The innervation of effector organs or target tissues by autonomic nerves differs from the innervation of skeletal muscle by somatic nerves. In contrast with skeletal muscles that display specifically localized postsynaptic regions, the effector neurons of the ANS have no discrete postsynaptic sites. Indeed, the postganglionic nerve endings possess multiple swellings, or varicosities, that contain vesicles filled with neurotransmitter substances that can diffuse for distances up to several hundred nanometers before they reach the effector organ. In consequence, a small number of motor fibers can control the function of significant masses of smooth muscle or glandular tissue simultaneously.[6] Additionally, specialized intercellular communications—the gap junctions that exist between cells of cardiac and smooth muscle—contribute to the spread of electrical activity, resulting in a response of the entire tissue, even though the effector tissue may have received the discharge of only a single autonomic nerve fiber.

Visceral efferent fibers may be described as:

- General visceral efferent (GVE) neurons that convey impulses from the CNS to smooth muscle, cardiac muscle, and glands, via spinal and cranial nerves. GVE fibers may be either parasympathetic or sympathetic. The GVE fibers located in the cranial nerves are parasympathetic. They include: the oculomotor nerve (CN III), the facial nerve (CN VII), the glossopharyngeal nerve (CN IX) and the vagus nerve (CN X). Other parasympathetic GVE neurons are found in the pelvic splanchnic nerves (S2–S4). The sympathetic GVE fibers are distributed via the thoracolumbar component of the ANS.
- Special visceral efferent (SVE) neurons that convey impulses from the CNS to skeletal muscles involved in facial expression and position of the jaw, neck, larynx, and pharynx via cranial nerves. In fact, they are the cranial

nerve fibers that supply muscles derived from the branchial arches: the trigeminal nerve (CN V), the facial nerve (CN VII), the glossopharyngeal nerve (CN IX), the vagus nerve (CN X) and the accessory nerve (CN XI).

# Divisions of the autonomic nervous system

The ANS consists of two anatomically and functionally distinct divisions: the sympathetic and parasympathetic systems. With the exception of peripheral vasculature, sweat glands of the trunk and extremities, and hair follicles that receive only sympathetic supply, normally every other tissue innervated by the ANS receives some nervous input from both the sympathetic and parasympathetic divisions at all times. The tonic activity of these two divisions allows precise regulation, enhancing or inhibiting physiology. On average, the sympathetic and the parasympathetic systems have opposing effects, with one system increasing its activity while at the same time the other system is decreasing its activity. It should, however, be kept in mind that this is not an antagonistic relationship, but rather results in the maintenance of a dynamic state of balance within the target tissues.

Overall the sympathetic nervous system prevails during emergency situations, when preparing the body for 'fight-or-flight.' Blood flow will increase in vital organs and skeletal muscle whereas visceral activity will decrease. On the contrary, the parasympathetic system is prominent during peaceful, resting conditions, increasing the activity of basic body functions such as digestion, and reducing heart rate and cardiac output.

## Sympathetic division
### Preganglionic sympathetic fibers

Preganglionic fibers of the sympathetic division have their cell bodies in the intermediolateral horn of the spinal cord between the first thoracic spinal segment and second lumbar segments (T1–L2). From the spinal cord, the preganglionic fibers travel in the ventral root of the spinal nerves, and then, through the white rami communicantes, they join the sympathetic ganglia which lie along each side

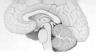

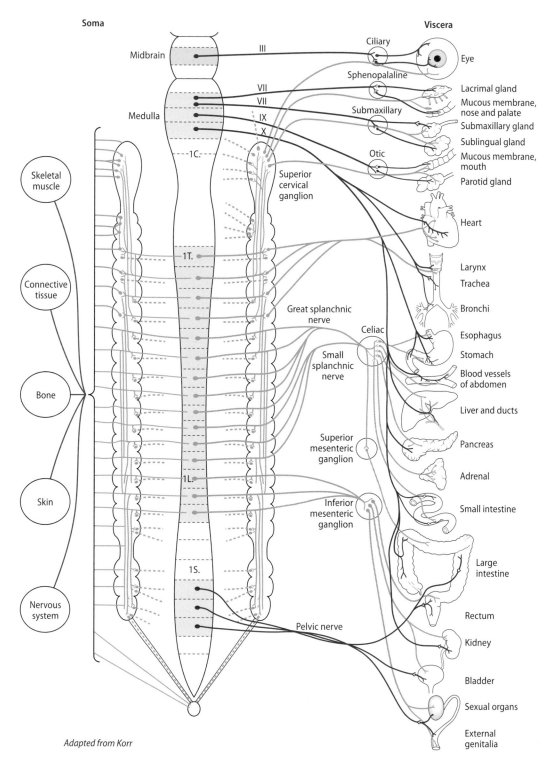

*Adapted from Korr*

**Figure 4.7.2:** Autonomic nervous system innervation, showing the sympathetic and parasympathetic systems

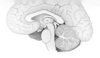
of the spinal cord, where they synapse with post-ganglionic neurons.

Preganglionic fibers may synapse with postganglionic fibers in a ganglion at their spinal segmental level of origin. They may also run superiorly or inferiorly to synapse with postganglionic neurons in ganglia of the paravertebral chain at other levels. As such, preganglionic neurons may synapse with several postganglionic neurons, and the ratio of pre- to postganglionic fibers is about 1:20. This results in a mass sympathetic discharge i.e., a coordinated sympathetic stimulation of tissues throughout the body, a characteristic not shared to the same degree by parasympathetic ganglia.

### Sympathetic ganglia

On either side of the spinal cord, adjacent to the spinal column, the sympathetic ganglia form a sympathetic chain, also called the sympathetic trunk or paravertebral chain. Each chain consists of 23 ganglia that extend from the cervical to the sacral regions: three in the cervical region, 10–12 in the thoracic region, four in the lumbar region, four or five in the sacral region and a single coccygeal ganglion.

Frequently, the middle and lower cervical ganglia are fused to form the stellate ganglion. Because preganglionic fibers arise between T1–L2, the corresponding ganglia are the only ones to receive white rami communicantes. Therefore, paravertebral ganglia situated above T1 or below L2 receive preganglionic fibers from spinal segments T1–L2. These preganglionic fibers pass through a ganglion at the same spinal cord level from which they arise and run superiorly or inferiorly along the paravertebral chain to reach ganglia located above or below T1–L2.

In the cervical region, the ganglia of the paravertebral chain are located anterior to the transverse processes of the cervical vertebrae. In the thorax, the sympathetic chain is anterior to the heads of the ribs. In the lumbar area, the ganglia are anterolateral to the bodies of the vertebrae, while in the pelvis they are anterior to the sacrum and medial to the anterior sacral foramina. In front of the coccyx, the two paravertebral chains converge and form a small, unpaired ganglion called the 'impar' ganglion. In most cases, sympathetic preganglionic fibers are short, because ganglia are close to their origin; postganglionic fibers, however, are likely to be longer.

### Postganglionic sympathetic fibers

Postganglionic fibers that supply structures in the head come from the superior sympathetic cervical ganglion, opposite the second and third cervical vertebrae. From there they travel along the branches of the carotid arteries to their targets in the head.

It should be stressed that these postganglionic fibers have already synapsed with preganglionic fibers derived from the T1–T4 spinal segments. Therefore, the cell bodies of these preganglionic fibers are located in the lateral horn of the upper thoracic cord. For this reason, when treating conditions of the head that manifest autonomic dysfunction, like sinusitis, as well as treating any upper thoracic dysfunction, it is important to also treat somatic dysfunction of the upper cervical region which can impact the superior cervical ganglion.

After synapsing in the ganglia, most postganglionic fibers travel with the arteries that supply the effectors. Some postganglionic fibers, however, may join the spinal nerves via the grey rami communicantes. In fact, a typical spinal nerve demonstrates about 8% sympathetic postganglionic axons. As a result, cervical and upper thoracic sympathetic postganglionic nerve fibers supply blood vessels, sweat glands, hair follicles, glands, and visceral organs of the head (eye, salivary glands, and mucus membranes of the nasal cavity) and the chest (heart and lungs). Anatomic studies indicate that the sympathetic innervation of the upper extremity emanates from the mid-thoracic region (T5–T7).[7] Clinical experience, however, demonstrates that somatic dysfunction in the upper to mid-thoracic region results in sympathetically-mediated symptoms affecting the upper extremity.[8] [9 10] Lower thoracic (T6 and lower) and lumbar sympathetic nerve fibers innervate peripheral blood vessels, sweat glands, and pilomotor smooth muscle of the lower torso and lower extremity, and the abdominal and pelvic viscera.

In several instances, preganglionic fibers traverse the sympathetic ganglia of the paravertebral chain without forming synaptic contact, to join a thoracic, lumbar, or sacral splanchnic nerve and synapse on neurons of the collateral ganglia, also called the

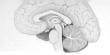

prevertebral ganglia. These collateral ganglia include the celiac ganglia, the superior and inferior mesenteric ganglia, and small ganglia spread within the pelvic plexus. They innervate the GI system and the accessory GI organs, including the pancreas and liver, and also provide sympathetic innervation for the kidneys, bladder, and genitalia.

An additional group of preganglionic fibers travels in the thoracic splanchnic nerves into the abdomen and synapses directly with the adrenal medulla. The cells of the adrenal medulla are developmentally and functionally related to postganglionic sympathetic neurons. However, as an endocrine gland, the adrenal medulla secretes adrenaline and noradrenaline into the circulatory system, reaching all of the effector tissues of the sympathetic system.

## Parasympathetic division

The parasympathetic division of the ANS supplies only viscera and the blood vessels of the head and neck, thorax, abdomen, and pelvis. The peripheral vasculature of the extremities and trunk does not receive parasympathetic innervation.

### Preganglionic parasympathetic fibers

Preganglionic fibers of the parasympathetic division arise from several nuclei of the brainstem and from the sacral region of the spinal cord (segments S2–S4). They exit the CNS to reach broadly dispersed ganglia where they synapse. Unlike the sympathetic system, where the ganglia are located at some distance from their target, the parasympathetic ganglia are located either on cranial nerves or they lie close to, embedded within, the visceral target organs. Thus, the axons of preganglionic neurons of the parasympathetic division are relatively long, and the postganglionic axons short.

The preganglionic parasympathetic nuclei within the brainstem, associated with cranial nerves, are: the Edinger-Westphal (CN III), the superior salivary (CN VII), the inferior salivary (CN IX), and the dorsal vagal and nucleus ambiguus (CN X). The preganglionic neurons that exit the brainstem do so via CNs III, VII, IX, and X.

Parasympathetic fibers arising from the lateral horn of the sacral portion of the spinal cord travel in the ventral roots of spinal nerves S2, S3, and S4. They enter the anterior primary rami of these nerves and travel in the pelvic splanchnic nerves to reach the inferior hypogastric plexus (pelvic plexus) before synapsing in ganglia close to, or within, the target viscera.

### Parasympathetic ganglia

Five small, paired peripheral ganglia are found in the cranial part of the parasympathetic system; they are:
- the ciliary ganglion, located in the orbit;
- the pterygopalatine ganglion, located in the pterygopalatine fossa;
- the otic ganglion, located in the inferior temporal fossa;
- the submandibular and sublingual ganglia, located in the floor of the mouth.
- Other parasympathetic ganglia are small intramural ganglia located within the organs they innervate.

### Postganglionic parasympathetic fibers

Postganglionic parasympathetic fibers are shorter than postganglionic sympathetic fibers. The cell bodies of postganglionic parasympathetic fibers are, typically, distant from the CNS, located either in distinct ganglia near the structures innervated, or in ganglia dispersed within the walls of the target viscera. Because of this proximity between the ganglia and the effector, divergence in the parasympathetic system is smaller than that of the sympathetic system, with an average ratio of pre- to postganglionic fibers of about 1:3. Consequently, the effects of the parasympathetic system are likely to be more isolated and localized in contrast to the sympathetic system where widespread discharge is possible.

Preganglionic fibers travelling through CNs III, VII, and IX project to postganglionic neurons in the ciliary, pterygopalatine, submandibular, and otic ganglia. Cranial nerve III innervates the eyes. Cranial nerve VII innervates the lacrimal gland, the salivary glands, and the mucus membranes of the nasal cavity. Cranial nerve IX innervates the parotid gland. Preganglionic fibers from the dorsal vagal nucleus project via CN X to postganglionic fibers embedded in thoracic and abdominal effectors. Cranial nerve X innervates the heart, lungs, stomach, liver, gall blad-

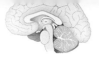

der, pancreas, small intestine, and upper half of the large intestine as far as the splenic flexure of the colon. Preganglionic fibers from the ventrolateral nucleus ambiguus project via CN X to postganglionic fibers and supply the principal parasympathetic innervation of the cardiac ganglia that innervate the heart, esophagus, and respiratory airways.

Most of the preganglionic fibers arising from spinal nerves S2, S3 and S4 project via the pelvic splanchnic nerves to the inferior hypogastric plexus to reach the urinary bladder, reproductive organs, and the rectum, while some traverse the inferior mesenteric plexus to reach the descending and sigmoid colon.

### Neurotransmitters of the autonomic nervous system

Neurons of the ANS release mainly acetylcholine and noradrenaline (norepinephrine). Acetylcholine is released by cholinergic fibers; they are the preganglionic and postganglionic fibers of the parasympathetic system, the preganglionic fibers of the sympathetic system, and the sympathetic postganglionic fibers innervating sweat glands. Noradrenaline and occasionally adrenaline (epinephrine) are released by adrenergic fibers; they include most sympathetic postganglionic fibers.

In order to have some effect, neurotransmitters must bind with particular receptors at target cells. Diverse sympathetic and parasympathetic receptors exist. Each of them determines a specific intracellular response. (See 'Table 7.1: Summary of the main functions of the autonomic nervous system,' p. 352.)

Acetylcholine released by preganglionic fibers binds to nicotinic receptors of the postganglionic fibers. Additionally, some neuropeptides such as enkephalin, somatostatin, and neurotensin, coexist with acetylcholine in the preganglionic fibers. Acetylcholine released by postganglionic fibers binds to muscarinic receptors, while noradrenaline released by sympathetic postganglionic fibers affects several types of adrenoreceptors ($\alpha1$, $\alpha2$, $\beta1$, $\beta2$), each with individual effect upon the postsynaptic cells.

In addition to the conventional acetylcholine and noradrenaline neurotransmitters, several other neuroactive substances have been demonstrated within the ANS. Some neurons do not use either acetylcholine or noradrenaline as their primary transmitter, but rather employ substances such as adenosine 5'-triphosphate (ATP), numerous peptides, and nitric oxide (NO).

# Functions of the autonomic nervous system

Classically, one of the two divisions of the ANS is described as dominant in different situations. The sympathetic system is activated during emergency 'fight-or-flight' reactions, while the parasympathetic system dominates during tranquil circumstances or 'rest and digest.' With this in mind, the effects of each division of the ANS are predictable.

During energetic physical activity or any stressful condition, the sympathetic nervous system predominates in order to accommodate to the situation. A widespread activation occurs. The constriction of cutaneous arteries results in an increased delivery of well-oxygenated, nutrient-rich blood to the heart, muscles, and brain while protecting the individual from excessive blood loss if cutaneous injury should occur. At the same time, vasoconstriction affects smooth muscle of the GI system and kidneys to reallocate the blood distribution in favor of active tissues and contracting muscles. Heart rate, myocardial contractility, blood pressure, and bronchodilatation are increased, while peristalsis slows down, and sphincters contract in order to mobilize body energy to face increased activity. Additionally, thermoregulation is controlled with sweating, and the ability to see at greater distance is increased through relaxation of the ciliary body allowing lens adaptation when the pupil dilates (mydriasis).

During 'rest and digest' circumstances, parasympathetic activity results in cardiac slowing and increased intestinal glandular and peristaltic activities, directed to conserve body energy. Gastrointestinal functions are stimulated: salivary and GI secretions augment and GI motility increases to facilitate absorption of food. Other glandular secretion from the lacrimal gland and glands of the respiratory tract increase while the stimulation of the ciliary body allows lens adaptation and the pu-

pil contract (miosis). In addition, parasympathetic innervation also allows emptying of the urinary bladder and the rectum.

### Table 7.1 Summary of the main functions of the ANS.

| Organ | | Parasympathetic stimulation | Sympathetic stimulation |
|---|---|---|---|
| Lungs | Bronchial muscles | Contraction | Relaxation |
| | Bronchial glands | Stimulation | Inhibition ($\alpha$) Stimulation ($\beta$) |
| Heart | Heart rate | Decreased | Increased |
| | Force of contraction | Decreased | Increased |
| | Conduction velocity | Increased | Decreased |
| Arteries | | Dilatation | Constriction ($\alpha$) Dilatation ($\beta$) |
| Veins | | | Constriction |
| Submandibular and parotid glands | | Watery salivary secretions | Viscous salivary secretions |
| Stomach | Motility | Increased | Decreased |
| | Sphincters | Relaxation | Contraction |
| | Secretion | Increased | Decreased |
| intestines | Motility | Increased | Decreased |
| | Sphincters | Relaxation | Contraction |
| | Secretion | Increased | Decreased |
| Liver | | Glycogen synthesis | Glycogenolysis Gluconeogenesis Lipolysis |
| Gall bladder | | Contraction | Relaxation |
| Pancreas | Exocrine | Increased enzyme secretion | Decreased enzyme secretion |
| | Endocrine | Increased insulin secretion | Decreased insulin secretion |
| Kidneys | | | Increased renin secretion |
| Adrenal medullae | | | Secretion of adrenaline and noradrenaline |
| Spleen | | | Contraction |
| Urinary bladder | Detrusor | Contraction | Relaxation |
| | Sphincter | Relaxation | Contraction |
| Uterus | | | Contraction of pregnant uterus ($\alpha$) Relaxation of pregnant and non-pregnant uterus ($\beta$) |
| Male genitals | | Erection | Ejaculation |
| Sweat glands | | | Increased sweating |
| Piloerector muscles | | | Contraction |
| Eyes | Pupil | Constriction | Dilatation |
| | Ciliary muscle | Contraction for near vision | Relaxation for far vision |
| | Lacrimal gland secretions | Increased | |

# Dysautonomia

Dysautonomia, or autonomic dysfunction, is an abnormal functioning of the ANS that can manifest as either acute or chronic overactivity, underactivity, or failure of the sympathetic or parasympathetic components of the ANS. Symptoms of this autonomic dysfunction can manifest as either irregular uncomfortable sensations or as more severe established diseases. Because the ANS is involved in the function of almost every organ system, ANS dysfunction may be associated with various diseases involving different medical disciplines such as cardiology, neurology, psychiatry, and endocrinology. Such diseases may be localized, as complex regional pain syndromes, or manifestations of whole-body pure autonomic failure such as in diabetes.

Multiple symptoms may exist in dysautonomia, with ample variation between patients, from mild discomfort to total disability. There may be excessive fatigue, polydipsia, dizziness or vertigo, anxiety or panic, arrhythmia, orthostatic hypotension occasionally associated with syncope, and GI dysfunctions such as irritable bowel syndrome, constipation, diarrhea, nausea, and gastroesophageal reflux. Sometimes, the multiplicity of symptoms can be diagnostically very confusing, and patients may end up as being misdiagnosed as having psychiatric conditions.

The dualism between body and mind is an old notion leading to the concept that disease must be either physical or mental. 'Cartesian dualism,' although different from the dualism proposed by Descartes himself, has been used to substantiate the body as a set of mechanistic, organic processes, which are quite separate from the mind.[11] This mind-body dichotomy has lead to a separation between the practice of psychiatry and the remainder of medical practice. In contrast, osteopathic philosophy and approach firmly grounded upon the concept of the triune body, mind and spirit (nature of humanity) is perfectly appropriate to provide an integrated approach to patients suffering with ANS dysfunctions. See below: 'The osteopathic contribution to the physical examination and treatment,' p. 366.

Much controversy exists in the explanation and classification of the different manifestations of dysautonomia. Indeed, because of the complexity of symptoms and unidentified causes, the actual mechanisms that explain dysautonomia are not well understood. One approach to the classification of dysautonomia is functional:

- Parasympathetic underactivity is associated with sympathetic dominance, with symptoms of '*fight*' or '*flight*' (opposite to '*rest*' and '*digest*'): increased pulse rate, decreased salivary and nasal secretion, decreased peristaltic activities, constipation, urinary problems, and impotence in men.
- Sympathetic underactivity is associated with parasympathetic dominance, with symptoms of '*rest*' and '*digest*' (opposite to '*fight*' or '*flight*'): decreased pulse rate, decreased blood pressure, orthostatic hypotension, and ejaculation disorders in men.

## Baroreflex

The neurophysiology of the baroreflex is strongly linked to the primary respiratory mechanism (PRM). (See also: 'Section 1: Osteopathy, fascia, fluid, and the primary respiratory mechanism,' p. 18.) One of the manifestations of dysautonomia—orthostatic hypotension, with resultant syncope, or near syncope—is under the control of baroreflex. The ANS maintains internal homeostasis and to do so, among other functions, it regulates blood pressure, fluid, and electrolyte balance and body temperature. Regulation of blood pressure includes regulation of responses to positional change. The baroreflex is one of the mechanisms involved in this regulation.

The baroreflex depends on the baroreceptors—sensory nerve endings that lie in the walls of the arteries and are stimulated when stretched. They are particularly profuse in the walls of the internal carotid arteries, just above the carotid bifurcation, i.e., the carotid sinus, and in the wall of the aortic arch at the origin of the right subclavian artery. They are also found in the walls of the cardiopul-

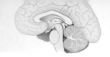

monary veins, and the atria, and the left ventricle of the heart.

Signals from the carotid sinus travel via Hering's nerves to CN IX, and to the first synapse located in the nucleus tractus solitarius (NTS) in the medullary area of the brainstem. Additionally, signals from the aortic arch are transmitted through the aortic depressor nerve that travels with CN X to the NTS. Cardiopulmonary receptors located in the heart and lungs project also through the vagus nerves to the NTS. Any small change in pressure triggers a change in the baroreflex signal with resultant adjustment of arterial pressure. Stretch of vascular walls augments baroreceptor discharge frequency, resulting in inhibition of sympathetic activity and stimulation of parasympathetic activity. The NTS projects to, and stimulates, the caudal ventrolateral medulla (CVLM). The activated CVLM sends fibers to the rostral ventrolateral medulla (RVLM) with an efferent path to the intermediolateral cell columns of the spinal cord. Parasympathetic activity originates in the nucleus ambiguus (NA) and the dorsal motor nucleus of the vagus (DMNV).[12]

Thus through the above mechanism, when blood pressure increases, the resultant stretch of the baroreceptors in the vascular wall causes an increase in their discharge frequency. Thus, sympathetic activity is decreased while parasympathetic activity is increased, leading to a reduction in blood pressure and heart rate. The reverse events occur with a decrease in blood pressure.[13]

## Orthostatic hypotension

Deregulation of blood pressure can result in orthostatic hypotension. The consensus statement on the definition of orthostatic hypotension is: "Orthostatic hypotension is a sustained reduction of systolic blood pressure of at least 20 mmHg or diastolic blood pressure of 10 mmHg within 3 minutes of standing or head-up tilt to at least 60° on a tilt table."[14]

With aging, the prevalence of orthostatic hypotension increases due to age-related changes in the cardiovascular system, additional diseases, and use of various medications. It is a clinical sign

that may be symptomatic or asymptomatic, and it happens in patients with neurodegenerative disorders, such as Parkinson's disease.

The symptoms of orthostatic hypotension include lightheadedness, dizziness, pre-syncope, and syncope. The loss of consciousness tends to be slow and gradual. Other signs are more global and include weakness, fatigue, cognitive slowing, leg buckling, visual blurring, headache, neck pain, orthostatic dyspnea, or chest pain.[15]

Under normal circumstances, between 25-30% of circulating blood is in the thorax. In the few seconds after assumption of upright posture, there is a shift of 300–800 ml of blood toward the lower extremities and the abdominal venous capacitance system. This quick redistribution of about 25% of the body's total blood volume produces a decline in venous return to the heart. As a consequence, cardiac filling pressure is reduced and stroke volume may decline by 40%. Less stretch is applied on baroreceptors resulting in a decrease of discharge. This change in baroreceptors firing to the brain produces an increase in the activity of the sympathetic nervous system with the release of noradrenaline that in turn activates receptors in blood vessel walls. The blood vessels constrict, increasing resistance to blood flow. The resultant increase in total peripheral resistance usually maintains normal blood pressure.

Baroreceptor physiology is of paramount importance for the initiation of an immediate reflex response in vascular tone during postural change. Conversely, an extreme fall of cardiac output or deficient vasoconstrictor mechanisms can result in the development of neurogenic orthostatic hypotension through insufficient release of noradrenaline from sympathetic vasomotor neurons and vasoconstrictor failure.[16]

## Larson's (functional vasomotor hemiparesthesia) syndrome and complex regional pain syndrome 1

Larson's (functional vasomotor hemiparesthesia) syndrome is a sympathetically dominated condition exhibiting increased vasomotor tone.[17] It shares many characteristics with complex regional

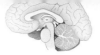

pain syndrome 1 (CRPS1), formerly called reflex sympathetic dystrophy, but typically presents without history of antecedent trauma.[18] The patient's skin will be up to 2° C cooler in the affected area.[19] In the complete syndrome the patient will complain of dysesthesia and paresthesias on one side of the body affecting the head, torso, and upper and lower extremities. Early in the course of the condition, the presentation is often limited to unilateral cervicothoracic pain in the area of the upper trapezius muscle. This pain pattern frequently extends to include the ipsilateral upper extremity and side of the head and neck. The primary somatic dysfunction affecting these patients is associated with upper thoracic paravertebral tissue texture change and tenderness that, when palpated, acts as a trigger point producing symptoms radiating into the area of the patient's complaint. The dysfunction is typically a vertebral, Fryette type II dysfunction, although it may result from a viscerosomatic reflex. The area of somatic dysfunction is most often found between T1 and T5. Etiologic dysfunctions, as low as T8 or T9, are occasionally encountered, often with symptoms referable to the ipsilateral lower extremity.

Larson's syndrome, in any of its presentations, responds, often dramatically, to treatment of the causative thoracic somatic dysfunction, either with specific osteopathic manipulative treatment (OMT), or, in the case of viscerosomatic reflexes, with the specific treatment of the underlying visceral condition. Because of the shared similarities between Larson's syndrome and CRPS1, from the perspective of the contribution of somatic dysfunction to the overall clinical presentation of these individuals, CRPS1 patients may be treated similarly when employing OMT. Physical changes within the CNS from longstanding CRPS1 often makes these patients more resistant to OMT. There is, however, no reason not to treat the somatic component of CRPS1 patients to alleviate, if not eliminate, their symptoms. [20]

Aside from the cutaneous manifestations, cool skin, and increased perspiration, the symptoms of Larson's syndrome are predominantly subjective. They are sensory complaints that rarely manifest as clinically demonstrable sensory deficits. The manifestation of hard neurological signs, including motor or sensory deficits, necessitates a complete medical evaluation to rule out potentially catastrophic pathology.

# Chronic fatigue syndrome

Fatigue is a frequent symptom among older patients, with up to half of the general population reporting fatigue. On average, the fatigue is temporary and can be explained. Nevertheless, for some persons, fatigue is persistent, debilitating, and cannot be explained by an apparent medical condition. These patients may suffer from chronic fatigue syndrome (CFS). CFS is defined by the Centers for Disease Control and Prevention (CDC) as "a debilitating and complex disorder characterized by profound fatigue that is not improved by bed rest and that may be worsened by physical or mental activity."[21]

The CDC criteria include severe fatigue lasting longer than six consecutive months that is not due to ongoing exertion or other medical conditions associated with fatigue, in addition to at least four of the following physical symptoms: postexertional malaise lasting more than 24 hours; unrefreshing sleep; impaired short-term memory or concentration; muscle pain; polyarthralgia without swelling or redness; new headaches; frequent or recurring sore throat; and tender lymph nodes in the neck or armpit.

The prevalence of CFS varies from 0.007–2.6% in the adult population, according to the population categories surveyed and the study methods.[22] [23] Women, minority groups, and persons with lower levels of education score the highest levels of CFS.

Although multiple theories for the pathophysiology of CFS have been proposed, no specific cause has been yet recognized. The etiology of CFS may be multifactorial. Different conditions that have been considered include: acute viral illness (such as Epstein-Barr virus, human herpes virus, HIV, enterovirus), toxins, immune disorders, stress, psychiatric disorder, sleep disorder, nutritional deficiency, and trauma. The association with some of the above conditions has been demonstrated, but they are, however, considered to be largely unique observations and the relationships among them are unexplored.[24]

A number of symptoms described by CFS patients seem to involve the CNS. They include: malaise following mental exertion, memory loss, impaired concentration or attention headache, brain fog, dizziness, balance problems or fainting, irritable bowel, chills and night sweats, visual disturbances (sensitivity to light, blurring, eye pain), and depression or mood problems (irritability, mood swings, anxiety, panic attacks). These observations have stimulated researchers to determine if the CNS may be involved in the pathophysiology of CFS, using structural and functional neuroimaging, cognitive testing, neuropeptide assays, and autonomic assessment. The overall significance of findings remains inconclusive and more research must be done.

# Fibromyalgia

Fibromyalgia (FM) is defined by the CDC as "a disorder of unknown etiology characterized by widespread pain, abnormal pain processing, sleep disturbance, fatigue, and often psychological distress."[29]

Fibromyalgia is most common among women, with a female to male ratio of roughly 3:1.[30] The prevalence rate of individuals who met FM criteria is estimated to be between 7.3% and 12.9% across different countries.[31] Prevalence rises steadily with age.

Since 1990, the American College of Rheumatology (ACR) has described criteria for the clinical diagnosis and classification of FM, a disease where the diagnosis of the somatic syndromes without objective physical or laboratory features or specific pathologic findings may be challenging.[32][33] The 2012 ACR classification criteria includes a greater recognition of the importance of cognitive problems and somatic symptoms. It also incorporates a widespread pain index (WPI), and a symptom severity (SS) scale.[34]

Interestingly, patients with CFS demonstrate symptoms similar to those found in functional illnesses such as fibromyalgia and irritable bowel syndrome. In a population of women with fibromyalgia, 58.0% of them demonstrate the full criteria for CFS, compared to 26.1% in the control group with widespread pain.[25]

Additionally, individuals with CFS show variations in measures of sympathetic and parasympathetic nervous system function.[26] Notably, when cognitively challenged, they demonstrate signs of diminished vagal activity: low and unresponsive heart rate variability (HRV), greater heart rate (HR) reactivity, and prolonged HR recovery.[27]

In fact, the imbalance of the ANS, characterized by a hyperactive sympathetic system and a hypoactive parasympathetic system, can critically influence the severity and outcome of a large spectrum of diseases such as CFS, fibromyalgia, sleep disorders, and irritable bowel syndrome. Ultimately, the extreme energy necessary to adjust continually to the imbalance of the ANS stresses the system and can influence aging and diseases.[28]

## Widespread pain index

The WPI is a measure of the number of painful body regions that correlates with the tender point count described in the previous 1990 ACR classification. Because many physicians rarely performed the previous tender point count in primary care, performed it incorrectly, or did not know how to examine for tender points,[35] the WPI seems more practical.

The WPI is obtained by counting the number of areas in which the patient has had pain over the previous week. The score is between 0 and 19, evaluating the following areas:
- Shoulder girdle left; shoulder girdle right
- Upper arm left; upper arm right
- Lower arm left; lower arm right
- Hip (buttock, trochanter) left; hip (buttock, trochanter) right
- Upper leg left; upper leg right
- Lower leg left; lower leg right
- Jaw left; jaw right

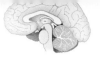
- Chest
- Abdomen
- Upper back
- Lower back
- Neck

## Symptom severity scale

The SS scale score evaluates three symptoms: fatigue, waking unrefreshed, and cognitive symptoms. For each of them, the level of severity over the past week is assessed, with a scale where 0 is no problem, 1 is mild problems, 2 is moderate, and 3 is severe.[36]

Additionally, somatic symptoms are evaluated as part of the process to obtain a SS scale score. Somatic symptoms are assessed with a scale where 0 is no symptom, 1 is a small number of symptoms, 2 is a moderate number of symptoms, and 3 is numerous symptoms. The list of somatic symptoms that the ACR suggests includes: "muscle pain, irritable bowel syndrome, fatigue/tiredness, thinking or remembering problem, muscle weakness, headache, pain/cramps in the abdomen, numbness/tingling, dizziness, insomnia, depression, constipation, pain in the upper abdomen, nausea, nervousness, chest pain, blurred vision, fever, diarrhea, dry mouth, itching, wheezing, Raynaud's phenomenon, hives/welts, ringing in ears, vomiting, heartburn, oral ulcers, loss of/change in taste, seizures, dry eyes, shortness of breath, loss of appetite, rash, sun sensitivity, hearing difficulties, easy bruising, hair loss, frequent urination, painful urination, and bladder spasms."[37]

The final SS scale score is obtained by adding the level of severity of the three first symptoms to the level of severity of the somatic symptoms, and should be between 0 and 12.

## Diagnostic criteria

Three conditions must be present to qualify for FM:
- A WPI greater than or equal to 7 and SS greater than or equal to 5, or WPI 3–6 and SS greater than or equal to 9;
- Symptoms must have been present at a comparable level for at least three months;
- The patient does not have a disorder that would otherwise account for the pain.

## Pathophysiology

The etiopathology of FM is not yet totally understood. Factors potentially contributing to the pathophysiology of FM include: genetic, neuroendocrinal, and immunological factors; dysfunction of the CNS and ANS; and environmental triggers such as exposure to stressors.

### Genetic factors

Genetic factors and familial predisposition may be part of the etiology of FM and chronic widespread pain.[38][39] Polymorphisms of genes in the serotonergic, dopaminergic and catecholaminergic systems seem to contribute to the etiopathogenesis of FM, and it may be that genetically predisposed individuals develop FM, when exposed to a host of environmental stressors.[40] Indeed, family members of patients with FM demonstrate a lower pain threshold to pressure stimulation, a sign of the involvement of genetic factors in the etiology of FM and pain sensitivity.[41] In addition, family members are also much more likely to have other syndromes, such as irritable bowel syndrome, Raynaud's phenomenon, headaches, and other regional pain syndromes.[42]

### Sensitization

Interestingly, individuals with FM demonstrate a lower pain threshold, not only when pressure stimulation is applied, but also with the application of heat, cold,[43] and electrical stimuli.[44] Fibromyalgia patients also exhibit decreased painful sound threshold.[45] Modification in central processing of sensory input seems to explain this enhanced sensitivity to stimuli. In fact, some patients with FM report pain sensations elicited by non-nociceptive stimuli, such as touch. This is defined as allodynia, a condition in which ordinarily non-painful stimuli induces pain, while hyperalgesia describes an extreme sensitivity to painful stimuli with a decreased threshold to nociceptive stimuli. Hyperalgesia may be further classified as primary—typically in areas of injury and inflammatory tissue changes—or secondary—outside the area of injury, and a response from central pain mechanisms.

Classically, hyperalgesia is considered to be the result of sensory input from nerve receptors where the stimulus applied is transmitted along primary afferent neurons (A-δ and C nerve fibers) to the dorsal horn of the spinal cord. Input is transmitted from there to second-order spinal neurons projecting to various regions in the brain such as the thalamus, somatosensory cortices, and the limbic system, resulting in the perception of pain.

In patients with FM, sensitization of nociceptors plays an important pathogenic role in the development of hyperalgesia. Sensitization results from repeated or sustained noxious input to the dorsal horn neurons that leads to increased neuronal responsiveness and abnormal pain processing. Initially, as a consequence of tissue injury and inflammation, tonic activity of nociceptive C fibers results in hyperexcitability of dorsal horn neurons. Next, the release of substance P and glutamate from primary afferent fibers contributes to sensitization of dorsal horn neurons.

The increased excitability of spinal cord neurons results in enlarged receptive field areas.[46] Another phenomenon, 'windup,' reflects the progressive increase in excitability of spinal cord neurons to successive stimuli-activating C fibers. As a result of sensitization and windup, stimuli of the same intensity are perceived as stronger. FM patients demonstrate abnormally excessive sensitization and windup as compared to controls.[47]

Descending inhibitory pain pathways normally inhibit the transmission of sensory input to the brain through the release of neurotransmitters, such as noradrenaline and serotonin, which are associated with changes in pain and mood. In FM patients, however, these processes may be impaired, thus increasing the effect of central sensitization.[48]

### Spinal glia

Central sensitization and modulation of pain transmission in the spinal cord seems to be facilitated by factors emanating from activated glia. The three main types of glial cells in the CNS i.e., the oligodendroglia, microglia, and astrocytes, act not only as supportive 'glue' between the different neuronal cell types, but are also functionally active. Glia have recently emerged as key contributors to pathological and chronic pain mechanisms.

It is now believed that dorsal horn glia are activated by various painful stimuli and the release of microglial stressors such as ATP, substance P, and various chemokines. Microglial activation releases proinflammatory cytokines, nitric oxide, prostaglandins, reactive oxygen species, and ATP, and contributes to changes in gene expression, central sensitization, neuroinflammation, and neuropathic pain.[49 50]

### Hypothalamic-pituitary-adrenal axis and sympathetic nervous system

"The function of the hypothalamic-pituitary physiology is of fundamental importance to the whole neuroendocrine system."[51]

Fibromyalgia is frequently described as a stress-related disorder associated with an altered stress reaction/response system. Stress can be defined as the result of physically injurious conditions (such as infections and myocardial infarction) and any state that tends to disturb one's normal physiological equilibrium. Stress can also have a psychological origin (such as anxiety, anger, and panic). Many aspects of human physiology may be involved in the response to stress, and therefore intensity of stress, psychoemotional status, and ability to deal with stress may affect health.

In fact, stress is quite often considered as a state of threatened homeostasis. In the 1930s, however, Hans Selye coined the terms "eustress" and "distress" to explain that not all states of stress, or challenges to homeostasis, were harmful. He thought, on the contrary, that minor, transitory, states of challenged homeostasis may act as positive stimuli and that only unmanageable circumstances of psychological and physical difficulty are harmful to health.[52]

Patients with FM frequently associate environmental triggers with the onset of their symptoms. In a study of 2,596 people with FM, about 79% of individuals indicated some triggering event occurring "around the same time that FM symptoms first became apparent."[53] Among them, over 73% reported emotional trauma or chronic stress. Acute illness and physical stressors, such as surgery, motor vehicle accidents, and other injuries, were the next most common events. Additionally, emotional distress was the main factor perceived to worsen the symptoms of FM.[54] In fact, women with FM were particularly susceptible to negative psychosocial stress, compared to osteoarthritis patients with similar levels of pain.[55]

The two major components of the stress system are the hypothalamic-pituitary-adrenal (HPA) axis and the ANS. They interact constantly with each another to maintain homeostasis, and dysfunction in this dynamic system leads to chronic diseases. Fibromyalgia patients demonstrate dysfunction of the stress response system, and both hypo- and hyperactivity of the HPA axis and ANS may exist in these individuals.[56]

The HPA axis is a complex feedback loop that involves the hypothalamus, the pituitary, and the adrenal glands. Interestingly, OMT, in particular cranial osteopathy, has long been suggested to affect the HPA axis: "The hypothalamic and pituitary bodies do have structural and functional interrelationship. Cerebrospinal fluid surrounds both of these tissues, and as the fluid can be effected in its movement and physiology from external manipulation, it follows that through the application of cranial technic (*sic*) we have the most efficient control of hypothalamic-pituitary activity."[57]

Major hormones activate the HPA axis: corticotropin-releasing hormone (CRH), arginine vasopressin (AVP) from the paraventricular nucleus of the hypothalamus, and adrenocorticotropin hormone (ACTH) from the anterior pituitary. The adrenal cortex is then stimulated by ACTH to secrete cortisol. Additionally, there is negative feedback caused by the release of cortisol upon the hypothalamus and pituitary. Among its different effects, the release of cortisol into the circulation increases blood glucose in response to increased metabolic demand. Cortisol also affects the immune system and prevents the release of immunotransmitters. The HPA axis is also under the influence of neuropeptides and neurotransmitters from other regions of the brain, such as the hippocampus and amygdala.

Under normal conditions, the secretion of cortisol, serotonin, melatonin, other hormones, and neurotransmitters is influenced by the circadian rhythm. A master pacemaker located in the supra-chiasmatic nucleus (SCN) of the hypothalamus regulates the circadian rhythm and synchronizes other cellular circadian oscillators within the body. The environmental light-dark cycle resets the circadian rhythm to a period of 24.18 hours.[58] Normally, cortisol levels are high in the morning and decreased at night, and the HPA axis is considered to be a closed-loop system, where the increase of cortisol secretion, following stress, is normalized in a 24 hour period. Studies show that HPA axis physiology is altered in FM patients, and that the rhythm of their hormonal secretion is disturbed, with the level of cortisol elevated in the evening.[59] It is hypothesized that the lack of circadian variation in basal hypercortisolemia demonstrates a declining ability of the HPA axis to return to baseline after a challenge.[60] Loss of resiliency of the HPA axis after activation occurs in the aging process as well, and may be the result of lifelong exposure to stress.[61]

When physical or emotional stimuli threaten homeostasis, and the organism is no longer capable of producing adaptive responses to stressors "stress turns into distress and homeostasis of the organism is no longer maintained."[62] As such, HPA alterations may play a role in the etiopathology of FM. Additionally, dysfunction of the ANS could be crucial in translating the resultant distress into pain.

The instinctive reaction of 'fight-or-flight' of the ANS, associated with fear, is a perfectly normal response. However, some individuals, as in post-traumatic stress disorder, have become sensitized to situations that unconsciously remind them of a strongly negative physical or emotional experience from their earlier life. They perceive danger in response to signals that remind them of that threat.[63] As such, certain stressors trigger the arousal reaction that would normally be triggered by danger. This then becomes a source of anxiety, a learned, but irrational fear reaction. Moreover, such recurrent 'fight-or-flight' reactions develop a continuous state of arousal without adequate recovery time.[64] This state of anxiety compromises the immune system, promotes inflammation, and increases risk for the early development of several diseases of aging.[65] Anxiety is associated with

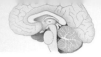

FM, and with other clinical symptoms also associated with FM, such as sleep disorders, pseudo-Raynaud's phenomenon, and intestinal irritability. All of these symptoms may be explained by relentless sympathetic hyperactivity. [66][67][68]

It is suggested that FM is a sympathetically maintained pain syndrome because the pain is submissive to sympathetic blockade and is re-awakened by noradrenaline injections.[69] Indeed, when compared to controls, FM patients, observed for 24 hours while performing their normal daily activities, demonstrate changes consistent with persistent sympathetic hyperactivity, that are particularly evident at night.[70][71] Normally, nocturnal sympathetic activity is less than diurnal sympathetic activity, while parasympathetic activity is dominant in the nocturnal period.[72]

It is of further interest to note that a significant decrease of nocturnal parasympathetic activity occurs with normal aging.[73] This results in the older patient being more susceptible to sympathetically maintained pain in a fashion similar to that seen in FM.

# Sleep disturbances

We spend about one-third of our lives asleep, and sleep disorders represent a major public health threat. About 35% of individuals 65 and older complain of insomnia that diminishes quality of life, decreases cognitive functioning, disturbs mood, and damages social interactions.[74] Sleep disorders have extreme and widespread effects on human health status, including increased risk of hypertension, diabetes, obesity, depression, heart attack, and stroke, in turn leading to significant healthcare costs.

## Normal sleep

Normal sleep consists of two types of sleep that alternate: non-rapid eye-movement (NREM) sleep and rapid eye-movement (REM) sleep. Non-rapid eye-movement sleep is further divided into stages 1, 2, and 3. Thus, a sleep cycle begins with a short phase of NREM stage 1, progressing through stage 2, followed by stages 3 and REM. However, sleep does not progress through these stages in sequence. After stage 1, 2, and 3, stage 2 is repeated before going on to REM sleep. This sequence of NREM and REM constitutes a single sleep cycle and can be repeated approximately four to six times a night, each cycle lasting about 90 to 110 minutes.[75]

Under normal conditions, each of the three stages of NREM sleep are related to distinctive brain activity and physiology such as more synchronous cortical neuron activity, stable auto-nomic function, variations in eye movements, and muscle tone. During these three stages arousal thresholds gradually increase.

- Stage 1 typically lasts one to seven minutes in the initial sleep cycle. It represents 2–5% of total sleep and is a relatively light stage of sleep that can be disrupted by noise.

- Stage 2 lasts about 10–25 minutes in the initial sleep cycle and progresses with each following cycle. During this stage, EEG demonstrates mixed-frequency activity with occasional series of high-frequency waves known as sleep spindles that are thought to be significant for memory consolidation.[76] Usually, they last 1-2 seconds and are generated by interactions between thalamic and cortical neurons. During stage 2, body temperature starts to decrease and heart rate begins to slow.

- Stage 3 corresponds to previous sleep stages 3 and 4, combined into a single stage 3 in 2008 by the American Academy of Sleep Medicine (AASM).[77] Stage 3 corresponds to the slow-wave sleep (SWS), the delta waves. It represents approximately 20–45% of sleep and is considered to be 'deep' and 'restorative' sleep. Indeed, stage 3 is associated with marked reductions in sympathetic activity resulting in stable breathing and decreased heart rate and blood pressure.[78] Reduced time in SWS is connected to hypertension risk in men over 65 years.[79] Typically, sleepwalking occurs during stage 3.

Rapid eye-movement sleep follows the three stages of NREM sleep. REM sleep was named 'paradoxical sleep' in 1959 by Michel Jouvet, because the EEG trace demonstrates faster waves of small amplitude, similar to that monitored in people who are awake.[80] Additionally, numerous rapid eye movements occur underneath the closed eyelids that give explanation for the name REM. Rapid eye-movement sleep accounts for 20–25% of total sleep—about 90–120 minutes of a night's sleep—and it is the stage of sleep in which our most detailed and strangest dreams occur. Normally, during REM, atonia of skeletal muscles and loss of reflexes protect individuals from 'acting out' their dreams or nightmares while sleeping. REM sleep may also be important for memory consolidation of emotional content.[81] With age, the amount of REM sleep varies greatly.

Regulation of sleep results from the interaction between two mechanisms: one that drives individuals to sleep (process S), and another that keeps them awake (process C). The homeostatic need to sleep builds up during the day, to reach its maximum at the end of the day, and disappears throughout the night. The longer one stays awake, the stronger the homeostatic need to sleep becomes and sleep inexorably occurs. When sleep debt accumulates, brief periods of sleep happen. They last 3-30 seconds, without awareness of the individual, and depending upon the activity of the person at the time they occur, are potentially dangerous.[82]

## Circadian rhythms

The sleep-wake cycle is under the significant influence of circadian rhythms, biological processes that display an endogenous, entrainable oscillation of approximately 24 hours. Besides the sleep-

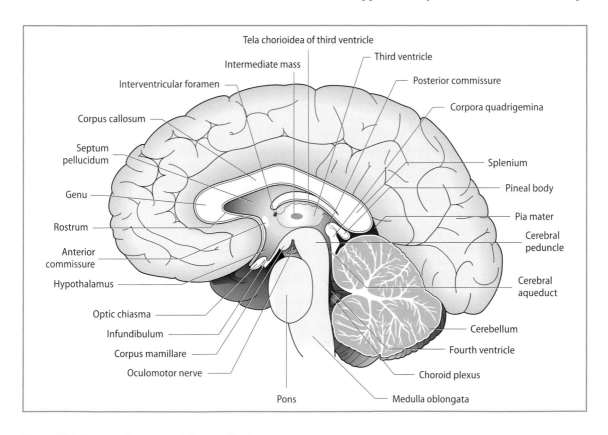

Figure 4.7.3: The hypothalamus and the pineal body

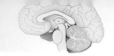

wake cycle, circadian rhythms regulate other functions such as locomotor activity, heartbeat frequency, blood pressure, body temperature, and endocrine release. Conversely, abnormal circadian rhythms are associated with sleep disorders, such as insomnia, and are also linked to obesity, diabetes, depression, bipolar disorder, and seasonal affective disorder.

Circadian rhythms—called the light entrainable oscillation—are driven by a CNS zeitgeber that is continuously reset by the environmental light-dark (LD) cycle.[83] The biological circadian clock was initially believed to be located exclusively in the SCN. Nevertheless, cloning of the 'clock' genes in the late 1990s demonstrated that they are expressed and oscillate with a circadian rhythm in each organ or cell, suggesting that each organ or cell has its own internal clock.[84] These clock systems are called the peripheral clocks, in contrast with the central clock in the SCN.[85] They are believed to interact through molecular pathways involving 'clock' genes. As a 'master clock,' the SCN coordinates all of the peripheral 'clocks' and maintains them in synchrony. The SCN consists of two small, bilateral groups of neurons located in the hypothalamus above the optic chiasma. Light is the most potent stimulus influencing circadian rhythms that turn genes in charge of peripheral clocks on or off. Photic information travels from the retina to the SCN, where circadian rhythms are generated, via the retinohypothalamic tract (RHT).[86]

The paraventricular neurons of the hypothalamus, responding to stimulus from the SCN, travel via the medial forebrain bundle to the intermediolateral column of the upper thoracic spinal cord. From the spinal cord, preganglionic fibers ascend to the superior sympathetic cervical ganglion. From there, postganglionic fibers travel along the carotid artery where some go on to reach the pineal gland. Noradrenaline released from these fibers—primarily during darkness when the SCN is electrically inactive—reaches the pineal cells by diffusion and increases the production of the hormone melatonin.[87] Levels of melatonin are low in the day and rise during the night helping to promote sleep. The importance of the cervical spinal cord in me-

latonin physiology is substantiated after cervical spinal cord injury that results in a loss of the normal melatonin cycle.[88] From an osteopathic point of view, the upper thoracic, upper cervical, and cranial areas must be free of any restriction and somatic dysfunction addressed to optimize circadian physiology. Sutherland described the motion of the pineal body as: "tipping backward when the sphenobasilar is in extension and tipping forward when it is in flexion."[89]

Besides light adjusting the phase of the SCN oscillator to the environmental light-dark cycle, other zeitgebers exist. These external signals from the environment represent fundamental entrainment cues for the peripheral clocks. Among them, daily fasting-feeding cycles are influential. Indeed, the timing of eating affects the expression profile of many circadian genes in peripheral organs, including the liver, kidney, pancreas, and heart.[90] A constant interaction exists between the SCN and peripheral oscillators to maintain circadian rhythms with a period of approximately 24 hours. The circadian pacemaker in association with sleep homeostasis plays fundamental roles in the control of one's state of vigilance.

## Sleep pattern change with age

From birth to maturity, sleep architecture changes significantly. Variations affect the initiation and maintenance of sleep, the importance of each stage of sleep, and sleep effectiveness. Typically, with aging, an increase of sleep disorders, such as sleep apnea and periodic leg movements during sleep, can affect one's sleep. However, sleep changes occur also in healthy individuals, and sleep disorders are not the only explanation for variations in sleep pattern of the aging individual.

With aging, increased stage 1 NREM sleep and a decrease in the number of rapid eye movements occurring during REM sleep are among the main changes in sleep patterns, the decrease of rapid eye movement being more important in men.[91] Additionally, aging of the hypothalamic nuclei that drive circadian rhythms may explain the decrease in the melatonin levels and irregularities in the sleep-wake cycle that occur with aging. As a result, the decrease in sleep homeostasis makes it difficult to

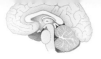
preserve long sleep episodes.[92] The importance of zeitgebers must be recognized here.[93] With aging, lifestyle changes occur including: decreased daylight exposure, irregular feeding times, nocturia, and decreased mobility associated with less physical activity. These factors all contribute to modification of external signals from the environment, compromising entrainment of the circadian clocks.

A complex biopsychosocial matrix is also part of the aging process, with the increase of nightly awakenings and daytime napping. Individuals who live with someone else often have earlier bedtimes, later wake-up times, and greater incidence of daytime napping. Regular sleep schedules seem to be more pronounced for individuals living with another person. Thus, cohabitation may protect against the noticeable chronobiological phase-advance of circadian rhythms classically attributed to the aging process. [94]

## Sleep disorders

The normal sleep duration for adults, including the elderly, is considered to be between seven to nine hours.[95] However, genetics may play an important role in regulating total daily sleep need.[96] Usually, sleep loss is identified when sleep duration lasts less than the average basal need of 7-8 hours per night. Sleep loss causes are multifactorial. Occupational or lifestyle reasons may be involved such as shift work with inconsistent sleep schedule, a poor sleep environment, excessive mental or physical stimulation in the hours before bedtime, and greater access to television and the internet. Other circumstances associated with sleep disorders include: insomnia, sleep apnea, and circadian rhythm disorders.

### Insomnia

Insomnia is usually considered to be difficulty falling asleep, staying asleep, or having adequate sleep duration. It is the most commonly reported sleep problem. Indeed, insomnia affects approximately 35% of the general population, with about 25% of persons reporting occasional insomnia and 9% regular sleep difficulty.[97 98] Insomnia may be associated with psychological stress and hyperarousal experienced throughout the day. Be-

cause insomnia patients demonstrate higher metabolic rates than control group, it is proposed that hyperarousal is associated to physiological or neurophysiological factors.[99] Chronic insomnia is related, as well, to a recurring activation of the stress response system in association with the HPA axis and the hypersecretion of cortisol.

### Obstructive sleep apnea

Obstructive sleep apnea (OSA) is said to be present when major pauses in breathing occur during sleep. (See further: 'Obstructive sleep apnea' in 'Section 4: Clinical considerations, Chapter 4: Respiratory dysfunctions,' p. 277.) Apneas result from full or partial collapse of the pharyngeal airway, which obstructs the intake of oxygen. Thus, blood oxygen saturation diminishes abruptly and intermittently, resulting in sleep arousal. Typically, the return of breathing takes place with noisy gasps and groans. Pharyngeal airway dysfunction is usually more prominent during REM sleep because of hypotonia of the upper-airway muscles occurring during this stage of sleep.[100]

Obstructive sleep apnea affects approximately 16% of men and 5% of women between 30 and 65 years of age, and its prevalence appears to increase with age.[101] Because of possible pathophysiological consequences such as hypertension, acute cardiovascular events, and insulin resistance, OSA should be diagnosed and treated.[102] Repeated arousals and intermittent hypoxemia associated with OSA are responsible for critical hemodynamic and autonomic dysfunction that promotes the development of hypertension.[103]

Besides a possible genetic basis,[104 105] two hypotheses are suggested to explain collapse of the pharyngeal airway in OSA. The neural hypothesis implies changes in neural activation mechanisms intrinsic to sleep,[106] while the anatomic proposition proposes a narrowing of the upper airway.[107] Airway obstruction can occur in areas of the nasopharynx, oropharynx, and hypopharynx. However, in apneic patients, the retropalatal region is significantly smaller, with airway narrowing in the lateral dimension.[108] Several factors are commonly proposed to explain the anatomic origin of the obstruction in a patient with OSA:

- narrowed pharynx[109]
- large tongue or dysfunctional tongue position[110]
- neck flexion and open bite[111]
- long soft palate or uvula, or both[112 113]
- enlarged tonsils[114]
- lowered hyoid bone[115]
- retroposition of the mandible and an increased cranial base flexure[116]

The craniomandibular differences found among OSA patients may explain some of the dysfunctions of soft tissues anchored on the skull and mandible. Sleep posture has also been studied, and more severe apneic events occur in the supine position than in the lateral position.[117] For all these reasons, OMT for somatic dysfunction affecting the cervical spine, cranial base, hyoid bone, and temporomandibular joints is appropriate for the treatment of patients with OSA.

Obesity is a major risk factor,[118] and in obese patients, increased adipose tissue in the neck may predispose the airway to narrowing.[119] Moreover, because sleep apnea is also associated with male gender, postmenopause, and systemic disorders such as hypertension and diabetes, some authors suggest that OSA is a systemic illness; a manifestation of obesity, or the associated inflammation and metabolic anomalies, or both; and not a local abnormality of the respiratory tract.[120] In this hypothesis, central neural mechanisms with hypofunctioning hypothalamic CRH play a key role in the pathogenesis of sleep apnea.

### Impact of sleep disorders

Loss of sleep has an adverse impact on health and quality of life, with multiple effects more or less common for all sleep disorders. Individuals suffering from sleep disorders have excessive daytime sleepiness, more risk for accidents, depressed mood, poor memory, concentration, or both, and increased healthcare utilization. Additionally, insomnia patients may develop a subsequent psychiatric disorder.[121]

Dysfunction of the ANS in cases of sleep loss is well documented. When compared to a control group, the average heart rates of insomnia patients are increased and heart rate variability is decreased in all stages of sleep. This implies that they may be at increased risk for the occurrence of disorders related to increased sympathetic nervous system activity, such as coronary artery disease.[122] Patients with autonomic disorders such as fibromyalgia or CFS also demonstrate sleep disorders, with an increased number of awakenings and nocturnal sympathetic hyperactivity.[123] Additionally, a significant decrease of nocturnal parasympathetic activity occurs with aging that may be observed with a constant decline of cardiac vagal modulation.[124]

Because of the strong connection between the circadian system and the sleep-wake cycle, sleep disorders are frequently associated with disruption of the circadian rhythm. The circadian system and the normal sleep and wake phases influence numerous physiological functions with fluctuating characteristics, such as the core body temperature and the secretion of cortisol. Cortisol, one of the principal human glucocorticoids, is a hormone released in stressful situations by the adrenal gland cortex. It regulates significant aspects of physiology, including cardiovascular, metabolic, immunologic, homeostatic, and even higher brain functions. Cortisol is referred to as the hormone of awakening. Its concentration starts to rise about 2-3 hours after sleep onset. It reaches a release peak in the morning at approximately 9 am. This is followed by a regular decrease as the day continues, until a nadir is reached around midnight.[125]

Circadian control of rhythmic glucocorticoid production and secretion implies the integrated activity of multiple regulatory mechanisms i.e., the central pacemaker (SCN), the peripheral clocks in the adrenal gland, and a central regulation mediated via the HPA axis and the ANS. Conversely, glucocorticoids send signals everywhere in the body to reset the peripheral clocks, contributing to circadian rhythms.

Circadian rhythms and sleep synchronization are essential for immune system reactivity, a system particularly altered in presence of chronic stress.[126] Indeed, loss of sleep interferes with immunosupportive functions within the body and modifies the nocturnal release of glucocorticoids. Sleep deprivation is a stressor that stimulates the activity of the neuroendocrine stress systems i.e., the HPA axis and the autonomic sympathoadre-

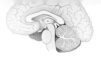

nal axis. Chronic sleep loss, therefore, promotes metabolic and endocrine alterations, increasing the gravity of age-related pathologies, such as diabetes and hypertension.[127] [128] In contrast, a large epidemiologic study of a population of chronic widespread pain subjects showed that, independent of changes in psychological factors, restorative sleep was associated with a resolution of symptoms and the return to musculoskeletal health.[129]

# Influence of the autonomic nervous system on menopause

Menopause is a normal biological process, not a disorder. It is the natural cessation of menstruation and fertility that usually occurs between the ages of 45 and 55. During menopause, a woman's ovaries stop releasing ova and produce less estrogen and progesterone. After 12 months of amenorrhea a woman is said to be postmenopausal. Multiple symptoms are typically associated with menopause. They include:

- Cessation of menstrual periods.
- Vasomotor instability: hot flashes, hot flushes, night sweats, and, in some people, cold flashes.
- Vascular instability: irregular heartbeat and headaches.
- Insomnia and lack of energy.
- Mood changes: irritability, depression, and anxiety.
- Genitourinary disorders: vaginal dryness, breast tenderness, and urinary incontinence.
- Muscle pains, joint pains, and osteoporosis.

Although many symptoms often occur together, this does not support the concept of a universal menopausal syndrome consisting of both vasomotor and psychological symptoms. Among the most frequent symptoms, while not universally reported, are hot flashes and night sweats. Furthermore, women who report vasomotor symptoms do not necessarily report other symptoms. In a large study of the prevalence of various symptoms in a multiethnic sample of American menopausal women, about 55% of them reported hot flashes or night sweats during late perimenopause, a number that declines to 44% in postmenopause.[130]

Multiple factors influence the prevalence and severity of menopausal symptoms including: race, ethnicity, and demographic and lifestyle aspects. A large intercultural disparity exists with regard to hot flashes. Studies have shown that vasomotor symptoms affect 0% of the Mayan women in Mexico, 18% of Chinese women, 70% of North American women, and 80% of Dutch women.[131] However, cultural sensitivity displays multiple subtleties. For instance, for Mayan women, menopause is not associated with physical or emotional symptomatology, and they have no terminology for hot flashes.[132] Across the United States, ethnicity also plays a part and vasomotor symptoms are more widespread in African-American and Hispanic women, and more frequent in women with greater BMI. Overall, hot flashes exhibit large variability in their frequency and severity.

Biocultural factors also affect the attitude of women towards menopause. When premenopausal women were asked if menopause had some positive aspects, 67.3% of women in Germany gave a positive answer, versus 95.2% in Papua New Guinea.[133] In general, women who have more negative attitudes report more symptoms during the menopausal transition.[134] Stress, lower income, and fear of aging also affect menopausal symptoms,[135] and there is constant epidemiological evidence to indicate that smoking increases the risk for hot flashes.[136]

Vasomotor symptoms, such as hot flashes are a sensation of warmth, often accompanied by cutaneous vasodilatation and skin flushing, with perspiration or profuse sweating. Heart rate may increase from 5-25 beats per minute. Sometimes, hot flashes are followed by a chill, when core body temperature drops, following the fast increase in heat loss caused by sweating and cutaneous vasodilatation. These symptoms can be sporadic or repeated, and they last from seconds to an hour. Frequent vasomotor symptoms can be a nuisance, affecting women's daily activities, social life, psychological health, sense of well-being, and ability to work, significantly decreasing their overall quality of life. Additionally, vasomotor symptoms can disturb sleep. The prevalence of symptoms of chronic insomnia increased

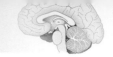

with the severity of hot flashes, carrying with them the adverse impact on health associated with loss of sleep.[137] Additionally, vasomotor symptoms represent a significant socioeconomic burden, with direct and indirect costs that include traditional pharmacotherapy as well as complementary and alternative medicine modalities.[138]

The pathophysiology of hot flashes is not yet fully understood. Many studies have focused on how diminished hormones and hormonal fluctuations that occur during the menopausal transition affect vasomotor symptoms in women. It is clear from multiple observations that estrogen plays some role, and estrogen has been used to treat hot flashes for over 60 years. However, studies evaluating the relation between estrogen levels and occurrence of hot flashes in symptomatic and asymptomatic women demonstrate conflicting results, and the mechanism explaining its action is still in question.[139] Although hot flashes clearly accompany the estrogen withdrawal at menopause, estrogen alone is not entirely responsible.

Transient dysregulation of the thermoregulatory system situated in the hypothalamus has also been implied as an etiology for vasomotor symptoms.[140] Estrogen and neurotransmitters, especially noradrenaline and serotonin, may play a major role in the altered homeostatic thermoregulatory mechanisms. More research, in several fields including endocrinology, neurophysiology, and thermoregulatory physiology, is necessary to better understand the pathophysiology of hot flashes.

Besides the diverse symptoms described, it is known that with the onset of menopause, women become at higher risk for cardiovascular disorders. This may be due to the decline in estrogen levels, to the aging process, or to dysregulation of the ANS. Usually, blood pressure (BP) is lower in premenopausal women than in men, but after menopause, the prevalence of hypertension is higher in women than in men. Hypertension is one of the significant cardiovascular risk factors that play a role in morbidity and mortality in postmenopausal women.[141] Regulation of BP is under the control of the renin-angiotensin system. The sympathetic component of the ANS is also a significant regulator of BP, and as such, a contributor to the pathogenesis of hypertension. In fact, through menopause, there is an increase in sympathetic nervous activity that may be related to impaired central modulation of baroreflex.[142]

Autonomic dysfunction, in fact, plays a role in hypertension as well as in menopausal hot flashes. The increase in heart rate, flushing, and sweating occurring throughout hot flashes are signs of ANS involvement. Furthermore, heart rate variability, an index of vagal control of heart rate, is significantly decreased during hot flashes, as compared to the minutes preceding and following hot flashes.[143 144]

## The osteopathic contribution to the physical examination and treatment

"The greatest and most direct conditioner of stress reactions are membranous articular strains in the craniosacral mechanism that lead to a disturbance of mobility and motility of the cranial articular mechanism, abnormal patterns of mobility of the reciprocal tension membrane, venous retardation, loss of mobility and motility of the pituitary gland within the sella turcica, disturbances of the hypothalamic areas, hyper and hypo irritability of the central innervation of the sympathetic and parasympathetic nervous systems, and hormonal changes that accompany all of this reaction to strain and stress."[145]

Osteopathic philosophy and its clinical application offer an integrated approach to patients suffering from ANS dysfunctions. The diagnosis of somatic dysfunction and application of OMT procedures should be taken into consideration when addressing dysfunctional imbalance between parasympathetic and sympathetic activity. OMT is, however, specifically used in the treatment of somatic dysfunction. It is not a specific treatment for organic pathology.

Following holistic principles, a complete physical examination is indispensable for a good diagnosis of ANS dysfunction. The osteopathically

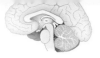

distinctive contribution to the physical examination is the evaluation of the neuromusculoskeletal system for somatic dysfunction both in the context of its local impact and its holistic implications. In order to obtain the best information during the examination and treatment, the patient must feel safe: "If neuroception identifies a person as safe, then a neural circuit actively inhibits areas in the brain that organize the defensive strategies of fight, flight, and freeze."[146]

In the standing position, observe the patient's posture. Pay particular attention to zones that may contribute to ANS dysfunction, such as the sacral, thoracic, and craniocervical areas. Palpation for function, with tests of listening, can be done in this position. See 'Observation and palpation in the standing position' in 'Section 2: Osteopathic Assessment,' p. 46. Complete the assessment with the patient seated, prone, and supine.

In each of the positions that the patient assumes during the examination, observe the posture that the patient spontaneously assumes, noting any asymmetries. The patient usually positions themselves in a release position consistent with their underlying dysfunctional pattern. Question about any areas of discomfort, and as appropriate address any such discomfort by repositioning the patient and, if necessary, by placing pillows to adjust the patient's position.

Observe the breathing pattern of the patient, and note any signs of nervousness. Listen to, and assess the pelvic area, the spine, the ribs, and thoracic inlet, and the cranial, thoracoabdominal, and pelvic diaphragms. Pay attention to the quality of connective tissue; this is of particular importance with FM patients. Treat identified dysfunctions. The treatment of the diaphragms with resultant synchronization of the frequencies of pulmonary and cranial respiration is particularly beneficial for patients with ANS dysfunction.

Sympathetic imbalance can result from somatic dysfunction between T1–L2 where preganglionic sympathetic fibers arise. If necessary, inhibition or stimulation procedures of these areas may be applied for a rapid effect. For a long lasting result, any somatic dysfunction of these areas should be addressed.

Parasympathetic imbalance may be the result of somatic dysfunction of the cranial base (the sphenoid, temporal bones, occiput, occipitomastoid sutures, and jugular foramina affecting CNs III, VII, IX, and X) and occipitoatlantal areas through CN X, and somatic dysfunction of the sacral region through the sacral nerves. These areas should be evaluated carefully and treated as necessary.

Venous and lymphatic drainage should also be considered when addressing autonomic dysfunction. Osteopathic procedures aim to promote fluid, electrolyte, and metabolic exchange within the tissues to facilitate drainage of edema compromising optimal function. Any treatment done employing the PRM facilitates these results.

With the patient supine, using a vault hold, examine the skull. Evaluate the quality of the PRM, and its palpable sensation, the cranial rhythmic impulse (CRI). Assess the power of the PRM and the frequency of the CRI. The potency of the PRM is usually decreased in patients with ANS dysfunctions. Look for somatic dysfunction affecting the motion of the skull and the PRM, which may include the structures of the skull, the cervical area, or somewhere lower in the body. The dysfunction acts as an anchor towards which all tissues seem to be attracted and the restriction of motility is indicative of the site of the dysfunction. Address any such somatic dysfunction.

Next, evaluate the membranous patterns of the cranial mechanism, paying close attention to the HPA axis. Below the hypothalamus, visualize the sella turcica, where the pituitary rests surrounded by dural expansions of the tentorium cerebelli, which also gives rise to the diaphragma sellae. Sutherland stated: "The hypothalamus, including the infundibulum and pituitary body, goes up and down rhythmically as the sphenoid circumrotates back and forth on its transverse axis."[147] Assess the poles of attachment of the tentorium cerebelli on the superior borders of the petrous portions of the temporal bones and the clinoid processes of the sphenoid bone. Assess the falx cerebri on the occipital squama, interparietal suture, and frontal bone.

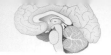

The meninges are in close relationship with the cerebrospinal fluid (CSF). Visualize and assess the ventricles and the CSF fluctuation. Cerebrospinal fluid flows from the lateral ventricles to the interventricular foramina, third ventricle, cerebral aqueduct, fourth ventricle, and through the foramen of Magendie and foramina of Luschka to the subarachnoid space over the brain and spinal cord. The third ventricle is above the sella turcica of the sphenoid that contain the pituitary gland, and in front of the pineal gland. The fourth ventricle is above and behind the back of the pons and medulla oblongata, and below the cerebellum. Remember that the CSF is reabsorbed by the arachnoid granulations mainly located in the calvaria, to then return to the vascular system, but that it also courses along the cranial and spinal nerves as they exit respectively from the skull and vertebral spine, to diffuse into the lymphatic channels. Follow the CSF and the tissues of the skull to a point of balanced membranous tension, or articular release, or both, and let the potency of the PRM attain a still point.

If necessary, employ specific procedures to accelerate (bilateral rotation of the temporal bones) or to temper (compression of the fourth ventricle – CV4) the PRM and the fluctuation of the CSF, which increases tone of the sympathetic or the parasympathetic systems respectively. According to Sutherland: "No one is too sick for fourth ventricle compression and in almost any case, if you do not know what else to do, compress the fourth ventricle."[148] Compression of the fourth ventricle is said to stimulate the HPA axis[149] and has been shown to affect the ANS through its affect upon baroreflex physiology.[150]

It should be recognized that any technique that relaxes the patient will be beneficial. That may, for instance, include massage of the back, the face, the feet, or the hands. It may also involve the use of global myofascial release techniques. However, in order to obtain a more prolonged and effective result, somatic dysfunction must be precisely diagnosed and addressed.

There is an intimate relationship between the ANS and the PRM. The dynamic exchange between sympathetic dominance and parasympathetic dominance is likely linked to the inspiratory flexion-external rotation and expiratory extension-internal rotation oscillatory phases of the PRM. As such, paying close attention to the inherent motility of the PRM and working in synchronicity with it will positively affect the treatment of ANS dysfunction.

The dosage of any OMT procedure is critical, particularly with the sensitive elderly patient who presents with dysfunction of the ANS. Procedures should be chosen wisely, and dosed according to the palpatory findings.

# Advice to the patient

An individualized program should be proposed to the patient, which may change over time according to the patient's responses. Explain to the patient that they should learn to 'listen' to their body and follow what it tells them. One of the goals is to promote parasympathetic activity which tends to decline in aging individuals. They should therefore try to avoid stressful events as much as possible, and try to learn to cope with stress.

Each patient with dysautonomia, CFS, FM, or those having disorders associated with sleep and menopause would benefit from relaxation techniques such as deep breathing, guided imagery, progressive muscle relaxation, or meditation. Regular exercise should be encouraged, but it should be adapted to the tolerance of the individual patient. Often, CFS individuals are too fatigued, and FM subjects in too much pain, to do anything. They will feel discouraged to be told one more time that they should exercise, when it means difficulty and pain. Here, you can explain to them that they can begin with breathing exercises and gentle stretches that can be done in bed. Slow, deep breathing is an excellent way to balance the ANS, trying progressively to comfortably reach six breaths per minute (inhale for four seconds and exhale and relax for six seconds). If the patient finds this respira-

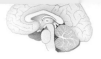

tory exercise overly difficult they can be encouraged to chant[151] or sing.[152] Women with menopausal vasomotor symptoms can practice slow breathing exercises whenever they perceive a hot flash starting to come on.

Teach your patients soft or light exercises such as the ones proposed with 'Autogenic Functional Balancing[SM]' or 'Senti Sur Soi.'[153] Insist on the fact that these exercises should bring pleasure and reconciliation with their body. Educate your patients to learn to stop before they begin to feel tired and encourage them to take frequent rest periods. Make them aware

that, as they feel better, they might be tempted to overdo their activity and as a result, experience regression. When possible, walking is an excellent exercise.

Educate your patients on the healing qualities of refreshing sleep. Insist on the necessity of a good night's sleep in a dark room to promote melatonin secretion, and as much as possible, regular bedtime and wake-up times to stay in synchrony with a beneficial circadian rhythm.

A good diet is part of the wellness program. A balanced diet must include a variety of vegetables, fruits, and whole grains

with limited saturated fats, oils, and sugars. Women with vasomotor symptoms should avoid spicy foods and alcohol that can trigger the symptoms. To reinforce a good circadian rhythm, meals should be taken at regular times of the day to entrain the peripheral clocks of the digestive tract. Encourage your patient to lose weight if necessary, particularly OSA patients, since obesity increases their symptoms.

For every patient, stress the positive benefits of the advice, not the mandatory aspect of it. Reinforce progress accomplished by your patient.

# References

1. Arouet FM. Lettre V. A Mr. l'Abbé Trublet. Lettres de M. de Voltaire à ses amis du Parnasse. Londres. Chez J. Nourse Libraire du Roi; 1766:42.

2. Pennazio S. Homeostasis: a history of biology. Riv Biol. 2009 May-Aug;102(2):253-71.

3. Gross CG. Claude Bernard and the constancy of the internal environment. Neuroscientist. 1998;4:380-5.

4. Enfield RE. Homeostasis. In: Weiner IB, Craighead WE, ed. The Corsini Encyclopedia of Psychology. Vol 2. 4th ed. Hoboken, NJ: John Wiley & Sons, Inc; 2010: 773.

5. Kandel ER, Schwartz JH, Jessell TM, eds. Chapter 49, The autonomic nervous system and the hypothalamus. In: Principles of Neural Science, 4th ed. New York: McGraw-Hill Medical, 2000: 961.

6. Kandel ER, Schwartz JH, Jessell TM, eds. Chapt. 49, The autonomic nervous system and the hypothalamus. In: Principles of Neural Science, 4th ed. New York: McGraw-Hill Medical, 2000: 961.

7. Willard FH. Chapt 10. Autonomic nervous system. In: Chila AG. ed. Foundations of Osteopathic Medicine. 3rd ed. Philadelphia: Wolters Kluwer/Lippincott Williams and Wilkins. 2011: 134-61.

8. Larson NJ. Functional vasomotor hemiparasthesia syndrome. Year Book of the Academy of Applied Osteopathy. American Academy of Osteopathy. Indianapolis, IN. 1970: 39-44.

9. Larson NJ. Osteopathic manipulation for syndromes of the brachial plexus. J Am Osteopath Assoc. 1972 Dec;72(4):378-84.

10. Walton FC. Chapt 23. The Patient with Larson's Functional Vasomotor Hemipares-

thesia Syndrome. In: Somatic Dysfunction in Osteopathic Family Medicine. Nelson KE, Glonek T, eds. Baltimore, MD: Lippincott, Williams & Wilkins; 2007:342-359.

11. Duncan G. Mind-body dualism and the biopsychosocial model of pain: what did Descartes really say? J Med Philos. 2000 Aug;25(4):485-513.

12. Robertson D, Diedrich A, Chapleau MW. Editorial on Arterial Baroreflex Issue. Auton Neurosci. 2012 Dec 24;172(1-2):1-3.

13. Robertson D, Diedrich A, Chapleau MW. Editorial on Arterial Baroreflex Issue. Auton Neurosci. 2012 Dec 24;172(1-2):1-3.

14. Freeman R, Wieling W, Axelrod FB, Benditt DG, Benarroch E, Biaggioni I, et al. Consensus statement on the definition of orthostatic hypotension, neurally mediated syncope and the postural tachycardia syndrome. Clin Auton Res. 2011 Apr;21(2):69-72.

15. Freeman R, Wieling W, Axelrod FB, Benditt DG, Benarroch E, Biaggioni I, et al. Consensus statement on the definition of orthostatic hypotension, neurally mediated syncope and the postural tachycardia syndrome. Clin Auton Res. 2011 Apr;21(2):69-72.

16. Freeman R, Wieling W, Axelrod FB, Benditt DG, Benarroch E, Biaggioni I, et al. Consensus statement on the definition of orthostatic hypotension, neurally mediated syncope and the postural tachycardia syndrome. Clin Auton Res. 2011 Apr;21(2):69-72.

17. Larson NJ. Functional vasomotor hemiparasthesia syndrome. Year Book of the Academy of Applied Osteopathy. American Academy of Osteopathy. Indianapolis, IN. 1970: 39-44.

18. Nelson KE. Osteopathic medical considerations of reflex sympathetic dystrophy. J Am Osteopath Assoc. 1997 May;97(5):286-9.

19. Kappler RE, Kelso AF. Thermographic studies of skin temperature in patients receiving osteopathic manipulative treatment for peripheral nerve problems. J Am Osteopath Assoc 1984;84(1):76-EOA.

20. Nelson KE. Osteopathic medical considerations of reflex sympathetic dystrophy. J Am Osteopath Assoc. 1997 May;97(5):286-9.

21. Chronic fatigue syndrome (CFS). Centers for Disease Control and Prevention. Available at http://www.cdc.gov/cfs/general/index.html. Accessed Dec 6, 2012.

22. Jason LA, Richman JA, Rademaker AW, Jordan KM, Plioplys AV, Taylor RR, McCready W, Huang CF, Plioplys S. A community-based study of chronic fatigue syndrome. Arch Intern Med. 1999 Oct 11;159(18):2129-37.

23. Ranjith G. Epidemiology of chronic fatigue syndrome. Occup Med (Lond). 2005 Jan;55(1):13-9.

24. Afari N, Buchwald D. Chronic fatigue syndrome: a review. Am J Psychiatry. 2003 Feb;160(2):221-36.

25. White KP, Speechley M, Harth M, Ostbye T. Co-existence of chronic fatigue syndrome with fibromyalgia syndrome in the general population. A controlled study. Scand J Rheumatol. 2000;29(1):44-51.

26. Freeman R, Komaroff AL. Does the chronic fatigue syndrome involve the autonomic nervous system? Am J Med. 1997 Apr;102(4):357-64.

27. Beaumont A, Burton AR, Lemon J, Bennett BK, Lloyd A, Vollmer-Conna U. Reduced car-

diac vagal modulation impacts on cognitive performance in chronic fatigue syndrome. PLoS One. 2012;7(11):e49518.

28. Thayer JF, Yamamoto SS, Brosschot JF. The relationship of autonomic imbalance, heart rate variability and cardiovascular disease risk factors. Int J Cardiol. 2010 May 28;141(2):122-31.

29. Fibromyalgia. Centers for Disease Control and Prevention. Available at http://www.cdc.gov/Arthritis/basics/fibromyalgia.htm. Accessed Dec 8, 2012.

30. White KP, Speechley M, Harth M, Ostbye T. The London Fibromyalgia Epidemiology Study: the prevalence of fibromyalgia syndrome in London, Ontario. J Rheumatol. 1999 Jul;26(7):1570-6.

31. Neumann L, Buskila D. Epidemiology of fibromyalgia. Curr Pain Headache Rep. 2003 Oct;7(5):362-8.

32. Wolfe F, Smythe HA, Yunus MB, Bennett RM, Bombardier C, Goldenberg DL, et al. The American College of Rheumatology 1990 Criteria for the Classification of Fibromyalgia. Report of the Multicenter Criteria Committee. Arthritis Rheum. 1990 Feb;33(2):160-72.

33. Wolfe F, Clauw DJ, Fitzcharles MA, Goldenberg DL, Katz RS, Mease P, et al. The American College of Rheumatology preliminary diagnostic criteria for fibromyalgia and measurement of symptom severity. Arthritis Care Res (Hoboken). 2010 May;62(5):600-10.

34. Wolfe F, Clauw DJ, Fitzcharles MA, Goldenberg DL, Katz RS, Mease P, et al. The American College of Rheumatology preliminary diagnostic criteria for fibromyalgia and measurement of symptom severity. Arthritis Care Res (Hoboken). 2010 May;62(5):600-10.

35. Buskila D, Neumann L, Sibirski D, Shvartzman P. Awareness of diagnostic and clinical features of fibromyalgia among family physicians. Fam Pract. 1997 Jun;14(3):238-41.

36. Buskila D, Neumann L, Sibirski D, Shvartzman P. Awareness of diagnostic and clinical features of fibromyalgia among family physicians. Fam Pract. 1997 Jun;14(3):238-41.

37. Wolfe F, Clauw DJ, Fitzcharles MA, Goldenberg DL, Katz RS, Mease P, et al. The American College of Rheumatology preliminary diagnostic criteria for fibromyalgia and measurement of symptom severity. Arthritis Care Res (Hoboken). 2010 May;62(5):600-10.

38. Buskila D, Neumann L, Hazanov I, Carmi R. Familial aggregation in the fibromyalgia syndrome. Semin Arthritis Rheum. 1996 Dec;26(3):605-11.

39. Kato K, Sullivan PF, Evengård B, Pedersen NL. Importance of genetic influences on chronic widespread pain. Arthritis Rheum. 2006 May;54(5):1682-6.

40. Buskila D, Sarzi-Puttini P, Ablin JN. The genetics of fibromyalgia syndrome. Pharmacogenomics. 2007 Jan;8(1):67-74.

41. Arnold LM, Hudson JI, Hess EV, Ware AE, Fritz DA, Auchenbach MB, et al. Family study of fibromyalgia. Arthritis Rheum. 2004 Mar;50(3):944-52.

42. Bellato E, Marini E, Castoldi F, Barbasetti N, Mattei L, Bonasia DE, Blonna D. Fibromyalgia syndrome: etiology, pathogenesis, diagnosis, and treatment. Pain Res Treat. 2012;2012:426130.

43. Petzke F, Clauw DJ, Ambrose K, Khine A, Gracely RH. Increased pain sensitivity in fibromyalgia: effects of stimulus type and mode of presentation. Pain. 2003 Oct;105(3):403-13.

44. Arroyo JF, Cohen ML. Abnormal responses to electrocutaneous stimulation in fibromyalgia. J Rheumatol. 1993 Nov;20(11):1925-31.

45. Gerster JC, Hadj-Djilani A. Hearing and vestibular abnormalities in primary fibrositis syndrome. J Rheumatol. 1984 Oct;11(5):678-80.

46. Li J, Simone DA, Larson AA. Windup leads to characteristics of central sensitization. Pain. 1999 Jan;79(1):75-82.

47. Staud R, Vierck CJ, Cannon RL, Mauderli AP, Price DD. Abnormal sensitization and temporal summation of second pain (wind-up) in patients with fibromyalgia syndrome. Pain. 2001 Mar;91(1-2):165-75.

48. Russell IJ, Michalek JE, Vipraio GA, Fletcher EM, Javors MA, Bowden CA. Platelet 3H-imipramine uptake receptor density and serum serotonin levels in patients with fibromyalgia/fibrositis syndrome. J Rheumatol. 1992 Jan;19(1):104-9.

49. O'Callaghan JP, Miller DB. Spinal glia and chronic pain. Metabolism. 2010 Oct;59 Suppl 1:S21-6.

50. Jha MK, Jeon S, Suk K. Glia as a Link between Neuroinflammation and Neuropathic Pain. Immune Netw. 2012 April; 12(2): 41-47.

51. Sutherland WG. Contributions of thought. Fort Worth, TX: Sutherland Cranial Teaching Foundation, Inc.; 1998:339.

52. Chrousos GP, Gold PW. The concepts of stress and stress system disorders. Overview of physical and behavioral homeostasis. JAMA. 1992 Mar 4;267(9):1244-52.

53. Bennett RM, Jones J, Turk DC, Russell IJ, Matallana L. An internet survey of 2,596 people with fibromyalgia. BMC Musculoskelet Disord. 2007 Mar 9;8:27.

54. Bennett RM, Jones J, Turk DC, Russell IJ, Matallana L. An internet survey of 2,596 people with fibromyalgia. BMC Musculoskelet Disord. 2007 Mar 9;8:27.

55. Davis MC, Zautra AJ, Reich JW. Vulnerability to stress among women in chronic pain from fibromyalgia and osteoarthritis. Ann Behav Med. 2001 Summer;23(3):215-26.

56. Williams DA, Clauw DJ. Understanding fibromyalgia: lessons from the broader pain research community. J Pain. 2009 Aug;10(8):777-91.

57. Cottrille WP. The management of hypothalmic-pituitary activity through the cranial concept. Year Book of the Academy of Applied Osteopathy. American Academy of Osteopathy. Indianapolis, IN. 1945:74.

58. Glonek T, Sergueef N, Nelson KE. Physiological Rhythms/Oscillations. Chapt 11. In: Chila AG. ed. Foundations of Osteopathic Medicine. 3rd ed. Philadelphia: Wolters Kluwer/Lippincott Williams and Wilkins. 2011:162-190.

59. Crofford LJ, Young EA, Engleberg NC, Korszun A, Brucksch CB, McClure LA, Brown MB, Demitrack MA. Basal circadian and pulsatile ACTH and cortisol secretion in patients with fibromyalgia and/or chronic fatigue syndrome. Brain Behav Immun. 2004 Jul;18(4):314-25.

60. Sapolsky RM, Krey LC, McEwen BS. The neuroendocrinology of stress and aging: the glucocorticoid cascade hypothesis. Endocr Rev. 1986 Aug;7(3):284-301.

61. Crofford LJ, Young EA, Engleberg NC, Korszun A, Brucksch CB, McClure LA, et al. Basal circadian and pulsatile ACTH and cortisol secretion in patients with fibromyalgia and/or chronic fatigue syndrome. Brain Behav Immun. 2004 Jul;18(4):314-25.

62. Schweinhardt P, Fitzcharles MA, Boomershine C, Vierck C, Yunus MB. Fibromyalgia as a disorder related to distress and its therapeutic implications. Pain Res Treat. 2012;2012:950602.

63. Lovy, A. Chapt 7, The Psychiatric Patient. In: Somatic Dysfunction in Osteopathic Family Medicine. Nelson KE, Glonek T, eds. Baltimore, MD: Lippincott, Williams & Wilkins; 2007:73-86.

64. Foxman P. Dancing with fear, 2nd ed. Alameda CA: Hunter House Inc. Publishers, 2007.

65. O'Donovan A, Slavich GM, Epel ES, Neylan TC. Exaggerated neurobiological sensitivity to threat as a mechanism linking anxiety with increased risk for diseases of aging.Neurosci Biobehav Rev. 2012 Nov 2;37(1):96-108.

66. Martinez-Lavin M. Biology and therapy of fibromyalgia. Stress, the stress response system, and fibromyalgia. Arthritis Res Ther. 2007;9(4):216.

67. Sarzi-Puttini P, Atzeni F, Cazzola M. Neuroendocrine therapy of fibromyalgia syndrome: an update. Ann N Y Acad Sci. 2010 Apr;1193:91-7.

68. Smith HS, Harris R, Clauw D. Fibromyalgia: an afferent processing disorder leading to a complex pain generalized syndrome. Pain Physician. 2011 Mar-Apr;14(2):E217-45.

69. Martinez-Lavin M. Fibromyalgia as a sympathetically maintained pain syndrome. Curr Pain Headache Rep. 2004 Oct;8(5):385-9.

70. Martinez-Lavin M. Fibromyalgia as a sympathetically maintained pain syndrome. Curr Pain Headache Rep. 2004 Oct;8(5):385-9.

71. Doğru MT, Aydin G, Tosun A, Keleş I, Güneri M, Arslan A, et al. Correlations between autonomic dysfunction and circadian changes and arrhythmia prevalence in women with fibromyalgia syndrome. Anadolu Kardiyol Derg. 2009 Apr;9(2):110-7.

72. Bonnemeier H, Richardt G, Potratz J, Wiegand UK, Brandes A, Kluge N, et al. Circadian profile of cardiac autonomic nervous modulation in healthy subjects: differing effects of aging and gender on heart rate variability. J Cardiovasc Electrophysiol 2003; 14: 791-9.

73. Furlan R, Colombo S, Perego F, Atzeni F, Diana A, Barbic F, et al. Abnormalities of cardiovascular neural control and reduced orthostatic tolerance in patients with primary fibromyalgia. J Rheumatol. 2005 Sep;32(9):1787-93.

74. McCrae CS, Wilson NM, Lichstein KL, Durrence HH, Taylor DJ, Riedel BW, Bush AJ. Self-reported sleep, demographics, health, and daytime functioning in young old and

old old community-dwelling seniors. Behav Sleep Med. 2008;6(2):106-26.

75. Luyster FS, Strollo PJ Jr, Zee PC, Walsh JK; Boards of Directors of the American Academy of Sleep Medicine and the Sleep Research Society. Sleep: a health imperative. Sleep. 2012 Jun 1;35(6):727-34.

76. Schabus M, Gruber G, Parapatics S, Sauter C, Klösch G, Anderer P, et al. Sleep spindles and their significance for declarative memory consolidation. Sleep. 2004 Dec 15;27(8):1479-85.

77. Schulz H. Rethinking sleep analysis. J Clin Sleep Med. 2008 Apr 15;4(2):99-103.

78. Luyster FS, Strollo PJ Jr, Zee PC, Walsh JK; Boards of Directors of the American Academy of Sleep Medicine and the Sleep Research Society. Sleep: a health imperative. Sleep. 2012 Jun 1;35(6):727-34.

79. Fung MM, Peters K, Redline S, Ziegler MG, Ancoli-Israel S, Barrett-Connor E, Stone KL; Osteoporotic Fractures in Men Research Group. Decreased slow wave sleep increases risk of developing hypertension in elderly men. Hypertension. 2011 Oct;58(4):596-603.

80. Mayet L. Interview de Michel Jouvet. Science et Avenir, Hors Série, le Rêve, Déc. 1996.

81. Groch S, Wilhelm I, Diekelmann S, Born J. The role of REM sleep in the processing of emotional memories: Evidence from behavior and event-related potentials. Neurobiol Learn Mem. 2012 Oct 30. pii: S1074-7427(12)00125-6.

82. Luyster FS, Strollo PJ Jr, Zee PC, Walsh JK; Boards of Directors of the American Academy of Sleep Medicine and the Sleep Research Society. Sleep: a health imperative. Sleep. 2012 Jun 1;35(6):727-34.

83. Inouye S-I T, Shibata S. Neurochemical organization of circadian rhythm in the suprachiasmatic nucleus. Neurosci Res. 1994;20(2):109-130.

84. King DP, Zhao Y, Sangoram AM, Wilsbacher LD, Tanaka M, Antoch MP, et al. Positional cloning of the mouse circadian Clock Gene. Cell. 1997;89(4):641-653.

85. Maemura K, Takeda N, and Nagai R. Circadian rhythms in the CNS and peripheral clock disorders: Role of the biological clock in cardiovascular diseases. J Pharmacol Sci. 2007;103:134-138.

86. Gooley JJ, Lu J, Chou TC, Scammell TE, Saper CB. Melanopsin in cells of origin of the retinohypothalamic tract. Nat Neurosci. 2001 Dec;4(12):1165.

87. Physiology of the pineal gland. Available at http://www.neuroradiology.ws/pinealosmasphysiology.htm. Accessed Dec 19, 2012.

88. Kneisley LW, Moskowitz MA, Lynch HG. Cervical spinal cord lesions disrupt the rhythm in human melatonin excretion. J Neural Transm Suppl. 1978;(13):311-23.

89. Sutherland WG. Contributions of thought. Fort Worth, TX: Sutherland Cranial Teaching Foundation, Inc.; 1998:337.

90. Dibner C, Schibler U, Albrecht U. The mammalian circadian timing system: organization and coordination of central and peripheral clocks. Annu Rev Physiol. 2010;72:517-49.

91. Wauquier A. Aging and changes in phasic events during sleep. Physiol Behav. 1993 Oct;54(4):803-6.

92. Dijk DJ, Duffy JF, Czeisler CA. Contribution of circadian physiology and sleep homeostasis to age-related changes in human sleep. Chronobiol Int. 2000 May;17(3):285-311.

93. Glonek T, Sergueef N, Nelson KE. Physiological Rhythms/Oscillations. Chapt 11. In: Chila AG. ed. Foundations of Osteopathic Medicine. 3rd ed. Philadelphia: Wolters Kluwer/Lippincott Williams and Wilkins. 2011:162-190.

94. Bliwise DL, Ansari FP, Straight LB, Parker KP. Age changes in timing and 24-hour distribution of self-reported sleep. Am J Geriatr Psychiatry. 2005 Dec;13(12):1077-82.

95. 'How Much Sleep Do We Really Need?' National Sleep Foundation. Available at http://www.sleepfoundation.org/article/how-sleep-works/how-much-sleep-do-we-really-need. Accessed Dec 23, 2012.

96. He Y, Jones CR, Fujiki N, Xu Y, Guo B, Holder JL Jr, et al. The transcriptional repressor DEC2 regulates sleep length in mammals. Science. 2009 Aug 14;325(5942):866-70.

97. Ancoli-Israel S, Roth T. Characteristics of insomnia in the United States: results of the 1991 National Sleep Foundation Survey. I. Sleep. 1999 May 1;22 Suppl 2:S347-53.

98. McCrae CS, Wilson NM, Lichstein KL, Durrence HH, Taylor DJ, Riedel BW, Bush AJ. Self reported sleep, demographics, health, and daytime functioning in young old and old old community-dwelling seniors. Behav Sleep Med. 2008;6(2):106-26.

99. Roth T. Insomnia: definition, prevalence, etiology, and consequences. J Clin Sleep Med. 2007 Aug 15;3(5 Suppl):S7-10.

100. Strollo PJ Jr, Rogers RM. Obstructive sleep apnea. N Engl J Med. 1996 Jan 11;334(2):99-104.

101. Ancoli-Israel S, Kripke DF, Klauber MR, Mason WJ, Fell R, Kaplan O. Sleep-disordered breathing in community-dwelling elderly. Sleep. 1991 Dec;14(6):486-95.

102. Pack AI. Advances in sleep-disordered breathing. Am J Respir Crit Care Med. 2006 Jan 1;173(1):7-15.

103. Strollo PJ Jr, Rogers RM. Obstructive sleep apnea. N Engl J Med. 1996 Jan 11;334(2):99-104.

104. Schwab RJ. Genetic determinants of upper airway structures that predispose to obstructive sleep apnea. Respir Physiol Neurobiol. 2005 Jul 28;147(2-3):289-98.

105. Song CM, Lee CH, Rhee CS, Min YG, Kim JW. Analysis of genetic expression in the soft palate of patients with obstructive sleep apnea. Acta Otolaryngol. 2012 Jun;132 Suppl 1:S63-8.

106. Ayappa I, Rapoport DM. The upper airway in sleep: physiology of the pharynx. Sleep Med Rev. 2003 Feb;7(1):9-33.

107. Sforza E, Bacon W, Weiss T, Thibault A, Petiau C, Krieger J. Upper airway collapsibility and cephalometric variables in patients with obstructive sleep apnea. Am J Respir Crit Care Med. 2000 Feb;161(2 Pt 1):347-52.

108. Schwab RJ, Gupta KB, Gefter WB, Metzger LJ, Hoffman EA, Pack AI. Upper airway and soft tissue anatomy in normal subjects and patients with sleep-disordered breathing. Significance of the lateral pharyngeal walls. Am J Respir Crit Care Med. 1995 Nov;152(5 Pt 1):1673-89.

109. Isono S, Remmers JE, Tanaka A, Sho Y, Sato J, Nishino T. Anatomy of pharynx in patients with obstructive sleep apnea and in normal subjects. J Appl Physiol. 1997 Apr;82(4):1319-26.

110. Schwab RJ, Pasirstein M, Pierson R, Mackley A, Hachadoorian R, Arens R, et al. Identification of upper airway anatomic risk factors for obstructive sleep apnea with volumetric magnetic resonance imaging. Am J Respir Crit Care Med. 2003 Sep 1;168(5):522-30.

111. Isono S, Tanaka A, Tagaito Y, Ishikawa T, Nishino T. Influences of head positions and bite opening on collapsibility of the passive pharynx. J Appl Physiol. 2004 Jul;97(1):339-46.

112. Jamieson A, Guilleminault C, Partinen M, Quera-Salva MA. Obstructive sleep apneic patients have craniomandibular abnormalities. Sleep. 1986 Dec;9(4):469-77.

113. Partinen M, Guilleminault C, Quera-Salva MA, Jamieson A. Obstructive sleep apnea and cephalometric roentgenograms. The role of anatomic upper airway abnormalities in the definition of abnormal breathing during sleep. Chest. 1988 Jun;93(6):1199-205.

114. Togeiro SM, Chaves CM Jr, Palombini L, Tufik S, Hora F, Nery LE. Evaluation of the upper airway in obstructive sleep apnoea. Indian J Med Res. 2010 Feb;131:230-5.

115. Fusco G, Macina F, Macarini L, Garribba AP, Ettorre GC. Magnetic resonance imaging in simple snoring and obstructive sleep apnea-hypopnea syndrome. Radiol Med. 2004 Sep;108(3):238-54.

116. Jamieson A, Guilleminault C, Partinen M, Quera-Salva MA. Obstructive sleep apneic patients have craniomandibular abnormalities. Sleep. 1986 Dec;9(4):469-77.

117. Oksenberg A, Khamaysi I, Silverberg DS, Tarasiuk A. Association of body position with severity of apneic events in patients with severe nonpositional obstructive sleep apnea. Chest. 2000 Oct;118(4):1018-24.

118. Pack AI. Advances in sleep-disordered breathing. Am J Respir Crit Care Med. 2006 Jan 1;173(1):7-15.

119. Schwab RJ. Pro: sleep apnea is an anatomic disorder. Am J Respir Crit Care Med. 2003 Aug 1;168(3):270-1; discussion 273.

120. Vgontzas AN. Does obesity play a major role in the pathogenesis of sleep apnoea and its associated manifestations via inflammation, visceral adiposity, and insulin resistance? Arch Physiol Biochem. 2008 Oct;114(4):211-23.

121. Roth T. Insomnia: definition, prevalence, etiology, and consequences. J Clin Sleep Med. 2007 Aug 15;3(5 Suppl):S7-10.

122. Bonnet MH, Arand DL. Heart rate variability in insomniacs and matched normal sleepers. Psychosom Med. 1998 Sep-Oct;60(5):610-5.

123. Becker S, Schweinhardt P. Dysfunctional neurotransmitter systems in fibromyalgia, their role in central stress circuitry and pharmacological actions on these systems. Pain Res Treat. 2012;2012:741746.

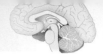

124. Furlan R, Colombo S, Perego F, Atzeni F, Diana A, Barbic F, et al. Abnormalities of cardiovascular neural control and reduced orthostatic tolerance in patients with primary fibromyalgia. J Rheumatol. 2005 Sep;32(9):1787-93.

125. Buckley TM, Schatzberg AF. On the interactions of the hypothalamic-pituitary-adrenal (HPA) axis and sleep: normal HPA axis activity and circadian rhythm, exemplary sleep disorders. J Clin Endocrinol Metab. 2005 May;90(5):3106-14.

126. Cutolo M, Buttgereit F, Straub RH. Regulation of glucocorticoids by the central nervous system. Clin Exp Rheumatol. 2011 Sep-Oct;29(5 Suppl 68):S-19-22.

127. Spiegel K, Leproult R, Van Cauter E. Impact of sleep debt on metabolic and endocrine function. Lancet. 1999 Oct 23;354(9188):1435-9.

128. Meerlo P, Sgoifo A, Suchecki D. Restricted and disrupted sleep: effects on autonomic function, neuroendocrine stress systems and stress responsivity. Sleep Med Rev. 2008 Jun;12(3):197-210.

129. Davies KA, Macfarlane GJ, Nicholl BI, Dickens C, Morriss R, Ray D, McBeth J. Restorative sleep predicts the resolution of chronic widespread pain: results from the EPIFUND study. Rheumatology (Oxford). 2008 Dec;47(12):1809-13.

130. Avis NE, Brockwell S, Colvin A. A universal menopausal syndrome? Am J Med. 2005 Dec 19;118 Suppl 12B:37-46.

131. Bachmann GA. Vasomotor flushes in menopausal women. Am J Obstet Gynecol. 1999 Mar;180(3 Pt 2):S312-6.

132. Beyene Y. Cultural significance and physiological manifestations of menopause. A biocultural analysis. Cult Med Psychiatry. 1986 Mar;10(1):47-71.

133. Kowalcek I, Rotte D, Banz C, Diedrich K. Women's attitude and perceptions towards menopause in different cultures. Cross-cultural and intra-cultural comparison of pre-menopausal and post-menopausal women in Germany and in Papua New Guinea. Maturitas. 2005 Jul 16;51(3):227-35.

134. Ayers B, Forshaw M, Hunter MS. The impact of attitudes towards the menopause on women's symptom experience: a systematic review. Maturitas. 2010 Jan;65(1):28-36.

135. Nosek M, Kennedy HP, Beyene Y, Taylor D, Gilliss C, Lee K. The effects of perceived stress and attitudes toward menopause and aging on symptoms of menopause. J Midwifery Womens Health. 2010 Jul-Aug;55(4):328-34.

136. Whiteman MK, Staropoli CA, Benedict JC, Borgeest C, Flaws JA. Risk factors for hot flashes in midlife women. J Womens Health (Larchmt). 2003 Jun;12(5):459-72.

137. Ohayon MM. Severe hot flashes are associated with chronic insomnia. Arch Intern Med. 2006 Jun 26;166(12):1262-8.

138. Utian WH. Psychosocial and socioeconomic burden of vasomotor symptoms in menopause: a comprehensive review. Health Qual Life Outcomes. 2005 Aug 5;3:47.

139. Kronenberg F. Menopausal hot flashes: a review of physiology and biosociocultural perspective on methods of assessment. J Nutr. 2010 Jul;140(7):1380S-5S.

140. Freedman RR. Core body temperature variation in symptomatic and asymptomatic postmenopausal women: brief report. Menopause. 2002 Nov-Dec;9(6):399-401.

141. Taddei S. Blood pressure through aging and menopause. Climacteric. 2009;12 Suppl 1:36-40.

142. Vongpatanasin W. Autonomic regulation of blood pressure in menopause. Semin Reprod Med. 2009 Jul;27(4):338-45.

143. Thurston RC, Sutton-Tyrrell K, Everson-Rose SA, Hess R, Matthews KA. Hot flashes and subclinical cardiovascular disease: findings from the Study of Women's Health Across the Nation Heart Study. Circulation. 2008 Sep 16;118(12):1234-40.

144. Thurston RC, Christie IC, Matthews KA. Hot flashes and cardiac vagal control: a link to cardiovascular risk? Menopause. 2010 May-Jun;17(3):456-61.

145. Becker RE. Diagnostic touch: its principles and application. Part IV. Trauma and stress. Year Book of the Academy of Applied Osteopathy. American Academy of Osteopathy. Indianapolis, IN. 1965; 2:174.

146. Porges SW. The Polyvagal Theory: Neurophysiological Foundations of Emotions, Attachment, Communication, and Self-regulation. New York:WW Norton and Company; 2011.

147. Sutherland WG. Contributions of thought. Fort Worth, TX: Sutherland Cranial Teaching Foundation, Inc.; 1998:338.

148. Magoun HI. Osteopathy in the cranial field. Kirksville, MO: The Journal Printing Company; 1951:82.

149. Magoun HI. Osteopathy in the cranial field. Kirksville, MO: The Journal Printing Company; 1951:85.

150. Nelson KE, Sergueef N, Glonek T. The effect of an alternative medical procedure upon low-frequency oscillations in cutaneous blood flow velocity. J Manipulative Physiol Ther. 2006 Oct;29(8):626-36.

151. Bernardi L, Sleight P, Bandinelli G, Cencetti S, Fattorini L, Wdowczyc-Sculc J, Lagi A. Effect of rosary prayer and yoga mantras on autonomic cardiovascular rhythms: Comparative study. Brit Med J 2001;323(7327):1446-9.

152. Niu NN, Perez MT, Katz JN. Singing intervention for preoperative hypertension prior to total joint replacement: a case report. Arthritis Care Res (Hoboken). 2011 Apr;63(4):630-2.

153. Sergueef N, Nelson KE, Glonek T. The effect of light exercise upon blood flow velocity determined by laser-Doppler flowmetry. J Med Eng Technol. 2004 Jul-Aug;28(4):143-50.

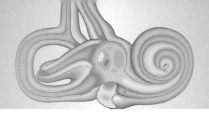

# Chapter 8

# Auditory and visual dysfunctions

## Auditory dysfunctions

Hearing or audition is the ability to perceive sound waves, to distinguish their frequencies, and to convey auditory information into the central nervous system (CNS). We will review two dysfunctions affecting hearing in the older patient: presbycusis (hearing loss) and tinnitus.

## Presbycusis

About 30% of 65 year old individuals have some degree of hearing loss, a number that increases to 47% after the age of 75. Indeed, hearing loss is the third most frequent chronic condition after hypertension and arthritis. In the United States, 17% of the adult population demonstrates some degree of hearing loss.[1]

The term presbycusis, also presbyacusis or presbyacousia, is derived from the Greek 'presbys' (elder) and 'akousis' (hearing), and indicates the loss of ability to perceive or discriminate sounds associated with aging. Initially, there is a diminished ability to understand speech and, afterward, the capacity to detect, identify, and localize sounds. Reduced hearing sensitivity usually starts with the highest sound frequencies, consonants such as 'S' and 'F', children's and women's voices, and then progress gradually to the lower frequencies. As hearing loss progresses, causing more difficulty in noisy environments, communication is affected, which can contribute to elder isolation, depression, and, in some cases, dementia. Furthermore, potential danger exists as the individual is no longer capable of detecting or localizing high-frequency warning sounds such as beepers and alarm signals.

Although aging is associated with presbycusis, there are other risk factors, including exposure to noise,[2] cigarette smoking,[3] ototoxic medication,[4] a genetic susceptibility stronger in women than in men,[5][6] and health co-morbidities such as atherosclerosis[7] and diabetes mellitus.[8] Indeed, presbycusis is caused by a combination of auditory stresses that can be cumulative over a lifetime. Exposure to noise, such as recreational noise, listening to loud music, shooting guns, or noise associated with some working conditions, has a deleterious effect on hearing. People living in industrialized societies are particularly at risk.[9]

### Presbycusis anatomopathology

The ear consists of three parts: the external ear, the middle ear, and the inner ear. Although there is a consensus that stresses the importance of the inner ear as the most prominent element in presbycusis, a review of the different parts of the ear is appropriate to understand the involved mechanisms.[10]

#### The external ear

The external ear consists of the auricle (pinna) and the auditory canal ending medially at the tympanic membrane or eardrum. Only vertebrates have an auricle and an external auditory canal. In other animals, such as the Galapagos iguana, the external tympanum appears on the lateral surface of the head.[11] The external ear identifies the direction of sound, reduces low frequencies, and acts as a resonator to increase the amplitude of the incoming sound wave within the range of frequencies for human speech.[12] Thereby, the auricle provides efficient sound transmission from the environment to the tympanic membrane.

Size and shape of the auditory canal differs between individuals. Usually sigmoid in shape, and about 2.5 cm in length, the auditory canal has rigid walls protecting the tympanic membrane and the

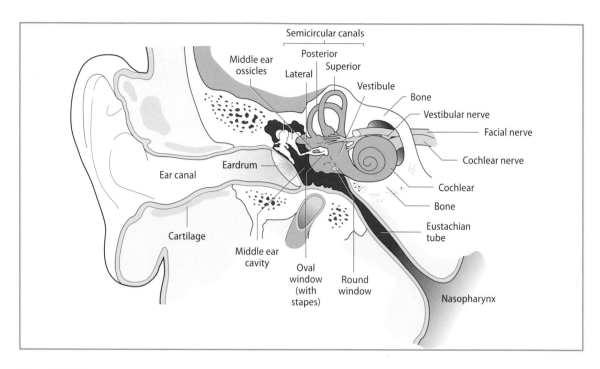

Figure 4.8.1: The ear

middle ear from direct injury. The outer third of the canal displays a stratified epithelium with specialized ceruminous glands. Cerumen cleans, lubricates, and protects the ear canal from bacteria and fungus.[13]

Still specifically used the understanding of cerumen as an example of the application of osteopathic principles to the practice of medicine, and he made an association between upper and lower respiratory tract illness and the presence of dessicated, impacted cerumen through neuro-reflex mechanisms, particularly involving the pneumogastric (vagus) nerve.[14] It is of interest to note that, because of the sensory innervation of the external auditory canal by the auditory branch of the vagus nerve, cerumen impaction is known to be associated with chronic cough.[15]

### Age-related changes to the external ear

As the individual ages, the production of large amounts of cerumen, associated with inadequate epithelial migration, may result in impacted cerumen that produces itching, tinnitus, vertigo, and hearing loss and may be a frequent cause of

hearing aid malfunction. Other changes that occur in the external ear with aging include hair growth in the external canal, especially in males, and enlargement of the auricles,[16] potentially affecting the transmission of sounds.

### The middle ear

The middle ear is an air-filled cavity in the petrous part of the temporal bone, located between the external canal and the labyrinth. Laterally, it is separated from the external canal by the tympanic membrane. Medially, it is separated from the inner ear by the round and oval windows. The middle ear communicates posteriorly with the mastoid air cells, and anteriorly with the nasopharynx via the pharyngotympanic (Eustachian or auditory) tube. Within the middle ear chamber are the three smallest bones in the body: the ossicles. They contribute to the transmission and amplification of the vibrations from the tympanic membrane to the inner ear.

The ossicles are:

- the malleus, or hammer, attached to the tympanic membrane;

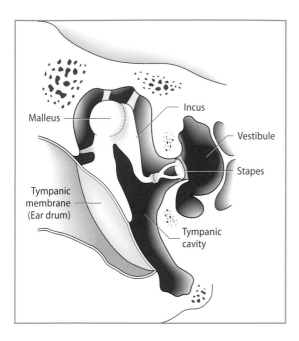

Figure 4.8.2: The ossicles of the middle ear

- the incus, or anvil, linked to the malleus;
- the stapes, or stirrup, connected to the incus and the lateral wall of the inner ear at the oval window.

Two muscles, the tensor tympani and the stapedius, are situated within the middle ear. They participate in the regulation of high intensity sounds.

The tensor tympani muscle arises from the cartilaginous portion of the pharyngotympanic tube, the adjoining part of the greater wing of the sphenoid, and from its bony canal, above the osseous part of the pharyngotympanic tube. It attaches to the upper part of the handle of the malleus. When it contracts, it draws the handle of the malleus medially, regulates the tension on the tympanic membrane, and thereby dampens sounds. Innervation of the tensor tympani is by a branch from the mandibular nerve (CN V3).

The stapedius muscle originates from a small projection on the mastoid wall of the middle ear and attaches to the posterior surface of the neck of the stapes. In response to loud noises, the stapedius muscle contracts, pulling the stapes posteriorly, preventing excessive oscillation.

Innervation of the stapedius is by a branch from the facial nerve (CN VII).

Besides these two muscles, the pharyngotympanic tube contributes also to the protection of the middle ear. It connects the tympanic cavity with the pharynx, and consequently equalizes external and internal pressures applied to the tympanic membrane.

## Middle ear function

Acoustic energy must be transmitted from the air of the external ear to the fluid-filled cochlea of the inner ear. Therefore, the middle ear has to match the impedance between an air environment and a fluid environment. If the sound pressure waves in the air were applied directly to the inner ear fluid, there would be a theoretical loss of 99.9% of the energy, equivalent to 30 dB, due to reflection. The middle ear functions as a pressure amplifier to increase auditory sensitivity.

The arrangement of the ossicular chain bony and ligamentous structures is involved in this process. Forces from sound waves striking the tympanic membrane are transmitted to the stapes footplate with an increased pressure, although with less motion in the stapes than in the malleus.

Normally, the tympanic membrane moves in and out, depending on the sound pressure. Because the malleus is connected to the tympanic membrane, every motion of the tympanic membrane causes the malleus and incus to rotate together, pushing the stapedial footplate towards the labyrinth and its perilymph. Inward movement of the stapes footplate is associated with a compensatory outward bulging of the secondary tympanic membrane (round window membrane). This stimulates the hair cells of the basilar membrane within the cochlea, allowing audition.

## Age-related changes to the middle ear

Opacification of the normally translucent tympanic membrane is commonly seen in older individuals. The tympanic membrane is also stiffer and thinner, with a loss of vascularity. The different components of the middle ear, and associated structures, undergo age-related changes as well. Normally, the levator veli palatini, tensor veli palatini (TVP), and salpingopharyngeus muscles open the pharyngotympanic tube to equalize pressure between the middle ear and the atmosphere. However, with aging they show histopathological changes, and their functions deteriorate.[17] [18] The TVP is particularly vulnerable to these changes. Changes occur also in the cartilaginous part of the pharyngotympanic tube, associated with the alteration of tubal compliance that lead to patulous or stenotic tubes.[19] [20] As a result, the pressure balance mechanism may be less efficient, modifying motion of the ossicles of the ear and contributing to temporary conductive hearing loss. Changes in the ossicular muscles may contribute to this deterioration of sound transmission.[21] The middle ear is also susceptible to inflammatory disease, and middle ear abnormalities and hearing loss are significantly more prevalent in patients with ossicular arthritis than in control patients.[22]

Somatic dysfunction of the temporal bone can also affect the function of the middle ear in the transmission of sounds. As stated by Sutherland: "When the petrous portion is held in internal rotation and the mouth of the auditory tube is held closed, the patient complains of a feeling like cotton stuffed in his ear."[23]

### The inner ear

Located, medially to the middle ear, in the petrous part of the temporal bone, the inner (internal) ear consists of a bony labyrinth that contains perilymph and a membranous labyrinth. The membranous labyrinth consists of a series of endolymph-filled membranous sacs and ducts, the vestibular apparatus, and the cochlear duct. (See further discussion of 'The vestibular sensory system' in 'Section 4: Clinical considerations, Chapter 2: Postural imbalance,' p. 216.)

The cochlear duct is a spiral tube that runs within the coiled bony cochlear portion of the bony labyrinth. The central position of the cochlear duct is the scala media. Above and below it are two chambers: the scala vestibuli above and the scala tympani below. The floor of the cochlear duct (the basilar membrane) contains the organ of Corti (the receptor organ of hearing) with its sensory hair cells.

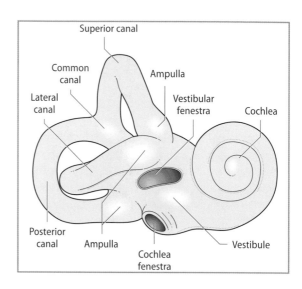

**Figure 4.8.3:** Right osseous labyrinth (lateral view)

The lateral wall of the cochlear duct consists of the spiral ligament that contains the stria vascularis. This has been referred to as the battery of the cochlea.[24] It contributes to ion concentrations in the endolymph and generation of endocochlear electrical potential.

### Inner ear function

When stimulated by sound waves striking the tympanic membrane, the ossicles of the middle ear move, transmitting vibrations to the cochlear fluid, producing oscillations of the sensory hair cells of the organ of Corti. In response, the mechanical stresses are transduced into nerve impulses in the vestibulocochlear nerve (CN VIII), which are transmitted to the auditory areas of the brain for processing.

### Age-related changes to the inner ear

The auditory hair cells of the organ of Corti are often damaged, following a lifetime exposure to loud sounds. Once damaged, mammals, unlike fish, birds, and reptiles, do not replace these hair cells.[25]

Decreased blood flow in the microvasculature of the stria vascularis is commonly seen with aging. This results in metabolic changes that lead to alterations of that tissue, which, in turn, significantly

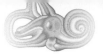

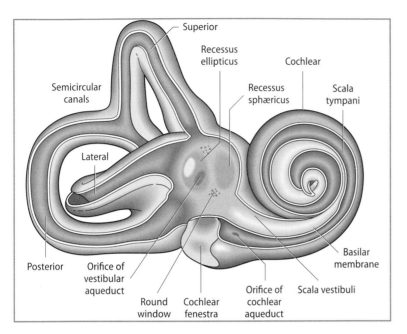

**Figure 4.8.4:** Right osseous labyrinth (interior)

Superior

Recessus
ellipticus

Cochlear

Semicircular
canals

Recessus
sphæricus

Scala
tympani

Lateral

Basilar
membrane

Posterior

Orifice of
vestibular
aqueduct

Round
window

Cochlear
fenestra

Orifice of
cochlear
aqueduct

Scala vestibuli

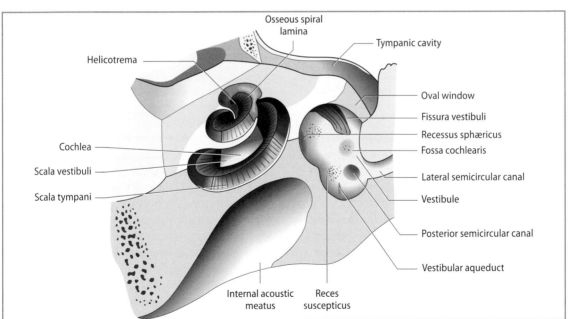

Osseous spiral
lamina

Tympanic cavity

Helicotrema

Oval window

Fissura vestibuli

Recessus sphæricus

Fossa cochlearis

Cochlea

Scala vestibuli

Lateral semicircular canal

Scala tympani

Vestibule

Posterior semicircular canal

Vestibular aqueduct

Internal acoustic
meatus

Reces
suscepticus

**Figure 4.8.5:** The cochlea and vestibule (viewed from above)

affect cochlear physiology and its role as an amplifier, resulting in hearing loss. Damage may be further increased by hypoxic circumstances resulting from the impaired cochlear blood supply due to atherosclerosis.[26] Additionally, oxidative stress is thought to induce apoptosis of the cochlear cells.

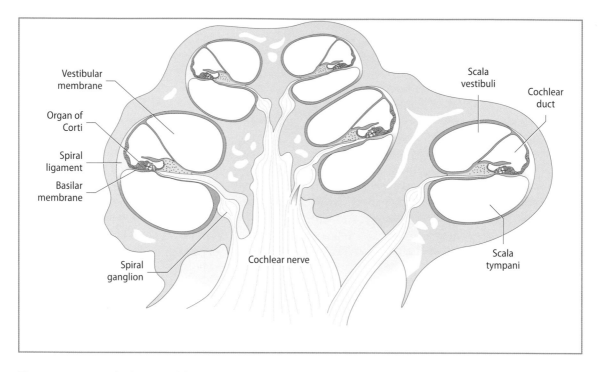

Figure 4.8.6: Longitudinal section of the cochlea

The effect of these stressors is damage or loss of sensory hair cells that results in a common type of hearing impairment classified as sensorineural hearing loss. Another cause of sensorineural hearing loss may be aging of CN VIII with increased thresholds of the compound action potential.

## The classification of presbycusis

Harold F. Schuknecht, a pioneer in the description of the light microscopic findings in the human inner ear, described four types of presbycusis based upon pathological findings: sensory, neural, metabolic, and cochlear conductive.[27] Hearing loss can now be categorized according to the portion of the auditory system that is damaged. Three basic types of hearing loss are identified: sensorineural hearing loss, conductive hearing loss, and mixed hearing loss.

Sensorineural hearing loss occurs when there is damage to the cochlear receptor organ, to the fibers of CN VIII, or to both. Indeed, the amount of hearing loss is associated with the degree of degeneration of the stria vascularis, spiral ganglion cells, and hair cells.[28]

Sensorineural hearing loss may also be associated with dysfunctions in the central auditory pathways. Although a decline in general cognitive processing speed is frequently associated with aging,[29] central hearing loss is often secondary after loss of sensory cells in the cochlea.[30] This process affects speech perception and is referred to as age-related auditory processing disorder.

When hearing loss is not associated with abnormal histopathology, it is referred to as conductive age-related hearing loss. First described by Schuknecht,[31] some authors debate its existence, asserting that modern histochemistry would demonstrate some histological change.[32] However, in conductive hearing loss, sounds reach the tympanic membrane but sound transmission fails to reach the inner ear. The problem can be in the external ear, the ossicular chain of the middle ear, or in the inner ear, where changes in physical properties of the cochlea can modify its mechanical response.[33]

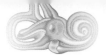

Interestingly, the ear has multiple connections with the temporal bone. The auricle is strongly attached to the temporal bone through extrinsic ligaments and is also connected to the skull and scalp through extrinsic auricular muscles. Further, both the middle and inner ears are lodged inside the petrous part of the temporal bone. It is worthy to note that the two joints located on each side of the petrous part of the temporal bone do not fuse as do other synchondroses of the cranial base. Anteriorly, the petrous portion articulates with the greater wing of the sphenoid bone resulting in the petrosphenoidal fissure. At the medial end of this suture, there is a large foramen—the foramen lacerum. Posteriorly, the petrous portion articulates with the basilar portion of the occipital bone at the petro-occipital suture. Normally, this suture remains patent throughout life and as such should demonstrate motility in all individuals. Observations have been made however, that when this suture does ossify, most often in older males, it is associated with age-related conductive hearing loss.[34] It appears that the petro-occipital suture dampens the transmission of forces transmitted to the skull from below, protecting the cochlear apparatus. Throughout a lifetime, physical stress and resulting somatic dysfunction affecting the upper body can restrict motion across the petro-occipital suture and thereby facilitate its ossification. For this reason, somatic dysfunction of the cranial base, particularly the temporal bones, thoracic inlet, and upper thoracic and cervical spine must be addressed.

# Tinnitus

Frequently, presbycusis is accompanied by tinnitus, the perception of noise in the ears. Tinnitus is classified into two categories: objective and subjective. Objective tinnitus is the result of sound generated within the body and transmitted to the ear. It can sometimes be heard by an observer, often by using a stethoscope and can be the result of blood flow turbulence. This is heard as a pulsatile sound from involved vessels including the large arteries and veins in the neck and base of the skull, and smaller vessels within the ear. Objective tinnitus

may also be associated with noises generated by musculoskeletal motion, often heard as clicking or popping sounds. Subjective tinnitus is heard only by the patient and is more often encountered. It tends to be a steady noise without frequent or regular changes in loudness. Because the severity of tinnitus is assessed by the patient and not measured objectively, epidemiologic studies report differing incidence, between 7.6% and 20.1%, for individuals over age 50.[35]

Described as a phantom sensation,[36] the perception of subjective tinnitus includes noises such as ringing, whistling, buzzing, hissing, roaring, and booming. It may be reported in one or both ears, and may be intermittent or continuous, varying from a low roar to a high squeal. Tinnitus often reduces quality of life and interferes with sleep and concentration.[37]

Several risk factors exist for tinnitus including age, exposure to noise, smoking, cardiovascular problems such as hypertension or atherosclerosis, certain medications such as non-steroidal anti-inflammatory drugs and diuretics, Ménière's disease, vestibular schwannoma, or head trauma. [38] [39] [40] Because tinnitus is a symptom of a myriad of clinical conditions, some potentially very serious, it should be assessed thoroughly before employing osteopathic manipulative treatment (OMT) as a sole treatment intervention.

## Tinnitus pathophysiology

In a large study of tinnitus, patients were asked what they believed had triggered their tinnitus, the answer was noise trauma (18%), followed by head and neck trauma (8%) and ear, nose, and throat infections (8%).[41] However, the cause of tinnitus is not always known and tinnitus may be qualified as idiopathic tinnitus.[42]

Many hypotheses have been suggested to explain the pathophysiological basis of tinnitus. The most common one involves the loss of cochlear hair cells causing afferent neurons to trigger aberrant auditory sensations.[43] An age-related deterioration of neural function or injury to CN VIII may also be the cause of tinnitus. Close contact between a vessel and a cranial nerve may alter neural conduction leading to hyperactive disorders and

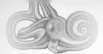

is thought to be the cause of some tinnitus,[44] although vascular loops with CN VIII are also found in patients with no tinnitus.[45] Additionally, multiple vascular etiologies, such as high jugular bulbus and aneurysm of, or an aberrant internal carotid artery, may cause transmission of pulsatile turbulent flow into the inner ear resulting in pulsatile objective tinnitus.[46]

Other sources of tinnitus are qualified as somatic. They are associated with mandibular disorders, such as temporomandibular joint (TMJ) syndrome,[47] or whiplash and head trauma. Following a whiplash injury, about 10% of individuals develop otological symptoms including tinnitus.[48] Displacement of the stapes has been reported after a rear-end collision and whiplash injury with consequent tinnitus.[49]

Considering somatic tinnitus from an osteopathic perspective, it is interesting to note that up to two-thirds of individuals with tinnitus can modulate the loudness or pitch of their tinnitus with jaw movements, craniocervical position change, or pressure applied to head and neck regions.[50] [51] [52] A possible interaction within the CNS between the central auditory nervous system and the central somatosensory system is hypothesized.[53] From clinical experience, however, somatic tinnitus can be improved by treating somatic dysfunctions present in the cranial base, temporal bone, craniocervical junction, cervical spine, and TMJ.[54] [55]

# Visual dysfunctions

The elimination or reduction of the influence of somatic dysfunction from a mechanical, neurophysiological, and circulatory perspective facilitates the body's inherent capacity for self-healing. Osteopathic manipulative treatment may be used for its complementary contribution to the treatment of visual dysfunction, after a complete medical diagnosis has been performed, with a thorough ocular examination, including cornea, lens, retina, and optic nerve, as well as the neurological status of the eye and extraocular muscles (EOM).

As the individual gets older, the prevalence of vision impairment and blindness increases significantly. In 2000, 2.76% of Americans were visually impaired, a number projected to be 3.6% by 2020.[56] Because decreased visual function is related with reduced quality of life and functional

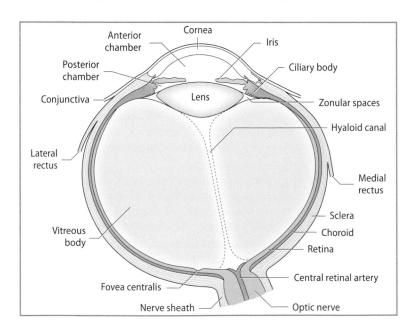

**Figure 4.8.7:** The eyeball (transverse section)

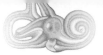

activities of living,[57] OMT should be considered as part of the prevention and treatment of visual impairment. Most common visual disorders include presbyopia, cataracts, glaucoma, and retinal detachment (RD).

## Dysfunctions of the lens

The lens is located between the anterior one-fifth of the eyeball and the posterior four-fifths. It is a biconvex shaped disc, with an anterior layer of epithelial cells covering a mass of elongated fiber cells that give the lens its transparency and refractive properties. A thick capsule surrounding and protecting the lens is attached circumferentially to the ciliary body via the zonular fibers. The ciliary body consists of the ciliary processes and the ciliary muscle. The ciliary muscle is responsible for the lens's refractive ability to maintain visual acuity accommodation. It adjusts the shape of the lens in order to change the focus of the eye. When the ciliary muscle contracts, it draws the ciliary body forward, thus reducing tension in the suspensory ligament. This results in a relaxation of the lens's capsule, with increased convexity of its surface, allowing the lens to adapt for short range focus. With the opposite mechanism, the decreased convexity of the lens adapts for long range focus. The ciliary muscle is controlled almost completely by parasympathetic nerve signals through CN III.

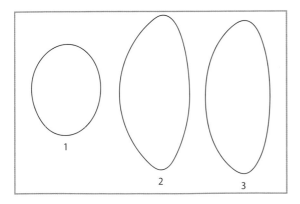

Figure 4.8.8: Profile views of the lens at different periods of life: 1) In the fetus, 2) In adult life, 3) In old age.

### Presbyopia

Accommodation—the change of the shape of the lens in order to focus the image of an external object on the retina—can only occur if the lens is sufficiently pliable. With aging, the lens becomes less elastic, to a certain extent, because of progressive denaturation of the lens's proteins. Its ability to change shape decreases, a condition identified as 'presbyopia,' with resulting blurred vision at a normal reading distance, and the need for the individual to wear bifocal glasses.

### Cataracts

Age-related cataracts refer to any opacification of the lens, the incidence of which is associated with increasing age. Its prevalence doubles with each decade of age after 40 years.[58] Cataracts remain the leading cause of blindness, responsible for 51% of the cases worldwide.[59] The main symptoms include: clouded, blurred, or dim vision; increasing difficulty with vision at night; sensitivity to light and glare; and fading of colors.

Age-related cataracts occur in diverse regions of the lens, described as nuclear, in the center of the lens (23.1%); cortical, involving the capsule of the lens (22.0%); and posterior subcapsular, at the back of the lens beneath the capsule (13.1%).[60] The different locations have different risk factors.[61] Exposure to ultraviolet-B radiation is associated with the development of cortical cataracts and perhaps posterior subcapsular cataracts.[62] Diabetes and smoking are also associated with cortical cataracts. Genetic and severe myopia appears to affect nuclear cataracts.[63][64] Posterior subcapsular cataracts are more prevalent in males, diabetic patients, and corticosteroid use.[65][66]

Initially, the proteins in some fibers of the lens are damaged. Progressively, they replace the normal transparent proteins, a pathogenic transformation that leads to lens opacification and blurred vision. Much of this damage may be linked to oxidative or free radical damage.[67] However, the pathogenic mechanisms underlying the development of cataracts are not completely understood. Surgery may be necessary, with removal of the lens, requiring the placement of a powerful convex lens in front of the eye, or implantation of an artificial lens.

# Glaucoma

Although the word glaukoma was employed as early as the fourth century BC by Hippocrates, it was not until 1626 that it was associated with an elevation of the intraocular pressure (IOP) recognizable by eyeball resistance, and only in the early 1700s that glaucoma became clearly differentiated from cataracts.[68] According to the World Health Organization, glaucoma is now the second leading cause of blindness in the world, after cataracts, and responsible for about 15% of the total burden of world blindness.[69] Prevalence varies with ethnic origin, with people of African or Hispanic ancestry and certain Asian populations most at risk.[70] Additional risk factors include advanced age, positive family history, myopia, and genetic factors. [71] [72] Because of the rapidly aging population demographics, the prevalence of glaucoma is increasing.[73] Thus, OMT for the elimination or reduction of the influence of somatic dysfunction from a mechanical, neurophysiological,

and circulatory perspective might be considered for its role in the prevention of glaucoma and as an adjunct treatment.[74] [75]

## Glaucoma anatomopathology

Besides anchoring the lens and adjusting its refractive ability, the ciliary body, through its ciliary processes, is the source of aqueous humour. Aqueous humour is derived from the plasma in the capillaries of the ciliary processes. It is secreted into the posterior chamber of the eyeball and then passes through the pupil into the anterior chamber, where most of it is drained through the trabecular meshwork of the iridocorneal angle into the canal of Schlemm and the episcleral veins.

### Glaucoma mechanical theory

Deficient drainage of aqueous humour results in the increased IOP that leads to glaucoma. If untreated, elevated IOP can damage the optic nerve and produce a progressive and permanent vision loss.

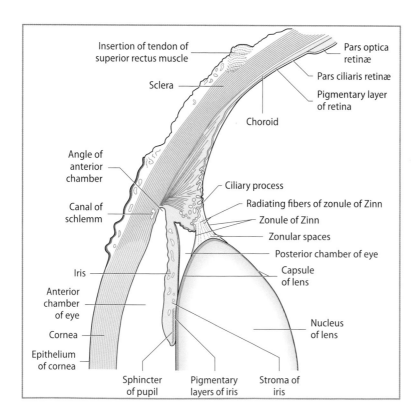

Figure 4.8.9: The upper half of the front of the eyeball (sagittal section)

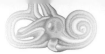

Glaucoma is either 'primary' or 'secondary' to a particular anomaly or disease of the eye. The two main types of primary glaucoma are 'closed-angle' and 'open-angle.' Closed-angle glaucoma, also called acute glaucoma, displays a closed or narrow iridocorneal angle. In that situation, drainage of the aqueous humour is blocked, resulting in a sudden rise in IOP that requires immediate medical attention. Symptoms include: severe eye pain, nausea, sudden visual disturbance, blurred vision with halos around lights, and reddening of the eye.

Open-angle glaucoma, the most common form—also called chronic glaucoma—results from reduced aqueous drainage following pathological changes within the trabecular meshwork of the iridocorneal angle. Although this angle remains wide and open, the IOP rises slowly, in a painless fashion, with visual symptoms of loss of peripheral vision, often appearing very late. Progressively increased IOP produces mechanical damage to retinal ganglion cell axons, impairment of the optic nerve head blood supply, or both, with gradual loss of vision.

### Glaucoma vascular theory

Besides elevated IOP as a major risk factor, there is increasing interest in altered ocular blood flow as a possible pathogenesis of glaucoma. Indeed, all patients with glaucomatous damage do not have an elevated IOP.[76] Normally, sufficient blood flow is necessary to provide oxygen and nutrients to all tissues of the body. However, a vascular dysregulation may exist in the eye, with an inappropriate arterial constriction, a vasospasm, or an inadequate dilation.[77] This vascular dysregulation may be part of a 'vasospastic syndrome' that can be secondary to other diseases, such as autoimmune diseases, or can exist as a primary vasospastic syndrome in response to stimuli like cold or emotional stress.[78] Vascular dysregulation may produce fluctuation in the optic nerve head perfusion with resultant axonal loss and remodeling changes in the optic nerve head.

Vascular regulation in the eye is complex, involving endothelial, neural, and glial cells, hormones, and autonomic innervation. The optic nerve head, retina, and choroid blood flow are under the control of endothelial cells. The vascular endothelium—the interface between the vessel wall and the blood—contributes substantially to angiogenesis, inflammatory responses, hemostasis, and control of vascular tone through the release of vasoactive substances, such as vasoconstrictors ET-1, angiotensin II and thromboxane, and vasodilators such as nitric oxide, prostacyclin, and hydrogen peroxide.[79] Endothelial cellular dysfunction may lead to ischaemia and vascular dysregulation.[80] Additionally, in glaucoma, endothelial dysfunction can affect the trabecular meshwork of the iridocorneal angle and the canal of Schlemm.

Normally, blood flow velocity in the optic nerve head demonstrates characteristics associated with vasomotion, breathing, and cardiac pulsation.[81] In glaucoma with normal IOP, however, most retrobulbar vessels demonstrate reduced blood flow velocities and higher resistive indices i.e., resistance to blood flow within the microvascular bed, distally.[82] Vascular dysregulation of the optic nerve may further make it more susceptible to IOP.

We have proposed that the 6–12 cpm (0.10–0.20 Hz) oscillation, associated with baroreflex and vagal physiology, is the Sutherland wave, or Becker's "fast tide," and that the 0.5–1.2 cpm (0.009–0.02 Hz) oscillation, associated with thermal regulation and endothelially-mediated vasomotion, is Becker's "slow tide." (See further: 'Section 1: Osteopathy, fascia, fluid, and the primary respiratory mechanism,' p. 18.) For these reasons, cranial osteopathy can be applied to contribute to the vascular regulation of the eye.

# Retinal detachment

Aging, extreme myopia, family history of RD, eye injury, RD in the other eye, and cataract surgery are all well-recognized risk factors for RD. A premature birth or other eye diseases or disorders, such as retinoschisis, uveitis, diabetic retinopathy, degenerative myopia, and inflammation are other less common risk factors.[83]

## *Retinal detachment anatomopathology*

The retina—the inner layer of the eyeball—is between 0.2 and 0.4 mm thick. It consists of two strata: the neurosensory retina or inner retina, and the

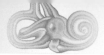

retinal pigment epithelium or outer retina. Light passes through the thickness of the retina before striking and activating the rods' and cones' photoreceptors. Afterward, the absorption of photons by the visual pigment of the photoreceptors is converted into a biochemical message and then an electrical message transmitted to the visual cortex of the brain through the optic nerve.

The retina receives its blood supply from two separate systems, both necessary and both derived from the ophthalmic artery, a branch of the internal carotid artery. The inner retina receives a direct blood supply through capillaries that connect branches of the central retinal artery and vein. The outer retina is avascular and depends on the vascular support provided by the choriocapillaris in the choroid, the connective tissue layer of the eye sandwiched between the retina and the protective outer layer of the eye (the sclera). Indeed, the choroid receives 80% of all ocular blood, and because the distance between the choriocapillaris and the photoreceptors is less than 20 μm, rapid diffusion is possible.

Retinal detachment is separation of the neurosensory retina from the underlying retinal pigment epithelium, and is classified into three groups: serous, tractional, and rhegmatogenous.

### Serous detachment

Serous pigment epithelial detachment occurs due to inflammation, injury, vascular abnormalities, or less often, neoplastic ocular tumors. Fluid accumulates between the neurosensory retina and the retinal pigment epithelium, but the retina remains intact.

### Tractional detachment

The vitreous structure changes with age, particularly after 60 years. Tractional detachment occurs when cells growing in the vitreous humour attach to the surface of the retina and contract. This fibrous or fibrovascular tissue, the 'vitreoretinal adhesions', pulls the neurosensory retina from the retinal pigment epithelium, creating a RD.

### Rhegmatogenous detachment

The most common form of RD arises from a break or tear across the retina, allowing the passage of liquefied vitreous humour through the retinal break. The accumulation of fluid under the retina that follows results in a detachment. Possible factors, such as weakened adhesive force between the retina and vitreous humour, and molecular changes at the vitreoretinal interface can predispose to focal areas of vitreoretinal traction and lead to posterior vitreous detachment.[84]

### Symptoms

Peripheral or central vision is decreased depending upon the type of detachment, its size, and location. Commonly, patients ignore the symptoms of detachments until they approach the macula and produce a defect in the visual field that cannot be ignored. It is often during an ocular examination that RD is discovered. Associated symptoms that should require medical attention include painless vision disturbances, changes in the peripheral visual field, decreased acuity, defective color vision, distorted vision, flashing lights, and increased floaters. Acute rhegmatogenous RD that threatens central vision is an emergency requiring immediate medical attention.

## Changes with age

With aging, changes in the soft tissues of the face occur at the same time that the shape of the facial skeleton remodels. Anterior cheek mass becomes less prominent and the frontal bone moves anteriorly and slightly inferiorly, while the midface rotates posteriorly and slightly superiorly.[85] Thus, the shape, size, and volume of the bony orbits change.[86] Additional cranial somatic dysfunction of any of the orbital structures will contribute to decreased motility of the eyeball, with diminished vascular and fluidic perfusion.

The rhythmic contractions of the intra- and EOM contribute to fluid exchange within the eye and with associated vasculature, and aging affects this system. In older individuals, there is a progressive increase in endomysial fibrosis, changes in myofibers with more variation in fiber size, and loss of the contractile elements in EOM.[87] Relative to the globe center, the lateral and medial recti muscles are located more inferiorly in the aging subject, resulting in more difficulty initiating and

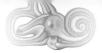

maintaining an upward gaze.[88] Effects from this diminished muscular activity, added to any postural changes, and somatic dysfunction in the craniocervical junction and cervical spine, ultimately contribute to diminished cervico-ocular and vestibulo-ocular reflexes. Visual stability may also be affected. A vicious circle is initiated with compensatory contraction of intra- and EOM resulting in increased ocular tension.

## The osteopathic contribution to the physical examination and treatment

Examination and treatment of any auditory and visual dysfunctions starts with a total-body examination. Postural dysfunctions are frequent in the aging patient and often associated with auditory and visual dysfunctions. In particular, upper thoracic and cervical spine somatic dysfunctions should be addressed because of their relations with the vascular, lymphatic, and autonomic nervous systems that may affect cephalic sensory functions. Myofascial structures attached on the upper thoracic and cervical spine, such as the sternocleidomastoid muscles, may also be responsible for restriction of mobility at the level of the temporal bones and cranial base.

Next, proceed to examine the neurocranium and viscerocranium. This is most easily accomplished with the patient in the supine position. Assess the sphenobasilar synchondrosis and the cranial base, with particular attention to the temporal bones. Visualize the temporal petrous parts, their relationship with the tentorium cerebelli, and the petro-occipital and petrosphenoidal sutures. Check the temporomandibular joints and the occlusal pattern of the patient. Address any dysfunction.

For auditory dysfunctions, remember Sutherland's statement: "Realize that the middle ear is an air sinus. When the petrous portion is held abnormally in external rotation and the mouth of the auditory tube is held open, you can hear the roar."[89] Also Magoun said: "With an external rotation lesion of the temporal, the tube may be held continuously open, and the patient complains of a low-pitched roar. With internal rotation, it may be held closed, accompanied by high-pitched humming or buzzing."[90]

Visualize the middle and inner ear structures within the petrous parts of the temporal bones.

The vascularity of the auditory system is very significant and impaired circulation affects hearing. By following and balancing the inherent motility of the inner ear, you may contribute to the circulation of perilymph and endolymph, and improve blood flow of the microvasculature.

Membranous dysfunctions, as well, are of importance for auditory and visual dysfunctions and should be diagnosed and treated. All of the cranial nerves establish intimate relations with the dura. Cranial nerve VIII does so at the level of the auditory meatus, and CNs III, IV, V1, and VI at the level of the laterosellar compartment (cavernous sinus). The dura forms the floor, roof, lateral, and medial walls of the laterosellar compartment in which these nerves travel, before passing through the superior sphenoidal fissure to enter the orbital cavity. A strong connection exists between the dura of the laterosellar compartment, its content, and the temporal and sphenoid bones.

The internal carotid artery also runs through the laterosellar compartment, before giving off the ophthalmic artery. Within this compartment, the internal carotid artery supplies the blood for the cranial nerves contained there within, and as such, any stasis inside the laterosellar compartment can compromise the vasa nervorum. Following the path of the internal carotid artery, coming from the superior cervical ganglion, on each side, there is also the internal carotid nerve that reaches the laterosellar compartment and supplies the eye.

Inside the laterosellar compartment, the cavernous sinus drains the blood from the superior and inferior ophthalmic veins into the superior and inferior petrosal sinuses, and ultimately through the jugular foramen. As such, the intracranial membranes, in particular the tentorium cerebelli, must be balanced to ensure good venous drainage from the orbits and the eyes, as Sutherland pointed out: "In the case of glaucoma, one may reason that the accumulation of fluid points to a condition somewhere back along the intracranial membranous wall of the cavernous sinus, or in the walls of the petrosal sinus, to a membranous restriction affecting the venous return, and back of that, the possibility of a cranial lesion as an etiological factor."[91] Also, compression of the fourth ventricle is "indicated for venous congestion such as the back pressure through the cavernous or petrosal sinuses in glaucoma and cataract."[92]

There is an anatomic continuity between the dura and the lining and structures of the orbital cavity, the eyeball, and the EOM. At the level of the superior orbital fissure, the endosteal layer of the dura extends through the fissure to blend with the orbital periosteum. Also, a tubular dural sheath from the meningeal layer of the dura encases the optic nerve as it passes through the optic canal. This dural layer blends with the ocular sclera and adheres closely to the common annular tendon of the four recti muscles. As such, any membranous dysfunction in the skull, as well as dysfunction at any distant point, through the core-link, may affect visual function and should be considered in the osteopathic treatment of visual dysfunctions.

The eyeball is contained within, and establishes intimate relationship with, the orbital cavity. One of the main osteopathic principles is that structure and function are interrelated at all levels. Structure determines function and is, in turn, influenced by function and dysfunction. Considering visual dysfunctions, the structures forming the orbital cavity may affect the ocular functions of sight, associated vascular and neurological aspects, and intra- and EOM activity. Therefore, it is appropriate to consider the protective case for the eye, i.e., the orbital cavity, and to see how its osseous components contribute to ocular dysfunction. Cranial flexion-external rotation is associated with a decrease of the orbital depth, whereas extension-internal rotation is associated with increased orbital depth. As such an extension-internal rotation dysfunction, by maintaining an increased anteroposterior orbital dimension, can increase mechanical stress applied upon the eyeball and its contents, contributing to visual dysfunctions.

A release of the ocular muscles is indicated to decrease tension on the eyeball, and to promote fluid exchange. Intraocular fluid stasis, as might contribute to chronic glaucoma, may also be addressed with intraocular fluid balancing. Note however, that acute glaucoma is an emergency requiring immediate medical attention.

## Advice to the patient

In both auditory and visual dysfunctions, managing stress is good advice. Explain to your patient how to relax and how to feel the release of tension in the shoulder and neck and in the auditory and orbital areas. If appropriate, help your patient to cope with decrease or loss of function.

The easiest way to relax both the ears and eyes is to yawn as much as possible. Most of the time, this will open the pharyngotympanic tube, promote drainage of the middle ear, and therefore sound transmission. Teach your patient how to relax the mandible and TMJ with simple motions, such as slowly opening and closing the mouth, without any effort, and gentle motions of diduction to the right and to the left. A sensation of relaxation of the temporal muscles in the temporal fossae should follow.

Patients with hearing loss may be fitted with a hearing aid that amplifies sound. Such devices have shown to be more effective in cases of conductive hearing loss, and have a positive effect on quality of life.[93] However, they often need an adjustment period, and some people find them uncomfortable. Cochlear prostheses have been developed to treat profound sensorineural hearing loss. New therapeutic approaches are currently under investigation to regenerate hair cells.[94]

Explain to your patient that one of the greatest risk factors for presbycusis is exposure to noise, and that deterioration of hearing can be reduced by avoidance of excessive noise exposure. A good diet rich in antioxidants, fruits, and vegetables is recommended. Avoidance of high lipid diets is

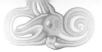

advised as they are associated with poor hearing.[95] There is some evidence, as well, of a significant relationship between systolic blood pressure and hearing loss in the speech frequencies.[96] Thus, acting to prevent hypertension should be considered. (See further: 'Section 4: Clinical considerations, Chapter 3: Cardiovascular dysfunctions,' p. 257.)

Explain to your patient with hearing difficulties that it is important to, as much as possible, maintain communication, and not to withdraw from social interactions. This requires effort and new habits, such as paying more attention, admitting when they don't understand and looking for visual cues, like facial expression and lip motion, when in conversation with others.

Patients with visual dysfunction will also benefit from a good diet. Encourage them to reduce caffeine that, in high amounts, may increase eye pressure. Moderate exercise should be encouraged for its contribution to ocular and perioccular fluid exchange. Also stress the importance of thorough annual visual examinations and the use of corrective eyeglasses that are the most accurate prescription possible.

# References

1. National Institute on Deafness and Other Communication Disorders. Quick Statistics. Available at http://www.nidcd.nih.gov/health/statistics/Pages/quick.aspx. Accessed April 04, 2013.
2. Goycoolea MV, Goycoolea HG, Farfan CR, Rodriguez LG, Martinez GC, Vidal R. Effect of life in industrialized societies on hearing in natives of Easter Island. Laryngoscope. 1986 Dec;96(12):1391-6.
3. Cruickshanks KJ, Klein R, Klein BE, Wiley TL, Nondahl DM, Tweed TS. Cigarette smoking and hearing loss: the epidemiology of hearing loss study. JAMA. 1998 Jun 3;279(21):1715-9.
4. Yorgason JG, Luxford W, Kalinec F. In vitro and in vivo models of drug ototoxicity: studying the mechanisms of a clinical problem. Expert Opin Drug Metab Toxicol. 2011 Dec;7(12):1521-34.
5. Gates GA, Couropmitree NN, Myers RH. Genetic associations in age-related hearing thresholds. Arch Otolaryngol Head Neck Surg. 1999 Jun;125(6):654-9.
6. Wolber LE, Steves CJ, Spector TD, Williams FM. Hearing ability with age in northern European women: a new web-based approach to genetic studies. PLoS One. 2012;7(4):e35500.
7. Yoshioka M, Uchida Y, Sugiura S, Ando F, Shimokata H, Nomura H, Nakashima T. The impact of arterial sclerosis on hearing with and without occupational noise exposure: a population-based aging study in males. Auris Nasus Larynx. 2010 Oct;37(5):558-64.
8. Lin SW, Lin YS, Weng SF, Chou CW. Risk of developing sudden sensorineural hearing loss in diabetic patients: a population-based cohort study. Otol Neurotol. 2012 Dec;33(9):1482-8.
9. Goycoolea MV, Goycoolea HG, Farfan CR, Rodriguez LG, Martinez GC, Vidal R. Effect of life in industrialized societies on hearing in natives of Easter Island. Laryngoscope. 1986 Dec;96(12):1391-6.
10. Gates GA, Mills JH. Presbycusis. Lancet. 2005 Sep 24-30;366(9491):1111-20.
11. Bluestone CD. Galapagos: Darwin, evolution, and ENT. Laryngoscope. 2009 Oct;119(10):1902-5.
12. Ballachanda BB. Theoretical and applied external ear acoustics. J Am Acad Audiol. 1997 Dec;8(6):411-20.
13. Roeser RJ, Ballachanda BB. Physiology, pathophysiology, and anthropology/epidemiology of human earcanal secretions. J Am Acad Audiol. 1997 Dec;8(6):391-400.
14. Still AT. Philosophy of Osteopathy. Kirksville, MO : A.T. Still ; 1899. Reprinted, Indianapolis, IN : American Academy of Osteopathy ; 1971:53-67.
15. McCarter DF, Courtney AU, Pollart SM. Cerumen impaction. Am Fam Physician. 2007 May 15;75(10):1523-8.
16. Tan R, Osman V, Tan G. Ear size as a predictor of chronological age. Arch Gerontol Geriatr. 1997 Sep-Oct;25(2):187-91.
17. Tomoda K, Morii S, Yamashita T, Kumazawa T. Histology of human eustachian tube muscles: effect of aging. Ann Otol Rhinol Laryngol. 1984 Jan-Feb;93(1 Pt 1):17-24.
18. Takasaki K, Sando I, Balaban CD, Haginomori S, Ishijima K, Kitagawa M. Histopathological changes of the eustachian tube cartilage and the tensor veli palatini muscle with aging. Laryngoscope. 1999 Oct;109(10):1679-83.
19. Kaneko A, Hosoda Y, Doi T, Tada N, Iwano T, Yamashita T.Tubal compliance--changes with age and in tubal malfunction. Auris Nasus Larynx. 2001 Apr;28(2):121-4.
20. Bodrova IV, Dobrotin VE, Kulakova LA, Fominykh EV, Pokoziï Ilu, Lopatin AS. Conductive hearing loss caused by eustachian tube dysfunction according to the data of functional computed tomography. Vestn Rentgenol Radiol. 2012 Jan-Feb;(1):127-36.
21. Baba Y. Degenerative changes in stapedius muscle morphology caused by aging. Nihon Jibiinkoka Gakkai Kaiho. 2000 Sep;103(9):993-1000.
22. Rawool VW, Harrington BT. Middle ear admittance and hearing abnormalities in individuals with osteoarthritis. Audiol Neurootol. 2007;12(2):127-36.
23. Sutherland WG. Teachings in the science of Osteopathy. Fort Worth, TX : Sutherland Cranial Teaching Foundation, Inc. ; 1991: 88.
24. Gates GA, Mills JH.Presbycusis. Lancet. 2005 Sep 24-30;366(9491):1111-20.
25. Chardin S, Romand R. Regeneration and mammalian auditory hair cells. Science. 1995 Feb 3;267(5198):707-11.
26. Yamasoba T, Lin FR, Someya S, Kashio A, Sakamoto T, Kondo K. Hear Res. 2013 Feb 16. pii: S0378-5955(13)00035-X. doi: 10.1016/j.heares.2013.01.021.
27. Schuknecht HF. Presbycusis. Laryngoscope. 1955 Jun;65(6):402-19
28. Nelson EG, Hinojosa R. Presbycusis: a human temporal bone study of individuals with downward sloping audiometric patterns of hearing loss and review of the literature. Laryngoscope. 2006 Sep;116(9 Pt 3 Suppl 112):1-12.
29. Tun PA, Williams VA, Small BJ, Hafter ER. The effects of aging on auditory processing and cognition. Am J Audiol. 2012 Dec;21(2):344-50.
30. Gates GA, Mills JH.Presbycusis. Lancet. 2005 Sep 24-30;366(9491):1111-20.
31. Schuknecht HF. Presbycusis. Laryngoscope. 1955 Jun;65(6):402-19.
32. Gates GA, Mills JH.Presbycusis. Lancet. 2005 Sep 24-30;366(9491):1111-20.
33. Chisolm TH, Willott JF, Lister JJ. The aging auditory system: anatomic and physiologic changes and implications for rehabilitation. Int J Audiol. 2003 Jul;42 Suppl 2:2S3-10.
34. Balboni AL, Estenson TL, Reidenberg JS, Bergemann AD, Laitman JT. Assessing age-related ossification of the petro-occipital fissure: laying the foundation for understanding the clinicopathologies of the cranial base. Anat Rec A Discov Mol Cell Evol Biol. 2005 Jan;282(1):38-48.
35. Møller AR. Tinnitus: presence and future. Prog Brain Res. 2007;166:3-16.
36. Jastreboff PJ. Phantom auditory perception (tinnitus): mechanisms of generation and perception. Neurosci Res. 1990 Aug;8(4):221-54.
37. Nondahl DM, Cruickshanks KJ, Dalton DS, Klein BE, Klein R, Schubert CR, Tweed TS, Wiley TL. The impact of tinnitus on quality of life in older adults. J Am Acad Audiol. 2007 Mar;18(3):257-66.

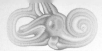

38. Møller AR. Tinnitus: presence and future. Prog Brain Res. 2007;166:3-16.

39. Nondahl DM, Cruickshanks KJ, Wiley TL, Klein BE, Klein R, Chappell R, Tweed TS. The ten-year incidence of tinnitus among older adults. Int J Audiol. 2010 Aug;49(8):580-5.

40. Kreuzer PM, Landgrebe M, Schecklmann M, Staudinger S, Langguth B; TRI Database Study Group. Trauma-associated tinnitus: audiological, demographic and clinical characteristics. PLoS One. 2012;7(9):e45599.

41. Henry JA, Dennis KC, Schechter MA. General review of tinnitus: prevalence, mechanisms, effects, and management. J Speech Lang Hear Res. 2005 Oct;48(5):1204-35.

42. Møller AR. Tinnitus: presence and future. Prog Brain Res. 2007;166:3-16.

43. Kaltenbach JA, Rachel JD, Mathog TA, Zhang J, Falzarano PR, Lewandowski M. Cisplatin-induced hyperactivity in the dorsal cochlear nucleus and its relation to outer hair cell loss: relevance to tinnitus. J Neurophysiol. 2002 Aug;88(2):699-714.

44. De Ridder D, Vanneste S, Adriaenssens I, Lee AP, Plazier M, Menovsky T, et al. Microvascular decompression for tinnitus: significant improvement for tinnitus intensity without improvement for distress. A 4-year limit. Neurosurgery. 2010 Apr;66(4):656-60.

45. Sirikci A, Bayazit Y, Ozer E, Ozkur A, Adaletli I, Cüce MA, Bayram M. Magnetic resonance imaging based classification of anatomic relationship between the cochleovestibular nerve and anterior inferior cerebellar artery in patients with non-specific neuro-otologic symptoms. Surg Radiol Anat. 2005 Dec;27(6):531-5.

46. Sonmez G, Basekim CC, Ozturk E, Gungor A, Kizilkaya E.Imaging of pulsatile tinnitus: a review of 74 patients. Clin Imaging. 2007 Mar-Apr;31(2):102-8.

47. Saldanha AD, Hilgenberg PB, Pinto LM, Conti PC. Are temporomandibular disorders and tinnitus associated? Cranio. 2012 Jul;30(3):166-71.

48. Tranter RM, Graham JR. A review of the otological aspects of whiplash injury. J Forensic Leg Med. 2009 Feb;16(2):53-5.

49. Träger V, Seidl RO, Ernst A. Displacement of a stapes piston as a consequence of whiplash injury with head impact. HNO. 2005 Feb;53(2):163-5.

50. Rubinstein B, Axelsson A, Carlsson GE. Prevalence of signs and symptoms of craniomandibular disorders in tinnitus patients. J Craniomandib Disord. 1990 Summer;4(3):186-92.

51. Pinchoff RJ, Burkard RF, Salvi RJ, Coad ML, Lockwood AH. Modulation of tinnitus by voluntary jaw movements. Am J Otol. 1998 Nov;19(6):785-9.

52. Simmons R, Dambra C, Lobarinas E, Stocking C, Salvi R. Head, Neck, and Eye Movements That Modulate Tinnitus. Semin Hear. 2008 Nov;29(4):361-370.

53. Levine RA, Abel M, Cheng H. CNS somatosensory-auditory interactions elicit or modulate tinnitus. Exp Brain Res. 2003 Dec;153(4):643-8.

54. Jensen OK, Nielsen FF, Vosmar L. An open study comparing manual therapy with the use of cold packs in the treatment of post-traumatic headache. Cephalalgia 1990;10:241-50.

55. de Felício CM, Melchior Mde O, Ferreira CL, Da Silva MA. Otologic symptoms of temporomandibular disorder and effect of orofacial myofunctional therapy. Cranio. 2008 Apr;26(2):118-25.

56. Congdon N, O'Colmain B, Klaver CC, Klein R, Muñoz B, Friedman DS, Kempen J, Taylor HR, Mitchell P; Eye Diseases Prevalence Research Group. Causes and prevalence of visual impairment among adults in the United States. Arch Ophthalmol. 2004 Apr;122(4):477-85.

57. Knudtson MD, Klein BE, Klein R, Cruickshanks KJ, Lee KE. Age-related eye disease, quality of life, and functional activity. Arch Ophthalmol. 2005 Jun;123(6):807-14.

58. Brian G, Taylor H. Cataract blindness – challenges for the 21st century. Available at http://www.who.int/bulletin/archives/79(3)249.pdf. Accessed April 12, 2013.

59. World Health Organization. Prevention of Blindness and Visual Impairment. Available at http://www.who.int/blindness/causes/priority/en/index1.html. Accessed April 12, 2013.

60. Koo E, Chang JR, Agrón E, Clemons TE, Sperduto RD, Ferris FL 3rd, et al. Ten-Year Incidence Rates of Age-Related Cataract in the Age-Related Eye Disease Study (AREDS): AREDS Report No. 33. Ophthalmic Epidemiol. 2013 Apr;20(2):71-81.

61. Beebe DC, Shui YB, Holekamp NM. Biochemical mechanisms of age-related cataract. Chapt 30. In: Levin LA, Albert DM. ed. Ocular Disease: Mechanisms and Management. Saunders/Elsevier. 2010.

62. McCarty CA, Taylor HR. A review of the epidemiologic evidence linking ultraviolet radiation and cataracts. Dev Ophthalmol. 2002;35:21-31.

63. Hammond CJ, Snieder H, Spector TD, Gilbert CE. Genetic and environmental factors in age-related nuclear cataracts in monozygotic and dizygotic twins. N Engl J Med. 2000 Jun 15;342(24):1786-90.

64. Beebe DC, Shui YB, Holekamp NM. Biochemical mechanisms of age-related cataract. Chapt 30. In: Levin LA, Albert DM. ed. Ocular Disease: Mechanisms and Management. Saunders/Elsevier. 2010.

65. Chang JR, Koo E, Agrón E, Hallak J, Clemons T, Azar D, et al. Risk factors associated with incident cataracts and cataract surgery in the Age-related Eye Disease Study (AREDS): AREDS report number 32. Ophthalmology. 2011 Nov;118(11):2113-9.

66. Fel A, Aslangul E, Le Jeunne C. Indications et complications des corticoïdes en ophtalmologie. Presse Med. 2012 Apr;41(4):414-21.

67. Truscott RJ. Human cataract: the mechanisms responsible; light and butterfly eyes. Int J Biochem Cell Biol. 2003 Nov;35(11):1500-4.

68. Messenger HK. Glaukoma and glaucoma. Arch Ophthalmol. 1964 Feb;71:264-6.

69. Thylefors B, Négrel AD. The global impact of glaucoma. Bulletin of the World Health Organization. 1994 72(3):323-6.

70. Javitt JC, McBean AM, Nicholson GA, Babish JD, Warren JL, Krakauer H. Undertreatment of glaucoma among black Americans. N Engl J Med. 1991 Nov 14;325(20):1418-22.

71. Resch H, Garhofer G, Fuchsjäger-Mayrl G, Hommer A, Schmetterer L. Endothelial dysfunction in glaucoma. Acta Ophthalmol. 2009 Feb;87(1):4-12.

72. Detry-Morel M. Facteurs de risque : la myopie. J Fr Ophtalmol. 2011 Jun;34(6):392-5.

73. Quigley HA, Broman AT. The number of people with glaucoma worldwide in 2010 and 2020. Br J Ophthalmol. 2006 Mar;90(3):262-7.

74. Ruddy TJ. Osteopathic manipulation in eye, ear, nose, and throat disease. Year Book of the Academy of Applied Osteopathy. American Academy of Osteopathy. Indianapolis, IN. 1962:133-40.

75. Feely RA, Castillo TA, Greiner JV: Osteopathic manipulative treatment and intraocular pressure. J Am Osteopath Assoc1982. 82:60,

76. Grieshaber MC, Flammer J. Blood flow in glaucoma. Curr Opin Ophthalmol. 2005 Apr;16(2):79-83.

77. Flammer J, Pache M, Resink T. Vasospasm, its role in the pathogenesis of diseases with particular reference to the eye. Prog Retin Eye Res. 2001 May;20(3):319-49.

78. Flammer J, Pache M, Resink T. Vasospasm, its role in the pathogenesis of diseases with particular reference to the eye. Prog Retin Eye Res. 2001 May;20(3):319-49.

79. Resch H, Garhofer G, Fuchsjäger-Mayrl G, Hommer A, Schmetterer L. Endothelial dysfunction in glaucoma. Acta Ophthalmol. 2009 Feb;87(1):4-12.

80. Resch H, Garhofer G, Fuchsjäger-Mayrl G, Hommer A, Schmetterer L. Endothelial dysfunction in glaucoma. Acta Ophthalmol. 2009 Feb;87(1):4-12.

81. Osuský R, Schoetzau A, Flammer J. Variations in the blood flow of the human optic nerve head. Eur J Ophthalmol. 1997 Oct-Dec;7(4):364-9.

82. Plange N, Remky A, Arend O.Colour Doppler imaging and fluorescein filling defects of the optic disc in normal tension glaucoma. Br J Ophthalmol. 2003 Jun;87(6):731-6.

83. National Eye Institute. Facts About Retinal Detachment. Available at http://www.nei.nih.gov/health/retinaldetach/retinaldetach.asp#c. Accessed April 17, 2013.

84. Mitry D, Fleck BW, Wright AF, Campbell H, Charteris DG. Pathogenesis of rhegmatogenous retinal detachment: predisposing anatomy and cell biology. Retina. 2010 Nov-Dec;30(10):1561-72.

85. Richard MJ, Morris C, Deen BF, Gray L, Woodward JA.Analysis of the anatomic changes of the aging facial skeleton using computer-assisted tomography. Ophthal Plast Reconstr Surg. 2009 Sep-Oct;25(5):382-6.

86. Kahn DM, Shaw RB Jr. Aging of the bony orbit: a three-dimensional computed tomographic study. Aesthet Surg J. 2008 May-Jun;28(3):258-64.

87. McKelvie P, Friling R, Davey K, Kowal L. Changes as the result of ageing in extraocular muscles: a post-mortem study. Aust N Z J Ophthalmol. 1999 Dec;27(6):420-5.

88. Clark RA, Demer JL. Effect of aging on human rectus extraocular muscle paths demonstrated by magnetic resonance imaging. Am J Ophthalmol. 2002 Dec;134(6):872-8.

89. Sutherland WG. Teachings in the science of Osteopathy. Fort Worth, TX: Sutherland Cranial Teaching Foundation, Inc. ; 1991: 87.

90. Magoun HI . Osteopathy in the cranial field . 2nd ed . Kirksville, MO: The Journal Printing Company ;1966 . p. 300.

91. Sutherland WG. Contributions of thought. Fort Worth, TX: Sutherland Cranial Teaching Foundation, Inc.; 1998:171.

92. Magoun HI. Osteopathy in the cranial field. Kirksville, MO: The Journal Printing Company; 1951:82.

93. Mulrow CD, Aguilar C, Endicott JE, Tuley MR, Velez R, Charlip WS, Rhodes MC, Hill JA, DeNino LA. Quality-of-life changes and hearing impairment. A randomized trial. Ann Intern Med. 1990 Aug 1;113(3):188-94.

94. Groves AK. The challenge of hair cell regeneration. Exp Biol Med (Maywood). 2010 Apr;235(4):434-46.

95. Rosen S, Olin P, Rosen HV. Diery prevention of hearing loss. Acta Otolaryngol. 1970 Oct;70(4):242-7.

96. Brant LJ, Gordon-Salant S, Pearson JD, Klein LL, Morrell CH, Metter EJ, Fozard JL. Risk factors related to age-associated hearing loss in the speech frequencies. J Am Acad Audiol. 1996 Jun;7(3):152-60.

# Index

Note: Page number followed by f and t indicates figure and table respectively.

## A

Abdominal aorta, 179
Abdominal prominence, 48–49
Abdominal scars, 14
Abducens nerve (CN VI), 221
Abductus angle, 241f
Abnormal soft tissue texture, 78
Acetylcholine, 351
Achilles tendonitis, 86–87, 87f
Acromion enthesopathy, 205
Active hand-passive hand test, 54
Adipocytes, 4
Adipose tissue, 7
Adson's test, 55–56, 56f
Aging. *See also specific disorder*
    connective tissues and, 14–15
    and musculoskeletal system
        deterioration, 1
    respiratory system, effect on, 274
    spine, effect on, 186
        degenerative disc disease,
          189–190
        facet joint osteoarthritis,
          188–189
        osteophytes, 187–188
        osteoporosis, 186–187
        spinal stenosis, 190–191
Airways, conducting, 272–273
Allodynia, 358
Alpha-gamma coactivation, 224
Ampulla, 218
Angiotensin I, 259
Angiotensin II, 259
Ankle sprains, 62
ANS. *See* Autonomic nervous system
    (ANS)
Anterior cervical fascial procedures
    alternative supine procedure,
        129–130, 130f
    hyoid bone procedure, 130f, 131
    indications for, 129
    laryngeal procedure, 131
    submandibular procedure, 130, 130f
    supine procedure, 129, 129f
Apnea-hypopnea index (AHI), 278
Arterial system, 22
Artery of Adamkiewicz, 179
Articulation, 80
Assessment, 37. *See also* Physical
examination; Somatic dysfunction;
specific dysfunction
    history examination in, 43–45
        chief complaint (CC), 43–44
        history of present illness (HPI), 44
        past family history (PFH), 45
        past medical history (PMH), 45
        review of systems (ROS), 44
        social history (SH), 45
    physical examination in, 45
        observation, 45
        palpation for function, 45
        palpation for structure, 45
        patient positions and, 45–46
Atlantoaxial procedure, 127, 127f
Atlas, 167–168, 168f
Auditory dysfunctions, 373
    patient, advice to, 386–387
    physical examination and
        treatment, 385–386
    presbycusis, 373–379
    tinnitus, 379–380
Autonomic nervous system (ANS), 259,
    265, 345–346
    afferent, 346
    chronic fatigue syndrome, 355–356
    dysautonomia, 353–355
    efferent, 346–347, 346f
    fibromyalgia, 356–360
    functions of, 351–352, 352t
    menopause, influence of, 365–366
    neurotransmitters of, 351
    parasympathetic division of, 347, 350
    patient, advice to, 368–369
    physical examination and
        treatment, 366–368
    postganglionic parasympathetic
        fibers, 350–351
    sleep disturbances, 360–365
    sympathetic division of, 347
        postganglionic sympathetic
          fibers, 349–350
        preganglionic sympathetic
          fibers, 347–349
        sympathetic ganglia, 349
Axis, 168, 168f

## B

Bacterial infections, and COPD, 275
Balanced ligamentous tension (BLT), 82
Baroreflex, 353–354
    and control of arterial BP, 258–259

tonic oscillation of, 263–264
Becker's slow and fast tides, 18, 19
Benign paroxysmal positional vertigo
    (BPPV), 229–232
Benign prostate disorders, 335–336,
    340–341
Biconcave deformities, spine, 187
Bilateral temporal bone release,
    147–148, 147f
Bipedal gait, 199
B lymphocytes, 5
BPPV. *See* Benign paroxysmal
    positional vertigo (BPPV)
Brain, motion of, 20

## C

Canalithiasis, 230
Cannon, Walter, 345
Cardiac orifice, 293
Cardiovascular diseases, 257
    congestive heart failure, 261–265
    hypertension, 257–260
    patient, advice to, 267–268
    physical examination and
        treatment, 265–267
Carpal tunnel syndrome, 209
    anatomopathology related to,
        209–210
    medical conditions associated
        with, 209
    patient, advice to, 212
    physical examination and
        treatment, 211–212
    prevalence of, 209
    and somatic dysfunction, 210–211
Cataracts, age-related, 381
Cellular respiration, 21–22
Central nervous system (CNS), motion
    of, 18, 20–21
Cerebrocerebellum, 226
Cerebrospinal fluid (CSF), fluctuation
    of, 20–21
Cerumen, 374
Cervical dysfunction, procedure for,
    127–128
    alternative supine procedure,
        128, 128f
    seated procedure, 128–129, 129f
    supine procedure, 128, 128f
Cervical procedures, 125
    anterior cervical fascial procedures,
        129–131, 130f